T0331106

Biology and Pathology of the Oocyte

Role in Fertility, Medicine, and Nuclear Reprogramming

Second Edition

Biology and Pathology of the Oocyte

Role in Fertility, Medicine, and Nuclear Reprogramming

Second Edition

Edited by

Alan Trounson

Californian Institute for Regenerative Medicine, San Francisco, CA, USA

Roger Gosden

Center for Reproductive Medicine and Infertility, Weill Medical College of Cornell University, New York, NY, USA

Ursula Eichenlaub-Ritter

Faculty of Biology, Institute of Gene Technology/Microbiology, University of Bielefeld, Bielefeld, Germany

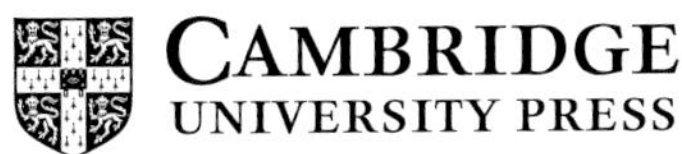

CAMBRIDGE
UNIVERSITY PRESS

University Printing House, Cambridge CB2 8BS, United Kingdom

One Liberty Plaza, 20th Floor, New York, NY 10006, USA

477 Williamstown Road, Port Melbourne, VIC 3207, Australia

314-321, 3rd Floor, Plot 3, Splendor Forum, Jasola District Centre, New Delhi - 110025, India

79 Anson Road, #06-04/06, Singapore 079906

Cambridge University Press is part of the University of Cambridge.

It furthers the University's mission by disseminating knowledge in the pursuit of education, learning and research at the highest international levels of excellence.

www.cambridge.org
Information on this title: www.cambridge.org/9781107021907

First published 2013

A catalogue record for this publication is available from the British Library

Library of Congress Cataloging in Publication data
Biology and pathology of the oocyte : role in fertility, medicine, and nuclear reprogramming / Alan Trounson, Californian Institute for Regenerative Medicine, San Francisco, CA, Roger Gosden, Center for Reproductive Medicine & Infertility, Weill Medical College of Cornell University, New York, NY, Ursula Eichenlaub-Ritter, University of Bielefeld, Faculty of Biology, Institute of Gene Technology/Microbiology, Bielefeld, Germany. – Second edition.
pages cm
Includes bibliographical references and index.
ISBN 978-1-107-02190-7 (hardback)
1. Ovum. I. Trounson, Alan. II. Gosden, R. G.
QM611.B45 2013
612.6′2 – dc23 2013016805

ISBN 978-1-107-02190-7 Hardback

Every effort has been made in preparing this book to provide accurate and up-to-date information which is in accord with accepted standards and practice at the time of publication. Although case histories are drawn from actual cases, every effort has been made to disguise the identities of the individuals involved. Nevertheless, the authors, editors and publishers can make no warranties that the information contained herein is totally free from error, not least because clinical standards are constantly changing through research and regulation. The authors, editors and publishers therefore disclaim all liability for direct or consequential damages resulting from the use of material contained in this book. Readers are strongly advised to pay careful attention to information provided by the manufacturer of any drugs or equipment that they plan to use.

In memory of Bob Edwards (1925–2013), mentor, colleague, friend

Contents

Contributor affiliations

Dasari Amarnath
Fels Institute for Cancer Research and Molecular Biology, Temple University School of Medicine, Philadelphia, PA, USA

Ellen Anckaert
Follicle Biology Laboratory, UZ Brussel, Brussels, Belgium

Valerie L. Baker
Department of Obstetrics and Gynecology, Reproductive Endocrinology and Infertility, Stanford School of Medicine, Palo Alto, CA, USA

Natalie Barbey
Infertility Center of St. Louis, St. Luke's Hospital, St. Louis, MO, USA

Tiziana A. L. Brevini
Laboratory of Biomedical Embryology, Centre for Stem Cell Research UNISTEM, Università degli Studi di Milano, Milan, Italy

Frank Broekmans
Department of Reproductive Medicine and Gynecology, University Medical Center, Utrecht, the Netherlands

Anne Grete Byskov
Laboratory of Reproductive Biology, Juliane Marie Center, Rigshospitalet, Copenhagen, Denmark

John Carroll
Department of Anatomy and Developmental Biology, School of Biomedical Sciences, Monash University, Melbourne, Australia

Rita P. Cervera
Division of Reproductive and Developmental Sciences, Oregon National Primate Research Center, Oregon Health and Science University, Beaverton, OR, USA

Jose Cibelli
Cellular Reprogramming Laboratory, Department of Animal Science, Michigan State University, East Lansing, MI, USA; LARCel, Programa Andaluz de Terapia Celular y Medicina Regenerativa, Andalucía, Spain

Paula E. Cohen
Department of Biomedical Sciences, College of Veterinary Medicine, Cornell University, Ithaca, NY, USA

Marco Conti
Center for Reproductive Sciences and The Eli and Edythe Broad Center of Regeneration Medicine and Stem Cell Research, Department of Obstetrics and Gynecology and Reproductive Sciences, University of California, San Francisco, CA, USA

Scott A. Coonrod
Baker Institute for Animal Health, College of Veterinary Medicine, Cornell University, Ithaca, NY, USA

David S. Cram
Department of Anatomy and Developmental Biology, Monash University, Clayton, Australia

Madeleine Dólleman
Department of Reproductive Medicine and Gynecology, University Medical Center, Utrecht, the Netherlands

Ursula Eichenlaub-Ritter
Faculty of Biology, Institute of Gene Technology/Microbiology, University of Bielefeld, Bielefeld, Germany

Anna P. Ferraretti
SISMeR, Reproductive Medicine Unit, Bologna, Italy

Tom P. Fleming
Centre for Biological Sciences, University of Southampton, Southampton General Hospital, Southampton, UK

Saiichi Furukawa
University of Tokyo, Tokyo, Japan

Fulvio Gandolfi
Laboratory of Biomedical Embryology, Centre for Stem Cell Research UNISTEM, Università degli Studi di Milano, Milan, Italy

Luca Gianaroli
SISMeR, Reproductive Medicine Unit, Bologna, Italy

Isabelle Gilbert
Université Laval, Quebec City, Quebec, Canada

Robert B. Gilchrist
Research Centre for Reproductive Health, Robinson Institute, School of Paediatrics and Reproductive Health, The University of Adelaide, Adelaide, Australia

Roger Gosden
Jamestowne Bookworks, Williamsburg, VA, USA

Alain Gougeon
CRCL, UMR INSERM and CNRS, Faculté de Médecine Laennec, Lyon, France

John B. Gurdon
Wellcome Trust/Cancer Research UK Gurdon Institute, University of Cambridge, Cambridge, UK

Karen E. Hemmings
Division of Reproduction and Early Development, Leeds Institute of Genetics, Health and Therapeutics, University of Leeds, Leeds, UK

Mary Herbert
Wellcome Trust Centre for Mitochondrial Research, Institute for Ageing and Health, Newcastle University, Bioscience Centre, International Centre for Life, Newcastle-upon-Tyne, UK

Hayden Homer
Mammalian Oocyte and Embryo Research Laboratory, Cell and Developmental Biology, Division of Biosciences and Reproductive Medicine Unit, Institute for Women's Health, UCL, London, UK

Aaron J. W. Hsueh
Program of Reproductive and Stem Cell Biology, Department of Obstetrics and Gynecology, Stanford University School of Medicine, Stanford, CA, USA

Karin Hübner
Department of Cell and Developmental Biology, Max Planck Institute for Molecular Biomedicine, Münster, Germany

Gayle M. Jones
GMJ A.R.T. Solutions, Melbourne, and Department of Anatomy and Developmental Biology, Monash University, Clayton, Australia

Kazuhiro Kawamura
Department of Obstetrics and Gynecology, St. Mariana University School of Medicine, Kawasaki, Japan

Boram Kim
Baker Institute for Animal Health, College of Veterinary Medicine, Cornell University, Ithaca, NY, USA

Keith E. Latham
Department of Animal Science, College of Agriculture, Michigan State University, East Lansing, MI, USA

Ruth Lathi
Department of Obstetrics and Gynecology, Reproductive Endocrinology and Infertility, Stanford School of Medicine, Palo Alto, CA, USA

Qinglei Li
Department of Veterinary Integrative Biosciences, Texas A&M University, College Station, TX, USA

M. Cristina Magli
SISMeR, Reproductive Medicine Unit, Bologna, Italy

Victoria L. Mascetti
Department of Surgery and Anne McLaren Laboratory for Regenerative Medicine, University of Cambridge, Cambridge, UK

Martin M. Matzuk
Departments of Molecular and Human Genetics, Pathology and Immunology, Molecular and Cellular Biology, and Pharmacology, Baylor College of Medicine, Houston, TX, USA

Serge McGraw
Departments of Pediatrics, Human Genetics, and Pharmacology and Therapeutics, McGill University and of the Research Institute of the McGill University Health Centre at the Montreal Children's Hospital, Montreal, Canada

Shoukhrat Mitalipov
Division of Reproductive and Developmental Sciences, Oregon National Primate Research Center and Departments of Obstetrics and Gynecology and Molecular and Medical Genetics, Oregon Stem Cell Center, Oregon Health and Science University, Beaverton, OR, USA

Kei Miyamoto
Wellcome Trust/Cancer Research UK Gurdon Institute, University of Cambridge, Cambridge, UK

Swapna Mohan
Department of Biomedical Sciences, College of Veterinary Medicine, Cornell University, Ithaca, NY, USA

Lawrence Nelson
Intramural Research Program on Reproductive and Adult Endocrinology, Integrative Reproductive Medicine Group, National Institute of Child Health and Human Development, National Institutes of Health, Bethesda, MD, USA

Robert J. Norman
The Robinson Institute Research Centre for Reproductive Health, School of Paediatrics and Reproductive Health, University of Adelaide, Adelaide, Australia

Roger A. Pedersen
Department of Surgery and Anne McLaren Laboratory for Regenerative Medicine, University of Cambridge, Cambridge, UK

Jia Peng
Departments of Molecular and Human Genetics, and Pathology and Immunology, Baylor College of Medicine, Houston, TX, USA

Melissa E. Pepling
Department of Biology, Syracuse University, Syracuse, NY, USA

Luca Persani
Department of Clinical Sciences and Community Health, University of Milan and Division of Endocrine and Metabolic Diseases, IRCCS Istituto Auxologico Italiano, Milan, Italy

Helen M. Picton
Division of Reproduction and Early Development, Leeds Institute of Genetics, Health and Therapeutics, University of Leeds, Leeds, UK

Carlos Plancha
Unidade de Biologia da Reprodução, Instituto de Histologia e Biologia da Deservolvimento, Faculdade de Medicina de Lisboa, Lisbon and Centro Médico de Assistência à Reprodução – CEMEARE, Lisbon, Portugal

Santhi Potireddy
Department of Biochemistry, Temple University School of Medicine, Philadelphia, PA, USA

Renee A. Reijo Pera
Center for Human Embryonic Stem Cell Research and Education, Institute for Stem Cell Biology and Regenerative Medicine, Department of Obstetrics and Gynecology, Stanford University School of Medicine, Palo Alto, CA, USA

Laura Rienzi
Centro GENERA, Clinica Valle Giulia, Rome, Italy

Rebecca L. Robker
The Robinson Institute Research Centre for Reproductive Health, School of Paediatrics and Reproductive Health, University of Adelaide, Adelaide, Australia

Heide Schatten
Department of Veterinary Pathobiology, University of Missouri, Columbia, MO, USA

Hans R. Schöler
Department of Cell and Developmental Biology, Max Planck Institute for Molecular Biomedicine and Medical Faculty, University of Münster, Münster, Germany

Stephanie Sherman
Department of Human Genetics, Emory University School of Medicine, Atlanta, GA, USA

David Silber
Infertility Center of St. Louis, St. Luke's Hospital, St. Louis, MO, USA

Sherman Silber
Infertility Center of St. Louis, St. Luke's Hospital, St. Louis, MO, USA and University of Amsterdam, Department of Obstetrics and Gynecology, Reproductive Endocrinology, Amsterdam, Netherlands

Marc-André Sirard
Université Laval, Quebec City, Quebec, Canada

Johan Smitz
Follicle Biology Laboratory, UZ Brussel, Brussels, Belgium

Dominic Stoop
Centre for Reproductive Medicine, UZ Brussel, Brussels, Belgium

Fumihiro Sugawa
Department of Cell and Developmental Biology, Max Planck Institute for Molecular Biomedicine, Münster, Germany

Koji Sugiura
University of Tokyo, Tokyo, Japan

Qing-Yuan Sun
State Key Laboratory of Reproductive Biology, Institute of Zoology, Chinese Academy of Sciences, Beijing, China

Karl Swann
Institute of Molecular and Experimental Medicine, Cardiff University School of Medicine, Cardiff, UK

Jeremy G. Thompson
Research Centre for Reproductive Health, Robinson Institute, School of Paediatrics and Reproductive Health, The University of Adelaide, Adelaide, Australia

Jacquetta M. Trasler
Departments of Pediatrics, Human Genetics, and Pharmacology and Therapeutics, McGill University and of the Research Institute of the McGill University Health Centre at the Montreal Children's Hospital, Montreal, Canada

Alan Trounson
Californian Institute for Regenerative Medicine, San Francisco, CA, USA

Helen A. L. Tuppen
Wellcome Trust Centre for Mitochondrial Research, Institute for Ageing and Health, Newcastle University Medical School, Newcastle-upon-Tyne, UK

Doug M. Turnbull
Wellcome Trust Centre for Mitochondrial Research, Institute for Ageing and Health, Newcastle University Medical School, Newcastle-upon-Tyne, UK

Miguel A. Velazquez
Centre for Biological Sciences, University of Southampton, Southampton General Hospital, Southampton, UK

Dagan Wells
Nuffield Department of Obstetrics and Gynaecology, Institute of Reproductive Sciences, Oxford, UK

Claus Yding Andersen
Laboratory of Reproductive Biology, Juliane Marie Centre, University Hospital of Copenhagen, and Faculty of Health Science, University of Copenhagen, Copenhagen, Denmark

Hang Yin
Center for Reproductive Medicine and Infertility, Weill Medical College of Cornell University, New York, NY, USA

Preface

When approached by Nick Dunton of Cambridge University Press to edit the second edition of *The Biology and Pathology of the Oocyte*, my response was an emphatic yes, providing my co-editor Roger Gosden could be enticed from retirement. He agreed and we both wanted Ursula Eichenlaub-Ritter to be the third editor because we admired her expertise in the basic biology of the oocyte and her ability to get the job done. There has been incredible progress in the knowledge of the oocyte and applications for medicine that have regularly appeared since the first edition. We considered the areas of reproductive technology – IVF – and the areas of reprogramming somatic cell phenotype as spin-offs of the progress made in oocyte biology. Both these areas received Nobel Prizes in the last few years and are included in the contributions for the second edition. We were fortunate to have John Gurdon open the second edition the year (2013) after he won the Nobel Prize in Physiology or Medicine. He and his coauthor set the scene for a rather different perspective of the power and influence of the oocyte in modern biology. The contributors invited for the second edition are exceptional in their areas of oocyte biology, pathology, and applications to biotechnology and medicine. We think they have captured the excitement of the fast-moving frontier of the oocyte field.

The second edition will enthuse the reader interested in how the oocyte is formed, its function, and the underlying mechanisms of what is the most extraordinary cell in the body. It remains the germinal link from generation to generation and must undergo the most elaborate series of changes to be ready to accept the

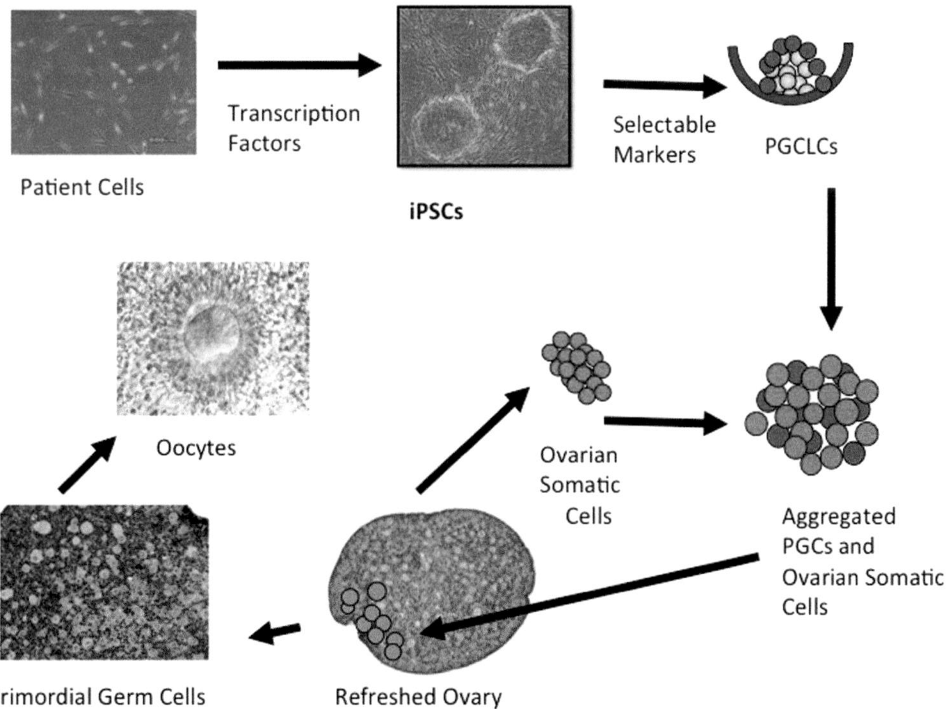

Figure P.1 A potential future strategy for generating viable new oocytes using technology to create iPSCs from adults, their germ cell differentiation and maturation in reconstructed ovaries. PGCLCs, primary germ cell-like cells; PGCs, primary germ cells. From Trounson [3].

genomic contribution of the most differentiated of all cells – the sperm. The oocyte must then enter the developmental program that enables an organism to arise with extremes in patterning and lineage differentiation consistent with the species of origin. In this exquisitely crafted program of development, it is possible to intervene to manipulate the oocyte for purposes of solving human infertility, to clone animals, develop pluripotent embryonic stem cells, and reprogram cell commitment in fully differentiated cells in animals including the human – so-called induced pluripotent stem cells (iPSCs). As a consequence we are able to address human infertility and avoid some of the worst inheritable genetic diseases, enable advances in selective animal breeding, and potentially address many human pathologies by using stem cell therapies.

While editing the second edition, we noted the astonishing reports of Hayashi *et al.* [1, 2] who were able to generate sperm and eggs in mice from embryonic stem cells (see Chapter 16). While it remains to be seen if other labs can replicate their observations, these could herald the ultimate method to derive new oocytes for research in the human and other species. Importantly, iPSCs derived from adult cells of female mice could be directed into primordial germ cells and selected for aggregation with fetal ovarian somatic cells to form viable follicles, oocytes, embryos, and live young – a possible future treatment for sterility (see Figure P.1). We would expect a considerable expansion of research in this area because of the implications for human sterility, animal reproduction, and conservation of threatened species. Perhaps other developments will arise around the germ cell and oocyte that will also accelerate the field in new directions. It is often difficult to predict what the next major advance will be. We hope funding bodies will continue to strongly support research on the oocyte as the NIH did with Dick Tasker's Egg Club.

We wish to thank all those contributors who selflessly gave their time to make the second edition a remarkable and very different book. We also thank Rob Sykes for all his assistance and enthusiasm in the publishing team and for Nick Dunton in getting us together. It has been a privilege to work with you all.

References

1. Hayashi K, Ohta H, Kurimoto K, Aramaki S, Saitou M. Reconstitution of the mouse germ cell specification pathway in culture by pluripotent stem cells. *Cell* 2011; **146**: 519–32.
2. Hayashi K, Ogushi S, Kurimoto K, *et al.* Offspring from oocytes derived from in vitro primordial germ cell-like cells in mice. *Science* 2012; **338**: 971–5.
3. Trounson A. A rapidly evolving revolution in stem cell biology and medicine. *Reprod Biomed Online* 2013; **26**(6), in press.

Alan Trounson, Roger Gosden, and
Ursula Eichenlaub-Ritter

Section 1 Historical perspective

Chapter 1

Insights into the amphibian egg to understand the mammalian oocyte

Kei Miyamoto and John B. Gurdon

Abstract

Amphibian eggs and oocytes have been widely used as a model system for understanding animal development. They have led to numerous major discoveries in cellular and developmental biology. These findings have greatly helped us to understand the physiology of mammalian oocytes. Amphibian eggs have also played an important role not only in revealing genomic conservation and plasticity historically, but also in gaining a mechanistic insight into nuclear reprogramming. This chapter summarizes major findings using amphibian eggs and oocytes, focusing on reprogramming aspects. We also discuss how *Xenopus* eggs can be used to study mammalian oocytes.

Introduction

For over 100 years, amphibian embryos have been the favored choice of material for research into mechanisms of early vertebrate animal development. This is because amphibian embryos are unusually large, being about 1 mm in diameter. The whole amphibian egg divides into an embryo whereas, in birds, for example, only a very small amount of material in the huge egg actually forms an embryo. All mammalian eggs are relatively inaccessible and are very small, usually 70–120 μm in diameter. European amphibia include the Urodeles (salamanders, newts, *Triturus*, etc.) as well as Anura (frogs, toads, *Rana*, *Bufo*). Members of these groups usually lay abundant eggs in natural pond water in the northern-hemisphere spring. The eggs are easy to culture. Their large size and consistency make them exceptionally favorable for microdissection and other manipulative experiments. This was the material used by Spemann, Hamburger, and Holtfreter and others.

The only disadvantage of most anuran species is that they produce eggs naturally only in the European spring, amounting to one or two months during the year. Soon after World War II, *Xenopus* became the favored choice for amphibian research. The interesting history of how this happened was largely coincidental [1]. The huge advantage of *Xenopus* is that it can be induced to lay eggs at any time of year, following an injection of mammalian pituitary hormone. The species is permanently aquatic, making its laboratory maintenance a great deal easier than for land-living amphibia. Since it naturally lives in highly infected pond water (in Africa) *Xenopus laevis* is exceptionally disease-free and easy to culture. Over the last 50 years, nearly all amphibian research has come to be conducted on *Xenopus* species.

The majority of experimental interventions now carried out on a range of vertebrate species, and especially in mammals, have their origin in work that started with amphibia. Moreover, many scientific discoveries and knowledge in amphibia have been extended to mammals. In this review, we trace back the origin of many experimental procedures and scientific findings that are now in widespread use in mammals, and find that these were first pioneered in amphibia.

Meiotic prophase germ line in *Xenopus laevis* and the mouse

In *Xenopus laevis*, the female germ cell, the so-called oocyte, is arrested in prophase of meiosis I (MI) in the ovary of the adult frog (Figure 1.1; stage I to VI). During this period, oocytes accumulate a stockpile of macromolecules and organelles that are required to support early embryonic development. Stage VI oocytes are fully grown and capable of reacting to progesterone from the surrounding follicle cells. They complete MI and are subsequently arrested in metaphase of meiosis II (MII). These matured

Biology and Pathology of the Oocyte, 2nd edn., ed. Alan Trounson, Roger Gosden, and Ursula Eichenlaub-Ritter.

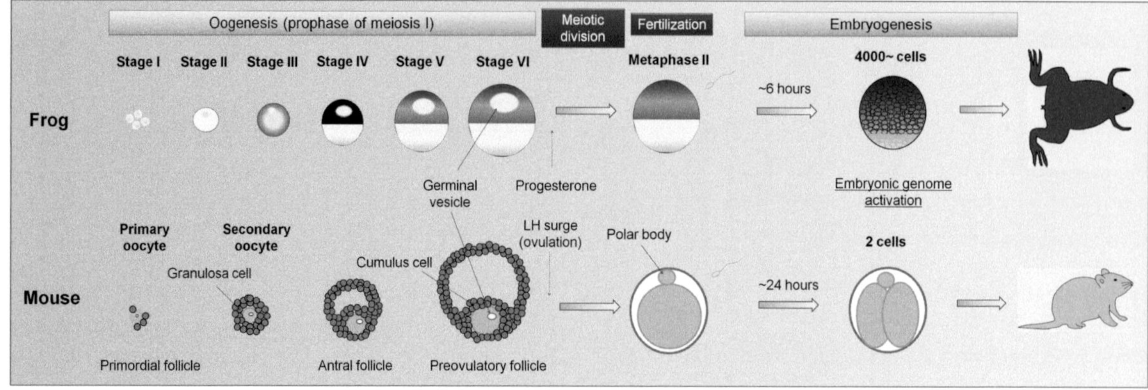

Figure 1.1 Oogenesis and embryogenesis in frog and mouse. Oocytes contain a giant nucleus referred to as the germinal vesicle. Upon resumption of meiosis, germinal vesicles are broken down and oocytes are matured to the metaphase II stage, followed by fertilization. Fertilized embryos undergo early cleavages directed by maternally stored factors without conspicuous transcription. Embryonic genome activation happens at the indicated cell stages, allowing embryos to develop further. LH, luteinizing hormone.

oocytes are then ovulated as unfertilized eggs (MII eggs). Upon fertilization, the egg is released from meiotic arrest and enters interphase. Early embryonic development is characterized by rapid progression through the cell cycle, consisting of repeated S- and M-phases. The stockpile of components present within the eggs supports this early development until the mid-blastula transition (MBT). Major embryonic gene activation starts at this MBT (Stage 8–8.5 embryos; 4000–8000 cells) and embryonic gene products then direct further embryonic development.

Mouse oocytes, as well as *Xenopus* oocytes, are arrested at prophase of MI in the ovary. During oogenesis, mouse oocytes increase their size from ~10 μm to 80 μm while actively transcribing the maternal genome for subsequent embryonic development (Figure 1.1). When the luteinizing hormone (LH) surge stimulates the resumption of meiosis, oocytes surrounded by cumulus cells are released from fully grown follicles. Oocytes are re-arrested at the MII stage until fertilization takes place. Major embryonic genome activation is first observed at the 2-cell stage.

As summarized above, maternal factors required for early embryonic development are accumulated in both *Xenopus* and mouse oocytes. During this oogenesis period, oocytes at the first meiotic prophase contain a giant nucleus referred to as the germinal vesicle (GV). The *Xenopus* GV reaches a diameter of 400 μm, which is more than 100 times larger than that of a mature mouse oocyte itself. It also stores huge amounts of macromolecules and nuclear organelles for intensive transcription; these include extrachromosomal nucleoli (~1500), Cajal bodies (50–100), and RNA polymerase II whose activity is sufficient for 100 000 somatic nuclei [2]. Notably, *Xenopus* GV oocyte genomes form so-called lampbrush chromosomes with actively transcribing chromatin loops and are found throughout chromosomes. Chromatin loops are maximally extended during early oogenesis and retracted towards the fully grown stage (stage VI). In the mouse, although lampbrush-like chromosomes have not been identified, oocyte genomes are also actively transcribed and produce a large stockpile of maternal RNA and protein. The chromatin structure of a mouse oocyte has been extensively studied. Follicular activation, at the beginning of oogenesis, is characterized by the loading of an oocyte-specific linker histone H1foo (closely related to the *Xenopus* histone B4) into the oocyte nucleus. Chromatin in growing mouse oocytes is initially decondensed and supports active transcription. As oogenesis proceeds, chromatin becomes progressively condensed and transcriptionally silenced, forming a heterochromatin rim around the oocyte nucleolus. Recent research suggests that histone-modifying enzymes play roles in the mouse oocyte chromatin remodeling associated with changes in transcriptional abilities [3]. Revealing mechanisms of oocyte transcription and its associated chromatin structure helps our understanding not only of germ cell development but also of the maternal contribution to early embryonic development.

Signaling in early embryogenesis

The first pivotal experiment which demonstrated signaling in development was that of Spemann and Mangold [4]. By transplanting tissue from one embryo into another (distinguished by pigment markers), it was proved that one set of cells can alter the fate of other cells placed near them. The Spemann signaling center exists in early amphibian embryos at the early gastrula stage. Subsequently, Nieuwkoop [5] demonstrated that signaling also occurs much earlier in development from the vegetal cells to the overlying animal cells. This Nieuwkoop center is the first known source of signaling in animal development and is responsible for the formation of the mesoderm layer.

In more recent years the mechanism of the Spemann signaling process has become greatly clarified. This is particularly due to the work of De Robertis [6] who has identified a number of signaling and other molecules that regulate the signaling process and in particular the distance in an embryo over which a signal factor acts. A network of such signaling centers and of the counteracting molecules that restrict the strength or distance of signaling has been identified [7].

Many such signaling processes work as morphogen gradients. This means that the concentration of signaling factor decreases with distance from its source. Most importantly, cells are able to sense the strength of the signal, at the position in which they lie, and differentiate in directions related to the strength of the signal that they receive. The mechanisms of morphogen gradient interpretation continue to attract wide interest [8]. The phenomenon is of great importance because the single source of signal can generate several different cell types according to the strength and duration of signal that a cell receives. The regulation of morphogen gradient interpretation is complex because it depends on the rate of movement of the morphogen, its stability, and particularly on the abundance of counteracting factors which can inactivate the morphogen [9].

Signaling in embryos is now well established in mammalian development. Gene ablation technologies and the availability of cultured pluripotent stem cells, such as embryonic and epiblast stem cells, in mice accelerated our understanding of how signaling pathways function in mammals [10, 11]. Signaling pathways that play a key role in early post-implantation development, such as Wnt and transforming growth factor beta (TGFβ), have been extensively studied [12].

Cell-free system

Components of amphibian eggs can be efficiently extracted by crushing them in an appropriate buffer. These cell-free extracts retain many egg proteins intact and as a result numerous cellular events, such as transcription, translation, cell-cycle progression, chromatin remodeling, and even reprogramming, are reproduced in the extracts to some extent. *Xenopus laevis* eggs have been widely used as a source of extracts due to their large size and abundance. Egg extracts are valuable for identifying molecules and molecular mechanisms involved in cellular events since many biochemical approaches can be applied to extracts. For example, specific proteins can be depleted from extracts by immunodepletion using antibodies in order to assess the roles of these proteins. To carry out such knockout experiments is very challenging in living embryos. In addition, the complexity of a live cell or egg can be somewhat simplified in extracts. We summarize below major discoveries and recent applications of egg extracts to understand reprogramming.

DNA replication

Xenopus egg extracts that are widely used at present were first reported by Lohka and Masui [13]. Unfertilized frog eggs are collected in a test tube and crushed by centrifugation. After centrifugation, the cytoplasmic fraction is used as an extract (Figure 1.2A). When demembranated sperm nuclei are incubated in this extract, these nuclei are immediately decondensed (Figure 1.2B) and start to form nuclear envelopes and pronuclei, accompanied by DNA replication. This is followed by breakdown of nuclear envelopes and chromosome condensation. This egg extract was further developed and could also replicate purified DNA [14]. Egg factors required for the DNA replication, such as Orc (origin recognition complex, subunit 2) [15], cdc6 (cell division cycle 6) [16], and MCMs (minichromosome maintenance proteins) [17], have been found and characterized in this system.

Cell-cycle analysis

Many important findings using *Xenopus* egg extracts have been achieved in the field of cell-cycle analysis. After the first egg extract, in which a single cell cycle is reproduced [13], Hutchison *et al.* [18] and Murray and Kirschner [19] developed and established the cycling extracts in which multiple cell cycles are reproduced. This led to the identification of cyclin-dependent protein kinase, CDK1, and cyclin B as necessary regulators for mitotic entry. CDK1 and cyclin B are also known as maturation-promoting factor (MPF). Molecules that modulate MPF activity have been extensively studied. Extracts have been also prepared from eggs arrested in

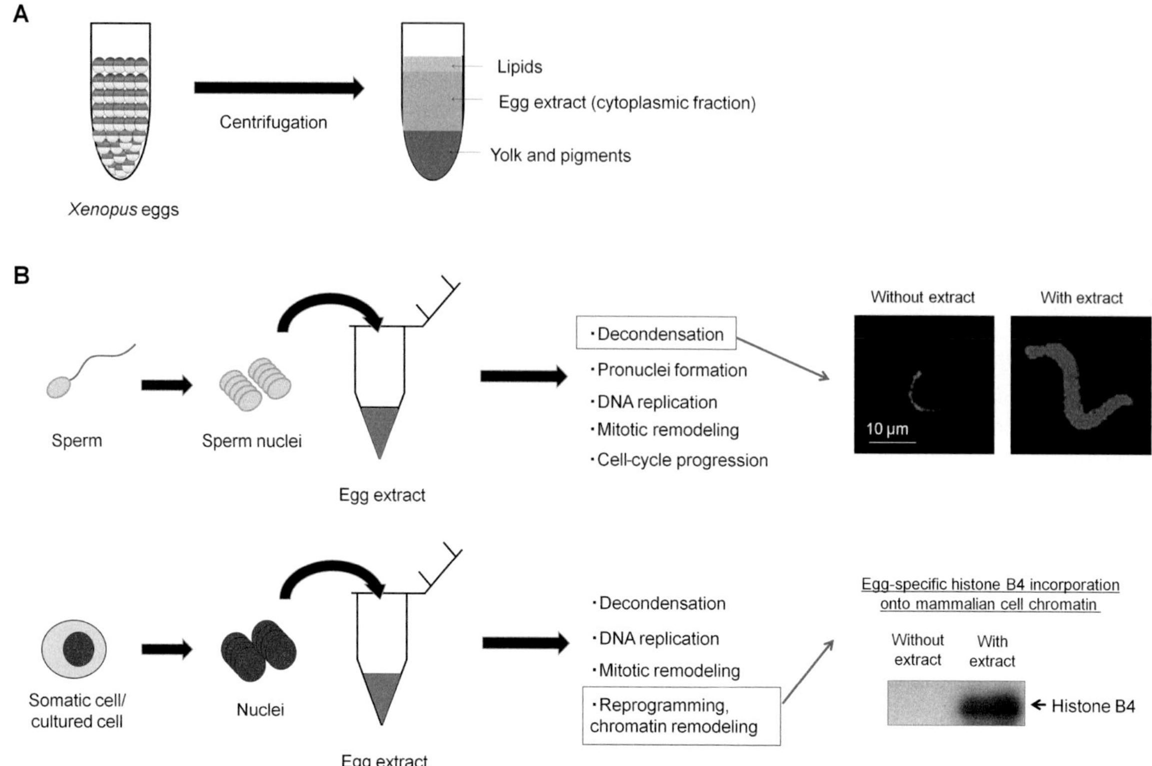

Figure 1.2 *Xenopus* egg extracts and their utility. (A) *Xenopus* eggs collected in a test tube are crushed by centrifugation and separated into three fractions. The middle fraction containing cytoplasm and membranes is used as an egg extract. (B) Various kinds of cellular and molecular events are reproduced in *Xenopus* egg extracts. When sperm nuclei are incubated in egg extracts, rapid decondensation of sperm nuclei is observed as shown. Egg extracts also induce several changes in somatic nuclei. Notably, a part of reprogramming, which includes oocyte linker histone B4 incorporation onto chromatin as revealed by the western blotting, is induced in somatic nuclei.

metaphase of the second meiotic division by an activity called cytostatic factor (CSF) [20]. CSF in connection with MPF activity plays an essential role in MII arrest to prevent parthenogenesis. Although some differences in molecular behavior between *Xenopus* and the mouse have been reported [21], the *Xenopus* egg cell-free system is a powerful tool to analyze biochemical interactions and signaling pathways involved in this meiotic arrest, egg activation, and early embryonic cell cycles.

Chromatin remodeling (sperm decondensation, mitotic remodeling and chromatin assembly)

As previously mentioned, sperm decondensation and male pronucleus formation were induced in frog egg extracts. By utilizing this property, nucleoplasmin in egg extracts was identified as a factor to decondense sperm nuclei and remove protamines from sperm nuclei [22, 23]. Oocyte linker histone B4 is also involved in sperm chromatin remodeling [24].

In addition to the above-mentioned replicating cell-cycle extracts, CSF extracts maintain the metaphase state so that they can induce nuclear envelope breakdown, chromosome condensation, and spindle assembly [20]. The roles of chromosomal proteins, such as topoisomerase IIα and histone H1, in mitotic chromosome assembly have been examined [25, 26]. Condensin necessary for mitotic chromosome condensation was identified using mitotic extracts [27].

Chromatin is formed when double-stranded or single-stranded plasmid DNA molecules are incubated in egg extracts [28, 29], providing unique opportunities to study chromatin assembly. Histones stored in eggs carry distinct patterns of histone modification [30]. Changes in histone modification are related to those of transcriptional activities in oocytes.

Therefore, it would be interesting to study chromatin structures in eggs/oocytes using this system.

Recapitulation of reprogramming in egg/oocyte extracts

Since *Xenopus* egg extracts mimic sperm nuclear remodeling after fertilization, it is reasonable to speculate that egg extracts, at least to some extent, can recapitulate somatic nuclear reprogramming that is induced after nuclear transplantation to eggs. Kikyo *et al.* [31] first reported that somatic nuclei incubated in *Xenopus* egg extracts are remodeled towards an embryonic state in which somatic proteins are lost, while egg proteins are incorporated into somatic chromatin. They have shown that the ATP-dependent chromatin remodeling factor ISWI plays a key role in this process. This system has also led to the identification of FRGY2a/b as a critical factor for nucleolar disassembly [32]. These are the first reports to identify actual egg factors involved in somatic cell reprogramming in vitro, proving that the egg cell-free system is a good route to manifest reprogramming mechanisms.

Subsequently, several reports have shown that reprogramming activities of egg extracts are conserved in mammalian somatic nuclei. The incorporation of *Xenopus* egg factors into mammalian chromatin was observed, including oocyte type lamin LIII [33] and histone B4 (Figure 1.2B) [34]. Moreover, the ability of egg extracts to trigger induction of mammalian embryonic gene expression has been shown [34, 35]. Egg and oocyte extracts from another amphibian species, the axolotl, also exhibit strong epigenetic reprogramming activities in mammalian nuclei [36]. These findings emphasize the utility of amphibian egg extracts as a tool to study reprogramming of mammalian nuclei, especially for the purpose of identifying egg factors with reprogramming activities.

Application of cell-free systems for understanding mammalian oocytes

The *Xenopus* egg cell-free system has greatly advanced molecular understanding of many cellular events, as mentioned above. Factors and mechanisms originally found in this system have been extensively tested and validated in mammalian in vivo systems. Therefore, the *Xenopus* cell-free system has served as a foundation for revealing molecular mechanisms. If a similar kind of cell-free system can be developed in mammals, our molecular understanding of mammalian oocytes may advance rapidly. This idea has been hampered by the fact that we cannot collect enough mammalian oocytes for making functional extracts. Nevertheless, some attempts to produce these have been made [37, 38], although further sophistication is needed. It might be a good idea to start first with one specialized oocyte extract that can reproduce only one aspect of cellular events.

Special manipulations

Nuclear transfer in eggs and oocytes

Spemann did an ingenious delayed nucleation experiment in which the nucleus of one of the first eight cells of an amphibian embryo was shown to lead to the formation of a normal embryo [39]. This demonstrated the totipotency of one of the first eight cells of an embryo, but did not test later stages. The first major success in nuclear transplantation was that of Briggs and King [40] when they were able to transplant the nuclei of *Rana pipiens* blastula cells into enucleated eggs of that species and obtain normal embryos. When they tried the same experiment using nuclei from slightly later stages, they were no longer able to obtain normal development [41]. They reached the entirely reasonable conclusion that, as development proceeds, the nuclei of somatic cells lose their totipotency. In 1958 nuclear transplantation had succeeded in *Xenopus*. A series of experiments culminated in the finding that totally normal, sexually mature adult animals could be obtained by transplanting the nuclei of embryo endoderm cells into enucleated eggs (Figure 1.3A) [42]. Subsequently it was found that the nuclei of differentiated intestinal epithelium cells could also yield normal, sexually mature animals. This was the proof that cell differentiation does not necessarily involve any loss of genetic totipotency. It is now generally accepted that, with very special exceptions like antibody-producing cells, all cells of the body have the same complete genome. In recent time, notably following the work of Takahashi and Yamanaka [43], the principle of totipotency of somatic cell nuclei has led to extensive work aiming to derive embryonic stem cells from adult tissue cells, with a view to drug testing and possibly cell replacement therapy.

For technical reasons, it was nearly 40 years after the first successful nuclear transplantation in amphibia

A. Nuclear transfer (NT)

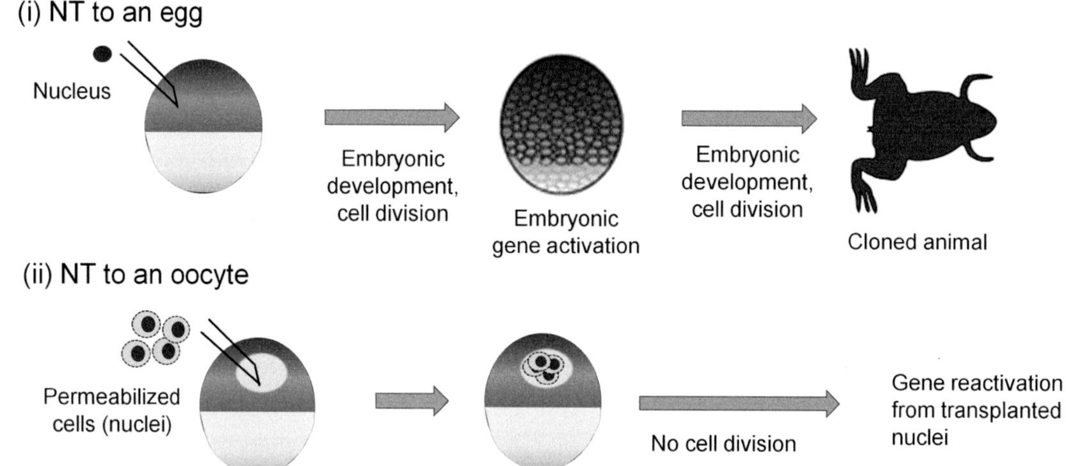

B. mRNA injection

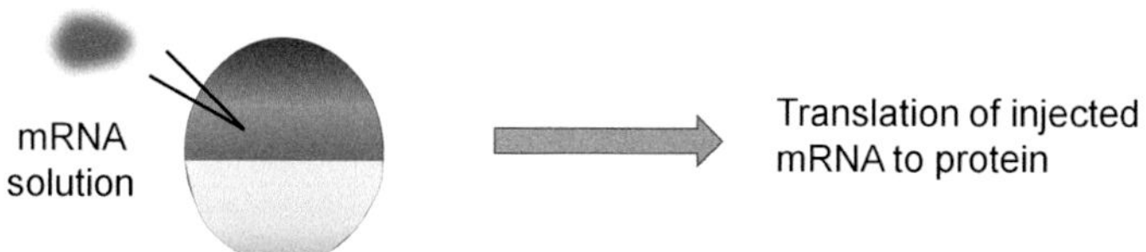

C. Single cell transplant

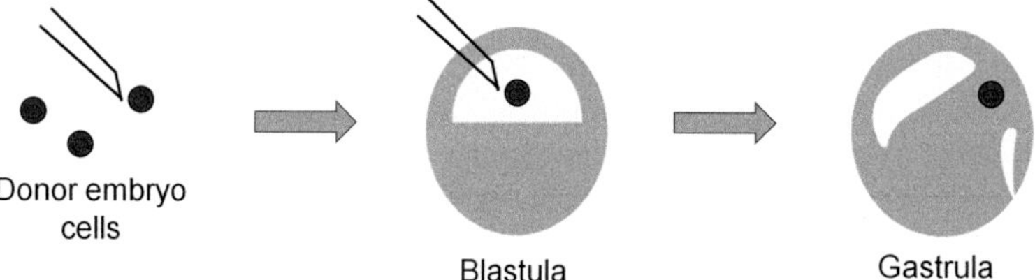

D. Community effect

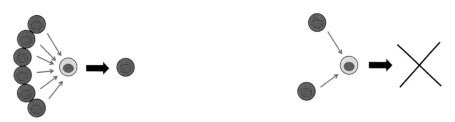

Figure 1.3 Special manipulations using *Xenopus* eggs and oocytes. (A) Two types of nuclear transfer (NT) are available in *Xenopus*. NT to MII eggs generates NT embryos, which finally give rise to cloned animals. Hundreds of nuclei can be injected into a nucleus of the *Xenopus* oocyte. Injected nuclei do not change to another cell type, but, instead, previously silenced genes are reactivated. Direct transcriptional reprogramming of somatic nuclei without the need for cell division is induced in this oocyte NT unlike NT to an egg, in which cell divisions are required before initiation of embryonic gene transcription. (B) In vitro synthesized mRNAs are injected into the cytoplasm of eggs/oocytes and are readily translated. (C) Embryo cells are separated from each other. A single cell is injected into the cavity of a blastula embryo and the fate of the injected cell can be traced. (D) Cell transplantation experiments led to the finding of the community effect, the phenomenon in which cells in close proximity to each other contribute some signal factor and receive more signals from their neighbors, thereby allowing efficient differentiation.

that Dolly the sheep was produced [44]. This demonstrated that a differentiated adult tissue, in this case mammary gland, could yield normal, fertile animals by nuclear transfer. Since then, nuclear transfer in a wide range of mammals has been successful. Byrne *et al.* has reported the successful derivation of embryonic stem cells from monkey nuclear transfer embryos [45]. Recently, Tachibana *et al.* have succeeded in establishing human embryonic stem cells from nuclear transfer embryos with high efficiency [46].

Nuclear reprogramming by the induced pluripotent stem (iPS) cell technology currently works at a low efficiency. There is a strong desire to understand the mechanism of this route towards deriving pluripotent stem cells from adult cells, in the hope that the efficiency of the procedure might be improved. By comparison, the transplantation of somatic nuclei to enucleated eggs, whether amphibian or mammalian, works at a much higher efficiency and therefore gives a special opportunity to understand the mechanism of this route towards nuclear reprogramming. Amphibian eggs and oocytes are very favorable for an analysis of nuclear reprogramming mechanisms. This is because a *Xenopus* egg is approximately 4000 times larger than a mouse or other mammalian egg, and one frog can provide as many as 25 000 eggs or oocytes. An attempt to make use of these conspicuous advantages has led to the development of nuclear transfer to oocytes (first meiotic prophase egg progenitors). Multiple somatic nuclei (including those of mammals) can be transplanted to the GV of an oocyte (Figure 1.3A). There is no DNA replication or cell division, characteristics which cause much of the abnormality in nuclear transfer to egg (second meiotic metaphase) experiments with amphibia. Somatic nuclei transplanted to oocytes undergo transcriptional reprogramming by inducing the expression of pluripotency genes characteristic of embryonic stem cells. A large number of new transcripts (~1000 *Sox2* transcripts per gene per day) are produced after transfer to the oocyte GV, and therefore provide a special opportunity to analyze mechanisms of transcriptional reprogramming. Work with oocytes has revealed some of the mechanisms by which the specialized state of a somatic nucleus can be reversed to allow reactivation of embryo-specific genes. This is the initial step of nuclear reprogramming. Current progress in this direction has recently been reviewed by Pasque *et al.* [47].

The oocyte route of nuclear reprogramming has not yet been extended to work with mammals, but some of the reprogramming factors identified in this oocyte system have been shown to be involved in reprogramming in mammalian oocytes. In conclusion, the success of Dolly the sheep, and subsequently of work with other mammals, was clearly initiated by work with amphibia some 40 years earlier. This is therefore an area in which early work with amphibia has helped to lead success with mammals.

Messenger RNA (mRNA) injection

The first success of injecting mRNA into living eggs was in 1971 (Figure 1.3B) [48]. This experiment was undertaken primarily because, in previous years, success had been achieved by injecting purified DNA into eggs as an attempt to analyze the mechanism of DNA replication that immediately follows nuclear transfer to eggs. Surprisingly, the mRNA injection experiment worked remarkably well. It was even possible to derive swimming *Xenopus* tadpoles in which as much as half of their soluble protein was derived from the injection of rabbit globin mRNA at the egg stage. The "transplanted" mRNA turned out to be very stable and translated with very high efficiency after injection into living eggs or oocytes. Evidently the microinjection of eggs and oocytes does not release any of the ribonuclease activity which is carefully sequestered in living eggs and embryos.

The use of mRNA injection into eggs and oocytes was much enhanced by the finding of Krieg and Melton [49] which showed that mRNA could be synthesized in vitro from any cloned gene and then overexpression of that gene achieved with high efficiency after mRNA injection into amphibian eggs or oocytes. This procedure has now become extensively used for the overexpression of any gene that might be important in development. In just the same way, the overexpression of dominant negative constructs is an effective way of knocking down the expression of genes that might be important in development.

In due course, this procedure for message injection was extended to mammals where it is also widely used for gene overexpression and cell tracing experiments [50].

Cell separation, reaggregation, and rearrangement

Much of what we now know about mechanisms of development has depended on experiments in which cells are moved from their normal in vivo environment to be cultured in vitro or transplanted to the vicinity of other kinds of cells. In general, groups of cells or tissues are explanted or transplanted. While informative, these experiments are not ideal. This is because a cell within a group will always be surrounded by other cells of the same source. Therefore, it is unclear whether an individual cell is truly surrounded by cells of another germ layer or by cells of its own origin. This uncertainty is compounded by the fact that most tissues consist of cells which are not identical. Therefore, interactions between cells of different kinds may continue even if the group of cells is now transplanted to an ectopic site or cultured in vitro. The most informative experiments are those in which a single cell is transplanted to a new environment.

Nowadays, it is not uncommon to carry out single cell transplants. It is therefore interesting to consider the origin of single cell transplant experiments. Looking back to the time of Spemann, Holtfreter, etc., much of the work published between 1900 and 1940 involved tissue, that is, multicell, transplants or explants [51]. The earliest experiments involving single cell isolation in vertebrates go back to a landmark paper by Townes and Holtfreter [52] that involved isolating embryo cells from different germ layers, mixing them together, and then reaggregating them to determine their fate. For an appreciation of this paper, see Steinberg and Gilbert [53].

The difference between rearranging whole multicellular tissues from embryos and separating single cells so that they can be transplanted or recombined is not trivial. For example, in 1953, Grobstein and Zwilling showed the so-called "mass effect" [54]. This meant that the differentiation of cells is much less successful when they are cultured as progressively smaller groups ranging from large pieces of tissue containing several 1000 cells to small groups of only 100 cells or less. Therefore, single cells do not like being cultured on their own. Furthermore, groups of cells are often heterogeneous and unknown interactions may take place between them. To accurately determine the state of determination or specification of cells requires that single cells are used.

An important paper was published by Heasman *et al.* [55], in which they implanted single amphibian cells of known germ layer origin into the *Xenopus* blastocoel cavity at the blastula stage (Figure 1.3C). The embryos were cultured and the fate of the transplanted single cell and its immediate descendants was determined. The results showed that endoderm cells become irreversibly committed (determined) remarkably early in development. However this experiment was not perfect. This is because, when dropping a cell into a blastocoel cavity, it is not certain to which host cells it will become attached. For example, in zebrafish experiments, a single transplanted cell tends to migrate back into its own tissue of origin, even if it has been transplanted to an ectopic position in an embryo. In amphibia, it was possible to transplant single embryonic cells into sandwiches of unlike cells so that they could not migrate back to their own preferred environment. This kind of experiment led to the description of the community effect (see below).

The concept of isolating, rearranging, and transplanting single cells was soon taken up by early mammalian embryologists. Notably Tarkowski [56, 57] was able to separate early mammalian cells and rearrange them into different embryo aggregates. By combining this kind of experiment with appropriate genetic markers, it was possible to analyze the fate and differentiation potential of single cells in mammalian embryos. Indeed, such a design of experiment was central to the pioneering work of Gardner [58] in which he transplanted single embryo cells into the blastocyst of an early mouse embryo. These experiments now form a central part of the whole field of mouse embryonic stem cells. Experiments of this kind are now routinely used in mammalian embryo and stem cell research.

Community effect

This phenomenon describes a situation in which like cells in proximity to each other each contribute a small amount of some signal factor. So long as many cells close to each other each contribute a low concentration of factor, the concentration of that factor in the cell group will increase to a higher level than could be achieved by the factor production from one single cell on its own (Figure 1.3D).

The community effect should not be confused with the so-called "mass effect." The community effect first came to light in experiments in which single cells were transplanted to different parts of an embryo (see above); even though not exposed to any artificial environment, single transplanted cells failed to differentiate in the way that members of a group did. A range of experiments was subsequently carried out and led to the conclusion that secreted signal factors account most readily for the community effect. In one case [59] there was evidence that a particular variety of basic fibroblast growth factor was the secreted factor involved. There are many instances in normal development when a community effect may apply. In any case where a group of cells needs to differentiate in a coordinated way, the building up of a sufficient concentration of factor by a group of cells, but not by single cells, would account for the effect. This applies to many tissues in embryos, such as muscle tissue.

Conclusions and perspectives

Xenopus research has been developed by taking advantage of large and abundant eggs and easy manipulation procedures. With this useful experimental material, many breakthrough discoveries have been achieved, such as signaling pathways that govern the cell fate decision, the egg cell-free system, tissue or cell grafts, mRNA injection, and nuclear transfer. Since the whole genome sequence of *Xenopus tropicalis* has been decoded, *Xenopus* research is now compatible with the genome-wide sequencing technology, making it possible to draw global views of gene expression and chromatin signature in early embryos. We will be able to envisage more detailed molecular networks underlying development. In addition, genetic approaches such as mutation screening for finding developmentally important genes can now be applied [60]. These useful features together with the state-of-the-art technologies can make it possible to answer questions that are currently difficult to answer using mammalian oocytes, such as the genome-wide ChIP-seq analysis of chromatin factor binding in early embryonic development. For using *Xenopus* eggs/oocytes as a model to understand mammalian oocytes, it is important to study conserved mechanisms between these species. In this sense, reprogramming is appropriate since many reprogramming factors that play a role in *Xenopus* have been also shown to work in mammalian systems. We therefore believe that *Xenopus* eggs work well together with mammalian oocytes to understand animal development and reprogramming.

Acknowledgments

We thank Marta Teperek for her careful reading of the manuscript. K.M. is supported by the Japan Society for the Promotion of Science (International Research Fellowship Program). Gurdon laboratory is supported by a grant from the Wellcome Trust (Grant RG54943) to J.B.G.

References

1. Gurdon JB, Hopwood N. The introduction of *Xenopus laevis* into developmental biology: of empire, pregnancy testing and ribosomal genes. *Int J Dev Biol* 2000; **44**: 43–50.
2. Sommerville J. Using oocyte nuclei for studies on chromatin structure and gene expression. *Methods* 2010; **51**: 157–64.
3. De La Fuente R. Chromatin modifications in the germinal vesicle (GV) of mammalian oocytes. *Dev Biol* 2006; **292**: 1–12.
4. Spemann H, Mangold H. Über Induktion von Embryonanlagen durch Implantation artfremder Organisatoren. *Wilhelm Roux's Arch Dev Biol* 1924; **100**: 599–638.
5. Nieuwkoop PD. Inductive interactions in early amphibian development and their general nature. *J Embryol Exp Morphol* 1985; **89** Suppl: 333–47.
6. De Robertis EM. Spemann's organizer and self-regulation in amphibian embryos. *Nat Rev Mol Cell Biol* 2006; **7**: 296–302.
7. De Robertis EM. Spemann's organizer and the self-regulation of embryonic fields. *Mech Dev* 2009; **126**: 925–41.
8. Rogers KW, Schier AF. Morphogen gradients: from generation to interpretation. *Annu Rev Cell Dev Biol* 2011; **27**: 377–407.
9. Muller P, Schier AF. Extracellular movement of signaling molecules. *Dev Cell* 2011; **21**: 145–58.
10. Goumans MJ, Mummery C. Functional analysis of the TGFbeta receptor/Smad pathway through gene ablation in mice. *Int J Dev Biol* 2000; **44**: 253–65.
11. Pera MF, Tam PP. Extrinsic regulation of pluripotent stem cells. *Nature* 2010; **465**: 713–20.
12. Tam PP, Loebel DA, Tanaka SS. Building the mouse gastrula: signals, asymmetry and lineages. *Curr Opin Genet Dev* 2006; **16**: 419–25.
13. Lohka MJ, Masui Y. Formation in vitro of sperm pronuclei and mitotic chromosomes induced by amphibian ooplasmic components. *Science* 1983; **220**: 719–21.
14. Blow JJ, Laskey RA. Initiation of DNA replication in nuclei and purified DNA by a cell-free extract of *Xenopus eggs*. *Cell* 1986; **47**: 577–87.

15. Carpenter PB, Mueller PR, Dunphy WG. Role for a *Xenopus* Orc2-related protein in controlling DNA replication. *Nature* 1996; **379**: 357–60.
16. Coleman TR, Carpenter PB, Dunphy WG. The *Xenopus* Cdc6 protein is essential for the initiation of a single round of DNA replication in cell-free extracts. *Cell* 1996; **87**: 53–63.
17. Chong JP, Mahbubani HM, Khoo CY, *et al.* Purification of an MCM-containing complex as a component of the DNA replication licensing system. *Nature* 1995; **375**: 418–21.
18. Hutchison CJ, Cox R, Drepaul RS, *et al.* Periodic DNA synthesis in cell-free extracts of *Xenopus* eggs. *EMBO J* 1987; **6**: 2003–10.
19. Murray AW, Kirschner MW. Cyclin synthesis drives the early embryonic cell cycle. *Nature* 1989; **339**: 275–80.
20. Lohka MJ, Maller JL. Induction of nuclear envelope breakdown, chromosome condensation, and spindle formation in cell-free extracts. *J Cell Biol* 1985; **101**: 518–23.
21. Perry AC, Verlhac MH. Second meiotic arrest and exit in frogs and mice. *EMBO Rep* 2008; **9**: 246–51.
22. Philpott A, Leno GH, Laskey RA. Sperm decondensation in *Xenopus* egg cytoplasm is mediated by nucleoplasmin. *Cell* 1991; **65**: 569–78.
23. Ohsumi K, Katagiri C. Characterization of the ooplasmic factor inducing decondensation of and protamine removal from toad sperm nuclei: involvement of nucleoplasmin. *Dev Biol* 1991; **148**: 295–305.
24. Dimitrov S, Dasso MC, Wolffe AP. Remodeling sperm chromatin in *Xenopus laevis* egg extracts: the role of core histone phosphorylation and linker histone B4 in chromatin assembly. *J Cell Biol* 1994; **126**: 591–601.
25. Adachi Y, Luke M, Laemmli UK. Chromosome assembly in vitro: topoisomerase II is required for condensation. *Cell* 1991; **64**: 137–48.
26. Ohsumi K, Katagiri C, Kishimoto T. Chromosome condensation in *Xenopus* mitotic extracts without histone H1. *Science* 1993; **262**: 2033–5.
27. Hirano T, Kobayashi R, Hirano M. Condensins, chromosome condensation protein complexes containing XCAP-C, XCAP-E and a *Xenopus* homolog of the *Drosophila* Barren protein. *Cell* 1997; **89**: 511–21.
28. Laskey RA, Mills AD, Morris NR. Assembly of SV40 chromatin in a cell-free system from *Xenopus* eggs. *Cell* 1977; **10**: 237–43.
29. Almouzni G, Mechali M. Assembly of spaced chromatin promoted by DNA synthesis in extracts from *Xenopus* eggs. *EMBO J* 1988; **7**: 665–72.
30. Nicklay JJ, Shechter D, Chitta RK, *et al.* Analysis of histones in *Xenopus laevis*. II. Mass spectrometry reveals an index of cell type-specific modifications on H3 and H4. *J Biol Chem* 2009; **284**: 1075–85.
31. Kikyo N, Wade PA, Guschin D, *et al.* Active remodeling of somatic nuclei in egg cytoplasm by the nucleosomal ATPase ISWI. *Science* 2000; **289**: 2360–2.
32. Gonda K, Fowler J, Katoku-Kikyo N, *et al.* Reversible disassembly of somatic nucleoli by the germ cell proteins FRGY2a and FRGY2b. *Nat Cell Biol* 2003; **5**: 205–10.
33. Alberio R, Johnson AD, Stick R, *et al.* Differential nuclear remodeling of mammalian somatic cells by *Xenopus laevis* oocyte and egg cytoplasm. *Exp Cell Res* 2005; **307**: 131–41.
34. Miyamoto K, Furusawa T, Ohnuki M, *et al.* Reprogramming events of mammalian somatic cells induced by *Xenopus laevis* egg extracts. *Mol Reprod Dev* 2007; **74**: 1268–77.
35. Hansis C, Barreto G, Maltry N, *et al.* Nuclear reprogramming of human somatic cells by *Xenopus* egg extract requires BRG1. *Curr Biol* 2004; **14**: 1475–80.
36. Bian Y, Alberio R, Allegrucci C, *et al.* Epigenetic marks in somatic chromatin are remodelled to resemble pluripotent nuclei by amphibian oocyte extracts. *Epigenetics* 2009; **4**: 194–202.
37. Miyamoto K, Tsukiyama T, Yang Y, *et al.* Cell-free extracts from mammalian oocytes partially induce nuclear reprogramming in somatic cells. *Biol Reprod* 2009; **80**: 935–43.
38. Bui HT, Wakayama S, Kishigami S, *et al.* The cytoplasm of mouse germinal vesicle stage oocytes can enhance somatic cell nuclear reprogramming. *Development* 2008; **135**: 3935–45.
39. Spemann H. *Embryonic Development and Induction.* New Haven: Yale University, 1938.
40. Briggs R, King TJ. Transplantation of living nuclei from blastula cells into enucleated frogs' eggs. *Proc Natl Acad Sci USA* 1952; **38**: 455–63.
41. Briggs R, King TJ. Changes in the nuclei of differentiating endoderm cells as revealed by nuclear transplantation. *J Embryol Exp Morphol* 1957; **100**: 269–312.
42. Gurdon JB, Elsdale TR, Fischberg M. Sexually mature individuals of *Xenopus laevis* from the transplantation of single somatic nuclei. *Nature* 1958; **182**: 64–5.
43. Takahashi K, Yamanaka S. Induction of pluripotent stem cells from mouse embryonic and adult fibroblast cultures by defined factors. *Cell* 2006; **126**: 663–76.

44. Wilmut I, Schnieke AE, McWhir J, *et al.* Viable offspring derived from fetal and adult mammalian cells. *Nature* 1997; **385**: 810–13.

45. Byrne JA, Pedersen DA, Clepper LL, *et al.* Producing primate embryonic stem cells by somatic cell nuclear transfer. *Nature* 2007; **450**: 497–502.

46. Tachibana M, Amato P, Sparman M, *et al.* Human embryonic stem cells derived by somatic cell nuclear transfer. *Cell* 2013; **153**: 1228–38.

47. Pasque V, Jullien J, Miyamoto K, *et al.* Epigenetic factors influencing resistance to nuclear reprogramming. *Trends Genet* 2011; **27**: 516–25.

48. Gurdon JB, Lane CD, Woodland HR, *et al.* Use of frog eggs and oocytes for the study of messenger RNA and its translation in living cells. *Nature* 1971; **233**: 177–82.

49. Krieg PA, Melton DA. Functional messenger RNAs are produced by SP6 in vitro transcription of cloned cDNAs. *Nucleic Acids Res* 1984; **12**: 7057–70.

50. Zernicka-Goetz M, Pines J, McLean Hunter S, *et al.* Following cell fate in the living mouse embryo. *Development* 1997; **124**: 1133–7.

51. Hamburger V. *The Heritage of Experimental Embryology: Hans Spemann and the Organizer*. New York: Oxford University Press, 1988.

52. Townes PL, Holtfreter J. Directed movements and selective adhesion of embryonic amphibian cells. *J Exp Zool* 1955; **128**: 53–120.

53. Steinberg MS, Gilbert SF. Townes and Holtfreter (1955): directed movements and selective adhesion of embryonic amphibian cells. *J Exp Zool A Comp Exp Biol* 2004; **301**: 701–6.

54. Grobstein C, Zwilling E. Modification of growth and differentiation of chorio-allantoic grafts of chick blastoderm pieces after cultivation at a glassclot interface. *J Exp Zool* 1953; **122**: 259–84.

55. Heasman J, Snape A, Smith J, *et al.* Single cell analysis of commitment in early embryogenesis. *J Embryol Exp Morphol* 1985; **89** Suppl: 297–316.

56. Tarkowski AK. Mouse chimaeras developed from fused eggs. *Nature* 1961; **190**: 857–60.

57. Tarkowski AK. Experiments on the development of isolated blastomers of mouse eggs. *Nature* 1959; **184**: 1286–7.

58. Gardner RL. Mouse chimeras obtained by the injection of cells into the blastocyst. *Nature* 1968; **220**: 596–7.

59. Standley HJ, Zorn AM, Gurdon JB. eFGF and its mode of action in the community effect during *Xenopus* myogenesis. *Development* 2001; **128**: 1347–57.

60. Harland RM, Grainger RM. *Xenopus* research: metamorphosed by genetics and genomics. *Trends Genet* 2011; **27**: 507–15.

Chapter 2

Ontogeny of the mammalian ovary

Anne Grete Byskov and Claus Yding Andersen

Introduction

Mammalian ovarian formation and differentiation takes place early in life, often before birth, but the ovary is not ready to fulfill its main purpose, that is, to ovulate a mature oocyte, until puberty. During early fetal development the germ cells populate the gonadal areas in close association with the mesonephros. The following developmental pattern of the ovary differs greatly among species, but one parameter is a must for all: each germ cell differentiates to an oocyte and becomes together with granulosa cells enclosed in a follicular entity. The pool of follicles is final and determines the length of the future reproductive lifespan. The finely tuned interaction between germ cells and somatic cells early in life is therefore crucial.

Formation of the sexually undifferentiated gonad

Origin and migration of primordial germ cells (PGCs) from the epiblast to the gonadal anlage: role of the autonomic nervous system

The classic concept of gonadal formation is that the PGCs arise in the proximal part of the yolk sac, the proximal epiblast [1], and migrate a relatively long distance within the hindgut that grows towards the area where the gonads will develop, around somite 16 [2]. Then the PGCs leave the hindgut and move towards the developing gonads at the ventral part of the mesonephros. Thus, the PGCs are first guided by the hindgut and thereafter by other mechanisms to the gonadal anlage. The importance of the hindgut for PGC movement was shown in *Sox17*-null mouse embryos in which the hindgut does not expand and the PGCs become immobilized in the hindgut [3].

According to Freeman, however, the relatively long migration by the PGCs may actually not take place [4]. He proposed that the PGCs most likely are passively translocated as the proximal end of the yolk sac develops into/becomes part of the hindgut during the embryonic lateral folding which in the human is completed by the fifth week of gestation (postconception – pc).

Specific signaling molecules, for example bone morphogenetic proteins like BMP4 and BMP8, are important for PGC formation and are responsible for expression of PGC markers like Stella and Blimp1 (reviews: [5, 6]). Moreover, the RNA-binding protein Lin28 is involved in PGC specification from their formation to their arrival in the gonadal ridges [7] while Prdm14–Klf2 together appear to enhance epigenetic changes in PGC formation [8]. The genes *Steel* (encoding Kit ligand or stem cell factor [SCF]) and *Kit* are also involved in PGC migration and survival [9]. The PGCs' directional migration may be facilitated by a specific plasma membrane localization of the receptor tyrosine kinase-like protein Ror2 that is stimulated by SCF, and is asymmetrically distributed in migrating PGCs [10]. It has been reported that retinoic acid (RA) acts as an anti-apoptotic and proliferative factor on murine PGCs [11]. Other genes such as *ZFX* (which encodes a putative zinc finger protein) play important roles in PGC proliferation and/or survival [12].

Nevertheless, the final journey from the developing hindgut to the future gonadal ridge is not clarified but is probably dependent on factors with attractive as well as repellent actions from the surrounding tissues and the germ cells themselves. A number of studies have identified germ cell-specific markers and chemoattractants in the surrounding tissues that

Biology and Pathology of the Oocyte, 2nd edn., ed. Alan Trounson, Roger Gosden, and Ursula Eichenlaub-Ritter.

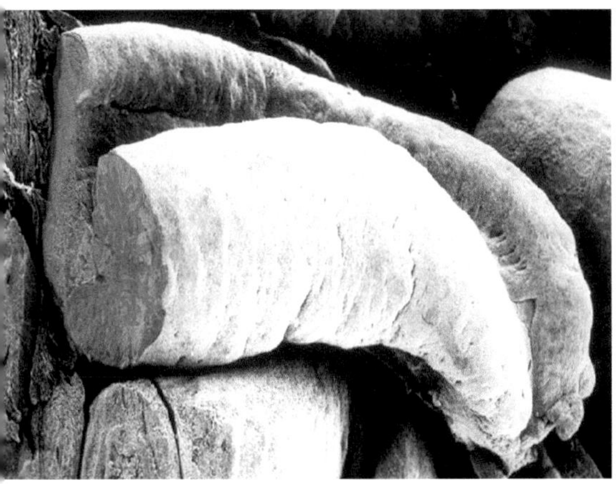

Figure 2.1 Cranial part of a human fetal ovarian–mesonephros complex, 12 weeks pc. The cutting edge is colored orange (ovary) and yellow (mesonephric remnants). The Wolffian and Müllerian ducts develop within the sausage-like structure along the ovary and are closely attached to the cranial part of the ovary. Scanning electron micrograph in collaboration with photographer Lennart Nilsson. ×90.

might direct germ cell migration towards the gonads [13]. It was recently shown that human PGCs migrate along autonomic nerve fibers and Schwann cells from the dorsal hindgut mesentery of embryos aged 29 days pc to 7 weeks pc to the gonadal ridge where they are delivered by a fine nerve plexus [14]. The nerve fibers and the PGCs were identified by their ultrastructure as well as by immunohistochemical markers such as cKIT and OCT4. Tiny nerve fibers remain in close contact to the migrating germ cells within the developing gonads (Figure 2.1). In the pig embryo at day 27 of gestation neurons originating in the neural crest cells have also been shown to invade the gonadal ridge [15]. In concordance with previous findings [14], we suggest that the neural–germ cell relationship as found in the human embryo and fetus is important for guiding the germ cells from the hindgut to the gonad and perhaps for further germ cell differentiation within the gonad (Figure 2.1).

The statement "Follow the fatty brick road: lipid signaling in cell migration" [16] thus reflects the PGCs' migration as they follow the myelin sheets of the neurons reaching from the hindgut to the gonadal anlage.

Once the PGCs arrive at the gonadal anlage early in life the ovary starts to develop in close connection with the second nephric organ, the mesonephros. The first sign of the developing gonad is the arrival of PGCs at the mesenchyme that covers the ventral cranial–medial part of the mesonephros. At this time the coelomic epithelium has not yet been defined, that is, an epithelial basement membrane is still lacking. In the human embryo the first PGCs populate this area from about 30 days pc and germ cells continue to invade this area during the next weeks [2]. It is, however, unknown when the last PGCs arrive at the gonadal anlage. Migrating female PGCs may, in principle, continue to invade the developing ovary as long as PGCs are present extragonadally. Since very few PGCs/oogonia are left in the human newborn ovary and none are seen after the second year of life [17] invasion probably stops sometimes during fetal life. In the embryonic testis the germ cells become enclosed in testicular cords during the sixth to seventh week pc although a few can be found between the testicular cords some time after sex differentiation. It is unlikely that more germ cells populate the developing testis and penetrate the basal membrane surrounding the testicular cords subsequent to sex differentiation. Meanwhile, PGCs are present extragonadally in the dorsal mesentery of both sexes also after week 7 pc [18]. Whether these PGCs will reach the gonadal anlage or become eliminated or trapped along their migration path after sex differentiation is not known.

Origin of the somatic cells

The somatic cells constituting the developing embryonic gonads originate in the mesonephric mesenchyme and mesonephric epithelial cells and the developing coelomic epithelium that covers this area. At this early developmental stage the coelomic epithelium is in fact a pseudo-epithelium lacking a basal membrane. A separation between the epithelium and the underlying tissues by an epithelial basement membrane is not formed until much later, dependent on the species (Figure 2.2). Thus, the invading PGCs find themselves in a morphologically undifferentiated mesenchyme in which the mesonephric structures are also embedded, more proximally. Concomitant with mesenchymal cells and PGCs other components such as nerve cells, blood vessels, and blood cells are also important components of the developing ovary, although often ignored.

The number of PGCs in the gonads increases by arrival of new germ cells and by their mitotic proliferation at the cranial, ventral area of the mesonephros, resulting in a gradually better-defined gonadal ridge.

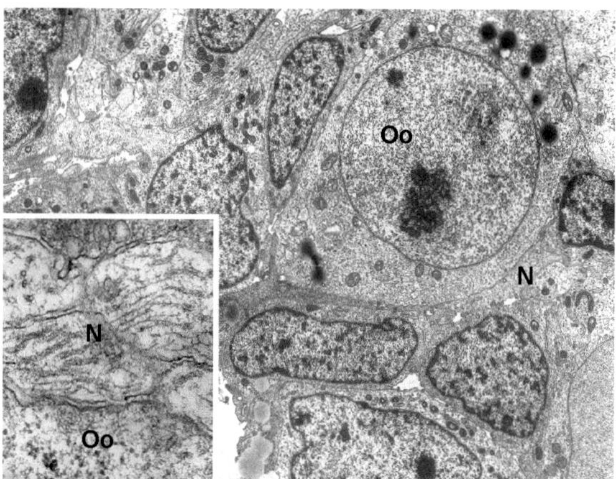

Figure 2.2 Electron micrograph of a section from the ovarian surface area of a human embryo, 28 days pc. An oogonium (Oo) is seen in the upper right-hand corner. A surface epithelium with a basement membrane is not yet formed. ×1900. Inset: Nerve cell cytoplasm with neurotubuli (N) in connection with the oogonium. ×32 000.

Proliferation of the PGCs within the developing gonad seems to be affected by several factors, for example neuropeptides (pituitary adenylate cyclase-activating polypeptide [PACAP]) [19]. During further development epithelial-derived cells from cranial–medial structures of the regressing mesonephros, that is, mesonephric tubules and/or the regressing Bowman's capsules, begin to invade the gonadal ridges [20–22]. It is conceivable that these cells undergo an epithelial–mesenchyme transition (EMT) as they migrate to the gonads where they retransform to epithelial-like cells and differentiate into extra-, connecting-, and intra-ovarian rete, the latter in connection with the developing granulosa cells.

The connections between the mesonephros and the developing gonad and the importance for gonadal formation have been recognized for a century (reviews: [23, 24]). In the male gonads the connections between the testicular cords and the rete testis – originating in the mesonephros – have long been recognized. Perhaps less appreciated is that a similar connection exists in female mammals during early ovarian formation as the rete ovarii and develops further into an endocrine organ in others.

Early ovarian development

Sexual differentiation of the gonads is genetically determined by expression of the Y-linked genes *Sry* and *Sox9* of somatic cells in the testis by initiating differentiation of Sertoli cells [11, 25, 26], whereas in the ovary the absence of Y genes and activation of XX-related genes, such as *Wnt4*, code for femaleness constitutively inducing ovarian differentiation in the absence of *Sry* [27].

From proliferating oogonia to oocytes in meiosis

As mentioned, the PGCs continue to proliferate after they have entered the gonadal ridge. This results in the formation of a cortex rich in oogonia and few somatic cells, and a central medulla with somatic cells relatively more abundant. During the first waves of oogonial proliferation the germ cells seem to undergo normal mitosis, that is, two separate cells are the result of one division. However, after some time – or perhaps after a certain number of divisions – the daughter cells remain interconnected through cell bridges [28]. Further incomplete divisions may result in a syncytium of oogonia, the so-called germ cell nests or germ cell cysts (reviewed by [29, 30]). "Germ cell cysts" may be a misleading term, since they do not contain a fluid-filled cavity. Perhaps "germ cell cluster" or "germ cell nest" or even better described as "germ cell syncytium," may be more appropriate. It is unknown what controls the formation of these syncytia and a possible importance for further germ cell development is not clear, but in the mouse these interconnections seem to be expendable [31].

During further development, again species specific, centrally placed oogonia of the syncytia leave the mitotic cycle and assume meiotic prophase. The switch from mitosis to meiosis finalizes germ cell proliferation and they are now termed oocytes. The mechanisms which control onset of meiosis are not yet clarified (see later).

Meiosis starts early in life, apparently unrelated to sex differentiation of the gonads and to the time of birth, but the timing is species specific. The first meiotic prophase exhibits four morphologically distinguishable transitory stages, preleptotene, leptotene, zygotene, and pachytene, followed by the diplotene stage, the "resting" stage in which meiosis is blocked with decondensed chromatin in the nucleus (germinal vesicle), also termed "dictyate stage." The germ cell syncytium mentioned above is visualized in the human ovary when the interconnected germ cells simultaneously pass through the different stages of meiosis (Figure 2.3). At diplotene stage, it is a prerequisite for

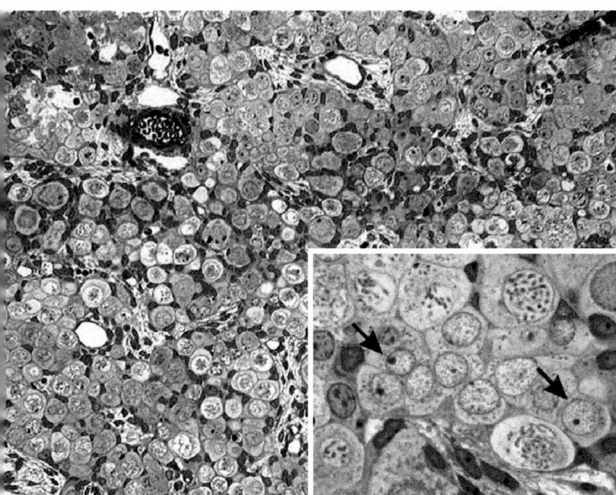

Figure 2.3 Cortex of a human ovary, 14 weeks pc, showing numerous oocytes in different transitory stages of the first meiotic division, as well as clusters of synchronously developing oogonia and oocytes, as seen in higher magnification of the inset. Nine nuclei, all in preleptotene stage, can be seen in this section; the arrows point at two of the preleptotene stages. One-μm-thick plastic section, ×220. Inset: ×650.

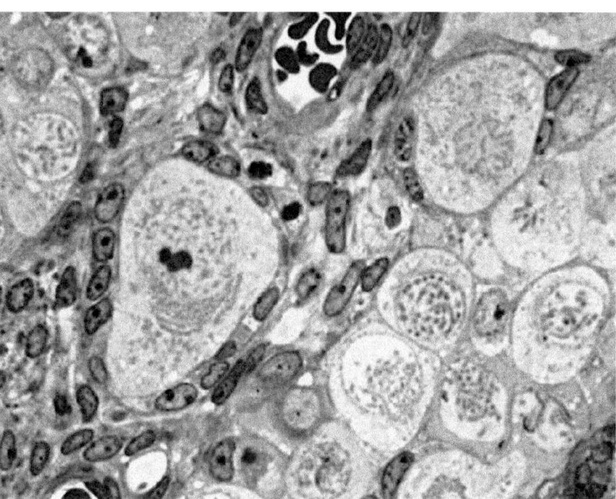

Figure 2.4 Inner part of the cortex of an ovary from a human fetus, 14 weeks pc, showing a very small follicle surrounded by darkly stained somatic cells, and groups of pachytene and pachytene/early diplotene oocytes. One-μm plastic section, ×750.

further survival of the diplotene/dictyate oocyte that it becomes surrounded by granulosa cells and sealed by a basement membrane, thus forming a follicle (Figure 2.4). No oocyte seems to continue to exist without being enclosed in its follicle. At a certain time the oocyte/follicle will begin to grow and possibly mature.

During all developmental stages, oogonia, oocytes, and follicles may become atretic and die. Actually, around two-thirds of germ cells in the human ovary die and become eliminated during fetal life (see the section on the first generations of follicles). The final pool of resting follicles is also termed the "ovarian reserve" and determines the future reproductive capacity (see the section on establishment of the follicle pool).

It has long been recognized that the mesonephros has a promoting effect on onset of meiosis in both male and female mammalian gonads [32, 33] and that this effect seems to be caused by mesonephric secretion of RA, the active form of vitamin A [34, 35]. The role of RA was recently evaluated in respect to meiotic initiation in fetal human gonads [30]. Interestingly, it was found that the enzymes needed for synthesizing RA (ALDH1A1, -A2, -A3) are present in both sexes in late first trimester gonads, at the time when the very first meiotic cells are found in the ovary [36]. However, RA within the fetal ovary is not degraded and is able to induce female meiosis, but RA in the human fetal testis is, unlike in the mouse, not degraded as in the ovary, and other mechanisms may act to prevent the meiotic action of RA in the testis in the human [30]. It seems likely that within the testicular cords a micromilieu is created that maintains the spermatogonia within their mitotic cycle. In fact, when spermatogonia are left outside the testicular cords in newly sex-differentiated fetal mouse testes they enter meiosis but only if placed close to the extragonadal mesonephric cords. This indicates that at early stages of testicular formation, mesonephric tubules secrete a substance that is able to induce meiosis in the male germ cells and that testicular cords produce a meiosis preventing factor within the testicular cords which is not present or active outside the cords [37]. A meiosis activating substance (sterol), MAS, was later shown to be present not only in adult testis and in fetal ovaries with meiosis ongoing but also in follicular fluids of preovulatory follicles of several species [38]. Although MAS is able to induce resumption of meiosis in fully grown oocytes this function may not be its main role in reproduction.

Surprisingly, only a few genes, such as *Stra8* (stimulated by RA), have been found to be involved in a direct stimulation of the onset of meiosis. In the mouse ovary with *Stra8* deficiency oogonia fail to enter meiosis [39]. A recent study suggests that the genes *Msx1* and *Msx2* are strongly expressed in the fetal mouse ovary and may be required for meiotic initiation [40]. In the mouse testis, Wnt4 signaling seems crucial for meiosis via the enzyme CYP26B1 that degrades RA and thus inhibits meiosis [41].

Meiosis in ovaries of many species; pig, sheep, mink, and more, is delayed, a phenomenon that is

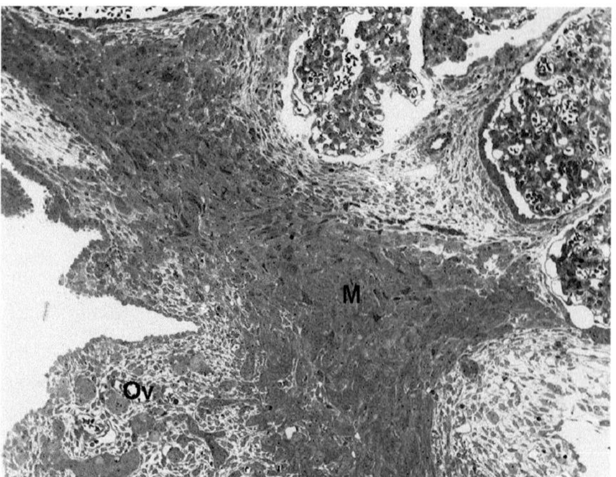

Figure 2.5 Part of a fetal pig ovary, 45 days pc, connected to the mesonephros (M) through broad darkly stained streams of mesonephric cells (connecting rete). Germ cell cords are seen in the ovary (Ov) at the lower, left-hand corner. One-μm plastic section, ×160.

closely related to the enclosure of the oogonia in well-defined cell cords, much like testicular cords (Figure 2.5). Only little mitotic activity seems to take place among the cord-enclosed germ cells during the delay period. Not until these cords/clusters begin to resolve – starting at the medullary part of the ovary – is mitotic activity accelerated or meiosis initiated – or is inhibition of meiosis prevented. It would be interesting to study the action of the meiotic-related enzymes/genes during the delay period in these species (see below).

Species differences in relation to onset of meiosis and steroid production

Although the mammalian gonad of all species studied forms along the ventral surface of the mesonephros, independent of sex, the male and female gonadal developmental pattern will soon take different morphological and functional pathways thus revealing the sex of the fetus. The dogma has been that in the male the enclosure of germ cells into cords with no sign of meiotic initiation characterizes the developing testis, whereas in the ovary germ cells form syncytia, where meiosis begins followed by follicular enclosure of individual oocytes. However, the pattern of early mammalian ovarian differentiation and onset of meiosis differs greatly among species. In some, the onset of meiosis is often preceded by a period where the oogonia become enclosed in cell cords and where meiosis is absent, but steroid synthesis occurs, quite similar to the coeval testes. This stage has been termed "delayed meiosis," for example this occurs in the pig, cat, mink, and sheep (Figure 2.6) [42]. In other species such as the mouse and hamster, meiosis in the ovary begins almost simultaneously with formation of cords in testis of the male siblings, that is, immediate meiosis. In the human, meiosis is also delayed, but obvious germ cell cords are not formed during the delay period. However, in ovaries with immediate or delayed meiosis, no or few steroids are synthesized when meiosis is initiated and proceeds (review: [43]).

In the human, testicular cords begin to form around week 6 pc, but in the coeval ovary mitotically dividing oogonia are scattered around somatic cells and only later become confined to germ cell syncytia as the mitotic divisions among oogonia often are unfinished in cytokinesis and leave the oogonia interconnected through cell bridges [28]. Meiosis in the human ovary is not recognized morphologically until week 9 pc, around 3 weeks later than testicular differentiation occurs [36]. Thus, the time of onset of female meiosis is not related to the time of gonadal sex differentiation, as defined by the time when germ cell cords of the coeval testis are morphologically recognizable. In all cases of ovarian development in mammals the first meiotic germ cells are situated towards the medulla and the oogonia in the cortical periphery are the last to enter meiosis.

The beginning of female meiosis in different mammalian species is also independent of the time of birth [43]. Although female meiosis of most species begins before birth (e.g., mouse, human, pig, sheep, and cow) oogonia of other species (e.g., hamster, rabbit, ferret, and dog) enter meiosis after birth, as late as 10 days after as in the ferret. Thus, onset of meiosis does not appear to be a landmark in respect to either gonadal sex differentiation or the time of birth. In contrast to early human fetal ovaries, fetal testes secrete steroids, in particular testosterone, from the time of sex differentiation [44]. In other species not only the testes but also the ovaries secret significant amounts of steroids during the delay period after gonadal sex differentiation and before meiosis begins, such as the sheep [45].

It is not known whether locally produced steroids in the developing ovary influence the onset and/or progression of meiosis. It would be interesting to know whether the enzyme CYP26B1, which converts RA into inactive metabolites in the developing testis and prevents onset of meiosis, is also involved in regulating meiotic delay in species with delayed meiosis [46].

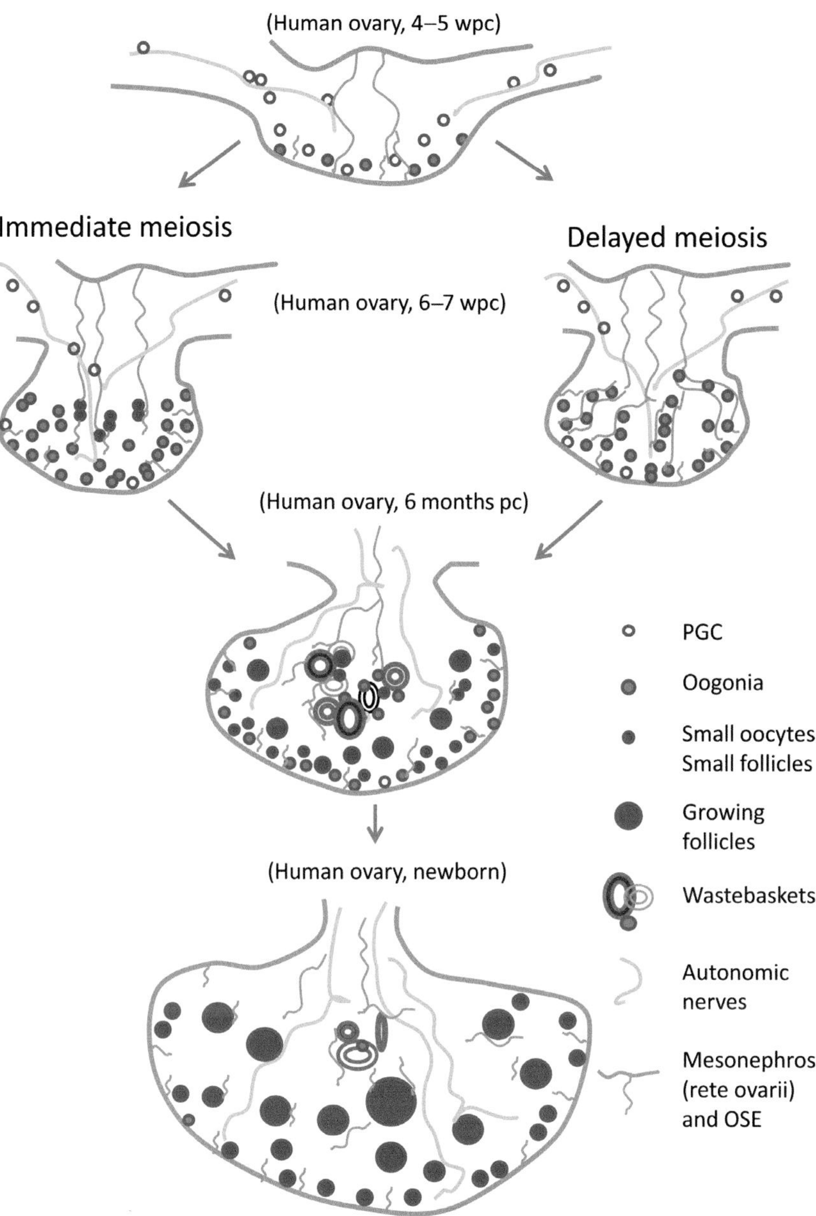

Figure 2.6 Schematic drawing of the developing mammalian ovary. Correspondence to the developing human ovary is indicated. The upper drawing depicts a very early sexually undifferentiated gonadal anlage. Indication of cell contributions to the somatic cells of developing ovary by the mesonephros and ovarian surface epithelium (OSE) are indicated by gray lines. Two patterns of early ovarian differentiation are shown: "immediate meiosis" and "delayed meiosis" (see text). Early folliculogenesis is indicated in the next drawing where the center of the ovary contains wastebaskets and the cortex may still contain some oogonia as well as small and growing follicles. The last drawing symbolizes the ovary exhibiting the well-known geographical distribution with small follicles at the periphery and growing follicles towards the center. Note that the autonomic nerve fibers are present throughout development. This drawing is a modification of Figure 2, Byskov AG, *Phys Rev*, **56**, 71–117, 1986 [43].

Formation of follicles

Onset of meiosis is a landmark of the germline fate and the ultimate stop for germ cell proliferation in both male and female germ cells. The female meiosis is arrested late in prophase, diplotene stage, of the first meiotic cell cycle and forms an oocyte. In order to survive the oocyte must become part of a follicle.

The diplotene/dictyate stage oocyte will spend most of its remaining lifetime within the follicle until it matures and resumes the first meiotic division or – more likely – becomes atretic and eliminated. Since almost all oogonia are converted to oocytes early in life without further ability to proliferate, the size of the oocyte/follicle pool is most important for the future reproductive life.

The process of follicle assembly and origin of granulosa cells

The crucial process that controls the enclosure of a single diplotene oocyte with a few granulosa cells into a follicle is not well known. By reaching diplotene stage the oocyte must be surrounded by somatic cells and sealed by a basement membrane, follicle formation or assembly, in order to survive. Entrance into meiosis and early follicle formation seem to be closely interrelated.

Since Baker's publication on the germ cell number in the fetal human ovary [47] it has repeatedly been reported that the developmental processes that lead germ cells from the oogonial stage through meiosis to follicle enclosure are tightly correlated to a hefty loss of oogonia/oocytes. However, the elimination processes of dying germ cells are presumably very fast since morphological signs of degeneration among oogonia and oocytes in transitory stages of meiosis are not frequently encountered in histological sections (Figure 2.3).

It has been proposed that a proper breakdown of the germ cell syncytium is a prerequisite for a successful follicle formation to follow (review: [48]). The exact mechanisms that control individual oocyte escape from the syncytium are unknown, but Foxl2, Nobox, and estrogens interfere with this process.

Recently it was found that in the fetal mouse ovary proliferating cell nuclear antigen (PCNA) promotes apoptosis in oocytes going from leptotene to pachytene and again later when follicles are formed, indicating a role in folliculogenesis [49]. This promotion of germ cell death may be important for individualizing the interconnected oocytes before follicle formation. Among many other factors (review: [50]), KIT and KIT ligand (SCF) are required not only for migration of PGC towards the gonads but also for the formation of follicles [18].

The origin of the granulosa cells of the follicles has been disputed for many years. Witschi and others claimed that two consecutive waves of ovarian surface epithelial migration provided granulosa cells for two generations of follicles: the first wave would not succeed and degenerate, whereas the second results in healthy follicles [22, 51]. Burns suggested that a first invasion of mainly mesonephric cells transdifferentiated to the granulosa cells of follicles that later degenerated and that the granulosa cells of a second and more successful follicle wave originated from the surface epithelium, as Witschi originally suggested [52]. Byskov and co-workers found that the main part of the granulosa cells derived in the mesonephros but that some also originated in the ovarian surface epithelium [53]. However, the close association between the mesonephric originated rete ovarii and the first cohorts of growing follicles indicates that granulosa cells originate from these cells. Recent data suggest that primordial follicle formation in mice occurs in two phases, with recruitment of granulosa cells from the proliferative ovarian surface epithelium prior to birth and from the surface epithelium perinatally (see below; [54]). In any case, follicle formation and growth always commence centrally in the ovary, often in cellular connection to mesonephric cells and far away from the surface epithelium (Figure 2.6). It seems conceivable that the outer cortex gradually acquires more coelomic epithelial cells than the medullary part, which on the other hand will get a higher concentration of mesonephric-derived cells.

The first generations of follicles

In the developing human ovary, as in many other species, the first generations of oocytes and follicles are often failures that will never succeed but become eliminated. In the human ovary some of these elimination processes can be followed over time in the second half of fetal life. As mentioned previously the first follicles seem to assemble around the oocytes that bud off from the germ cell syncytium. However, in the human ovary this process is frequently associated with errors and strange developmental patterns are often seen. From around week 16 pc single follicle-like structures may enclose one or more oocytes, oogonia, and somatic cells. Often some of the germ cells appear to be pyknotic/necrotic. Single follicles, small and growing ones, may contain many oogonia in the granulosa layer (Figure 2.7). These structures have been termed

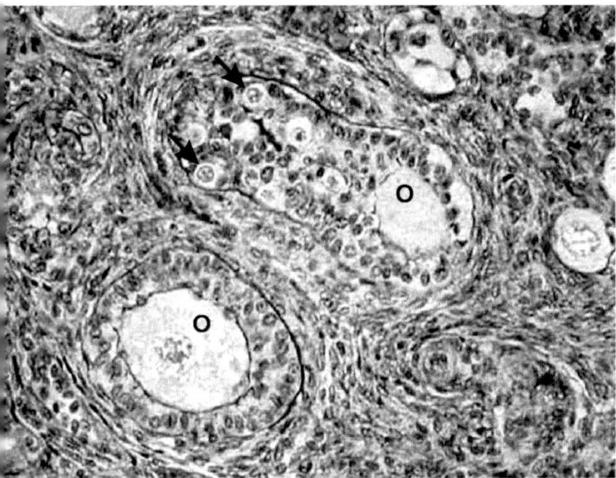

Figure 2.7 Inner part of cortex from a fetal human ovary, 32 weeks pc. A normal growing follicle with a growing oocyte (O) and another growing, but deformed, follicle containing one oocyte (O) and several oogonia within the granulosa layer. The basement membranes are stained red (periodic-hematoxylin staining). Five-μm paraffin section, ×310.

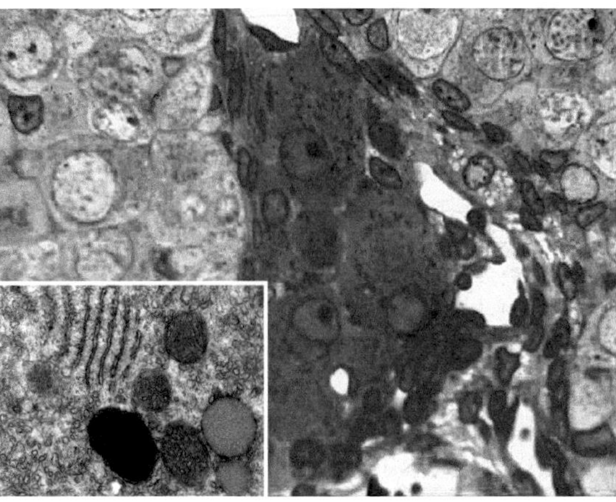

Figure 2.8 Endocrine-like interstitial cells in the middle part of the cortex of a human fetal ovary, 14 wpc, in a 1-μm plastic section. These cells are in close association with germ cells in meiosis and blood vessels (empty irregular "holes" between the endocrine-like cells). ×600. The inset shows an electron micrograph of one of these cells with cytoplasmatic characteristics of steroid-producing cells, such as tubular mitochondria, smooth endoplasmic reticulum, and fat droplets. ×22 000.

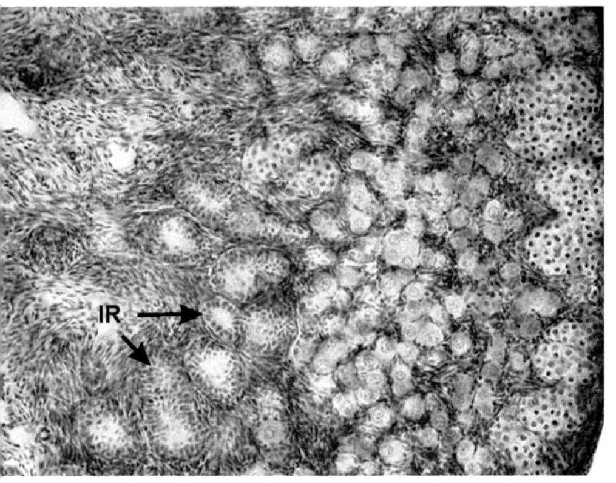

Figure 2.9 Newborn pig ovary showing the geographical distribution of oogonia and oocytes of the cortex. Most peripherally is a layer of oocytes in transitory stages of the first meiotic division appearing as dark dots on a clear background. Towards the center larger groups of early diplotene oocytes are recognized as a clear zone. More centrally are the prominent intraovarian rete cords (IR) in close association with the diplotene oocyte layer. Forty-μm-thick paraffin section, ×160.

wastebaskets, WBs [18, 55]. The third trimester human ovarian medulla may contain hundreds of WBs, which gradually become eliminated and are absent in the child's ovary after the age of 2 years [55]. Perhaps the drastic decrease in number of germ cells in the ovary during the second half of gestation as reported by Baker [47] may be related to this strange elimination pattern. Simultaneously, other follicles successfully develop and grow to early antral stages. However, the lack of gonadotropins hinders further development until new cohorts of follicles develop at puberty. In the meanwhile the peripheral placed oogonia in the fetal human ovary proliferate and gradually enter meiosis and at the time of birth almost all oogonia are transformed to oocytes enclosed in primordial follicles. These late generations of oocytes/follicles seem to escape the WB formations.

None or very few steroids can be detected in the embryonic and fetal human ovary, but mRNAs encoding steroidogenic enzymes and steroid receptors increase during the second trimester. This activity seems to be confined to pregranulosa cells and small groups of cells among the oocyte nests [56]. The ultrastructure of these cells exhibits close similarities to the steroid-producing Leydig cells of the testes (Figure 2.8) [23].

In many species with delayed meiosis the first follicles arises as part of the mesonephric-derived intraovarian rete cell cords. The germ cells enclosed in these cords assume meiosis in the usual medullary–cortical direction (Figure 2.9). Follicles are then pinched off from these prominent rete cords and formation of prominent WBs, as in the human ovary, seem to be rather inconspicuous in these species.

Establishment of the follicle pool, the "ovarian reserve"

Folliculogenesis, that is, enclosure of the diplotene oocyte with granulosa cells by a basement membrane, is controlled by a multitude of growth factors and signaling molecules (review: [57]). It is conceivable that the oocyte itself is the master regulator that signals to the surrounding somatic cells when it reaches diplotene stage.

The follicle is one of the most well-defined stem cell niches in the body. No cells intrude or exit the niche except during follicle death or at ovulation. The integrity of the follicle niche is required for the interaction between the granulosa cells and the oocyte and the subsequent differentiation of the surrounding cells into the hormone-producing theca cells.

The germ cell number in ovaries of human and monkey during fetal life was originally determined by Baker using volumetric counting methods of germ cells and somatic cells [47, 58]. In the past 10 years stereological studies showed that the number of germ cells in human fetal ovaries up to 4.5 months old increased more than indicated by Baker's original studies (review: [59]). Baker found that the number of germ cells per ovary peaked at midgestation at 3.5 million and thereafter decreased to 1 million at the time of birth. However, using stereology Fowler *et al.* counted approximately 6.5 million germ cells per ovary around 4 to 5 months pc [60]. Stereological counting of the number of germ cells in older female fetuses or newborns has not yet been performed and the dramatic loss of germ cells during the last half of fetal life remains unconfirmed. It is possible that BMP4 signaling may play a differentiated role in promoting germ cell apoptosis at least during the first half of pregnancy [61].

Another strategy for eliminating oogonia and very early diplotene oocytes is the extrusion of these cells through the ovarian surface epithelium as observed in mouse [62] and human [63]. In the mouse ovary around 10% of small oocytes are found in the periovarian space on day 3 post-partum. Whether the exit of oogonia/oocytes from the human ovarian surface epithelium is of comparable magnitude is not known. The mouse ovary is enclosed by a bursa ovarii where the extruded germ cells can be found for some time whereas a bursa ovarii does not exist in the human.

In mammals an accepted concept has been that all germ cells enter meiosis to become oocytes enclosed in follicles early in life, a concept that was challenged by Johnson *et al.* [64]. Actually, small pockets of oogonia are still present in the cortex of pubertal or even adult ovaries of some mammalian species, for example monkey and dog, and sometimes meiosis is recognized in such pockets [65]. However, a different concept has been promoted that germ stem cells exit in the adult mammalian ovary, in particular in the ovarian surface epithelium; when retrieved from the epithelium these cells can differentiate in culture and express mRNA known to be specific to PGCs, such as NANOG, OCT-4, and SOX-2 [66]. Recent reports suggest that there may be oogonial stem cells (OSCs) also in human ovary that can be isolated, enriched, and induced to form oocyte-like cells after transplantation [67]. Production of offspring was obtained from such germline stem cells from mice. There are, however, still vigorous discussions on the physiological relevance of OSCs and whether formation of viable follicles and oocytes is possible and applicable in humans, although they may offer unique opportunities for research [68–70]. From mouse studies it appears that RSPO1 signaling together with WNT4 is important to maintain granulosa cell specification and represses Sox9 expression because females deficient in these genes initially possess ovaries which after birth acquire Sertoli-like cells and testis cords (review: [71]).

In all circumstances genetic models in mice and mutations in humans suggest that the size of the pool of small follicles determines the natural length of the fertile period and precocious loss can induce premature ovarian insufficiency (POI), for instance when defects in germ cell cyst breakdown occur [72]. Furthermore, at all times a number of small follicles leave the pool and begins to grow (see other chapters). The pool will be exhausted around menopause in humans. A recent model depicts the number of non-growing follicles from conception to menopause [73].

Time will show whether it will be possible to harvest and culture germ stem cells from the human ovary and produce oocytes that are safe for use in human reproduction in the future.

Acknowledgments

The competent help with the photographic work by photographer John Post is greatly appreciated. The authors also appreciate the fruitful discussions of this manuscript with Professor Ursula Eichenlaub-Ritter.

References

1. Wylie CC. The biology of primordial germ cells. *Eur Urol* 1993; **23**(1): 62–6.
2. Witschi E. Migration of the germ cells of human embryos from the yolk sac to the primitive gonadal folds. *Contrib Embryol* 1948; **209**: 67–80.
3. Hara K, Kanai-Azuma M, Uemura M, *et al.* Evidence for crucial role of hindgut expansion in directing proper migration of primordial germ cells in mouse early embryogenesis. *Dev Biol* 2009; **330**(2): 427–39.
4. Freeman B. The active migration of germ cells in the embryos of mice and men is a myth. *Reproduction* 2003; **125**(5): 635–43.
5. Saitou M, Payer B, O'Carroll D, Ohinata Y, Surani MA. Blimp1 and the emergence of the germ line during development in the mouse. *Cell Cycle* 2005; **4**(12): 1736–40.
6. Nichols J, Smith A. The origin and identity of embryonic stem cells. *Development* 2011; **138**(1):3–8.
7. West JA, Viswanathan SR, Yabuuchi A, *et al.* A role for Lin28 in primordial germ-cell development and germ-cell malignancy. *Nature* 2009; **460**(7257): 909–13.
8. Gillich A, Bao S, Grabole N, *et al.* Epiblast stem cell-based system reveals reprogramming synergy of germline factors. *Cell Stem Cell* 2012; **10**(4): 425–39.
9. Dolci S, Williams DE, Ernst MK, *et al.* Requirement for mast cell growth factor for primordial germ cell survival in culture. *Nature* 1991; **352**(6338): 809–11.
10. Laird DJ, Altshuler-Keylin S, Kissner MD, Zhou X, Anderson KV. Ror2 enhances polarity and directional migration of primordial germ cells. *PLoS Genet* 2011; 7(12): e1002428.
11. Koshimizu U, Watanabe M, Nakatsuji N. Retinoic acid is a potent growth activator of mouse primordial germ cells in vitro. *Dev Biol* 1995; **168**(2): 683–5.
12. Luoh SW, Bain PA, Polakiewicz RD, *et al.* Zfx mutation results in small animal size and reduced germ cell number in male and female mice. *Development* 1997; **124**(11): 2275–84.
13. Richardson BE, Lehmann R. Mechanisms guiding primordial germ cell migration: strategies from different organisms. *Nat Rev Mol Cell Biol* 2010; **11**(1): 37–49.
14. Møllgård K, Jespersen A, Lutterodt MC, *et al.* Human primordial germ cells migrate along nerve fibers and Schwann cells from the dorsal hind gut mesentery to the gonadal ridge. *Mol Hum Reprod* 2010; **16**(9): 621–31.
15. Dees WL, Hiney JK, McArthur NH, *et al.* Origin and ontogeny of mammalian ovarian neurons. *Endocrinology* 2006; **147**(8): 3789–96.
16. Renault AD, Lehmann R. Follow the fatty brick road: lipid signaling in cell migration. *Curr Opin Genet Dev* 2006; **16**(4): 348–54.
17. Byskov AG, Hoyer PE, Yding AC, *et al.* No evidence for the presence of oogonia in the human ovary after their final clearance during the first two years of life. *Hum Reprod* 2011; **26**(8): 2129–39.
18. Hoyer PE, Byskov AG, Mollgard K. Stem cell factor and c-Kit in human primordial germ cells and fetal ovaries. *Mol Cell Endocrinol* 2005; **234**(1–2): 1–10.
19. Pesce M, Canipari R, Ferri GL, Siracusa G, De Felici M. Pituitary adenylate cyclase-activating polypeptide (PACAP) stimulates adenylate cyclase and promotes proliferation of mouse primordial germ cells. *Development* 1996; **122**(1): 215–21.
20. Zamboni L, Bézard J, Mauléon P. The role of mesonephros in the development of the sheep fetal ovary. *Ann Biol Anim Biochim Biophys* 1979; **19**(4B): 1153–78.
21. Byskov AG. The anatomy and ultrastructure of the rete system in the fetal mouse ovary. *Biol Reprod* 1978; **19**(4): 720–35.
22. Juengel JL, Sawyer HR, Smith PR, *et al.* Origins of follicular cells and ontogeny of steroidogenesis in ovine fetal ovaries. *Mol Cell Endocrinol* 2002; **191**(1): 1–10.
23. Byskov AG, Høyer PE. Embryology of mammalian gonads and ducts. In: Knobil E, Neill JD, eds. *The Physiology of Reproduction*, 2nd edn. New York: Raven Press, Ltd. 1994; 487–540.
24. Wrobel KH, Suss F. The significance of rudimentary nephrostomial tubules for the origin of the vertebrate gonad. *Anat Embryol (Berl)* 2000; **201**(4): 273–90.
25. Koopman P, Gubbay J, Vivian N, Goodfellow P, Lovell-Badge R. Male development of chromosomally female mice transgenic for Sry. *Nature* 1991; **351**(6322): 117–21.
26. Vidal VP, Chaboissier MC, de Rooij DG, Schedl A. Sox9 induces testis development in XX transgenic mice. *Nat Genet* 2001; **28**(3): 216–17.
27. Vainio S, Heikkila M, Kispert A, Chin N, McMahon AP. Female development in mammals is regulated by Wnt-4 signalling. *Nature* 1999; **397**(6718): 405–9.
28. Gondos B, Zamboni L. Ovarian development: the functional importance of germ cell interconnections. *Fertil Steril* 1969; **20**(1): 176–89.
29. Pepling ME, Spradling AC. Female mouse germ cells form synchronously dividing cysts. *Development* 1998; **125**(17): 3323–8.

30. Childs AJ, Cowan G, Kinnel HL, Anderson RA, Saunders PT. Retinoic acid signalling and the control of meiotic entry in the human fetal gonad. *PLoS One* 2011; **6**(6): 1–6.

31. Chen Y, Jefferson WN, Newbold RR, Padilla-Banks E, Pepling ME. Estradiol, progesterone, and genistein inhibit oocyte nest breakdown and primordial follicle assembly in the neonatal mouse ovary in vitro and in vivo. *Endocrinology* 2007; **148**(8): 3580–90.

32. Byskov AG. Does the rete ovarii act as a trigger for the onset of meiosis? *Nature* 1974; **252**(5482): 396–7.

33. Byskov AG, Grinsted J. Feminizing effect of mesonephros on cultured differentiating mouse gonads and ducts. *Science* 1981; **212**(4496): 817–18.

34. Menke DB, Koubova J, Page DC. Sexual differentiation of germ cells in XX mouse gonads occurs in an anterior-to-posterior wave. *Dev Biol* 2003; **262**(2): 303–12.

35. Koubova J, Menke DB, Zhou Q, *et al.* Retinoic acid regulates sex-specific timing of meiotic initiation in mice. *Proc Natl Acad Sci USA* 2006; **103**(8): 2474–9.

36. Bendsen E, Byskov AG, Andersen CY, Westergaard LG. Number of germ cells and somatic cells in human fetal ovaries during the first weeks after sex differentiation. *Hum Reprod* 2006; **21**: 30–5.

37. Byskov AG. The meiosis inducing interaction between germ cells and rete cells in the fetal mouse gonad. *Ann Biol Anim Biochim Biophys* 1978; **18**(2): 327–34.

38. Byskov AG, Andersen CY, Nordholm L, *et al.* Chemical structure of sterols that activate oocyte meiosis. *Nature* 1995; **374**(6522): 559–62.

39. Baltus AE, Menke DB, Hu YC, *et al.* In germ cells of mouse embryonic ovaries, the decision to enter meiosis precedes premeiotic DNA replication. *Nat Genet* 2006; **38**(12): 1430–4.

40. Le Bouffant R, Souquet B, Duval N, *et al.* Msx1 and Msx2 promote meiosis initiation. *Development* 2011; **138**(24): 5393–402.

41. Naillat F, Prunskaite-Hyyrylainen R, Pietila I, *et al.* Wnt4/5a signalling coordinates cell adhesion and entry into meiosis during presumptive ovarian follicle development. *Hum Mol Genet* 2010; **19**(8): 1539–50.

42. Byskov AG. Regulation of meiosis in mammals. *Ann Biol Anim Biochim Biophys* 1979; **19**(4B): 1251–61.

43. Byskov AG. Differentiation of mammalian embryonic gonad. *Physiol Rev* 1986; **66**(1): 71–117.

44. George FW, Wilson JD. Sex determination and differentiation. In: Knobil E, Neill JD, eds. *The Physiology of Reproduction*. New York: Raven Press Ltd., 1988; 3–25.

45. Lun S, Smith P, Lundy T, *et al.* Steroid contents of and steroidogenesis in vitro by the developing gonad and mesonephros around sexual differentiation in fetal sheep. *J Reprod Fertil* 1998; **114**(1): 131–9.

46. Bowles J, Koopman P. Retinoic acid, meiosis and germ cell fate in mammals. *Development* 2007; **134**(19): 3401–11.

47. Baker TG. A quantitative and cytological study of germ cells in human ovaries. *Philos Trans R Soc Lond B* 1963; **158**: 417–33.

48. Tingen C, Kim A, Woodruff TK. The primordial pool of follicles and nest breakdown in mammalian ovaries. *Mol Hum Reprod* 2009; **15**(12): 795–803.

49. Xu B, Hua J, Zhang Y, *et al.* Proliferating cell nuclear antigen (PCNA) regulates primordial follicle assembly by promoting apoptosis of oocytes in fetal and neonatal mouse ovaries. *PLoS One* 2011; **6**(1): e16046.

50. Monget P, Bobe J, Gougeon A, *et al.* The ovarian reserve in mammals: a functional and evolutionary perspective. *Mol Cell Endocrinol* 2012; **356**(1–2): 2–12.

51. Witschi E. Embryogenesis of the adrenal and the reproductive glands. *Horm Res* 1951; **6**: 1.

52. Burns RK. Role of hormones in the differentiation of sex. In: Young WC, ed. *Sex and Internal Secretions*, 3rd edn. Baltimore: The Williams and Wilkins Co. 1961; 76–158.

53. Byskov AG, Skakkebaek NE, Stafanger G, Peters H. Influence of ovarian surface epithelium and rete ovarii on follicle formation. *J Anat* 1977; **123**(1): 77–86.

54. Mork L, Tang H, Batchvarov I, Capel B. Mouse germ cell clusters form by aggregation as well as clonal divisions. *Mech Dev* 2012; **128**(11–12): 591–6.

55. Byskov AG, Hoyer PE, Yding AC, *et al.* No evidence for the presence of oogonia in the human ovary after their final clearance during the first two years of life. *Hum Reprod* 2011; **26**(8): 2129–39.

56. Fowler PA, Anderson RA, Saunders PT, *et al.* Development of steroid signaling pathways during primordial follicle formation in the human fetal ovary. *J Clin Endocrinol Metab* 2011; **96**(6): 1754–62.

57. Pepling ME. Follicular assembly: mechanisms of action. *Reproduction* 2012; **143**(2): 139–49.

58. Baker TG. A quantitative and cytological study of oogenesis in the rhesus monkey. *J Anat* 1966; **100**(4): 761–76.

59. Mamsen LS, Lutterodt MC, Andersen EW, Byskov AG, Andersen CY. Germ cell numbers in human embryonic and fetal gonads during the first two trimesters of pregnancy: analysis of six published studies. *Hum Reprod* 2011; **26**(8): 2140–5.

60. Fowler PA, Flannigan S, Mathers A, *et al.* Gene expression analysis of human fetal ovarian primordial

follicle formation. *J Clin Endocrinol Metab* 2009; **94**(4): 1427–35.

61. Childs AJ, Kinnell HL, Collins CS, *et al.* BMP signaling in the human fetal ovary is developmentally regulated and promotes primordial germ cell apoptosis. *Stem Cells* 2010; **28**: 1368–78.

62. Byskov AG, Rasmussen G. Ultrastructural studies of the developing follicle. In: Peters H, ed. *International Congress Series 267.* Amsterdam: Excerpta Medica. 1973; 55–62.

63. Motta PM, Makabe S. Elimination of germ cells during differentiation of the human ovary: an electron microscopic study. *Eur J Obstet Gynecol Reprod Biol* 1986; **22**(5–6): 271–86.

64. Johnson J, Canning J, Kaneko T, Pru JK, Tilly JL. Germline stem cells and follicular renewal in the postnatal mammalian ovary. *Nature* 2004; **428**(6979): 145–50.

65. Byskov AG, Faddy MJ, Lemmen JG, Andersen CY. Eggs forever? *Differentiation* 2005; **73**(9–10): 438–46.

66. Virant-Klun I, Zech N, Rozman P, *et al.* Putative stem cells with an embryonic character isolated from the ovarian surface epithelium of women with no naturally present follicles and oocytes. *Differentiation* 2008; **76**(8): 843–56.

67. White YA, Woods DC, Takai Y, *et al.* Oocyte formation by mitotically active germ cells purified from ovaries of reproductive-age women. *Nat Med* 2012; **18**(3): 413–21.

68. Zhang H, Zheng W, Shen Y, *et al.* Experimental evidence showing that no mitotically active female germline progenitors exist in postnatal mouse ovaries. *Proc Natl Acad Sci USA* 2012; **109**(31): 12580–5.

69. Telfer EE, Albertini DF. The quest for human ovarian stem cells. *Nat Med* 2012; **18**(3): 353–4.

70. Oatley J, Hunt PA. Of mice and (wo)men: purified oogonial stem cells from mouse and human ovaries. *Biol Reprod* 2012; **86**(6): 196.

71. Liu CF, Liu C, Yao HH. Building pathways for ovary organogenesis in the mouse embryo. *Curr Top Dev Biol* 2010; **90**: 263–90.

72. Lechowska A, Bilinski S, Choi Y, *et al.* Premature ovarian failure in nobox-deficient mice is caused by defects in somatic cell invasion and germ cell cyst breakdown. *J Assist Reprod Genet* 2011; **28**(7): 583–9.

73. Wallace WH, Kelsey TW. Human ovarian reserve from conception to the menopause. *PLoS One* 2010; **5**(1): e8772.

Section 2 Life cycle

Chapter 3

Gene networks in oocyte meiosis

Swapna Mohan and Paula E. Cohen

Introduction

In the current era of the genome, the amount of information available about gene expression, protein products, their interactions and pathways in almost any physiological system has become quite overwhelming. The processes of mammalian meiosis and oocyte development are no exception. Most of these data have been generated using high throughput genomic and proteomic screening systems. However, various experimental approaches over several decades, such as targeted mutagenesis, modification/suppression of specific genes both in vivo and in vitro, have also contributed greatly to our understanding of the genetic basis for meiotic processes and oogenesis [1]. Such studies have also been greatly enhanced using comparative analyses of these processes across the animal kingdom, allowing us to identify key genetic pathways that are functionally conserved in germ cells. With all the available information from multiple online databases, gaining an understanding of a complex process like meiosis, which spans several years and involves numerous cellular pathways, is challenging. It is especially difficult when trying to obtain a view that encompasses the cellular events of meiosis, yet also puts these processes in the context of the overall physiology and systems biology of the ovary. Representation of biological interactions within the cell in terms of gene networks provides an accurate and explanatory basis for studying cellular events. In addition, creating gene networks, by its very nature, helps us to define common processes amongst many different species, allowing us to appreciate both the similarities and the differences in these processes across the animal kingdom. At the same time, we can identify commonalities among cellular processes in terms of the networks that they utilize.

Table 3.1. Common interactions in a network

Physical interactions	
Interaction type	**Example**
• Between components found in the same cellular compartment	Membrane fusion proteins and cargo binding proteins in secretory vesicles
• Part of the same macromolecular structure	Structural proteins forming the meiotic spindle
• Produced at about the same time in the cell cycle	Proteins required for gap junction closure in cumulus–oocyte complex and proteins for phosphodiesterase activity in the oocyte
Functional interactions	
Interaction type	**Example**
• Found in the same cellular pathway	DNA repair proteins
• Genetic interactions	Proteins involved in the epigenetic reprogramming of the oocyte during development
• Producing similar tissue expression patterns (in analogous processes across cell types or between species)	Retinoic acid response elements expression in testicular tissue
• Taking part in the same functional process	Chemotactic proteins and extracellular matrix proteins both regulating germ cell migration

Gene networks are defined as graphs showing multiple genes as intersection points of lines that represent the interaction between these points [2]. These can represent direct gene product interactions, such as protein–protein interactions, or indirect interactions corresponding to successive steps of a metabolic pathway (Table 3.1). Interactions can also arise between

Biology and Pathology of the Oocyte, 2nd edn., ed. Alan Trounson, Roger Gosden, and Ursula Eichenlaub-Ritter.
Published by Cambridge University Press. © Cambridge University Press 2013.

Table 3.2. Commonly used databases for observing biological themes in expression patterns

Database	Description
Gene ontology http://www.geneontology.org/	Gene and gene product functions across species at biological, cellular, and molecular levels
NCBI Gene Entrez http://www.ncbi.nlm.nih.gov/gene	Gene and protein sequences, structures, chromosome maps, references
Kyoto Encyclopdia of Genes and Genomes (KEGG) http://www.genome.jp/kegg/	Genomes, biological pathways, molecular interactions, diseases, and drug development
OMIM http://www.ncbi.nlm.nih.gov/omim	Catalog of human diseases with known genetic components
UniProt database http://www.uniprot.org/	Protein function, cellular localization, interactions, expression patterns, domains

genes themselves causing an up-regulation or suppression of activity (protein–DNA interaction). These interactions can be useful in predicting changes in expression patterns and/or change in metabolic pathways of other genes that are closer in the network to the gene of interest. This is extremely useful in creating a detailed biological model of cell–cell interactions, pathways, and roles of genes in specific cellular pathways within a tissue without having to determine the action of each individual gene one by one [3]. Networks can also be used to predict the function of previously unknown genes if they are identified to be a part of known gene clusters with high-confidence interconnections [4].

A gene network is created by integrating many different criteria such as temporal gene expression, physical interaction of products, protein domains, comparative expression patterns in taxonomically close organisms (phylogeny), contribution to similar pathology, and participation in connected biological processes (gene ontology) [4]. Some of these criteria are obtained by wet-bench experimentation (expression profiles, etc.), while others can be obtained *in silico* (by computational means: gene similarities, common functional motifs, etc.). Many databases are becoming available for collating such data across large gene sets, often linked to the genome browser sites (Table 3.2). Collectively, all these features are assigned quantitative values and their combined measurement gives an idea of the strength of functional association of a group of genes. Such data sets are then analyzed by different methods like cluster analysis, correlation analysis, and analysis of mutual information [5]. The resulting data are then used as a resource to highlight groups of genes over-represented in a particular cell type at specific times and subsequently to understand the mechanisms driving the development and function of that cell type/tissue.

Germ cell development

The formation of germ cells and their commitment to either one of two sex-specific developmental pathways (oogenesis or spermatogenesis) occurs during fetal life in mammalian species. In the mouse and human, cells in the germ cell lineage arise from the epiblast region of the embryo, closest to the extraembryonic ectoderm [6]. These cells acquire the competence to form primordial germ cells (PGCs) but only a subset of them actually go on to become PGCs [7]. Competence to enter the PGC specification pathway occurs under the influence of factors such as bone morphogenetic protein 4 (BMP4) and BMP8b, which are expressed by cells of the surrounding extraembryonic ectoderm [6, 8]. These factors induce the expression of genes in the Fragilis family, such as *Ifitm3* (*Fragilis*), *Ifitm1* (*Fragilis2*), and *Ifitm2* (*Fragilis3*), in the PGC precursor cells, which may play a role in germ cell adhesion and specification [7]. A subset of the PGC precursor cells also begins expression of *Blimp1* (*Prdm1*). It is these cells specifically that are destined for the PGC fate [9]. BLIMP1 is a key factor in regulating PGC specification of cells characterized by the repression of somatic genes and up-regulation of germ cell-specific genes such as *Prdm14, Ssea1, Tnap,* and *Tiar.*

Ifitm3 and *1* are responsible for the production of Fragilis family of proteins in the mouse, which then induce the expression of a germ cell-specific gene *Stella* (*Dppa3*) that is involved in chromosome organization, RNA processing and allows the PGCs to retain pluripotency [9]. Retention of pluripotency in the PGCs is accompanied by the expression of stem cell-associated markers, including *Nanog, Oct4,* and *Sox2,* which are initially seen only in the very early embryo, and which are then re-expressed in the mouse PGCs by embryonic day 7.25 (E7.25) [9]. However, transcripts of *Oct4* have been detected in the mouse epiblast as early as E6.5. *Oct4*, in addition to

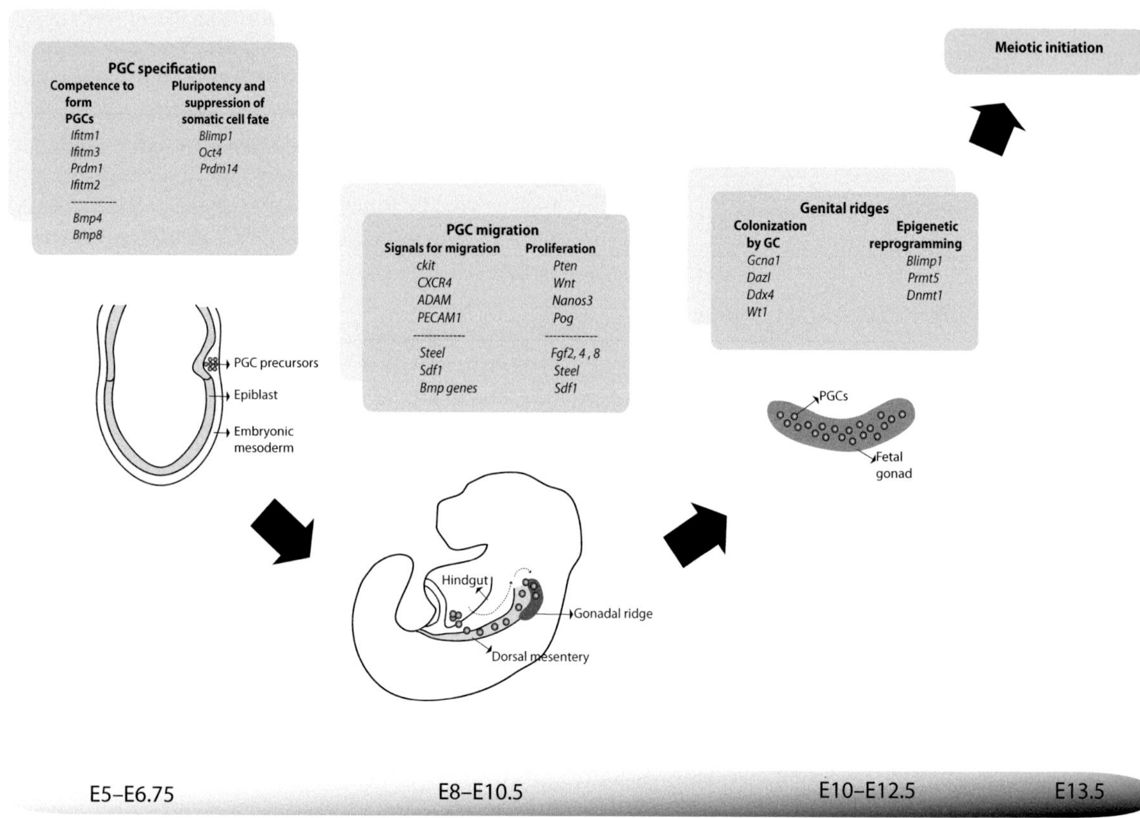

Figure 3.1 Genes expressed for primordial germ cell (PGC) development in the mouse. Gene names above the dotted line are expressed in the germ cell and below the dotted line are observed in the somatic cell population. Germ cell specification begins in the extraembryonic ectoderm when cells in the proximal epiblast acquire competence to form PGCs (PGC precursor cells). A subset of these cells then goes on to have PGC fate later on in development. Both these steps of specification are the effect of paracrine signals from the surrounding cells of the extraembryonic ectoderm such as proteins from TGFβ, BMP, and SMAD families. These signals induce the expression of genes involved in the germline fate allocation of the cells expressing them. Simultaneously, the PGCs also express genes required for maintaining the pluripotency potential and for suppression of a somatic cell fate. The next step in PGC development is their migration from the specification site along the hindgut through the dorsal mesentery to the genital ridges on either side. This process is mediated by somatic cell-derived signals for motility such as Kit-Ligand factor (encoded by *Steel*) and signals for chemotaxis such as SDF1 (encoded by *Sdf1*), and adhesion molecules such as those of the ADAM family. Colonization of the genital ridges is mediated by the expression of germ cell-specific factors (*Gcna1*, *Ddx4*), which is followed by epigenetic reprogramming (*Blimp1*, *Prmt5*) which sends the germ cells to a fate of meiotic competence. The timescale is as per embryonic development in the female mouse.

maintaining pluripotency, is needed for the survival of the PGCs, which may explain its relatively early expression [10]. In addition to this, *Blimp1* and *Smad1* expression has been implicated in suppression of genes required for setting up somatic cell lineage, such as *Hoxb*, *Fgf8*, and *Snail* [11].

The PGCs migrate from the extraembryonic mesoderm to the urogenital ridge of the embryo at E10 in mice and about the third week of gestation in humans [8] (Figure 3.1; see also Chapter 2). This migration is mediated by the interaction between cKit, a tyrosine kinase receptor located on the surface of PGCs, and its ligand, KitL, located on the somatic cells along the migratory pathway. The expression of *cKit/W* in the PGCs and *Kitl* in the somatic cells, therefore, is high at this time [12] as are several somatic cell signals necessary to regulate PGC motility, such as stromal cell-derived factor-1 (SDF1) and PECAM1 [7]. At the same time, the PGCs themselves express a variety of genes, including *Mvh*, *Dnd*, *Dazl1*, and *Nanos3*, all of which assist in maintaining germ cell lineage during this migration [10, 13].

After migration to, and colonization of, the genital ridges, new interactions with the surrounding somatic cells of the indifferent gonad induce expression of genes encoding adhesion molecules (ADAM family) in the germ cells (Figure 3.1) [11]. The PGCs proliferate rapidly under the influence of several proliferation signals from genes such as *Cxcr4, Pin1, Ssea1, Wt1, Nanos3,* and leukemia inhibiting factor (LIF) receptor [7, 14]. Surrounding somatic cells also initiate several paracrine mechanisms with factors such as tumor necrosis factor alpha (TNFα), SDF1, fibroblast growth factor 2 (FGF2), FGF4, and FGF8 to ensure the survival and proliferation of the PGCs in their new environment [7]. Expression of some germ cell markers decreases (*Tnap, Prdm1, Ssea1*) at this time, accompanied by a reduction in ability to form pluripotent stem cells in culture [11, 14]. Concomitantly, however, expression analysis on fetal gonads in mice (E11–18) shows higher expression of a group of 37 genes, which include known pluripotency markers such as *Dppa2, Nanog, Oct4,* and *Sox2,* along with other genes that regulate meiotic entry and germ cell differentiation, including *Ddx4, Gcna1, Dazl,* and *Gcl* [14]. These expression changes are accompanied by widespread epigenetic reprogramming in the form of genome demethylation and chromatin remodeling [14], with some 100 or so genes undergoing this type of imprinting in the females. At this time the non-germ cell populations in the gonad are bipotential, having the ability to develop into Sertoli or granulosa cells [11].

The germ cells colonizing the female gonadal ridges (now known as the oogonia at around E9.5 in mice) are initially present as cell clusters connected by cytoplasmic bridges, which after complete cytokinesis become surrounded by pregranulosa cells, thereby forming the first primordial follicles. *Figα* expression in the oogonia is shown to be required for this process [11]. Gene network analysis of mouse oogonia showed overexpression of some 500 or so genes at this stage of development. GO annotation analysis revealed their involvement in biological processes such as germ cell development, DNA methylation, ovarian follicle development, and meiosis [14].

Sex determination

Mouse fetal gonads at E12 start showing sexual dimorphism, which is initiated by the somatic cell environment of the germ cells. Sexual differentiation of the somatic component of the gonad is followed by differentiation of the germ cells, which involves an up-regulation of several genes in both the male and female gonad. About 250 of these genes are germ cell specific while close to 1700 genes are in the somatic cells. Of these genes, female bias is shown by a group containing *Bmp2, Fst,* and *Wnt4* genes whereas *Sox9, Amh,* and *Cyp26b1* show male-biased expression. After E12 some 60 or 50 genes have been shown to have female-specific expression. Some of these are meiosis-specific genes like *Dmc1* and *Spo11,* indicating the achievement of meiotic competence in female germ cells immediately after colonizing the gonads [11]. Furthermore, this same group of genes was highly expressed in postnatal testis only at the beginning of spermatogenesis although both XX and XY germ cells have been shown to be meiotically competent in culture at this stage [11, 14].

Entry into and progression through meiotic prophase I during fetal life

In female mouse embryos, entry into meiosis is marked by, and dependent on, up-regulation of retinoic acid (RA) response genes, including *Stra8* [11], while PGCs from male embryos express genes that are required for RA degradation, thus preventing meiotic entry at this time [15]. In females, germ cells at this stage are called primary oocytes. *Stra8* expression is required for pre-meiotic DNA replication and chromosome condensation and occurs at E12–13 in mice and 8–13 weeks of gestation in humans [11]. At the same time, the RNA-binding factor, *Dazl,* is also expressed, and this appears to be essential for germ cell specification in both males and females [16]. *Dazl* expression is coincident with expression of at least 13 other genes, including some that code for translation factors (*Eif3g, Eif4b, Eif4h*), and other RNA-binding proteins (*Igf2bp1, Cpeb2*) [17], collectively suggesting a requirement for RNA involvement and/or control of translation in germ cell specification. Here, once again, gene ontology can provide vital clues as to the functional requirements for a given process.

RA is a metabolite of vitamin A, and is essential for the development of several tissues in the embryo [18]. RA is synthesized by the oxidative metabolism of retinol by retinaldehyde dehydrogenases. It acts through two nuclear receptors, RAR (retinoic acid receptor) and RXR (retinoic X receptor), to activate RA response elements (RARE) in target genes to modulate their transcriptional activity [11, 18]. RA is degraded by enzymes in the cytochrome P450 family (CYP26A1, CYP26B1, CYP26C1), which help to regulate RA levels within a tissue [11]. One of the main gene targets of RA within the gonad is *Stra8,* which is expressed in the mouse fetal ovary as early as E12.5 whereas its expression in the testis is delayed until 10 dpp (10 days post-partum). Up until that time, endogenous RA is constantly degraded in the testis by CYP26B1 [11]. Studies performed on embryonic mouse gonads show that both exogenous and endogenous RAs as well as several RARs (RARα, RARβ, RARγ) can induce *Stra8* expression in vitamin A-deficient mice, indicating the role of RA in regulating *Stra8* function [15, 18].

Stra8 is upstream of pre-meiotic DNA replication, and analysis of *Stra8* null mice demonstrates its requirement in meiotic initiation during both spermatogenesis and oogenesis [19]. However, *Stra8* is only one of the genes in the transcriptome profile of RA response genes in mouse gonads. While this list contains genes known to be involved in meiosis, such as *Slc25a31*, *Tex15*, and *Rad51*, other genes with as yet unknown functions in meiosis (*Esco2*, *Setdb2*, *Uba6*) have been found to be highly up-regulated directly or indirectly in response to RA [20]. ESCO2 is involved in sister chromatid cohesion, whereas SETDB2 and another SET family protein SUV39H2 have been implicated in chromatin remodeling in germ cells [20]. UBA6 is a protein in the ubiquitylation pathway [20]. These genes have been implicated in meiotic initiation only in the male germ cells so far and their functions in females are yet to be identified. However, their presence downstream of RA in males, together with the timing of expression would, in predictive network analysis, make them solid candidates for oocyte RA responses too.

There appears to be some crosstalk between the RA response pathway and other pathways for meiotic initiation.The homeobox transcription factors *Msx1* and *Msx2,* which are up-regulated by RA, along with BMP4 and BMP2, regulate *Stra8* expression in mouse fetal ovary, but not in the testis [21]. The DM domain gene *Dmrt1* known to be required for testicular differentiation is required for transcriptional activation of *Stra8* in the mouse fetal ovary; however, the process maybe independent of RA [22].

Meiotic prophase I initiates soon after meiotic S-phase DNA replication, and is subdivided into five stages – leptonema, zygonema, pachynema, diplonema, and diakinesis (Figure 3.2). Prophase I encompasses all the defining features of meiosis, namely the pairing and physical association (or synapsis) of homologous chromosomes, formation of the synaptonemal complex (SC), and the initiation of recombination events between them (crossing over). The SC, the most characteristic feature of prophase I, is a tripartite proteinaceous structure that binds homologous chromosomes together to aid recombination events between them [23]. In the perinatal female mouse, oocytes then enter a prolonged diakinesis state known as dictyate arrest, in which meiosis I halts, only to resume following puberty in response to the luteinizing hormone (LH) surge that triggers ovulation [23, 24].

Prophase I begins with chromosomes searching for their homologous partner based on DNA sequence homology [25]. While it is thought that synapsis of homologous chromosomes is brought about by formation of single-strand overhangs that then find the homology sequence in the partner chromosome, it is believed that a physical congregation of chromosomes into a structure known as the "*telomere bouquet,*" and the attachment of their telomeres to the nuclear envelope facilitates the initial alignment of homologous chromosomes with each other [23]. In mammals, *Unc84a*/*Sun1* expression is believed to play a role in the formation of these telomeric clusters at the nuclear envelope, while other organisms express genes that are orthologous to the SUN/KASH domain genes [26].

The initial localization of SC proteins SYCP2 and SYCP3 to form axial elements of the SC also serves in bringing homologous chromosomes closer [23]. These associations culminate in synapsis, where the two homologous chromosomes are physically held together along their entire lengths by means of the central element. The SC components assemble sequentially, starting with the axial elements, which form foci along each homolog, and these foci then coalesce to form a filament that eventually spans the entire length of the chromosome, with DNA loops extending perpendicularly from the core. The foci of axial elements are formed by grouping of SC-specific proteins like SYCP2 and SYCP3. Complexes of cohesion proteins containing both mitotic and meiosis-specific cohesins such as SMC1B, REC8, and STAG3 localize to the axial elements and are believed to play a structural role in the assembly of the axial element [23]. Once pairing is established and confirmed, the central element then assembles, with appropriate density of double-strand break (DSB)-induced DNA–DNA interactions between homologs. The central element of the SC is formed by SYCP1, SYCE1, SYCE2, and TEX12, which are also meiosis specific [23]. HORMAD1 and

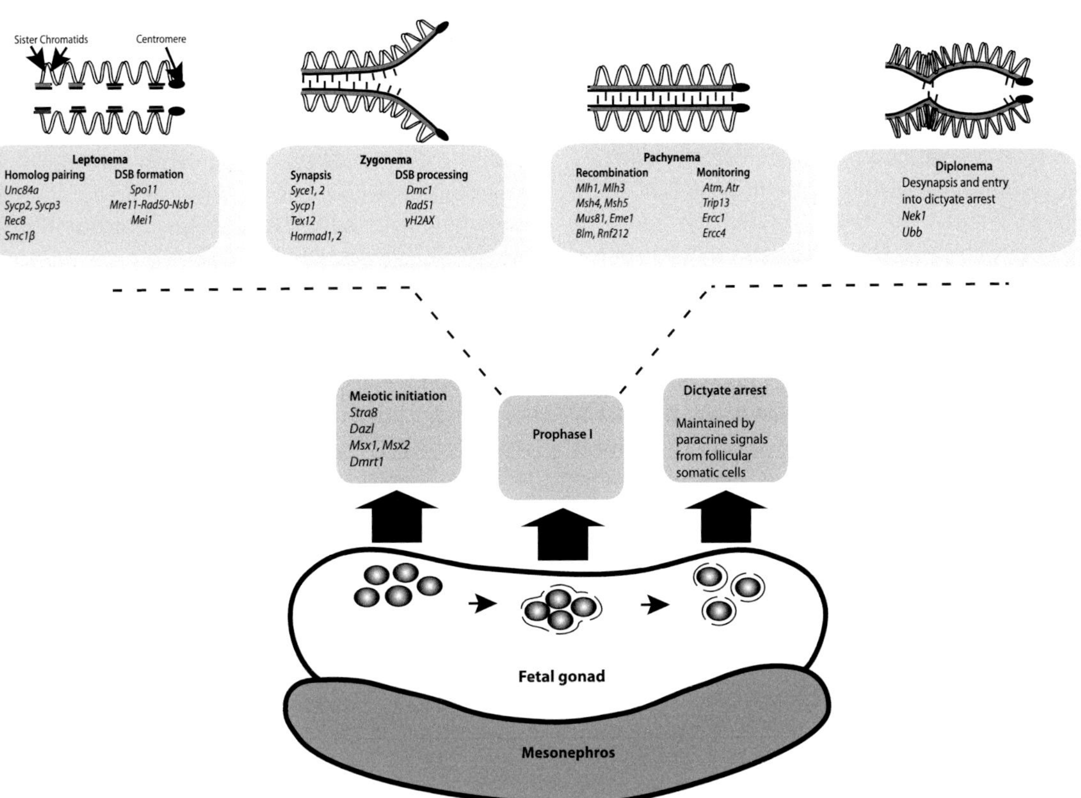

Figure 3.2 Gene expression during meiosis in the mammalian fetal germ cell. In response to retinoic acid production from somatic cells in female embryonic gonad, there is an up-regulation of retinoic acid response genes in the germ cells, such as *Stra8* and other related genes such as *Msx1*, *Msx2*, and *Dmrt1*, which facilitate the entry into meiosis in the germ cells. Other genes expressed at this time include *Dazl* as well as 13 other genes, which code for translation factors and RNA-binding proteins. Genes expressed at this time are involved in pre-meiotic DNA replication, after which the germ cells enter prophase I of meiosis. Homologous chromosomes are brought together by the action of *Unc84a*, which helps tether the chromosomes to the nuclear envelope. The products of genes such as *Spo11*, *Xrs2* (*Nbs1*), *Rad50*, *Mre11*, and *Mei1* are involved in production of double-strand breaks (DSBs). DMC1 and RAD51 proteins bind to the single-stranded overhangs and cause interaction between homologous chromosomes and facilitate strand invasion along with several other proteins that aid RAD51 localization. These foci are processed through various crossover and non-crossover pathways involving protein products of genes such as *Msh4*, *Msh5*, *Mlh1*, *Mlh3*, *Mus81*, and *Eme1*. Several gene products such as those of *Atr*, *Trip13*, *Atm*, *Ercc4*, and *Ercc1* are implicated in the pachytene checkpoint mechanism as well as supplementing the action of mismatch repair components in the repair of insertions/deletions that are large in size. RNA transcripts of *Nek1* have been reported to be present in mammalian oocytes from late pachytene stage onwards indicating a possible role at the end of prophase. *Ubb*-deficient oocytes show defects including inability to exit prophase prior to meiotic resumption. In males, after completion of recombination events, *Nek1* and *Ubb* are believed to be involved in cohesin removal and exit from prophase I. It is possible that they carry out similar functions at the prophase to metaphase transition in oocytes in the adult female.

HORMAD2 are present in unsynapsed regions of axial element and may play a role in the regulation of homolog interactions and synapsis [23, 27], as well as in quality control to eliminate asynaptic oocytes [28].

Homolog pairing occurs around the same time as the formation of the DSBs that are the precursors for meiotic recombination and which, in mammals at least, precedes the process of synapsis (the physical tethering of paired homologous chromosomes). Recombination between homologs in a chromosome pair is under the control of several serially expressed genes responsible for specific events in the recombination pathway and, in its simplest form, represents a highly regulated DNA repair process involving many components of the DNA damage repair (DDR) machinery. Not surprisingly, therefore, genes that participate in DDR events are all expressed at high levels during prophase I, and many share overlapping functions with canonical repair events in somatic cells.

DSB formation is catalyzed by the highly conserved topoisomerase SPO11 [27]. A SPO11 dimer creates DSBs in the two strands of DNA and each monomer then attaches to the 5′ terminus of each strand break from where it is cleaved away by endonucleases [29].

SPO11-induced DSB formation is found in almost all meiotic species studied to date. In *Saccharomyces cerevisiae* Spo11 requires at least nine other gene products in order to produce DSBs, only a handful of orthologs of which have been identified in mammals. These include components of the mammalian Mre11 complex (*Xrs2, Rad50, Mre11*), collectively known as the MRX/N complex, which tethers DNA to coordinate events at the two ends of the DSB [27, 30]. Apart from the MRX/N complex *Mei1* has also been implicated in DSB formation and interaction with SPO11 in the mouse [31, 32].

Following DSB formation in early leptonema, the breaks are then processed through several common precursor steps, for a number of possible recombination pathways. Firstly, 3′ overhangs are generated following 5′ end resection by an exonuclease whose identity is uncertain in mammals, but which appears to be primarily Exo1 in yeast [33]. The RecA homologs, DMC1 and RAD51, bind to the single-stranded overhangs and cause interaction between homologous chromosomes and facilitate strand invasion [27]. In addition the protein BRCA2 is also known to be involved in DSB processing and strand invasion, perhaps by interacting with RAD51 and DMC1 and allowing correct positioning of RAD51–DMC1 foci [25]. Among the other accessory proteins in mammals that assist the formation and function of RAD51–DMC1 foci is the HOP2–MND1 dimer that stabilizes these foci and promotes their ability to associate with DNA; and RAD54B, which is thought to promote that strand invasion activity of DMC1 [27]. In addition, mammals possess several *Rad51* paralogs that are expressed in cells exhibiting recombination such as *Rad51b, Rad51c, Rad51d, Xrcc2,* and *Xrcc3*. All these genes are expressed widely during homologous recombination [34]. In vitro these proteins form a complex known as the BCDX2 that binds to DSBs and is believed to aid RAD51 localization there [34].

The next step in meiotic recombination is the processing of strand exchange by either CO (crossover) or NCO (non-crossover) pathways. Importantly, the number of CO events in mammals is about 10% of the number of initiating DSB events, suggesting that most of these DSBs are resolved by NCO, but that both CO and NCO events arise from common precursors. Briefly, following DSB formation and 3′ overhang strand invasion, DNA synthesis takes place from this 3′ end using the other chromatid as a template [23]. A double Holliday junction (dHJ) is formed as a result of a ligation that is then resolved. The products can be either CO or NCO depending on how the Holliday junctions are resolved, but this process is extremely biased towards CO fates, leading researchers to speculate on the existence of temporally and functionally distinct NCO pathways that can account for the over-abundance of NCO events. Evidence for this earlier NCO pathway, which utilizes a process known as synthesis-dependent strand annealing (SDSA), exists in *S. cerevisiae* [35]. CO events correspond to "*chiasmata,*" which represent physical tethers that are essential for holding the two homologous chromosomes together and ensure proper segregation during anaphase [27]. The number and distribution of COs are strictly regulated by a process known as CO interference; hence only a fraction of DSBs are repaired to CO products [23, 35]. In *S. cerevisiae,* two components of the SC axial elements, Red1 and Hop1, are involved in prevention of COs between sister chromatids. The mammalian orthologs of these, HORMAD1 and HORMAD2, are also found in the axial region and are believed to perform the same function [23].

Of the several gene products that are active in the CO pathway in mammals, the mammalian orthologs of yeast ZMM proteins (a group of seven collaborating proteins) are involved in CO formation. MSH4 and MSH5 are proteins from this group that bind Holliday junctions as a heterodimer, presumably encircling the DNA duplex and stabilizing it [27]. This heterodimer, named MutSγ, is thought to participate in the CO bias for dHJ repair. However, the number of MSH4–MSH5 foci in the mouse exceeds the number of actual CO sites. Two other proteins that are downstream, MLH1 and MLH3, are recruited sequentially to MSH4–MSH5 foci for CO events [36]. Only those foci that are stabilized by MLH1 and MLH3 go on to become COs, indicating that the interactions of these four proteins may influence CO interference [35]. The fate of the other foci is not known, but these could be processed through NCO pathways, or through a second pathway regulated by the MUS81–EME1 complex.

Given the existence of other DSB processing pathways, it is not surprising that other genes are important for progression of prophase I events in mammals. These genes include the aforementioned *Mus81* and *Eme1*, which are thought to participate in another minor CO pathway that is interference independent and that does not require MLH1 and MLH3 [37].

BLM, a RecQ helicase, is also essential for limiting CO events and possibly for mediating crosstalk between CO pathways [27]. More recently, ubiquitin ligase genes, such as *Rnf212,* have been identified which determine recombination "hotspots" in the genome [27, 37]. The protein dimer XPF–ERCC1 supplements the action of mismatch repair components in the repair of insertions/deletions that are large in size [35]. Several gene products such as those of *Atr, Trip13,* and *Atm* are implicated in a checkpoint mechanism that monitors DSB repair and synapses of chromosomes at pachynema [23].

Much of our understanding of meiotic recombination comes from studies of yeast and other organisms. However, since many of the genes and their functions in prophase I are highly conserved, we can be confident that the pathways may be similar from yeast to human. In fact, gene co-expression networks constructed using gene profiles from meiotic prophase microarray data in yeast, mouse, and humans show several conserved gene modules that fall into GO categories like recombination, cohesion, transcription, SC assembly, and pachytene [38]. Also, not all genes forming a network in meiotic prophase are meiosis specific. Known non-meiosis-specific genes such as *Rad21, Smc3, Smc1, Mad2l1, Espl1, Ccna1,* and *Rad51* are seen to be interacting with meiosis-specific genes during several steps of the recombination pathway [17]. *Rad21, Smc1a,* and *Smc3* are involved in chromatin cohesion whereas *Mad2l1* participates in spindle assembly during both mitosis and meiosis [17]. The rest are involved in homologous recombination and mismatch repair. In a network constructed of genes conserved between human and mouse, several connections are found with non-meiotic genes. For instance, *Sycp2* is shown to be connected with genes such as *Tex11, Tex15, Hspa41, Hsf2bp,* and *Hormad2* [39]. Of these *Hspa41* and *Hsf2bp* are heat-shock proteins while the others have unknown functions but have been shown to associate with unsynapsed chromosomes. Similarly, *Msh4* has been shown to be connected with *Mtl5,* a gene encoding metallothionein protein, in this network [39]. These observations underscore the importance of using gene regulatory networks in studying specifics of prophase I and also concomitant mechanisms such as nuclear organization, DNA repair, and so on.

In contrast to the high degree of conservation among species at the genetic and functional level, it is important to note that humans exhibit an unusually high (10–25%) rate of aneuploidy, resulting in high rates of embryonic defects and fetal demise. Unusual distribution of recombination events, such as formation of COs close to the telomere, presence of two or more COs in close proximity, etc., have been associated with aneuploidy in the human oocyte [40]. The number of MLH1 and MLH3 foci is highly heterogeneous in human oocyte chromosomes as compared to the mouse, suggesting that the natural occurrence of achiasmatic chromosomes (and, therefore, aneuploidy) is more frequent [41]. Moreover, the placement and frequency of COs are different in males and females, with male COs being more peritelomeric than females, which might explain higher non-disjunction rates in the latter. These differences are believed to be tied to the length of the SC in pachynema, though the exact mechanism is not understood [42]. Maternal age has been the primary focus of studies on the risk of human aneuploidy, along with environmental pollutants such as bisphenol A [40, 43]. Both factors have been linked with heterogeneity of MLH1 foci as well. Studies on heat-shock proteins such as HSF1 and HSF2, whose activity is regulated by environmental stressors, show that they are powerful transcriptional regulators of several gene networks in the meiotic pathway. This indicates that meiosis, through the action of heat-shock proteins, is heavily modulated by environmental conditions [44]. Moreover, data from both mouse and humans indicate the involvement of less stringent checkpoint mechanisms in the female leading to a higher tolerance to errors [45]. This implies that in humans the already high tendency towards aneuploidy, combined with exposure to environmental risk factors and reduced regulatory control, may contribute to the high incidence of meiotic errors, thereby affecting the quality of reproductive health in women.

Meiotic resumption after birth

By the end of pachynema the SC begins to disassemble, allowing the homologs to move apart during diplonema. After this the oocytes enter what is known as the dictyate arrest (E20), which is a quiescent form of diplonema, and remain in this state until puberty when meiosis is resumed in cohorts of oocytes, under the influence of gonadotropins [11, 46]. Meiotic resumption is triggered by LH-induced epidermal growth factor receptor (EGFR) pathway signals from cumulus cells resulting in germinal vesicle breakdown (GVBD) in the oocytes followed by

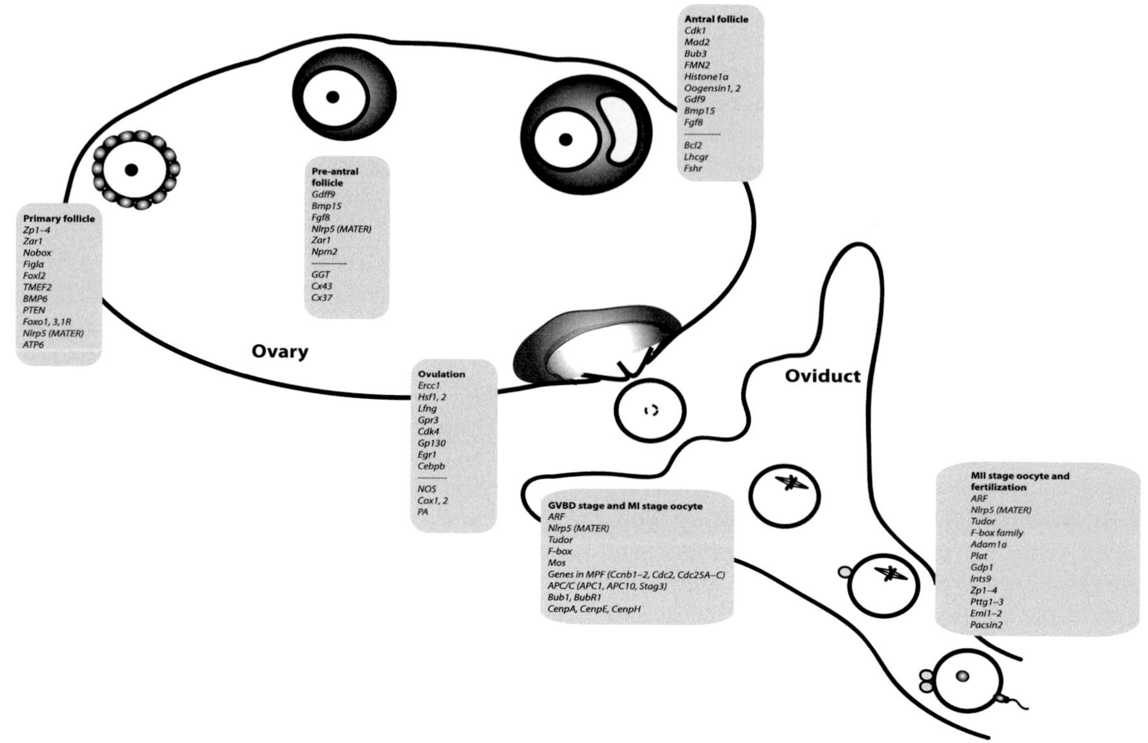

Figure 3.3 Genes expressed during different stages of mammalian oocyte development and function. Genes above the dotted line are expressed in the oocyte and below the dotted line are observed in the somatic cell population of the follicle. Oocytes within primary follicles in the ovary have up-regulation of specific transcription factors required for folliculogenesis (*Figla, Nobox*), zona pellucida formation (*Zp1, Zp2, Zp3, Zp4*) and post-fertilization development (*Zar1*). In the preantral follicles, several oocyte-expressed genes like *Gdf9, Bmp15*, etc. are involved in regulation of follicle development, proliferation, and differentiation of granulosa cells. Within the antral follicles several new genes are expressed in oocytes in preparation for meiotic resumption (*Cdk1, Mad2, Bub3*), cell-cycle progression (*FMN2* required for polymerization of actin), and GVBD (*Histone1α* required for chromatin remodeling). In the cumulus cells of the antral follicle, up-regulation of genes required for hormone response (*Lhcgr, Fshr*) and regulation of follicular atresia (*Bcl2*) is observed. Ovulation, being similar to an inflammatory response, shows an up-regulation of mediators of inflammation such as *NOS* (nitric oxide synthase) and *Cox* (cyclo-oxygenases). Genes up-regulated in GVBD and MI oocytes are required for participating in MPF (*Ccnb1, Ccnb2, Cdc2, Cdc25A, Cdc25B, Cdc25C*), signaling (*Mos, Bmp6, Gdf9, Fgf9, Kit, GPR family, Zp1, Zp2, Zp3, Zp4*), spindle assembly (*Bub1, BubR1, CenpA, CenpE, CenpH, Mad2L1*), and anaphase-promoting complex (*APC1, APC10, Stag3*). In addition to these, MII oocytes show up-regulation of genes that play a role in cell-cycle regulation (*Pttg1, Pttg3, Emi1*), fertilization (*Adam1a*), and early cleavage divisions (*MATER, Pacsin2*).

condensation of chromatin into chromosomes [47]. GVBD marks the exit of the oocyte from the first meiotic arrest, which is then followed by completion of meiosis I, where asymmetric cytokinesis after telophase I results in the formation of a small polar body that is then extruded [47]. The oocyte then enters meiosis II, progresses to metaphase II (MII), where it is arrested a second time. Exit from this arrest occurs only after fertilization followed by completion of meiosis II and extrusion of a second polar body [47]. These events are used to categorize oocytes into three important and physiologically distinct stages of post-prophase development; namely, GV stage (prior to onset of meiotic resumption), MI (during completion of meiosis; "reactivated" oocytes), and MII (at arrest prior to fertilization) [13]. Developing GV stage oocytes accumulate resources required for the resumption from dictyate arrest and completion of meiosis whereas the MII stage oocyte accumulates resources required for fertilization, oocyte-to-zygote transition, and early cleavage divisions of the embryo. Transcriptome profiling of these different stages provides great insight into the processes regulating development of an immature oocyte and its transformation to an embryo [48].

Developing oocytes in growing follicles accumulate mRNA transcripts and proteins required for later functions during fertilization and first cleavage divisions (Figure 3.3). Transcriptional activity is lower in oocytes that have reached their maximum size and progressively decreases with each step of the oocyte maturation, with the lowest gene expression in the MII oocyte [49]. Of the many genes in the same GO categories expressed in both GV and MII stages, such as metabolism and cell communication, the proportion of genes in individual categories is higher in the GV stage [49, 50]. However, oocytes undergoing meiotic resumption have been shown to have gene expression profiles that are stage specific. A stage-by-stage analysis of human oocyte mRNA transcripts and their GO categorization showed the total number of expressed genes declined from 10 869 in GV oocytes to 9682 in MI and 5633 in MII oocytes. While a large number of genes (444) were overexpressed in MII oocytes, there was an increase in the number of genes that were underexpressed (803) specifically at this stage. This demonstrates that the transcriptional activity is higher in oocytes earlier in meiotic resumption, leading to production and storage of transcripts required for completion of meiosis, fertilization, and early cleavage divisions.

Similar global gene expression analysis from mRNA transcripts of bovine oocytes undergoing meiotic resumption and maturation showed over 800 genes that are differentially expressed between GV and MII oocytes out of a total of 8000 expressed genes [50]. With mouse oocytes, the global gene expression patterns showed about 2000 genes differentially express between GV and MII [51]. While the differential expression between GV and MI oocytes is very minor in all mammalian species, a large number of modifications to mRNA transcripts occur after MI before entering MII and may be responsible for the widespread change in protein composition and abundance that accompanies fertilization and transition from oocyte to embryo [49]. For example, genes that encode the F-box family of proteins are over-represented in oocytes at different stages, are involved in the ubiquitin-linked protein degradation pathway, and have been implicated in this extensive change in protein profile along with proteins involved in epigenetic modifications, such as methylases, demethylases, and acetylases [13]. PADI6, another well-known histone demethylase, is involved in ribosome storage and embryonic genome activation and its transcript is present in the oocyte after the MI stage [52].

Studies on human oocytes collected at different stages of maturation and analyzed for gene expression levels using microarray and cluster analysis of specific marker and related genes showed that GV oocytes have a higher expression of genes involved in protein formation and metabolism, cell-cycle regulation, electron transport, and production of cytoskeletal elements whereas MII oocytes have an over-representation of genes involved in DNA replication and repair, cell proliferation, lipid and amino acid metabolism, formation of G protein-coupled receptors (GPCR) and other signaling molecules [51, 53] (see also other chapters). Gene networks constructed from mouse oocytes using an IPA database (Ingenuity Pathway Analysis – http://www.ingenuity.com/products/ipa) of MII-specific genes such as *Plat, Gdp1, Ints9, Gdf9,* and *Sic23a* revealed GO function categories of cellular movement, cellular assembly, and organization; cell-cycle regulation; DNA replication, recombination, and repair; lipid metabolism; and apoptosis [54]. In addition, genes up-regulated in mammalian oocytes can be subdivided into various post-prophase I meiotic events, including those participating in maturation-promoting factor (MPF) (*Ccnb1, Ccnb2, Cdc2, Cdc25A, Cdc25B, Cdc25C*), signaling (*Mos, Bmp6, Gdf9, Fgf9, Kit, GPR family, Zp1, Zp2, Zp3, Zp4*), spindle assembly (*Bub1, BubR1, CenpA, CenpE, CenpH, Mad2L1*), anaphase-promoting complex (*APC1, APC10, Stag3*), transcription factors (*Sox30, Sox15*), and cell-cycle regulation (*Pttg1, Pttg3, Emi1*) (Figure 3.3) [13, 49–51].

Results similar to the IPA were shown by proteome analysis of mouse oocytes [13]. In general, proteome profiles give a more accurate representation of regulatory networks, as non-translation of transcripts and activation of proteins within the cell cannot be assessed by transcriptome profiles alone. In the oocyte proteome profile about 2800 GV-specific proteins and 3000 MII-specific proteins were identified and a GO annotation analysis showed that GV oocytes specifically contain proteins related to metabolism, oocyte function, and maturation [13]. For example, several protein families involved in molecular transport across oocyte and cumulus cell membranes were found to be in abundance in the GV oocytes, such as the amino acid transporters of the solute carrier (SLC) family, gap junction proteins, and adhesion proteins [13]. Proteins involved in the DNA replication and recombination pathway are seen in MII oocytes in higher levels than the GV oocytes. MII oocytes, in addition to possessing proteins for cell-cycle regulation, show abundance of specific transcription factors such as SIN3a and TRIM28 that prevent stem cell differentiation and T-cell leukemia (TCL) family of proteins that are involved in reprogramming of cells to pluripotency. Both stages of oocytes (GV and MII) show high expression of protein families like ARF (ADP ribosylation factor), MATER (maternal antigen that embryos require), Tudor, and F-box family which are required for cell-cycle regulation and self-renewal. The ARF family of proteins is also involved in the asymmetric division of oocytes [13]. Other over-represented genes in the MII oocytes are part of the mitogen-activated protein kinase (MAPK) pathway and transforming growth factor beta (TGFβ) pathway, which are involved in oocyte activation, and cell differentiation and cell proliferation, respectively. For instance, *Map2k1* and *Pacsin2* are two genes whose products are involved in cell signaling pathways and are highly expressed after the GV stage. PACSIN2 belongs to a family of proteins known to participate in oocyte maturation, fertilization, and early embryonic divisions [51]. Products of another gene, *Adam1a,* are expressed in MII and are known to play a role in fertilization. However, zona pellucida (ZP) proteins, also known to be required for fertilization, are formed as early as GV stage oocytes, as seen by high expression of *Zp1*, *Zp2*, and *Zp3* genes in GV oocytes, indicating a possible role of these proteins in interactions with cumulus cells [51].

The role of cumulus cells in oocyte maturation and meiotic resumption has been further illuminated by gene expression analysis. Genome-wide expression analysis in human oocytes using oligonucleotide-based microarrays reveals significant differences in expression profiles for many genes between oocyte and cumulus cells (Figure 3.3). Some of these genes are known to be oocyte specific (*Zp1, Zp2, Zp3, Zp4, Gdf9*), and others are known to be specific to the meiotic pathway within the oocyte (*AurkC, Cdc25A, Cdc25B, Cdc25C*) [49]. Many genes involved in signaling pathways mediated by cumulus cells are overexpressed at all stages of development within the oocyte. For instance, genes encoding growth factor receptors (*Bmpr2, Kit, Erbb4*) and GPCRs (*Gpr37, Gpr39, Gpr51, Gpr126*) are overexpressed in oocytes, suggesting the role of their cumulus cell-derived ligands in regulating oocyte maturation [49]. Of the genes that are overexpressed in cumulus cells, 24% are involved in extracellular signals and membrane structure, indicating the highly supportive role that the cumulus cell plays in oocyte development [49].

Cumulus cells also play a major role in ovulation, and several gene networks spanning the entire cumulus–oocyte complex are involved in this process [55]. Hormonal stimulation of the ovary sets in motion a series of events that lead to the expulsion of the now viable (and fertilization competent) oocyte from the follicle. Gene profiles from mature follicles reveal gene networks comprising of several progesterone-regulated genes, such as *Adamts1, Edn2, Pparγ, Il6,* and *Ptgs2,* which code for proteins such as proteases, cell adhesion components, transcription factors, regulators of vascular activities, and inflammation regulators [55]. Each of these networks is involved in the damage and repair events that characterize the ovulation process [55].

Transcriptome profiles of human oocytes between the MII (unfertilized) stage and the 4-cell embryo stage revealed that while a large number of transcripts show an overall decreasing expression, there is an increase in the expression of a specific set of genes encoding proteins localized in the nucleus and on ribosomes. GO analyses identified these proteins as being required for RNA processing and metabolism, indicating that they are probably involved in the transition from maternal to zygote genome. The overall reduction in transcripts at this stage could be due to degradation of maternal transcripts that accompany this transition [48]. The oocyte-derived transcripts at this stage might be responsible for the extensive reprogramming of a terminally differentiated cell (the oocyte) to a pluripotent cell (the zygote). Study of gene networks involved in this unique process has great value in induced pluripotent stem cell (iPSC) research and therapy [13].

Role of the oocyte in ovarian development

While oocytes are progressing through prophase I of meiosis during fetal life, the somatic cells in the ovary surround the germ cell clusters and the whole gonad itself begins to be delineated into cortical and medullary regions due to differential gene expression in the cells [11]. For instance, cortical cells show a marked increase in *Bmp2* expression while medullary cells have higher *Wnt4* and *Fst* expression. While the exact function of *Bmp2* in the cortex cells is not known, follistatin (the protein product of the *Fst* gene) is known to be involved in activin-mediated regulation of ovary function. *Rspo1* expression activates the Wnt signaling pathway in the ovary, which, in turn, suppresses both endothelial cell migration and the formation of testis-specific vasculature in the ovary [11,

56]. Not surprisingly, therefore, GO biological process analysis of *Wnt4* shows its involvement in commitment to cell fate in primary germ layers and in branching and patterning of blood vessels [11, 56].

Somatic cells, as expected, influence follicle formation greatly in the postnatal ovary. *Foxl2* is required for normal follicle formation and is expressed by pregranulosa cells in the gonad (E12.5), and then later on by the granulosa cells of the early follicles [11]. However, the oocytes themselves are also important for folliculogenesis, since loss of oogonia at different stages of development has been shown to disrupt follicle and ovarian development [11]. In the absence of oogonia, somatic cells can still form clusters; however, they seem unable to form follicles and the cell clusters start regressing in a few days [11]. Two oogonia-specific genes, *Figla* and *Nobox,* have been implicated in the oocyte-driven control of folliculogenensis at this stage of development. Loss of oocytes in the meiotic stages of development produces a transdifferentiation of pregranulosa cells of the early follicles to Sertoli-like cells, indicating that oocytes play an important role in maintaining the female-specific differentiation pathway at this stage. *Wnt4, Rspo1,* and *Amh* expressed in the oocyte have been implicated in this part of ovarian development [6]. Even in much later stages of the female reproductive life, loss of oocytes can be detrimental to ovarian function. For instance, oocyte loss from preovulatory follicles in the adult ovary causes luteinization of the follicle. *Bmp15* and *Gdf9* expression in the oocyte has been shown to be responsible in preventing this disintegration and for maintaining proper follicle function prior to ovulation [11].

Conclusion

Our understanding of cellular processes has been aided greatly by a more complete picture of the genetic networks that regulate these events, and the oocyte is no exception. Indeed, the similarities in gene expression profiles between oocytes and somatic cells in terms of their proliferative and differentiation programs, and between oocytes during meiosis and the DDR (already described on page 29) program in somatic cells, will be useful in elucidating common mechanisms and in predicting genes that are likely to play important roles in one or both pathways. Indeed, as our ability to perform high throughput sequencing advances, and with the emergence of technologies capable of allowing transcriptome profiling of single oocytes, the scope and resolution of these gene networks is likely to improve dramatically.

References

1. Martin AC, Drubin DG. Impact of genome-wide functional analyses on cell biology research. *Curr Opin Cell Biol* 2003; **15**: 6–13.
2. Rapaport F, Zinovyev A, Dutreix M, Barillot E, Vert JP. Classification of microarray data using gene networks. *BMC Bioinformatics* 2007; **8**: 35.
3. D'Haeseleer P. How does gene expression clustering work? *Nat Biotechnol* 2005; **23**: 1499–501.
4. Cohen PE, Holloway JK. Predicting gene networks in human oocyte meiosis. *Biol Reprod* 2010; **82**: 469–72.
5. Hallinan JS, James K, Wipat A. Network approaches to the functional analysis of microbial proteins. *Adv Microb Physiol* 2011; **59**: 101–33.
6. Acevedo N, Smith GD. Oocyte-specific gene signaling and its regulation of mammalian reproductive potential. *Front Biosci* 2005; **10**: 2335–45.
7. Ewen KA, Koopman P. Mouse germ cell development: from specification to sex determination. *Mol Cell Endocrinol* 2010; **323**: 76–93.
8. Amleh A, Dean J. Mouse genetics provides insight into folliculogenesis, fertilization and early embryonic development. *Hum Reprod Update* 2002; **8**: 395–403.
9. Hayashi K, de Sousa Lopes SM, Surani MA. Germ cell specification in mice. *Science* 2007; **316**: 394–6.
10. Oktem O, Urman B. Understanding follicle growth in vivo. *Hum Reprod* 2010; **25**: 2944–54.
11. Combes A, Spiller C, Koopman P. Sex determination and gonadal development. In: Verlhac M-H, Villeneuve A, eds. *Oogenesis: The Universal Process.* Chichester: John Wiley & Sons. 2010; 27–78.
12. Zheng P, Dean J. Oocyte-specific genes affect folliculogenesis, fertilization, and early development. *Semin Reprod Med* 2007; **25**: 243–51.
13. Wang S, Kou Z, Jing Z, *et al.* Proteome of mouse oocytes at different developmental stages. *Proc Natl Acad Sci USA* 2010; **107**: 17639–44.
14. Rolland AD, Lehmann KP, Johnson KJ, Gaido KW, Koopman P. Uncovering gene regulatory networks during mouse fetal germ cell development. *Biol Reprod* 2011; **84**: 790–800.
15. Koubova J, Menke DB, Zhou Q, *et al.* Retinoic acid regulates sex-specific timing of meiotic initiation in mice. *Proc Natl Acad Sci USA* 2006; **103**: 2474–9.
16. Gill ME, Hu YC, Lin Y, Page DC. Licensing of gametogenesis, dependent on RNA binding protein

DAZL, as a gateway to sexual differentiation of fetal germ cells. *Proc Natl Acad Sci USA* 2011; **108**: 7443–8.

17. Zheng P, Griswold MD, Hassold TJ, *et al.* Predicting meiotic pathways in human fetal oogenesis. *Biol Reprod* 2010; **82**: 543–51.
18. Griswold MD, Hogarth CA, Bowles J, Koopman P. Initiating meiosis: the case for retinoic acid. *Biol Reprod* 2012; **86**: 35.
19. Anderson EL, Baltus AE, Roepers-Gajadien HL, *et al.* Stra8 and its inducer, retinoic acid, regulate meiotic initiation in both spermatogenesis and oogenesis in mice. *Proc Natl Acad Sci USA* 2008; **105**: 14976–80.
20. Hogarth CA, Mitchell D, Evanoff R, Small C, Griswold M. Identification and expression of potential regulators of the mammalian mitotic-to-meiotic transition. *Biol Reprod* 2011; **84**: 34–42.
21. Le Bouffant R, Souquet B, Duval N, *et al.* Msx1 and Msx2 promote meiosis initiation. *Development* 2011; **138**: 5393–402.
22. Krentz AD, Murphy MW, Sarver AL, *et al.* DMRT1 promotes oogenesis by transcriptional activation of Stra8 in the mammalian fetal ovary. *Dev Biol* 2011; **356**: 63–70.
23. Handel MA, Schimenti JC. Genetics of mammalian meiosis: regulation, dynamics and impact on fertility. *Nat Rev Genet* 2010; **11**: 124–36.
24. Morelli MA, Cohen PE. Not all germ cells are created equal: aspects of sexual dimorphism in mammalian meiosis. *Reproduction* 2005; **130**: 761–81.
25. Li W, Ma H. Double-stranded DNA breaks and gene functions in recombination and meiosis. *Cell Res* 2006; **16**: 402–12.
26. Hiraoka Y, Dernburg AF. The SUN rises on meiotic chromosome dynamics. *Dev Cell* 2009; **17**: 598–605.
27. Santucci-Darmanin S, Baudet F. Meiotic combination in mammals. In: Verlhac M-H, Villeneuve A, eds. *Oogenesis: The Universal Process*. Chichester: John Wiley & Sons. 2010; 141–77.
28. Kogo H, Tsutsumi M, Ohye T, *et al.* HORMAD1-dependent checkpoint/surveillance mechanism eliminates asynaptic oocytes. *Genes Cells* 2012; **17**: 439–54.
29. Keeney S. Spo11 and the formation of DNA double-strand breaks in meiosis. *Genome Dyn Stab* 2008; **2**: 81–123.
30. Keeney S. Mechanism and control of meiotic recombination initiation. *Curr Top Dev Biol* 2001; **52**: 1–53.
31. Munroe RJ, Bergstrom RA, Zheng QY, *et al.* Mouse mutants from chemically mutagenized embryonic stem cells. *Nat Genet* 2000; **24**: 318–21.
32. Kumar R, Bourbon HM, de Massy B. Functional conservation of Mei4 for meiotic DNA double-strand break formation from yeasts to mice. *Genes Dev* 2010; **24**: 1266–80.
33. Neale MJ, Pan J, Keeney S. Endonucleolytic processing of covalent protein-linked DNA double-strand breaks. *Nature* 2005; **436**: 1053–7.
34. Masson JY, Tarsounas MC, Stasiak AZ, *et al.* Identification and purification of two distinct complexes containing the five RAD51 paralogs. *Genes Dev* 2001; **15**: 3296–307.
35. Ehmsen K, Heyer W-D. Biochemistry of meiotic recombination: formation, processing, and resolution of recombination intermediates. In: Egel R, Lankenau D-H. *Recombination and Meiosis* Vol. **3** *Models Means, and Evolution (Genome Dynamics and Stability)*. Berlin Heidelberg: Springer. 2008; 91–164.
36. Kolas NK, Svetlanov A, Lenzi ML, *et al.* Localization of MMR proteins on meiotic chromosomes in mice indicates distinct functions during prophase I. *J Cell Biol* 2005; **171**: 447–58.
37. Holloway JK, Booth J, Edelmann W, McGowan CH, Cohen PE. MUS81 generates a subset of MLH1-MLH3-independent crossovers in mammalian meiosis. *PLoS Genet* 2008; **4**: e1000186.
38. Li Y, Lam KS, Dasgupta N, Ye P. A yeast's eye view of mammalian reproduction: cross-species gene co-expression in meiotic prophase. *BMC Syst Biol* 2010; **4**: 125.
39. Su Y, Li Y, Ye P. Mammalian meiosis is more conserved by sex than by species: conserved co-expression networks of meiotic prophase. *Reproduction* 2011; **142**: 675–87.
40. Garcia-Cruz R, Roig I, Caldes MG. Maternal origin of the human aneuploidies. Are homolog synapsis and recombination to blame? Notes (learned) from the underbelly. *Genome Dyn* 2009; **5**: 128–36.
41. Lenzi ML, Smith J, Snowden T, *et al.* Extreme heterogeneity in the molecular events leading to the establishment of chiasmata during meiosis I in human oocytes. *Am J Hum Genet* 2005; **76**: 112–27.
42. Lynn A, Schrump S, Cherry J, Hassold T, Hunt P. Sex, not genotype, determines recombination levels in mice. *Am J Hum Genet* 2005; **77**: 670–5.
43. Hunt PA, Koehler KE, Susiarjo M, *et al.* Bisphenol A exposure causes meiotic aneuploidy in the female mouse. *Curr Biol* 2003; **13**: 546–53.
44. Le Masson F, Rasak Z, Kaigo M, *et al.* Identification of heat shock factor 1 molecular and cellular targets during embryonic and adult female meiosis. *Mol Cell Biol* 2011; **31**: 3410–23.

45. Nagaoka SI, Hodges CA, Albertini DF, Hunt PA. Oocyte-specific differences in cell-cycle control create an innate susceptibility to meiotic errors. *Curr Biol* 2011; **21**: 651–7.

46. Cohen PE, Pollack SE, Pollard JW. Genetic analysis of chromosome pairing, recombination, and cell cycle control during first meiotic prophase in mammals. *Endocr Rev* 2006; **27**: 398–426.

47. Sun QY, Miao YL, Schatten H. Towards a new understanding on the regulation of mammalian oocyte meiosis resumption. *Cell Cycle* 2009; **8**: 2741–7.

48. Zhang P, Zucchelli M, Bruce S, *et al.* Transcriptome profiling of human pre-implantation development. *PLoS One* 2009; **4**: e7844.

49. Assou S, Anahory T, Pantesco V, *et al.* The human cumulus–oocyte complex gene-expression profile. *Hum Reprod* 2006; **21**: 1705–19.

50. Fair T, Carter F, Park S, Evans AC, Lonergan P. Global gene expression analysis during bovine oocyte in vitro maturation. *Theriogenology* 2007; **68** Suppl 1: S91–7.

51. Cui XS, Li XY, Jin XJ, *et al.* Maternal gene transcription in mouse oocytes: genes implicated in oocyte maturation and fertilization. *J Reprod Dev* 2007; **53**: 405–18.

52. Yurttas P, Vitale AM, Fitzhenry RJ, *et al.* Role for PADI6 and the cytoplasmic lattices in ribosomal storage in oocytes and translational control in the early mouse embryo. *Development* 2008; **135**: 2627–36.

53. Gasca S,Pellestor F, Assou S, *et al.* Identifying new human oocyte marker genes: a microarray approach. *Reprod Biomed Online* 2007; **14**: 175–83.

54. Jincho Y, Kono T. Dynamism in the gene expression profile after oocyte activation in mice. *J Mamm Ova Res* 2008; **25**: 150–62.

55. Kim J, Bagchi IC, Bagchi MK. Control of ovulation in mice by progesterone receptor-regulated gene networks. *Mol Hum Reprod* 2009; **15**: 821–8.

56. Yao HH, Matzuk MM, Jorgez CJ, *et al.* Follistatin operates downstream of Wnt4 in mammalian ovary organogenesis. *Dev Dyn* 2004; **230**: 210–15.

Section 2 Life cycle

Chapter 4

Follicle formation and oocyte death

Melissa E. Pepling

Introduction

This chapter will focus on the development of primordial germ cells (PGCs) into oocytes and their subsequent assembly into primordial follicles that is essential for reproductive success (Figure 4.1). In the mouse, PGCs migrate to the genital ridge and begin dividing rapidly by mitosis [1]. These oogonia remain connected, through incomplete cytokinesis, in clusters of synchronously dividing cells known as germline cysts [2]. The oogonia then begin to enter meiosis and arrest in the diplotene stage of prophase I. Around the same time, germ cell cysts begin to break apart [3]. As these cysts separate, many oocytes are lost by apoptosis while others are surrounded by a single layer of granulosa cells, forming primordial follicles [4]. It is believed that improper regulation of cyst breakdown and primordial follicle formation can lead to fertility disorders such as premature ovarian insufficiency and primary amenorrhea, where an early depletion of oocytes leads to infertility [5, 6]. In addition, aberrant regulation of oocyte death as primordial follicles form may be the underlying cause of ovarian dysgerminoma, or germ cell tumors [7]. Little is known about what molecules regulate cyst breakdown, primordial follicle formation, and oocyte death. Elucidation of mechanisms regulating cyst breakdown, oocyte numbers, and primordial follicle formation is important because it will lead to the development of early screening and interventions for infertility and germ cell cancers.

The process of follicle formation

Germ cells

The PGCs arrive at the ovary at approximately 10.5 days postcoitum (dpc) in the mouse and in humans at about 28 days of gestation [8, 9]. Once the PGCs reach the ovary, they undergo several rounds of mitosis. These mitotically dividing germ cells are called oogonia and develop in groups of cells known as clusters or nests. In the mouse, the germ cell clusters are also referred to as germ cell cysts because they have been shown to possess characteristics similar to *Drosophila* germline cysts [2]. The formation of germline cysts from germline stem cells in the *Drosophila* ovary has been well studied [10]. The germline stem cell divides to form a daughter stem cell and a cystoblast or cyst-forming cell. The cystoblast divides synchronously four times to form a 16-cell cyst. Cytokinesis at the end of each division is incomplete, leaving the cyst cells connected by intercellular bridges that in *Drosophila* are also called ring canals. Only one of the cells develops into a true oocyte. The other cells of the cyst become nurse cells and provide mRNAs, proteins, and organelles to the oocyte through the ring canals. The nurse cells eventually die by the process of programmed cell death.

Mouse germ cell clusters share several characteristics of germ cell cysts [2]. They undergo synchronous divisions although the synchrony appears to be lost in older cysts. They have been shown by electron microscopy to be connected by intercellular bridges that appear similar in structure to *Drosophila* ring canals. While many protein components of *Drosophila* ring canals have been identified, only a few have been found in mouse intercellular bridges. The first bridge component identified in mammalian intercellular bridges connecting male germ cells was testes-expressed gene 14 (TEX14) [11] and it was subsequently found in bridges connecting female germ cells as well [12]. Surprisingly, while *Tex14* knockouts are male sterile, females remain fertile though they have a reduced number of oocytes. Several other proteins

Biology and Pathology of the Oocyte, 2nd edn., ed. Alan Trounson, Roger Gosden, and Ursula Eichenlaub-Ritter.
Published by Cambridge University Press.

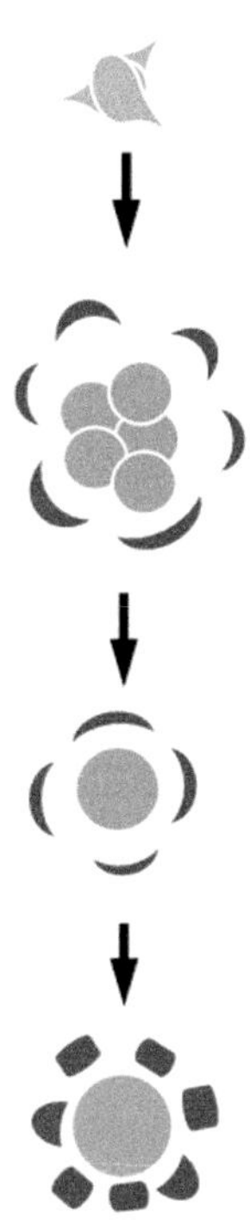
1 PGCs arrive at gonad
2 Oogonia divide by mitosis, forming germ cell cysts
3 Germ cells enter meiosis and become oocytes
4 Germ cell cysts break down and follicles form
5 First wave of follicles begins to develop

Figure 4.1 Events leading to formation and development of primordial follicles in the mouse. (1) PGCs migrate to the genital ridge starting at 10.5 days postcoitum (dpc). (2) After arriving at the genital ridge the oogonia undergo mitosis without complete cytokinesis and remain connected by intercellular bridges, forming germ cell cysts. (3) Starting at 13.5 dpc germ cells enter meiosis and develop as oocytes. They progress through prophase I of meiosis and arrest at the diplotene stage. (4) Late in fetal development germ cell cysts begin to break apart and individual oocytes are surrounded by granulosa cells, forming primordial follicles. Many oocytes are lost as follicles form. (5) Some primordial follicles begin to develop immediately after forming and progress to the primary follicle stage.

have been identified as components of the male intercellular bridges but only one other protein, KIF23, has been detected in female intercellular bridges so far [12]. KIF23 is a member of the kinesin family of microtubule motors. While mouse germ cell clusters can form by incomplete cytokinesis, recent work using chimeras shows that clusters can also form by aggregation [13]. Morphological studies of human fetal ovaries showing synchronously dividing germ cells connected by intercellular bridges support the idea that human oogonia and oocytes also develop in cysts [14].

The germ cells begin to enter meiosis at 13.5 dpc and become oocytes [15]. Meiotic entry occurs in a wave from anterior to posterior of the ovary in the mouse [16, 17] and is promoted by retinoic acid [18, 19]. Retinoic acid is present in both male and female embryonic gonads. However, males express an enzyme called cytochrome P450, family 26, subfamily B (CYP26B1) which degrades retinoic acid and prevents male germ cells from entering meiosis. In females, retinoic acid is not degraded and upregulates stimulated by retinoic acid gene 8 (STRA8), which in turn promotes entry into meiosis [20]. Subsequently, oocytes progress through pre-meiotic S-phase and the stages of prophase I that include leptotene, zygotene, and pachytene and arrest in the final stage of prophase I, diplotene. Arrest in diplotene occurs as early as 17.5 dpc in some oocytes while not all the oocytes reach this phase until several days after birth [21]. It is interesting to note that in the male but not in the female, asynapsed chromosomes lead to an arrest at the pachytene stage of meiosis I and subsequent loss of germ cells, leading to infertility. This is evidenced by the phenotype of the *Hormad 1* knockout mice where homologous chromosome pairing is disrupted and both males and females are infertile but only male germ cells arrest at the pachytene stage [22]. Oocytes develop normally and are able to be ovulated and fertilized. However, these embryos are aneuploid and do not develop past the blastocyst stage.

In the mouse, the germ cell cysts break apart perinatally [4]. The oocytes must become individualized and then surrounded by granulosa cells to form primordial follicles. The mechanisms involved in cyst breakdown are not completely understood. Concurrent with cyst breakdown, many oocytes are lost through programmed cell death. In the mouse it is estimated that two-thirds of the oocytes die and why this occurs is unknown. One model is that programmed cell death is required to break the cysts apart. It was proposed that one oocyte dies and this causes the large cyst to be split into two smaller cysts. The process would be repeated until only a few individual oocytes remain. This model is supported by mutant analysis of a cell death regulator and will be discussed in more detail later in the chapter.

Somatic cells

As the germ cell cysts form, they become loosely surrounded by somatic cells forming ovigerous cords which are surrounded by a basement membrane [23]. These somatic cells are pregranulosa cells that will eventually be the granulosa cells that surround each oocyte to form primordial follicles. There are three possible sources of pregranulosa cells in the mouse, the rete ovarii that connects the ovary to the mesonephrous, mesenchymal cells of the ovary, and ovarian surface epithelium [24]. Recent work had identified the ovarian surface epithelium as the main source of granulosa cells in the mouse [25]. However, there appear to be two waves of granulosa cells that form. Sertoli cells and granulosa cells are believed to arise from a common progenitor cell present before gonads become committed to develop into either an ovary or testis. These bipotential supporting cells are epithelial in origin and are located at the surface of the gonad. Mork and colleagues use lineage tracing to show that these cells develop into granulosa cells [25]. However, these cells are only found in the primordial follicles that develop in the medulla of the ovary. These follicles are the first to form and also begin to grow immediately. The granulosa cells of the primordial follicles that form in the cortex of the ovary and remain quiescent until sexual maturity are also derived from ovarian surface epithelium but form later.

During follicle formation, the ovigerous cord structure of the ovary must be reorganized into individual primordial follicles. In rodents, the epithelial pregranulosa cells begin to extend cytoplasmic processes in between the tightly associated oocytes which are thought to physically separate oocytes [4, 26]. As the granulosa cells enclose each oocyte, the basement membrane that was surrounding the ovigerous cords is remodeled to encircle each follicle. This remodeling involves proteases from the matrix metalloproteinase and plasmin families [27]. Supporting this, follicle formation is blocked in cultured neonatal rat ovaries exposed to serine protease inhibitors. The process of follicle formation likely involves communication between oocytes and granulosa cells and potential signals are discussed later in the chapter.

Oocyte death during follicle formation

As mentioned earlier in the chapter, cyst breakdown is accompanied by programmed cell death of approximately two-thirds of the oocytes in mammals. Human females are estimated to generate almost 7 million germ cells by 20 weeks of development but this number drops to 2 million by birth [28]. In mice, a similar drop in oocyte number is observed from about 6000 oocytes per ovary to about 2000 in the CD1 strain, although exact counts vary depending on the strain, counting method, and laboratory [3, 4, 29]. Reports also vary as to when the oocyte loss begins as well as the rate of loss though there is general agreement that loss begins during the fetal period [3, 30, 31]. Cysts begin to break down and follicles start to form first in the medullary region of the ovary and programmed cell death is also first observed in the central region of the ovary [3, 32].

It is not known why so many oocytes are made and then lost during early development. Several reasons for oocyte death have been suggested including that the death is necessary for germ cell cysts to break apart, that the dying cells serve as nurse cells for the surviving oocytes, that the dying oocytes have defective genomes and the process is part of a mechanism to select the highest quality mitochondria for the surviving oocytes [29]. The current model is that oocyte loss helps to individualize the surviving oocytes [4]. One oocyte of a large cyst dies and this separates the cyst into two. This process is repeated until there are a few single oocytes. Supporting this idea, dying oocytes are found where new basement membrane is forming during follicle assembly [27]. It is not known if the dying oocytes serve a function analogous to nurse cells of *Drosophila*. In the fly, as the nurse cells transport material to the oocyte, the oocyte volume increases greatly [10]. This does not appear to happen in the mouse though further studies are necessary. The idea that oocytes with defective nuclei or mitochondria are lost also warrants investigation.

Most studies have focused on apoptosis as the mechanism by which oocytes are lost during early mammalian oogenesis [33, 34]. Recently, however, autophagy has been implicated as another mechanism controlling oocyte death in the developing mouse ovary [34, 35]. Morphologically, apoptosis is characterized by nuclear condensation and DNA cleavage [36]. Autophagy is distinct from apoptosis and is identified by the formation of cytoplasmic vesicles

Table 4.1. Oocyte-expressed factors implicated in follicle formation

Gene	Protein/function	Evidence for role in follicle formation	References
Bmp15	Bone morphogenetic protein 15, TGFβ family member	Mutants have multiple oocyte follicles	[41]
Ctgf	Connective tissue growth factor, CCN protein family member	Promotes follicle formation	[45]
E-cadherin	Cell adhesion molecule	Neutralization in hamster organ culture results in accelerated follicle formation	[51]
ERβ	Estrogen signaling	Estrogen blocks cyst breakdown	[54]
Figla	Factor in the germline alpha, folliculogenesis-specific basic helix loop helix	Mutants are defective in follicle formation and exhibit perinatal oocyte loss	[46]
Gdf9	Growth differentiation factor 9, TGFβ family member	Mutants have multiple oocyte follicles	[41]
Jag1	Notch ligand	Inhibition of Notch signaling reduces follicle formation	[49]
Nobox	Newborn ovary homeobox-encoding gene	Mutants have delayed follicle formation and oocyte loss	[47]
Ntrk2	Receptor for NT4 and BDNF, neurotrophin signaling	Follicle formation and germ cell number is reduced in mutants	[48]

BDNF, brain-derived neurotrophic factor; NT4, neurotrophin 4; TGFβ, transforming growth factor beta.

called autophagosomes that enclose cytoplasm and organelles. Eventually, the autophagosome fuses with the lysosome and its contents are degraded. Autophagy can function as a protective mechanism resulting in cell survival under stressful conditions or in cell death [37]. In studies investigating fetal and neonatal apoptosis in the mouse ovary, though there is a significant loss of germ cells, the percent of apoptotic germ cells observed was low, suggesting another mechanism might also be involved [4, 38]. Rodrigues and colleagues [39] found increased lysosomal activation in newborn mouse oocytes as well as other indications that autophagy might be active during neonatal oocyte development.

Regulation of follicle formation

Follicle formation requires changes in both oocytes and surrounding pregranulosa cells as well as interactions between these two cells types. The factors involved in these changes are beginning to be identified. Some of these molecules are expressed in the oocyte while others are localized to somatic cells. In addition, some proteins with potential roles in follicle formation are found in more than one cell type. Finally, the cellular localization of some factors has not been determined.

Oocyte-specific factors

There is evidence that several oocyte-specific factors play roles in follicle formation (Table 4.1). These include transcription factors that would regulate genes important for controlling follicle formation and signaling molecules that would be important for communication between oocytes as well as between oocytes and somatic cells. Two signaling molecules of the transforming growth factor beta (TGFβ) superfamily, bone morphogenetic protein 15 (BMP15) and growth differentiation factor 9 (GDF9), are expressed in oocytes and mutants in either gene have multiple oocyte follicles (MOFs) [40, 41]. MOFs are abnormal follicles containing more than one oocyte and are believed to be derived from oocyte cyst cells that did not properly separate during cyst breakdown and follicle formation [42, 43]. The involvement of GDF9 in follicle formation is supported by organ culture studies in the hamster where addition of GDF9 promotes the formation of follicles [44]. Another TGFβ family member, TGFβ1, itself does not appear to play a role in follicle assembly but does interact with connective tissue growth factor (CTGF), an oocyte-specific protein that promotes follicle assembly in rat ovary organ culture [45].

A number of oocyte-expressed proteins have potential roles in promoting follicle assembly, with this process defective when they are either disrupted by mutation or blocked in organ culture. Mutants of two oocyte-specific transcription factors, factor in the germline alpha (FIGLA) and Nobox, have reduced follicle formation and more oocyte loss. The *Figla* gene encodes a basic helix-loop-helix (bHLH) protein. *Figla* mutants lose oocytes at birth and any remaining oocytes are not enclosed in primordial follicles [46]. Similarly, mutation of *Nobox,* encoding a homeobox-containing protein, results in increased oocyte loss and a delay in cyst breakdown [47]. Neurotrophic tyrosine kinase receptor type 2 (NTRK2) is also expressed in oocytes and serves as a receptor for neurotrophins, neurotrophin 4 (NT4) and brain-derived neurotrophic factor (BDNF) [48]. *Ntrk2* mutants have a phenotype similar to *Figla* and *Nobox*. Primordial follicle formation is reduced in organ culture when Notch signaling is inhibited [49]. One Notch ligand, Jagged1 (JAG1), is expressed in oocytes. However, *Jag1* mutants are embryonic lethal and oocyte-specific mutants have not yet been examined.

The oocytes within cysts are likely also held together by cell adhesion molecules (CAMs). This is supported by expression of E-cadherin on the surface of the developing germ cells [50]. One idea is that CAMs such as E-cadherin would need to be down-regulated for cysts to break apart. Supporting this, blocking E-cadherin function in hamster ovary organ culture resulted in accelerated follicle formation, suggesting that normally E-cadherin is involved in maintaining oocytes in cysts [51].

Estrogen signaling may play a role in regulating cyst breakdown and follicle formation. Treatment with estradiol (E_2) or with estrogenic compounds blocks both cyst breakdown and formation of follicles [42, 52, 53]. The model of estrogen action in the neonatal ovary is that high E_2 levels in the fetal ovary normally keep oocytes in cysts and that late in fetal development E_2 levels drop, resulting in separation of oocytes [52]. When ovaries are exogenously exposed to estrogens, cyst breakdown is inhibited. One estrogen receptor, ERβ, is expressed in a subset of oocytes during cyst breakdown and estrogens may affect oocyte development through this receptor [54]. However, *ER*β knockouts have no effect on neonatal oocyte development (F. Tang and M. Pepling, unpublished observations, 2011). These results suggest that estrogen signals through another receptor to maintain oocytes in cysts.

Somatic cell-specific factors

A few factors have been identified that are expressed specifically in ovarian somatic cells that may be involved in regulating follicle formation (Table 4.2). So far one transcription factor has been identified that is specifically expressed in granulosa cells and may play a role in follicle formation. Mutants in *Foxl2,* which encodes a winged-helix forkhead transcription factor, are female sterile. In these mutants, germ cell cysts do not break apart and granulosa cells do not enclose oocytes [55]. Two members of the Notch signaling pathway are expressed in granulosa cells during cyst breakdown and follicle formation. The first member, Lunatic fringe (LFNG), belongs to the Fringe family of proteins that regulates Notch signaling [56]. *Lfng* mutants are sterile and have ovaries with MOFs, supporting the idea that Notch signaling is important for cyst breakdown. The second member present in the granulosa cells is Notch2, which serves as a receptor in the Notch pathway [49]. As mentioned earlier, blocking Notch signaling in cultured neonatal ovaries results in defective cyst breakdown. Based on the expression of the Notch ligand JAG1 in neonatal oocytes and the Notch receptor Notch2 in granulosa cells, it is likely that the oocytes signal to the granulosa cells in order for cyst breakdown and follicle formation to occur. It should be noted that two other Notch signaling proteins, JAG2 and Notch1, are detected in the neonatal ovary by RT-PCR but their cellular localization has not been examined. Like the *Jag1* mutants, *Jag2, Notch1,* and *Notch2* mutants are embryonic lethal and further investigation awaits the generation of tissue-specific knockouts.

Another granulosa-specific protein, stem cell factor (SCF), when added to hamster ovary organ culture promotes follicle formation, while blocking SCF inhibits the process [44]. SCF is the ligand for the Kit receptor tyrosine kinase (KIT) that is expressed in oocytes. The Kit signaling pathway has been well studied at other times of ovarian development. The organ culture results suggest that SCF is a signal sent from granulosa cells to oocytes that is important for follicle formation but the role of the KIT receptor in follicle formation has not yet been elucidated.

The TGFβ family member anti-Müllerian hormone (AMH) is expressed in somatic cells and has been implicated in follicle assembly. In newborn rat ovaries treated with AMH, primordial follicle

Table 4.2. Somatic cell-expressed factors implicated in follicle formation

Gene	Protein/function	Evidence for role in follicle assembly	Expressed in	References
Amh	Anti-Müllerian hormone, TGFβ family member	Follicle formation is reduced and oocyte number increased in mutants	Stromal cells	[57]
ERα	Estrogen signaling	Estrogen blocks cyst breakdown		[54]
Foxl2	Forkhead box L2, winged-helix transcription factor	Mutants are defective in follicle formation	Granulosa cells	[55]
Lnfg	Regulator of Notch signaling	Mutants have multiple oocyte follicles	Granulosa cells	[56]
Notch2	Notch receptor	Inhibition of Notch signaling reduces follicle formation	Granulosa cells	[49]
Scf	Stem cell factor, Kit signaling	Promotes follicle formation in hamster	Granulosa cells	[44]

assembly and oocyte loss is reduced [57]. This suggests that AMH normally maintains oocytes in cysts and then must be down-regulated before follicle formation. Strikingly, AMH is the only factor so far with a potential role in follicle formation that is expressed in stromal cells.

ERα is expressed in granulosa cells during cyst breakdown [54]. As discussed earlier, estrogenic compounds block cyst breakdown. Estrogens may be able to signal to oocytes through ERβ and to granulosa cells through ERα. However, like the *ERβ* mutants, *ERα* mutants undergo cyst breakdown normally (F. Tang and M. Pepling, unpublished observations, 2011). Estrogens may be able to signal through another ER. In fact, E_2 can signal at the membrane to block cyst breakdown, supporting the idea that a membrane receptor might be involved, though the identity of the receptor is unknown [54].

Factors expressed in both oocytes and somatic cells

Some factors that may be involved in follicle formation are expressed in both oocytes and somatic cells and it is unclear if they are important in one or both cell types (Table 4.3). The TGFβ family member activin is expressed in oocytes and granulosa cells in the neonatal ovary [58]. Neonatal injection of recombinant activin results in an increased number of primordial follicles. Conversely, mice that overexpress inhibin β, an activin antagonist, have more MOFs, supporting the idea that activin is important in primordial follicle formation [59]. The ovarian cell types that express inhibin have not yet been determined. Follistatin, another activin antagonist, is expressed in oocytes, granulosa cells, and stromal cells [60]. *Follistatin* mutants that lack two of three isoforms also have a delay in cyst breakdown and follicle formation though how this relates to activin function is unclear.

AKT is another potential regulator of primordial follicle formation that is expressed in both oocytes and granulosa cells. AKT is activated by signaling through the phosphatidylinositol 3-kinase (PI3K) pathway. When activated, AKT can phosphorylate several target proteins, including tuberous sclerosis complex (TSC1/2), mammalian target of rapamycin (mTOR), FOXO3, and p27. *Akt1* mouse mutants have more MOFs, suggesting a role for the PI3K pathway in cyst breakdown [61]. Further, p27 expression is reduced and FOXO3a phosphorylation is decreased when AKT is inhibited in neonatal rat ovary organ culture [62]. In addition, oocyte apoptosis is also reduced. However, *Foxo3a* knockouts undergo normal primordial follicle formation so it is unlikely that FOXO3a is involved in cyst breakdown [63]. Primordial follicle formation is accelerated in *p27* mutants and p27 is expressed in both oocytes and in somatic cells surrounding cysts [64]. Few studies have examined the role of TSC1/2 and mTOR in follicle development, but recently *Tsc1* knockout mice were generated and exhibited defects in primordial follicle activation [65]. Oocyte-specific knockouts of *Tsc1* or *Pten* (a negative regulator of PI3K signaling) undergo normal primordial follicle formation [65, 66]. However, the promoter used to drive Cre recombinase in oocytes is not active until postnatal day (PND)3 after most cysts have already broken down [67]. The role of the PI3K pathway in cyst breakdown needs further study.

Several proteins in the neurotrophin signaling pathway are expressed in both oocytes and

Table 4.3. Factors implicated in follicle formation that are expressed in oocytes and somatic cells

Gene	Protein/function	Evidence for role in follicle assembly	References
Activin A	TGFβ family member	Promotes follicle formation	[58]
Ahr	Aryl hydrocarbon receptor, basic helix-loop-helix transcription factor	Primordial follicle formation is accelerated in mutants	[70, 71]
Akt1	Serine/threonine kinase, also known as protein kinase B (PKB)	Multiple oocyte follicles	[61]
Follistatin	Activin antagonist, TGFβ family member	Mutants that express only one of three isoforms have reduced follicle formation	[60]
Hnrnpk	Heterogeneous nuclear ribonucleoprotein K	siRNA knockdown in rat ovary organ culture caused a block in cyst breakdown and follicle formation	[72]
Ngf	Nerve growth factor, neurotrophin signaling	Follicle formation is reduced in mutants	[68]
Ntrk1	NGF receptor, neurotrophin signaling	Follicle formation is reduced in mutants	[48]
p27	Cyclin-dependent kinase inhibitor 1, downstream of PI3K signaling	Primordial follicle formation is accelerated in mutants	[64]

PI3K, phosphatidylinositol 3-kinase.

granulosa cells and have also been implicated in primordial follicle formation. Nerve growth factor (NGF) signals through its receptor, neurotrophic tyrosine kinase receptor, type 1 (NTRK1). Both *Ngf* and *Ntrk1* mutants have fewer primordial follicles and more oocytes still in germ cell cysts [48, 68]. These two proteins are expressed in both oocytes and granulosa cells, suggesting there may be reciprocal signaling between the two cell types using this pathway. As noted earlier, NT4 and BDNF are two growth factors related to NGF and both signal through NTRK2. It is not known which cell types in the ovary NT4 and BDNF are expressed in though blocking NT4 or BDNF in organ culture results in reduced neonatal oocyte survival [69]. As mentioned earlier, NTRK2 is expressed in the oocyte and may receive signals sent by other cell types in the ovary.

Two nuclear proteins with putative roles in follicle formation, aryl hydrocarbon receptor (AHR) and heterogeneous nuclear ribonucleoprotein K (HNRNPK), are found in both oocytes and somatic cells in the neonatal ovary. The AHR protein is a bHLH transcription factor and mutants form follicles at a faster rate than normal, suggesting that AHR is a negative regulator of follicle formation [70, 71]. HNRNPK functions as a transcription factor as well as by several other mechanisms. RNA interference (RNAi) knockdown of HNRNPK in rat ovary organ culture caused a block in cyst breakdown and follicle formation though whether it is acting by transcriptional regulation is unknown [72].

Control of oocyte death

Caspase activation during programmed cell death

Caspase activation is the main step leading to programmed cell death and two major pathways activate caspases (Figure 4.2) [73, 74]. The first pathway is referred to as the extrinsic or death receptor-dependent pathway and it is activated by factors such as Fas ligand and tumor necrosis factor (TNF) that bind to cell surface death receptors. Activation of the death receptor pathway results in activation of caspase 8. The second pathway is the intrinsic or death receptor-independent pathway and is activated by cellular stresses such as DNA damage, lack of growth factors, and hypoxia. The intrinsic death pathway is regulated by B-cell lymphoma/leukemia-2 (BCL2) family proteins and leads to caspase 9 activation.

Caspases function as cysteine proteases and are present in cells as inactive precursors which are activated by cleavage. They are usually classified into two groups, initiator caspases and effector caspases. The initiator caspases such as caspase 9 associate with apoptotic protease-activating factor 1 (APAF1) and cytochrome c to form the apoptosome, which activates effector caspases such as caspase 3, 6, and 7. One caspase, caspase 2, specifically affects oocyte cell death. *Caspase 2* mutants have a greater number of primordial follicles than wild-type mice [75]. In addition, when neonatal ovaries are exposed to ionizing

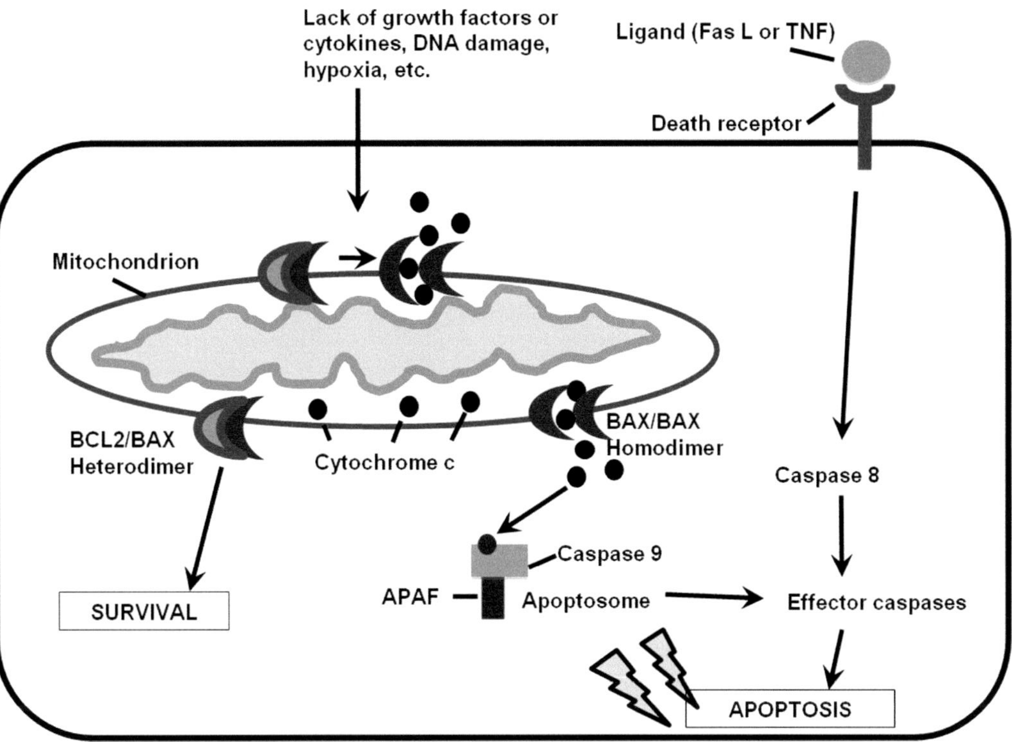

Figure 4.2 General pathways of programmed cell death. There are two major pathways leading to apoptosis. The extrinsic or death receptor-dependent pathway is activated when a ligand binds to a death receptor at the cell membrane. Subsequently, the initiator caspase, caspase 8, is activated, which in turn activates downstream effector caspases leading to cell death. The intrinsic or death receptor-independent pathway is activated by a lack of growth factors or cytokines, DNA damage, hypoxia or other cellular stresses. Prior to activation, BCL2 and other anti-apoptotic BCL2 family proteins located in the mitochondrial membrane bind to pro-apoptotic BCL2 family members such as BAX, keeping them inactive. Upon activation, the pro-apoptotic proteins form homodimers that serve as pores in the mitochondrial membrane. The pores allow cytochrome c into the cytoplasm. The apoptosome then forms consisting of cytochrome c, APAF, and caspase 9. The apoptosome then activates downstream effector caspases and activates apoptosis. APAF, apoptotic protease-activating factor; BCL2, B-cell lymphoma/leukemia-2; TNF, tumor necrosis factor.

radiation, caspase 2 is up-regulated as oocytes die [76]. Caspase 2 shares similarities with both initiator and effector caspases and its specific role in the apoptotic pathway is unclear [77].

BCL2 family of cell death regulators

The BCL2 protein family is important for the regulation of apoptosis [78]. In mammals, there are over 25 BCL2 family members sharing at least one BCL2 homology (BH) domain. These proteins can be divided into two groups, pro-apoptotic (such as BAX, BAK, and BAD) and anti-apoptotic (such as BCL2, BCLx, and MCL1) [79]. It is thought that the balance of pro- and anti-apoptotic BCL2 family proteins serves to regulate programmed cell death [80]. The current model is that anti-apoptotic BCL2 proteins guard the mitochondrial membrane against pro-apoptotic proteins. Following activation of programmed cell death, pro-apoptotic proteins such as BAX dimerize and increase mitochondrial membrane permeability by forming channels or interacting with existing pores to form larger channels. This allows the release of cytochrome c from the mitochondria and formation of the apoptosome. The combination of BCL2 proteins important in regulation of perinatal oocyte death is not known although some members have been implicated in oocyte survival as discussed below.

Examination of two *Bcl2* transgenic mouse strains suggests that BCL2 may be involved in regulating programmed cell death during cyst breakdown. Adult *Bcl2* female knockout mice have fewer total oocytes and follicles containing degenerating oocytes or lacking oocytes [81]. It is not known exactly when during development the oocytes are lost but it may be during cyst breakdown. The *Bcl2* mutants were initially reported to be fertile and have normal litter sizes. However, most *Bcl2* homozygous knockout mice die by 2 or 3 weeks of age, making fertility difficult to study [82]. In contrast, females that ectopically express BCL2 in germ cells have more oocytes than normal at PND8 [83]. By PND60, the *Bcl2* transgenic mice have the same number of oocytes as control mice, indicating that these extra germ cells are not maintained in the adult. It is not known if BCL2 levels affect cyst breakdown.

There is also evidence that the pro-apoptotic protein BAX plays a role in oocyte programmed cell death. Adult female homozygous mutants lacking the *Bax* gene have three times as many oocytes as wild-type females [84]. There is no difference in the number of oocytes at birth, suggesting that fewer oocytes are lost during postnatal development. Supporting this idea, *Bax* mutants have significantly more oocytes at PND7 compared to wild-type mice [85]. In addition, cyst breakdown is reduced, supporting the model that programmed cell death is required for cyst breakdown. The complete set of pro- and anti-apoptotic BCL2 family members involved in neonatal oocyte survival and death has not yet been determined.

Regulation of autophagy

As mentioned earlier in the chapter, an alternative pathway controlling oocyte death that may be active during follicle formation is autophagy. Disruption of two different genes encoding proteins involved in autophagy causes a greater loss of oocytes, supporting the role of autophagy in the regulation of oocyte survival [86]. The first autophagy protein is Beclin1 (BECN1), which is important in formation of autophagosomes. Oocyte number during follicle formation cannot be determined in *Becn1* homozygous mutants because they are embryonic lethal. However, PND1 *Becn1* heterozygotes have only half the number of oocytes of wild-type animals. The second autophagy protein that affects oocyte death is autophagy-related 7 (ATG7). ATG7 is important for expansion of vesicles during autophagy. At PND1, *Atg7* mutant ovaries contain no identifiable germ cells. Thus, autophagy, like apoptosis, is also important in regulating neonatal germ cell numbers.

Conclusions

Headway is being made in understanding the mechanisms involved in formation of primordial follicles. Oocyte death is an important process during follicle formation but how cell death in the neonate is selectively regulated so that some oocytes survive while others die remains a mystery. Several factors that appear to play a role in regulating oocyte numbers have been identified but a more complete picture will require further study. Understanding how oocyte death is controlled during primordial follicle assembly will be important in the development of potential therapeutic targets for infertility and ovarian cancer.

References

1. Peters H. Migration of gonocytes into the mammalian gonad and their differentiation. *Philos Trans R Soc Lond B Biol Sci* 1970; **259**: 91–101.
2. Pepling ME, Spradling AC. Female mouse germ cells form synchronously dividing cysts. *Development* 1998; **125**: 3323–8.
3. Pepling ME, Sundman EA, Patterson NL, *et al.* Differences in oocyte development and estradiol sensitivity among mouse strains. *Reproduction* 2010; **139**: 349–57.
4. Pepling ME, Spradling AC. The mouse ovary contains germ cell cysts that undergo programmed breakdown to form follicles. *Dev Biol* 2001; **234**: 339–51.
5. Kezele P, Skinner MK. Regulation of ovarian primordial follicle assembly and development by estrogen and progesterone: endocrine model of follicle assembly. *Endocrinology* 2003; **144**: 3329–37.
6. Yen SSC, Jaffe RB. *Reproductive Endocrinology: Physiology, Pathophysiology, and Clinical Management,* 3rd edn. Philadelphia: Saunders, 1991.
7. Berek JS, Novak E. *Berek & Novak's Gynecology*, 14th edn. Philadelphia: Lippincott Williams & Wilkins, 2007.
8. Monk M, McLaren A. X-chromosome activity in foetal germ cells of the mouse. *J Embryol Exp Morphol* 1981; **63**: 75–84.
9. Witschi E. Migration of the germ cells of human embryos from the yolk sac to the primitive gonadal folds. In: *Contributions to Embryology*,Vol. **32**. Washington DC: Carnegie Institution. 1948; 67–80.
10. de Cuevas M, Lilly MA, Spradling AC. Germline cyst formation in *Drosophila. Annu Rev Genet* 1997; **31**: 405–28.
11. Greenbaum MP, Yan W, Wu MH, *et al.* TEX14 is essential for intercellular bridges and fertility in male mice. *Proc Natl Acad Sci USA* 2006; **103**: 4982–7.
12. Greenbaum MP, Iwamori N, Agno JE, Matzuk MM. Mouse TEX14 is required for embryonic germ cell

intercellular bridges but not female fertility. *Biol Reprod* 2009; **80**: 449–57.

13. Mork L, Tang H, Batchvarov I, Capel B. Mouse germ cell clusters form by aggregation as well as clonal divisions. *Mech Dev* 2012; **128**: 591–6.

14. Gondos B, Bhiraleus P, Hobel CJ. Ultrastructural observations on germ cells in human fetal ovaries. *Am J Obstet Gynecol* 1971; **110**: 644–52.

15. McLaren A. Germ and somatic cell lineages in the developing gonad. *Mol Cell Endocrinol* 2000; **163**: 3–9.

16. Bullejos M, Koopman P. Germ cells enter meiosis in a rostro-caudal wave during development of the mouse ovary. *Mol Reprod Dev* 2004; **68**: 422–8.

17. Menke DB, Koubova J, Page DC. Sexual differentiation of germ cells in XX mouse gonads occurs in an anterior-to-posterior wave. *Dev Biol* 2003; **262**: 303–12.

18. Bowles J, Knight D, Smith C, *et al.* Retinoid signaling determines germ cell fate in mice. *Science* 2006; **312**: 596–600.

19. Koubova J, Menke DB, Zhou Q, *et al.* Retinoic acid regulates sex-specific timing of meiotic initiation in mice. *Proc Natl Acad Sci USA* 2006; **103**: 2474–9.

20. Baltus AE, Menke DB, Hu YC, *et al.* In germ cells of mouse embryonic ovaries, the decision to enter meiosis precedes premeiotic DNA replication. *Nat Genet* 2006; **38**: 1430–4.

21. Borum K. Oogenesis in the mouse. A study of the origin of the mature ova. *Exp Cell Res* 1961; **45**: 39–47.

22. Shin YH, Choi Y, Erdin SU, *et al.* Hormad1 mutation disrupts synaptonemal complex formation, recombination, and chromosome segregation in mammalian meiosis. *PLoS Genet* 2010; **6**: e1001190.

23. Byskov AG. Differentiation of mammalian embryonic gonad. *Physiol Rev* 1986; **66**: 71–117.

24. Liu CF, Liu C, Yao HH. Building pathways for ovary organogenesis in the mouse embryo. *Curr Top Dev Biol* 2010; **90**: 263–90.

25. Mork L, Maatouk DM, McMahon JA, *et al.* Temporal differences in granulosa cell specification in the ovary reflect distinct follicle fates in mice. *Biol Reprod* 2012; **86**: 37.

26. Merchant-Larios H, Chimal-Monroy J. The ontogeny of primordial follicles in the mouse ovary. *Prog Clin Biol Res* 1989; **296**: 55–63.

27. Mazaud S, Guyot R, Guigon CJ, *et al.* Basal membrane remodeling during follicle histogenesis in the rat ovary: contribution of proteinases of the MMP and PA families. *Dev Biol* 2005; **277**: 403–16.

28. Baker TG. Oogenesis and ovarian development. In: Balin H, Glasser S, eds. *Reproductive Biology*. Amsterdam: Excerpta Medica. 1972; 398–405.

29. Pepling ME. From primordial germ cell to primordial follicle: mammalian female germ cell development. *Genesis* 2006; **44**: 622–32.

30. De Felici M, Di Carlo A, Pesce M, *et al.* Bcl-2 and Bax regulation of apoptosis in germ cells during prenatal oogenesis in the mouse embryo. *Cell Death Differ* 1999; **6**: 908–15.

31. McClellan KA, Gosden R, Taketo T. Continuous loss of oocytes throughout meiotic prophase in the normal mouse ovary. *Dev Biol* 2003; **258**: 334–48.

32. Nandedkar T, Dharma S, Modi D, Dsouza S. Differential gene expression in transition of primordial to preantral follicles in mouse ovary. *Soc Reprod Fertil Suppl* 2007; **63**: 57–67.

33. Coucouvanis EC, Sherwood SW, Carswell-Crumpton C, Spack EG, Jones PP. Evidence that the mechanism of prenatal germ cell death in the mouse is apoptosis. *Exp Cell Res* 1993; **209**: 238–47.

34. Lobascio AM, Klinger FG, Scaldaferri ML, Farini D, De Felici M. Analysis of programmed cell death in mouse fetal oocytes. *Reproduction* 2007; **134**: 241–52.

35. De Felici M, Lobascio AM, Klinger FG. Cell death in fetal oocytes: many players for multiple pathways. *Autophagy* 2008; **4**: 240–2.

36. Edinger AL, Thompson CB. Death by design: apoptosis, necrosis and autophagy. *Curr Opin Cell Biol* 2004; **16**: 663–9.

37. Codogno P, Meijer AJ. Autophagy and signaling: their role in cell survival and cell death. *Cell Death Differ* 2005; **12** Suppl 2: 1509–18.

38. Pesce M, Farrace MG, Amendola A, Piacentini M, De Felici M. Stem cell factor regulation of apoptosis in mouse primordial germ cells. In: Tilly J, Strauss JF, eds. *Cell Death in Reproductive Physiology*. New York: Verlag. 1997; 19–31.

39. Rodrigues P, Limback D, McGinnis LK, Plancha CE, Albertini DF. Multiple mechanisms of germ cell loss in the perinatal mouse ovary. *Reproduction* 2009; **137**: 709–20.

40. Elvin JA, Yan C, Matzuk MM. Oocyte-expressed TGF-beta superfamily members in female fertility. *Mol Cell Endocrinol* 2000; **159**: 1–5.

41. Yan C, Wang P, DeMayo J, *et al.* Synergistic roles of bone morphogenetic protein 15 and growth differentiation factor 9 in ovarian function. *Mol Endocrinol* 2001; **15**: 854–66.

42. Jefferson W, Newbold R, Padilla-Banks E, Pepling M. Neonatal genistein treatment alters ovarian differentiation in the mouse: inhibition of oocyte nest

breakdown and increased oocyte survival. *Biol Reprod* 2006; **74**: 161–8.

43. Kent HA. Polyovular follicles and multinucleate ova in the ovaries of young mice. *Anat Rec* 1960; **137**: 521–4.

44. Wang J, Roy SK. Growth differentiation factor-9 and stem cell factor promote primordial follicle formation in the hamster: modulation by follicle-stimulating hormone. *Biol Reprod* 2004; **70**: 577–85.

45. Schindler R, Nilsson E, Skinner MK. Induction of ovarian primordial follicle assembly by connective tissue growth factor CTGF. *PLoS One* 2010; **5**: e12979.

46. Soyal SM, Amleh A, Dean J. FIGalpha, a germ cell-specific transcription factor required for ovarian follicle formation. *Development* 2000; **127**: 4645–54.

47. Rajkovic A, Pangas SA, Ballow D, Suzumori N, Matzuk MM. NOBOX deficiency disrupts early folliculogenesis and oocyte-specific gene expression. *Science* 2004; **305**: 1157–9.

48. Kerr B, Garcia-Rudaz C, Dorfman M, Paredes A, Ojeda SR. NTRK1 and NTRK2 receptors facilitate follicle assembly and early follicular development in the mouse ovary. *Reproduction* 2009; **138**: 131–40.

49. Trombly DJ, Woodruff TK, Mayo KE. Suppression of Notch signaling in the neonatal mouse ovary decreases primordial follicle formation. *Endocrinology* 2009; **150**: 1014–24.

50. Di Carlo A, De Felici M. A role for E-cadherin in mouse primordial germ cell development. *Dev Biol* 2000; **226**: 209–19.

51. Wang C, Roy SK. Expression of E-cadherin and N-cadherin in perinatal hamster ovary: possible involvement in primordial follicle formation and regulation by follicle-stimulating hormone. *Endocrinology* 2010; **151**: 2319–30.

52. Chen Y, Jefferson WN, Newbold RR, Padilla-Banks E, Pepling ME. Estradiol, progesterone, and genistein inhibit oocyte nest breakdown and primordial follicle assembly in the neonatal mouse ovary in vitro and in vivo. *Endocrinology* 2007; **148**: 3580–90.

53. Karavan JR, Pepling ME. Effects of estrogenic compounds on neonatal oocyte development. *Reprod Toxicol* 2012; **34**: 51–6.

54. Chen Y, Breen K, Pepling ME. Estrogen can signal through multiple pathways to regulate oocyte cyst breakdown and primordial follicle assembly in the neonatal mouse ovary. *J Endocrinol* 2009; **202**: 407–17.

55. Uda M, Ottolenghi C, Crisponi L, *et al.* Foxl2 disruption causes mouse ovarian failure by pervasive blockage of follicle development. *Hum Mol Genet* 2004; **13**: 1171–81.

56. Hahn KL, Johnson J, Beres BJ, Howard S, Wilson-Rawls J. Lunatic fringe null female mice are infertile due to defects in meiotic maturation. *Development* 2005; **132**: 817–28.

57. Nilsson EE, Schindler R, Savenkova MI, Skinner MK. Inhibitory actions of anti-Mullerian hormone (AMH) on ovarian primordial follicle assembly. *PLoS One* 2011; **6**: e20087.

58. Bristol-Gould SK, Kreeger PK, Selkirk CG, *et al.* Postnatal regulation of germ cells by activin: the establishment of the initial follicle pool. *Dev Biol* 2006; **298**: 132–48.

59. McMullen ML, Cho BN, Yates CJ, Mayo KE. Gonadal pathologies in transgenic mice expressing the rat inhibin alpha-subunit. *Endocrinology* 2001; **142**: 5005–14.

60. Kimura F, Bonomi LM, Schneyer AL. Follistatin regulates germ cell nest breakdown and primordial follicle formation. *Endocrinology* 2011; **152**: 697–706.

61. Brown C, LaRocca J, Pietruska J, *et al.* Subfertility caused by altered follicular development and oocyte growth in female mice lacking PKB alpha/Akt1. *Biol Reprod* 2010; **82**: 246–56.

62. Liu H, Luo LL, Qian YS, *et al.* FOXO3a is involved in the apoptosis of naked oocytes and oocytes of primordial follicles from neonatal rat ovaries. *Biochem Biophys Res Commun* 2009; **381**: 722–7.

63. John GB, Shirley LJ, Gallardo TD, Castrillon DH. Specificity of the requirement for Foxo3 in primordial follicle activation. *Reproduction* 2007; **133**: 855–63.

64. Rajareddy S, Reddy P, Du C, *et al.* p27kip1 (cyclin-dependent kinase inhibitor 1B) controls ovarian development by suppressing follicle endowment and activation and promoting follicle atresia in mice. *Mol Endocrinol* 2007; **21**: 2189–202.

65. Adhikari D, Zheng W, Shen Y, *et al.* Tsc/mTORC1 signaling in oocytes governs the quiescence and activation of primordial follicles. *Hum Mol Genet* 2010; **19**: 397–410.

66. Reddy P, Liu L, Adhikari D, *et al.* Oocyte-specific deletion of Pten causes premature activation of the primordial follicle pool. *Science* 2008; **319**: 611–13.

67. Lan ZJ, Xu X, Cooney AJ. Differential oocyte-specific expression of Cre recombinase activity in GDF-9-iCre, Zp3cre, and Msx2Cre transgenic mice. *Biol Reprod* 2004; **71**: 1469–71.

68. Dissen GA, Romero C, Hirshfield AN, Ojeda SR. Nerve growth factor is required for early follicular development in the mammalian ovary. *Endocrinology* 2001; **142**: 2078–86.

69. Spears N, Molinek MD, Robinson LL, *et al.* The role of neurotrophin receptors in female germ-cell survival in mouse and human. *Development* 2003; **130**: 5481–91.

70. Benedict JC, Lin TM, Loeffler IK, Peterson RE, Flaws JA. Physiological role of the aryl hydrocarbon receptor in mouse ovary development. *Toxicol Sci* 2000; **56**: 382–8.

71. Robles R, Morita Y, Mann KK, *et al.* The aryl hydrocarbon receptor, a basic helix-loop-helix transcription factor of the PAS gene family, is required for normal ovarian germ cell dynamics in the mouse. *Endocrinology* 2000; **141**: 450–3.

72. Wang N, Zhang P, Guo X, Zhou Z, Sha J. Hnrnpk, a protein differentially expressed in immature rat ovarian development, is required for normal primordial follicle assembly and development. *Endocrinology* 2011; **152**: 1024–35.

73. Fuchs Y, Steller H. Programmed cell death in animal development and disease. *Cell* 2011; **147**: 742–58.

74. Conradt B. Genetic control of programmed cell death during animal development. *Annu Rev Genet* 2009; **43**: 493–523.

75. Bergeron L, Perez GI, Macdonald G, *et al.* Defects in regulation of apoptosis in caspase-2-deficient mice. *Genes Dev* 1998; **12**: 1304–14.

76. Hanoux V, Pairault C, Bakalska M, Habert R, Livera G. Caspase-2 involvement during ionizing radiation-induced oocyte death in the mouse ovary. *Cell Death Differ* 2007; **14**: 671–81.

77. Troy CM, Shelanski ML. Caspase-2 redux. *Cell Death Differ* 2003; **10**: 101–7.

78. Hsu SY, Hsueh AJ. Tissue-specific Bcl-2 protein partners in apoptosis: an ovarian paradigm. *Physiol Rev* 2000; **80**: 593–614.

79. Kim MR, Tilly JL. Current concepts in Bcl-2 family member regulation of female germ cell development and survival. *Biochim Biophys Acta* 2004; **1644**: 205–10.

80. Cory S, Adams JM. The Bcl-2 family: regulators of the cellular life-or-death switch. *Nat Rev Cancer* 2002; **2**: 647–56.

81. Ratts VS, Flaws JA, Klop R, Sorenson CM, Tilly JL. Ablation of *bcl-2* gene expression decreases the number of oocytes and primordial follicles established in the postnatal female mouse gonad. *Endocrinology* 1995; **136**: 3665–8.

82. Veis DJ, Sorenson CM, Shutter JR, Korsmeyer SJ. Bcl-2-deficient mice demonstrate fulminant lymphoid apoptosis, polycystic kidneys, and hypopigmented hair. *Cell* 1993; **75**: 229–40.

83. Flaws JA, Hirshfield AN, Hewitt JA, Babus JK, Furth PA. Effect of bcl-2 on the primordial follicle endowment in the mouse ovary. *Biol Reprod* 2001; **64**: 1153–9.

84. Perez GI, Robles R, Knudson CM, *et al.* Prolongation of ovarian lifespan into advanced chronological age by Bax-deficiency. *Nat Genet* 1999; **21**: 200–3.

85. Greenfeld CR, Pepling ME, Babus JK, Furth PA, Flaws JA. BAX regulates follicular endowment in mice. *Reproduction* 2007; **133**: 865–76.

86. Gawriluk TR, Hale AN, Flaws JA, *et al.* Autophagy is a cell survival program for female germ cells in the murine ovary. *Reproduction* 2011; **141**: 759–65.

Section 2 Life cycle

Chapter 5

The early stages of follicular growth

Alain Gougeon

Introduction

Since the first edition of *Biology and Pathology of the Oocyte*, the use of technologies such as transgenic mouse models and microarray analyses has significantly increased our knowledge of early stages of follicular growth. In the present chapter, we will show that activation of resting follicles as well as early follicular growth are regulated by local factors produced by ovarian cell types (oocyte, granulosa, theca, and stroma) that mediate a dialog between neighbor follicles. Although it is now widely accepted that early stages of follicular growth are minimally gonadotropin-dependent, the role of follicle-stimulating hormone (FSH) will be revisited in the light of early studies suggesting that FSH might be, either directly or indirectly, involved in these processes. Nevertheless, identification of factors governing early folliculogenesis remains difficult because of the multiplicity of signaling pathways and molecules of unknown function, as revealed by microarray analyses, whereas the exact role played by specific factors is very complex to determine because of the presence within the ovary of a mixture of arrested and developing follicles.

The ovarian reserve

Aging changes

In the human ovary, primordial follicles begin to form during the fourth month of fetal life and although some of these follicles start to grow almost immediately, most of them remain in a resting stage. The stock of dormant follicles constitutes the ovarian reserve. In humans at birth, each ovary contains between 250 000 and 500 000 resting follicles (reviewed in [1]). In all mammalian species, resting follicles leave the stock in a continuous stream, either by apoptosis or by entry into the growth phase, thus depleting the ovarian reserve. Atresia of resting follicles is difficult to quantify because of the very quick disappearance of apoptotic oocytes. However, it can be estimated that apoptosis is responsible for approximately 90% of the ovarian reserve attrition. In physiological conditions, the factors triggering the onset of the apoptotic cascade in resting follicles remain unknown and, therefore, require further promising studies. The depletion rate of the ovarian reserve, which may be variable between subjects, accelerates, either continuously [2] or from approximately 38 years of age, leading to a stock at menopause estimated at less than 100 (see [1]). The "dogma" that the ovarian reserve is fixed at birth in most mammals was challenged, 8 years ago, by Tilly's team [3], who claimed that neo-oogenesis takes place in the adult ovary in both mouse and human species. According to the authors, the "germline stem cells," which continuously regenerate the stock of resting follicles, were firstly localized in the ovarian surface epithelium, then in the bone marrow and circulating blood. In a recent article, these authors have isolated germinal pre-meiotic cells, named "oogonia stem cells" (OSC) from murine and human ovaries. These cells, which are present in very low number, are able to proliferate in culture then to differentiate into presumptive primordial (human) or fertilizable mature oocytes (mouse) [3]. Although these data seem to be convincing, even though they require further confirmation, it cannot be excluded that OSC are residual oogonia that failed to transform into primordial oocytes during fetal life.

Biology and Pathology of the Oocyte, 2nd edn., ed. Alan Trounson, Roger Gosden, and Ursula Eichenlaub-Ritter. Published by Cambridge University Press.

Distinction between resting and early growing follicles

From the morphological aspect of their granulosa cells (GCs), very small follicles can be classified as primordial, intermediary, and primary follicles. Distinction between early growing follicles and resting follicles remains controversial, especially for follicles possessing both flattened and cuboidal GCs (named either intermediary, transitory, or early primary follicles) (reviewed in [4]). In rats, several authors, having observed the presence of at least one proliferating GC within these follicles, assumed that when at least one GC is either cuboidal or proliferative, the follicles have entered the growth phase (reviewed in [4]). However, in humans, primordial, intermediary, and primary follicles have a similar mean diameter of their oocyte and its nucleus, and 33% of follicles are intermediary, while in cattle, more than 82.5% of primordial follicles contain at least one cuboidal GC. After 5′-bromodeoxyuridine (BrdU) infusion in the rat, 57% of intermediary follicles are still labeled even 150 days after the removal of the BrdU source, thus demonstrating that these follicles must be considered non-growing. Finally, recent studies have shown that FOXO3a, a strong inhibitor of resting follicle activation, is expressed mainly in the oocyte nucleus of primordial and early primary follicles and that its expression in oocytes of larger primary follicles and further developed follicles is dramatically down-regulated (reviewed in [4, 5]). Taken together, these data show that primordial, intermediary, and small primary follicles must be considered resting follicles.

Activation of resting follicles

The mechanisms triggering activation of resting follicles remain poorly understood despite new exciting findings. Several working hypotheses have been proposed to elucidate this process. They imply circulating hormones or local factors, produced by either the resting follicle itself, ovarian stroma, or neighbor follicles. The most documented hypothesis is that primordial follicles are held at the resting stage by an inhibitory signal originating from growing follicles. Nevertheless, this hypothesis cannot explain the absence of global initiation when growing follicles are absent, for example during the late fetal life in humans or the perinatal life in mice. This implies the existence of another diffusible source of inhibition that can come from the resting follicles themselves as recently shown in the juvenile mouse [6]. However, multiple studies have shown that resting follicles can be stimulated to enter the growth phase by a variety of molecules, suggesting that initiation of follicular growth cannot simply be considered as the removing of an inhibitory signal.

A role for molecules binding a tyrosine kinase receptor (TrkR) (Figure 5.1)

Phenotypic observations of mice bearing spontaneous mutations of the *Steel* locus coding for the Kit ligand (KL), after treatment with an antibody against the receptor cKit, in in vitro culture of neonatal ovaries in the presence of KL, have shown that KL activates resting follicles and that its absence leads to a blockade of folliculogenesis at the primary follicle stage. In addition to KL, other local factors produced by ovarian cells (reviewed in [7]) stimulate activation of resting follicles. Microarray analyses have shown that alterations in the ovarian transcriptome occur in response to treatment of rat ovaries with FGF2 (fibroblast growth factor 2 or basic fibroblast growth factor), GDNF (glial-derived neurotrophic factor), KGF (keratinocyte growth factor), KL, and PDGF (platelet-derived growth factor) [8]. However, some of these factors present a species-specific effect. For example, FGF2 activates resting follicles in mice, but not in humans [9]. Finally, transgenic mice models and culture of neonatal rat ovary have shown that insulin [10], neurotrophin 3 (NT3) [11], nerve growth factor (NGF), and NT4/BDNF (brain-derived neurotrophic factor) [12] can promote initiation of follicle growth.

The common thread between all these factors is that they bind to a tyrosine kinase receptor (TrkR) present at the oocyte cell surface. The binding of the ligand to its TrkR activates the oocyte 3-phosphatidylinositol-dependent protein kinase 1 (PI3K) pathway [5] and leads to activation of the resting follicle. The PI3K pathway is composed, among others, of activating enzymes such as the serine threonine kinases PDK1 and Akt (also called protein kinase B), and of inhibiting molecules (phosphatase and tensin homolog 1 – PTEN, FOXO3, tumor suppressor tuberous sclerosis complex – TSC1, 2). When the latter are removed by deletion of the gene coding

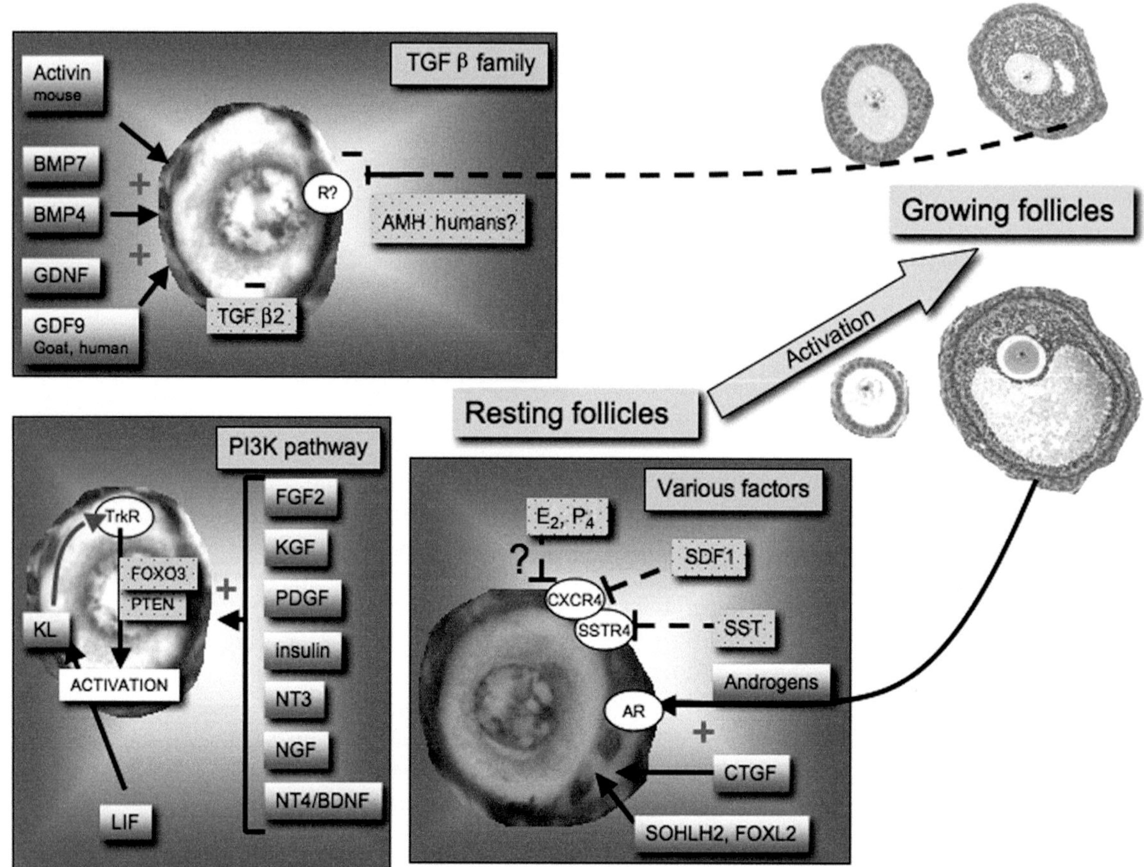

Figure 5.1 Factors that are or may be involved in activation of resting follicles. Most peptides belonging to the TGFβ superfamily stimulate activation of resting follicles, while AMH inhibits this process. All factors activating the PI3K pathway, either directly or indirectly via stimulation of KL production, promote transition of resting follicles to the growing stage.

for their synthesis, a dramatic increase of resting follicle activation can be observed. So, once activated, the PI3K pathway is under the control of inhibitory proteins preventing a premature exhaustion of the ovarian reserve in response to an excessive stimulation (reviewed in [5]). Regarding this issue, the treatment of human ovarian cortical fragments with an inhibitor of PTEN, followed by the xeno-transplantation to immunodeficient mice for 6 months, allowed the development of primordial follicles to the selectable stage with oocytes capable of undergoing nuclear maturation [13]. Surprisingly, hepatocyte growth factor (HGF), which stimulates KL production by GCs, and epidermal growth factor (EGF), which also binds to a TrkR, do not promote primordial follicle transition in the neonatal rat ovary system [10, 14], suggesting that all ligands of TrkR are not necessarily involved in resting follicle activation.

A role for molecules belonging to the transforming growth factor beta (TGFβ) superfamily (Figure 5.1)

As mentioned above, primordial follicles might be held at the resting stage by an inhibitory signal originating from growing follicles. Anti-Müllerian hormone (AMH) may be this inhibitory signal. In rodents, AMH inhibits initiation of follicular growth but its site of action on resting follicles remains to be determined [7, 15]. In rats, AMH acts by down-regulating cKit, KL, and KGF expression, as well as FGF2 receptor 1 synthesis [7]. It also decreases the TGFβ pathway signaling into processes such as cell differentiation and cell-cycle regulation, and down-regulates Akt, a key step in the stimulatory PI3K pathway [5]. So, AMH may use various mechanisms to suppress the primordial to primary follicle transition. However, its action in humans is debated since AMH either inhibits [16] or stimulates

[17] activation of resting follicles despite very few (1 of 17) primordial follicles containing mRNA for AMH-RII [18].

When growing follicles are absent, AMH action cannot explain that follicles remain at the dormant stage. Among the possible inhibitors produced by the resting follicles, transforming growth factor beta2 (TGFβ2) might be a good candidate [7]. Indeed, in monkeys, TGFβ2 is present in GCs from resting follicles and is absent in GCs from early growing follicles, while both TGFβ-RI and -RII are present in GCs and oocytes at all stages of follicular development [19]. Since TGFβ1 inhibits both marrow stromal cell expression of KL and hematopoietic progenitor cell expression of cKit (reviewed in [19]), it cannot be excluded that TGFβ2 may act as an inhibitor of the Kit system and subsequently may inhibit follicular growth initiation in primates. However, to our knowledge, TGFβ2 has not yet been tested for its action on resting follicle activation.

Whereas AMH and TGFβ are possible inhibitors of initiation, other members of the TGFβ family that are produced by various ovarian cell types (reviewed in [7]) promote activation of resting follicles. In addition to GDNF and bone morphogenetic protein 4 (BMP4), both altering the ovarian transcriptome in rats [8], BMP7, produced by theca interstitial cells (TICs) of antral follicles and interacting with extracellular matrix components, stimulates activation of resting follicles in the neonatal rat ovary cultured for 2 weeks (see [7]). While activin shows the same effect in the mouse ovary cultured in similar conditions [20], growth differentiation factor 9 (GDF9) has no effect on initiation of follicular growth in the cultured neonatal rat model [21], but stimulates it in the goat ovary [22] as well as in cultured pieces of human ovarian cortex [23].

A role for various molecules (Figure 5.1)

Analysis of the ovarian transcriptome and culture of neonatal rat ovaries have shown that leukemia inhibitory factor (LIF), which stimulates KL production by GCs [8], and connective tissue growth factor (CTGF) promote activation of resting follicles [8]. Conversely, the chemoattractive cytokine stromal cell-derived factor-1 (SDF1), its receptor CXCR4 being present in the resting oocyte, inhibits their activation (see [5]). When stimulated by androgens, prepubertal monkeys exhibit an increased activation of resting follicles [24], and in humans, it has been proposed that androgens stimulate follicular growth, either directly via androgen receptors, ARs, which are present as soon as the intermediate stage, or indirectly via local factors [18]. On the contrary, estradiol and progesterone might slow down initiation (see [5]). Somatostatin (SST), which is a potent inhibitor of cAMP generation in most epithelial cells, inhibits KL production in rat Sertoli cells (see [25]). As a SST receptor antagonist, like KL, promotes resting follicle growth in the neonatal mouse ovary cultured during 15 days [25], SST may be considered, at least partly, as an inhibitor of resting follicle activation. Finally, certain transcription factors are involved in initiation of follicular growth. FOXL2 and SOHLH2 are essential for the differentiation of flattened into cuboidal GCs [5, 26], and deletion of *FoxL2* leads to a dramatic depletion of the ovarian reserve [26]. In humans, a mutation of *FoxL2* leads to a premature ovarian insufficiency in patients suffering from a blepharophimosis, ptosis, and epicanthus inversus syndrome (BPES) [27]. Finally, by using various models of knockout mice for various oocyte-specific transcription factors, it has been shown that newborn ovary homeobox-encoding gene (*Nobox*), spermatogenesis, and oogenesis-specific basic helix-loop-helix1 (Sohlh1), and LIM homeobox protein 8 (Lhx8) may be involved in resting follicles' activation by down-regulating gene expression of factors previously shown to be involved in this process (see [5]).

Are gonadotropins involved in activation of resting follicles?

A role for FSH in initiation of the follicular growth has long been debated (reviewed in [4]). In hypogonadal *hpg* mice suffering from a deletion of the *Gnrh* gene, the number of early growing follicles is reduced; it can be restored to its normal number by treatment with FSH (see [4]). Hypophysectomy slows the loss of resting follicles in mice, while in aged rats, unilateral ovariectomy increases the concentration of FSH and is associated with increased loss of primordial follicles (see [4]). Taken together, these data suggest that gonadotropins may be involved in activation of resting follicles. However, several pieces of evidence suggest that FSH is not the primary motor of this process. In humans, all primordial and 66% of primary follicles do not express FSH receptor (FSHR) mRNA (see [4]). In mice, rats, cattle, and baboons, initiation of follicular growth can occur in vitro in the absence of FSH (see

[4]). In both FSH β subunit- and FSHR-null female mice, resting follicles can be activated and grow into preantral follicles (see [4]). Similarly, in a woman presenting a mutated FSH β-subunit, follicles can grow up to the selectable stage (reviewed in [28]). However, no quantitative data are available and it cannot be concluded that folliculogenesis is quantitatively normal in these models.

Thus, there are conflicting data concerning a possible role for gonadotropins in the process of resting follicle activation. Nevertheless, we assume that these data are conflicting only in appearance. As shown above, local factors can activate resting follicles, explaining why activation can occur in gonadotropin-deprived situations. But gonadotropins may act on neighbor growing follicles to either up-regulate production of stimulatory factors or down-regulate production of inhibiting factors, thus explaining the accelerated depletion of the ovarian reserve when circulating levels of gonadotropins are increased.

Conclusions

Whether activation of resting follicles can be initiated separately in the two compartments of the follicle, that is, the oocyte and GCs, remains intriguing. Certain factors promote transition of resting to growing follicles by acting at the oocyte level, either by stimulating KL production or by binding to a TrkR, thus activating the PI3K pathway. Neverthless, in various experimental or normal conditions, some follicles can be observed in which the oocyte has increased in diameter, while surrounding GCs are either still flattened or do not constitute a complete ring of cuboidal GCs. This is the case in the mouse ovary near the hilar part of the ovary, in ovarian cortex of the baboon ovary cultured in medium containing 10% serum, and in both *Sohlh*- and *Foxl2*-null mice (reviewed in [4, 5]). This suggests that the primordial to primary follicle transition can be initiated separately in the two follicular compartments and that a coordinated growth of the oocyte and GCs is required. This implies that more than one signal is involved in resting follicle activation and, since this process is essential for reproduction, it has a set of compensatory factors that have evolved such that loss of any one will still allow the process to proceed. So, while the exact pattern by which various factors control resting follicle activation remains unknown, this process may be envisioned as a multiphased process, tightly regulated by biological molecules acting, either directly or indirectly, at different follicular levels. However, further investigation is needed to elucidate certain issues such as: why a given resting follicle is activated whereas others, located in the same area, remain at the resting stage? how many follicles leave the stock every day? Finally, elucidation of the regulatory mechanisms involved in initiation of follicular growth might provide potential therapeutic targets to manipulate the ovarian reserve. A delay in resting follicle activation leading to a maintenance of the ovarian reserve could delay the onset of menopause and extend the reproductive lifespan of a female. In addition, the ability to inhibit initiation of follicular growth would provide a treatment for premature ovarian failure, while the stimulation of resting follicle activation by various molecules might treat certain forms of female infertility.

Early follicular growth

When follicles start to grow, they enlarge, both by proliferation of GCs and by increase in size of the oocyte. A zona pellucida begins to be laid down around the oocyte shortly after activation of resting follicles. Progressively (Figure 5.2), follicles become secondary (two complete layers of GCs), and some stroma cells near the basal lamina become aligned parallel to each other. As the follicle enlarges, the surrounding connective tissue stratifies and differentiates into two parts. The outer part, the theca externa, is composed of cells similar to those of the undifferentiated theca. In the inner part, the theca interna (TI), some fibroblast-like precursor cells change into polyhedral cells also referred to as epithelioid cells [1]. During the late preantral stage, multiple foci of fluid accumulate, possibly in the spaces left by degenerated GCs, and as these expand and coalesce, a larger centrally located antrum develops. Identification of factors promoting the appearance of the antrum is very complex since they can be confused with factors stimulating follicle growth. However, it would appear that synthesis of osmotically active molecules, such as versican, can be regulated by FSH and steroid hormones [29]. Thus, at the beginning of the follicle growth, the oocyte enlarges, GCs proliferate, and TICs differentiate, then proliferate. These various facets of early follicle development occur at the same time; they are mainly regulated by inter- and intrafollicular signaling molecules that mediate a dialog between the different follicular compartments. However, at various times during

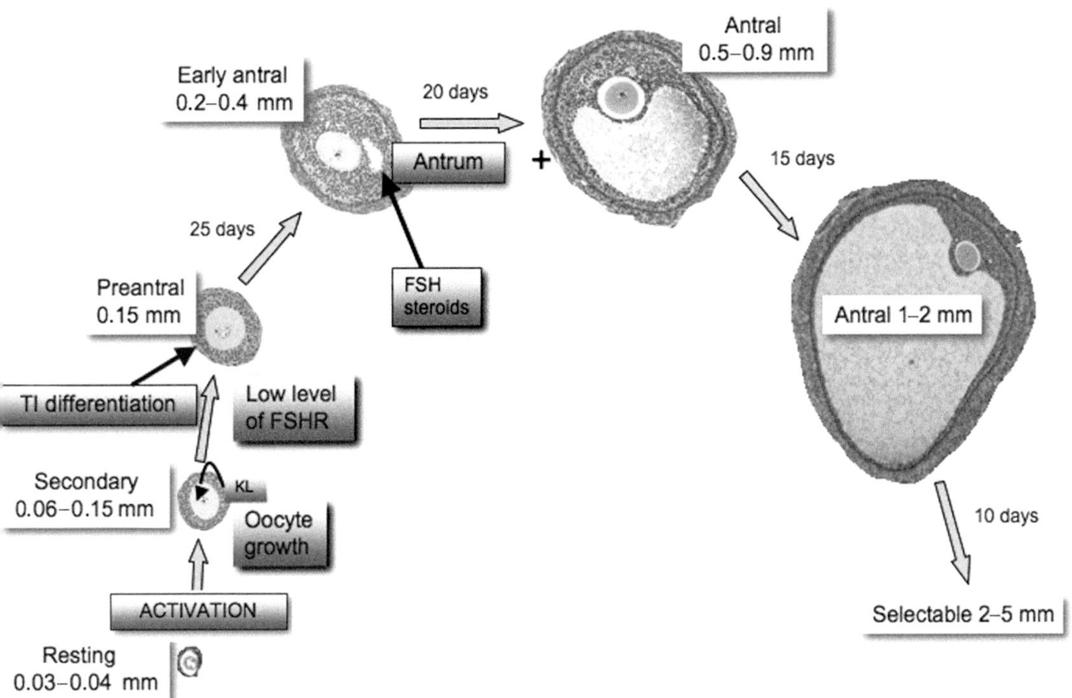

Figure 5.2 The different steps of early follicle growth in the human ovary.

growth, some follicles undergo atresia, then degenerate. Atresia of primary and secondary follicles is very low in humans (see [1]), but the percentages of atretic follicles increase at preantral and early antral stages, to peak at 30% and 32%, respectively. These percentages decrease to 15–16% in antral follicles smaller than 2 mm (see [1]), but strongly increase for FSH-responsive follicles (75–100% during the midluteal phase of the menstrual cycle). The low level of atresia in early growing follicles could be due to the lack of a Ca/Mg-sensitive endonuclease [30] that appears when GCs become fully responsive to FSH, that is, in follicles larger than 2 mm. This also could explain why in atretic small growing follicles, the oocyte degenerates while the incidence of GC apoptosis is still low [1].

Oocyte growth

It is during early follicular development that the oocyte grows at the quickest rate. In humans its diameter increases from approximately 40 μm in primary follicles to around 100 μm in early antral follicles. Beyond this stage, the increase in size of the oocyte is much slower since its diameter will reach approximately 140 μm in preovulatory follicles. Large primary and early secondary oocytes start to secrete factors, such as GDF9 and BMP15. These molecules will play a crucial role during folliculogenesis; firstly during oocyte growth since the latter is regulated by an ultra-short loop between KL and GDF9 [31], leading to the coordinated development of the oocyte and somatic follicular cells. Oocytes are coupled to neighbor GCs by gap junctions that allow bidirectional communications essential for the development and function of both follicular compartments [32].

Granulosa cell proliferation and differentiation

In the mouse, GCs are probably derived from the intraovarian rete and from approximately five precursor cells (see [33]). Throughout its development, the follicle is constructed by the non-random, radial proliferation of GC clones, which form long, thin, unbranched columns across the follicle wall, cumulus and mural GCs having a common origin [33]. Whether GCs derived from the different clones are in similar numbers remains unknown. However, it cannot be excluded that follicles of similar size may exhibit different proportions of GCs derived from individual clones and, consequently, may display differences in their developmental potentialities and capacities for synthesizing molecules that affect their own growth and differentiation [1].

What role does FSH play during early follicular growth?

When the early growing follicles become vascularized, they are directly exposed to factors circulating in the blood, especially gonadotropins. FSH is the primary pituitary regulator of ovarian folliculogenesis. However, similarly to the situation observed for activation of resting follicles, the role of FSH in sustaining early follicular growth remains unclear despite it being widely accepted that early folliculogenesis is FSH independent. Nevertheless, very little is known about the stage of follicular development at which GCs become responsive to FSH.

In vitro and in serum-free conditions, treatment of preantral follicles with FSH alone neither induces growth nor prevents apoptosis despite these follicles possessing FSHR on their GCs. In addition, FSH alone is unable to increase expression of its own receptor in rat GCs cultured without serum (reviewed in [4]). In humans, FSHR are present on GCs in only 33% of primary and small secondary follicles, and follicles smaller than 2 mm do not display any change of their GC proliferation in response to cyclic changes of FSH. In various pathological (hypogonadotropic hypogonadism, hypophysectomy) situations, selectable follicles were observed despite extremely low levels of gonadotropins, and in patients bearing an inactivating mutation of the FSHR gene, follicles can grow up to a size of several millimeters but cannot reach the ovulatory size. Taken together, these observations indicate that in the presence of very low levels of FSH activity, folliculogenesis can take place until the selectable stage (≥2 mm) even though some pieces of evidence indicate that folliculogenesis is quantitatively altered (reviewed in [4]). A possible explanation for these situations might be that factors, either present in the serum or locally produced by the ovary, sustain follicle growth when FSH is absent. Indeed, in laboratory rodents, many local factors such as activin A, EGF, TGFβ, FGF2, KGF, HGF, GDF9, and BMP15, all being produced by follicular tissues and oocytes, have been shown to stimulate GC proliferation in the absence of FSH (Figure 5.3) (reviewed in [4]).

However, many experiments show that FSH can stimulate early growing follicles in vivo. Transplantation of neonatal rat ovaries into recipient females either hypophysectomized or ovariectomized, shows that FSH sustains preantral follicle development in transplanted ovaries. In hypophysectomized rats and mice, hypogonadal mice, and gonadotropin-releasing hormone (GnRH) antagonist-treated juvenile rats, healthy preantral follicles are present but either in lower number than in controls or with structural abnormalities. In these situations, early follicular growth is not abolished but impaired and, in all these cases, exogenous FSH restores the normal aspect of early growing follicles and increases their number (reviewed in [4]). The positive effects of FSH on early follicular growth in vivo, despite the absence of effect of FSH alone on follicle proliferation in vitro, might be that FSH acts in synergy with locally produced factors (Figure 5.3).

Growth of preantral follicles isolated from immature rats is enhanced by both KGF and GDF9 acting in synergy with FSH. In adult hamsters, both EGF and TGFβ2 synergize with FSH to stimulate GC proliferation from preantral follicles. Although activin A alone can induce FSHR in cultured rat GCs in the absence of FSH, this effect is enhanced by FSH. Finally, TGFβ1 can induce the FSH responsiveness of preantral follicles from 11-day-old juvenile mice, although neither FSH nor TGFβ1 alone has a significant effect when administered separately (reviewed in [4]). Estrogens synergize with FSH to stimulate follicular growth in rodents and studies with αERKO, βERKO, and ArKO mice have shown that estrogens are primordial for early follicle development in the mouse [34]. In humans, early growing follicles acquire AR before FSHR [18]. Androgens sustain early follicular development in monkeys [24], an effect that can be due to their ability to increase FSHR mRNA in all follicle stages [35]. Additionally, FSH-treated monkeys show a marked induction in AR mRNA expression in primary follicles but not larger follicles, suggesting a potential physiological mechanism whereby FSH may promote early follicular development [35]. Studies in AR-null mice have shown that KL is a direct downstream target of androgen signaling, leading to a down-regulation of BMP15, GDF9, and HGF gene expression when AR are absent and to a strongly impaired folliculogenesis [36]. FSH might also stimulate ovarian production of factors known to support early folliculogenesis. TGFβ-RI and stimulatory

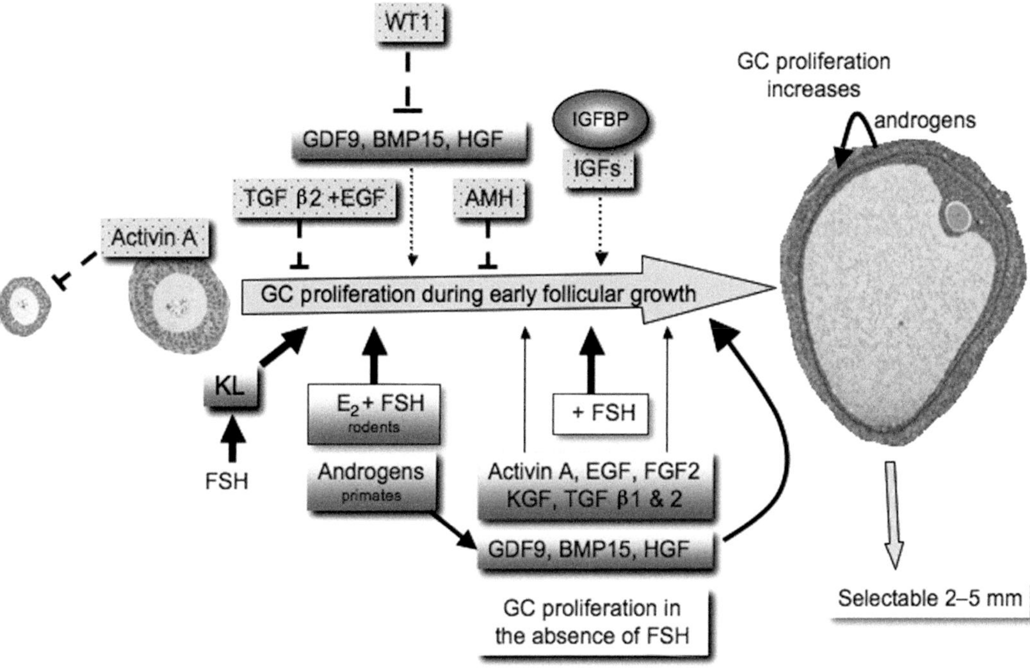

Figure 5.3 Factors acting on GC proliferation during early follicular growth. Some factors, acting alone or in synergy with FSH, stimulate follicular development (under the arrow), whereas others inhibit, at least partly, GC proliferation (above the arrow).

SMADS as well as several of the key ligands, including BMP15, GDF9, TGFβ2, and inhibin, are regulated in part by FSH [37, 38]. In addition, FSH may indirectly stimulate follicular growth via KL production by GCs, since in cattle, GC-derived KL stimulates theca-derived KGF and HGF, which in turn stimulate GC proliferation [14].

Taken together, these observations indicate that in conditions of FSH deprivation, the development of early growing follicles can be sustained by local signaling molecules; however, it appears likely that these factors are less efficient at sustaining growth than they are when they act in synergy with FSH.

Follicles grow at a slow, but increasingly faster rate during basal follicular growth

Recent reports have confirmed that early follicular growth is a very long process in humans (Figure 5.2). Approximately 30 days are required for a preantral follicle to reach a size of around 715 μm [39], a time very close to the calculated 35 days required by a follicle to pass through the classes 2 and 3 [1]. Follicles around 3 mm in diameter are observed 6 months after transplantation of frozen human cortex (96% primordial and 4% primary follicles) under the kidney capsule of ovariectomized immunodeficient mice [13]. In patients submitted to chemotherapy for cancer pathology, grafting of frozen ovarian cortex is followed within 3.5 to 6.5 months by appearance of a preovulatory follicle [40]. So, despite the positive role played by FSH and local factors on their development, early developing follicles grow slowly, but at an increasing rate during the late steps before the selectable stage [1]. Consequently, it is possible that during early folliculogenesis, inhibitory factors, produced by either the follicle itself or neighbor follicles, may partly counteract FSH- and local factor-induced GC proliferation (Figure 5.3).

Although both EGF and TGFβ2 are mitogenic for GCs when each of them acts in the presence of FSH, TGFβ2 can inhibit GC proliferation in the same cell type when EGF is present. Similarly, in rat GCs, TGFα suppresses the TGFβ-induced increase of FSHR, and activin A, produced by large preantral/early antral follicles, and maintains secondary follicles (100–120 μm) at a quiescent stage (reviewed in [4]). Additionally, WT1, a zinc-finger transcription factor that is highly expressed in preantral follicles over a range of species, may delay follicle growth by repressing

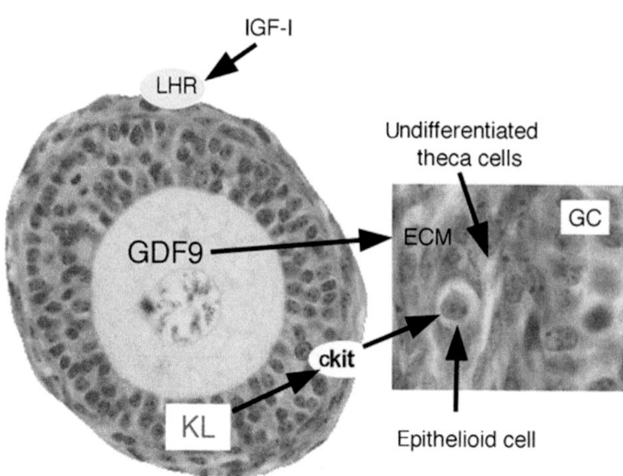

Figure 5.4 Factors involved in transformation of undifferentiated stromal theca cells into epithelioid theca interna cells.

the transcriptional activity of genes encoding FSHR and local factors, including TGFβ, PDGF, insulin-like growth factor-II (IGF-II), or their receptors [41]. In rats, AMH inhibits follicle growth by repressing synthesis of factors involved in GC proliferation such as GDF9, BMP15, activin receptor 1, and KL as well as the TGFβ signaling pathway [7]. However, in humans, mRNA for AMHRII is rarely expressed in small follicles since only 2 of 52 preantral follicles were AMHR mRNA positive [18]. This challenges the hypothesis that AMH exerts an inhibitory effect on follicles at this stage; the increasing levels of androgens produced by TICs might then explain why follicles grow faster when their size increases.

Granulosa cells are undifferentiated during basal follicular growth

Another characteristic of early growing follicles is that their GCs are undifferentiated, that is, they express neither steroidogenic enzymes nor luteinizing hormone receptor (LHR) (reviewed in [4]). In GCs, the transcription factor FOXO1 acts as a potent negative regulator of genes involved in cholesterol synthesis [42]. Whereas some local factors promote GC proliferation, they also inhibit their FSH-induced differentiation. EGF and FGF2 in the rat, and GDF9 and BMP15 in the mouse, inhibit *Fshr* mRNA expression and subsequent GC differentiation during early follicular growth. In the rat, HGF and KGF as well as BMP2 and BMP4 inhibit basal or hormone-stimulated aromatase activity and progesterone production by GCs (reviewed in [4]). In a number of mammalian species, IGF-I receptors (IGF-IR) are present on GCs in early growing follicles. Consequently, both IGF-I (rodents, porcine) and IGF-II (humans), may act on preantral follicles to stimulate both proliferation and differentiation (reviewed in [43]). Nevertheless, IGF-binding proteins (IGFBP)-2 and -5 are highly expressed in rat primary and secondary follicles [43]. Since IGFBPs are known to inhibit IGFs' action on follicular cells by decreasing their bioavailability, it can be hypothesized that in early growing follicles, the high expression of IGFBPs could be partly responsible for the slow growth rate of these follicles and their poor GC differentiation.

Taken together, these data show that early growing follicles are under the control of factors that are not only able to slow their growth, but are also able to inhibit the gonadotropin-induced differentiation of their GCs.

Theca cell proliferation and differentiation

In humans, early antral follicles exhibit a slight steroidogenic activity, as illustrated by a low expression of P450c17 in theca interna cells (TICs) [28], which are the primary site of androstenedione synthesis and bind luteinizing hormone (LH) at all stages from the preantral stage (see [1]). The origin of TICs is still obscure, and many questions about the mechanism leading to their differentiation remain to be answered. LH has been considered to be the primary hormone regulating the differentiation of TICs. IGF-I, by stimulating the initial expression of LHR during the early stages of thecal differentiation, may be acting as a differentiation factor for TICs (Figure 5.4). However, other factors are also involved in differentiation of TICs (Figure 5.4). GDF9 may play a key role in the theca genesis, since in GDF9-deficient mice there is no layer of undifferentiated theca cells around follicles [44] and no extracellular matrix on which theca cells can attach [45]. TICs express cKit and therefore may respond to GC-derived KL, which is the only known GC-derived growth factor that can stimulate both androstenedione production by TICs and their proliferation in the absence of gonadotropins. Consequently, KL as well as EGF/TGFα have been postulated to act as "granulosa-derived theca cell organizers" by attracting stroma cells around the follicle then stimulating their proliferation and their differentiation [4, 46].

Summary and conclusions

In summary, the present review confirms that both activation of resting follicles and early follicle growth are regulated by local factors produced by the different ovarian cell types and acting through multiple signal transduction pathways. Although studies in transgenic mice have shown that both processes can occur in the absence of FSH, it appears that most of the involved factors are more efficient when they act in synergy with FSH. More importantly, available data show that oocyte-produced factors, such as GDF9 and BMP15, play a crucial role during early follicular development by allowing a synchronous growth between the oocyte and GCs, and by stimulating GC proliferation either in the absence of or in synergy with FSH. Moreover, GDF9 and BMP15 are targets for signaling pathways of both androgen and AMH, while GDF9 is a key factor for TIC differentiation. So, according to Eppig *et al.* [32], the oocyte plays a central role in the orchestration and coordination of the early stages of follicular development.

The present review also shows why the mechanisms governing the key steps of folliculogenesis are so difficult to elucidate. Mixture of arrested and developing follicles, multiplicity of factors acting through different signaling pathways, and developmental changes of the follicular receptivity to such or such hormone or local factor constitute significant obstacles for a better understanding of folliculogenesis. Regarding this last issue, gene bionetwork analysis and microRNAs constitute very promising tools to identify novel factors and cellular processes involved in the various steps of ovarian follicular development [8]. Finally, new insights into knowledge of resting follicle activation and early follicular growth might provide new opportunities for reproductive medicine, including manipulation of the rate at which the ovarian reserve depletes and major improvement of follicular culture allowing a resting follicle to reach the development stage when its oocyte becomes fertilizable.

References

1. Gougeon A. Regulation of ovarian follicular development in primates: facts and hypotheses. *Endocr Rev* 1996; **17**: 121–55.
2. Wallace WH, Kelsey TW. Human ovarian reserve from conception to the menopause. *PLoS One* 2010; **5**: e8772.
3. White YA, Woods DC, Takai Y, *et al.* Oocyte formation by mitotically active germ cells purified from ovaries of reproductive-age women. *Nature Med* 2012; **18**: 413–21.
4. Gougeon A. The early stages of follicular growth. In: Trounson AO, Gosden RG, eds. *Biology and Pathology of the Oocyte: Role in Fertility and Reproductive Medicine.* Cambridge: Cambridge University Press, 2003; 29–43.
5. Adhikari D, Liu K. Molecular mechanisms underlying the activation of mammalian primordial follicles. *Endocr Rev* 2009; **30**: 438–64.
6. Da Silva-Buttkus P, Marcelli G, Franks S, *et al.* Inferring biological mechanisms from spatial analysis: prediction of a local inhibitor in the ovary. *Proc Natl Acad Sci USA* 2009; **106**: 456–61.
7. Nilsson E, Rogers N, Skinner MK. Actions of anti-Mullerian hormone on the ovarian transcriptome to inhibit primordial to primary follicle transition. *Reproduction* 2007; **134**: 209–21.
8. Nilsson EE, Savenkova MI, Schindler R, *et al.* Gene bionetwork analysis of ovarian primordial follicle development. *PLoS One* 2010; **5**: e11637.
9. Garor R, Abir R, Erman A, *et al.* Effects of basic fibroblast growth factor on in vitro development of human ovarian primordial follicles. *Fertil Steril* 2009; **91**(Suppl): 1967–75.
10. Kezele PR, Nilsson EE, Skinner MK. Insulin but not insulin-like growth factor-1 promotes the primordial to primary follicle transition. *Mol Cell Endocrinol* 2002; **192**: 37–43.
11. Nilsson E, Dole G, Skinner MK. Neurotrophin NT3 promotes ovarian primordial to primary follicle transition. *Reproduction* 2009; **138**: 697–707.
12. Ojeda SR, Romero C, Tapia V, *et al.* Neurotrophic and cell-cell dependent control of early follicular development. *Mol Cell Endocrinol* 2000; **163**: 67–71.

13. Li J, Kawamura K, Cheng Y, *et al.* Activation of dormant ovarian follicles to generate mature eggs. *Proc Natl Acad Sci USA* 2010; **107**: 10280–4.

14. Parrott JA, Skinner MK. Developmental and hormonal regulation of keratinocyte growth factor expression and action in the ovarian follicle. *Endocrinology* 1998; **139**: 228–35.

15. Durlinger AL, Gruijters MJ, Kramer P, *et al.* Anti-Mullerian hormone inhibits initiation of primordial follicle growth in the mouse ovary. *Endocrinology* 2002; **143**: 1076–84.

16. Carlsson IB, Scott JE, Visser JA, *et al.* Anti-Müllerian hormone inhibits initiation of growth of human primordial ovarian follicles in vitro. *Hum Reprod* 2006; **21**: 2223–7.

17. Schmidt KL, Kryger-Baggesen N, Byskov AG, *et al.* Anti-Müllerian hormone initiates growth of human primordial follicles in vitro. *Mol Cell Endocrinol* 2005; **234**: 87–93.

18. Rice S, Ojha K, Whitehead S, *et al.* Stage-specific expression of androgen receptor, follicle-stimulating hormone receptor, and anti-Müllerian hormone type II receptor in single, isolated, human preantral follicles: relevance to polycystic ovaries. *J Clin Endocrinol Metab* 2007; **92**:1034–40.

19. Gougeon A, Busso D. Morphologic and functional determinants of primordial and primary follicles in the monkey ovary. *Mol Cell Endocrinol* 2000; **163**: 33–41.

20. Oktay K, Karlikaya G, Akman O, *et al.* Interaction of extracellular matrix and activin-A in the initiation of follicle growth in the mouse ovary. *Biol Reprod* 2000; **63**: 457–61.

21. Nilsson EE, Skinner MK. Growth and differentiation factor-9 stimulates progression of early primary but not primordial rat ovarian follicle development. *Biol Reprod* 2002; **67**: 1018–24.

22. Martins FS, Celestino JJ, Saraiva MV, *et al.* Growth and differentiation factor-9 stimulates activation of goat primordial follicles in vitro and their progression to secondary follicles. *Reprod Fertil Dev* 2008; **20**: 916–24.

23. Hreinsson JG, Scott JE, Rasmussen C, *et al.* Growth differentiation factor-9 promotes the growth, development, and survival of human ovarian follicles in organ culture. *J Clin Endocrinol Metab* 2002; **87**: 316–21.

24. Vendola KA, Zhou J, Adesanya OO, *et al.* Androgens stimulate early stages of follicular growth in the primate ovary. *J Clin Invest* 1998; **101**: 2622–9.

25. Gougeon A, Delangle A, Arouche N, *et al.* Kit ligand and the somatostatin receptor antagonist, BIM-23627, stimulate in vitro resting follicle growth in the neonatal mouse ovary. *Endocrinology* 2010; **151**: 1299–309.

26. Schmidt D, Ovitt CE, Anlag K, *et al.* The murine winged-helix transcription factor FOXL2 is required for granulosa cell differentiation and ovary maintenance. *Development* 2004; **131**: 933–42.

27. Méduri G, Bachelot A, Duflos C, *et al.* FOXL2 mutations lead to different ovarian phenotypes in BPES patients: Case report. *Hum Reprod* 2010; **25**: 235–43.

28. Gougeon A. Human ovarian follicular development: from activation of resting follicles to preovulatory maturation. *Ann Endocrinol* 2010; **71**: 132–43.

29. Rodgers RJ, Irving-Rodgers HF. Formation of the ovarian follicular antrum and follicular fluid. *Biol Reprod* 2010; **82**: 1021–9.

30. Zeleznik AJ, Ihrig LL, Basseti SG. Developmental expression of Ca^{++}/Mg^{++}-dependent endonuclease activity in rat granulosa and luteal cells. *Endocrinology* 1989; **125**: 2218–20.

31. Elvin JA, Yan C, Matzuk MM. Oocyte-expressed TGF-beta superfamily members in female fertility. *Mol Cell Endocrinol* 2000; **159**: 1–5.

32. Eppig JJ, Wigglesworth K, Pendola FL. The mammalian oocyte orchestrates the rate of ovarian follicular development. *Proc Natl Acad Sci USA* 2002; **99**: 2890–4.

33. Boland NI, Gosden RG. Clonal analysis of chimaeric mouse ovaries using DNA in situ hybridization. *J Reprod Fert* 1994; **100**: 203–10.

34. Britt KL, Findlay JK. Estrogen actions in the ovary revisited. *J Endocrinol* 2002; **175**: 269–76.

35. Weil S, Vendola K, Zhou J, *et al.* Androgen and follicle-stimulating hormone interactions in primate ovarian follicle development. *J Clin Endocrinol Metab* 1999; **84**: 2951–6.

36. Shiina H, Matsumoto T, Sato T, *et al.* Premature ovarian failure in androgen receptor-deficient mice. *Proc Natl Acad Sci USA* 2006; **103**: 224–9.

37. Guéripel X, Brun V, Gougeon A. Oocyte bone morphogenetic protein 15, but not growth differentiation factor 9, is increased during gonadotropin-induced follicular development in the immature mouse and is associated with cumulus oophorus expansion. *Biol Reprod* 2006; **75**: 836–43.

38. Kobayashi N, Orisaka M, Cao M, *et al.* Growth differentiation factor-9 mediates follicle stimulating hormone-thyroid hormone interaction in the regulation of rat preantral follicular development. *Endocrinology* 2009; **150**: 5566–74.

39. Xu M, Barrett SL, West-Farrell E, *et al.* In vitro grown human ovarian follicles from cancer patients

support oocyte growth. *Hum Reprod* 2009; **24**: 2531–40.

40. Donnez J, Silber S, Andersen CY, *et al.* Children born after autotransplantation of cryopreserved ovarian tissue. a review of 13 live births. *Ann Med* 2011; **43**: 437–50.

41. Chun SY, McGee EA, Hsu SY, *et al.* Restricted expression of wt1 messenger ribonucleic acid in immature ovarian follicles: uniformity in mammalian and avian species and maintenance during reproductive senescence. *Biol Reprod* 1999; **60**: 365–73.

42. Richards JS, Pangas SA. The ovary: basic biology and clinical implications. *J Clin Invest* 2010; **120**: 963–72.

43. Monget P, Bondy C. Importance of the IGF system in early folliculogenesis. *Mol Cell Endocrinol* 2000; **163**: 89–93.

44. Dong J, Albertini DF, Nishimori K, *et al.* Growth differentiation factor-9 is required during ovarian early folliculogenesis. *Nature* 1996; **383**: 531–5.

45. Burns KH, Owens GE, Fernandez JM, *et al.* Characterization of integrin expression in the mouse ovary. *Biol Reprod* 2002; **67**: 743–51.

46. Parrott JA, Skinner MK. Kit ligand actions on ovarian stromal cells: effects on theca cell recruitment and steroid production. *Mol Reprod Dev* 2000; **55**: 55–64.

Chapter 6

Follicle and oocyte developmental dynamics

Aaron J. W. Hsueh and Kazuhiro Kawamura

Introduction

Mammalian follicle development starts during fetal (for human) or neonatal (for rodents) stages when primordial follicles are formed. Throughout reproductive life, most of this large but finite pool of ovarian primordial follicles remains dormant and only a small fraction of them initiates growth (Figure 6.1, initial recruitment) by uncharacterized intraovarian mechanisms [1]. Human follicles begin development during the fourth month of fetal life, and each human ovary contains ≈400 000 follicles at birth. Unknown intraovarian mechanisms activate a small number of dormant primordial follicles at a rate of ≈1000 per month to initiate growth, and follicle depletion occurs at menopause when <1000 follicles remain [2]. For follicles not activated, the default pathway is to remain dormant for years or decades. The onset of menopause is associated with the near depletion of ovarian follicles. Although the menarche time for modern girls has advanced due to improved health and other environmental factors, the menopause time for women has remained constant at ~51 years of age.

Once started to grow, the activated primordial follicles with a single layer of flattened granulosa cells surrounding the primordial oocytes develop into primary follicles, secondary follicles, and then antral follicles. During follicle growth, multiple layers of granulosa cells are formed and the oocytes are enlarged in size. Throughout the reproductive life, primordial follicles undergo initial recruitment to enter the growing pool of primary follicles (Figure 6.1, initial recruitment). In the human ovary, more than 120 days are required for the primary follicles to reach the secondary follicle stage, whereas approximately 70 days are needed to grow from the secondary to the early antral stage [3].

Once initiated to enter the growing pool, ovarian follicles progress to reach the antral stage and minimal follicle loss is found until the early antral stage. Although multiple early antral follicles are present during each reproductive cycle, exposure to increasing levels of pituitary follicle-stimulating hormone (FSH) leads to the selection of a single (for human) or limited number of (for rodents) large preovulatory follicles (Figure 6.1, cyclic recruitment) destined for ovulation for each cycle. Follicles exposed to insufficient circulating FSH undergo atresia mediated by the apoptosis of granulosa cells [4]. Once selected, follicles develop an antral cavity filled with follicle fluid. Inside the antrum, an oocyte is surrounded by cumulus cells which are connected through gap junctions to mural granulosa cells. Due to an oocyte-secreted morphogenic gradient of growth factors, granulosa cells in the tertiary or preovulatory follicle differentiate into four distinct subtypes: corona radiate, which surrounds the zona pellucida of the oocyte, membrana granulosa, which is interior to the basal lamina, periantral granulosa cells, which are adjacent to the antrum, and cumulus oophorus, which connects the membrana and corona radiata granulosa cells together.

During each menstrual cycle, a mid-cycle surge of serum luteinizing hormone (LH) is released by the anterior pituitary to induce the rupture of the preovulatory follicle, to initiate the final meiotic maturation of the preovulatory oocyte, and to start the luteinization of granulosa and thecal cells of the preovulatory follicle for the formation of the corpus luteum, which is essential for progesterone biosynthesis and successful pregnancy. During cyclic recruitment (Figure 6.1), increases in circulating FSH allow a cohort of antral follicles to escape apoptotic demise [5]. Among this cohort, a leading follicle emerges as dominant

Biology and Pathology of the Oocyte, 2nd edn., ed. Alan Trounson, Roger Gosden, and Ursula Eichenlaub-Ritter. Published by Cambridge University Press.

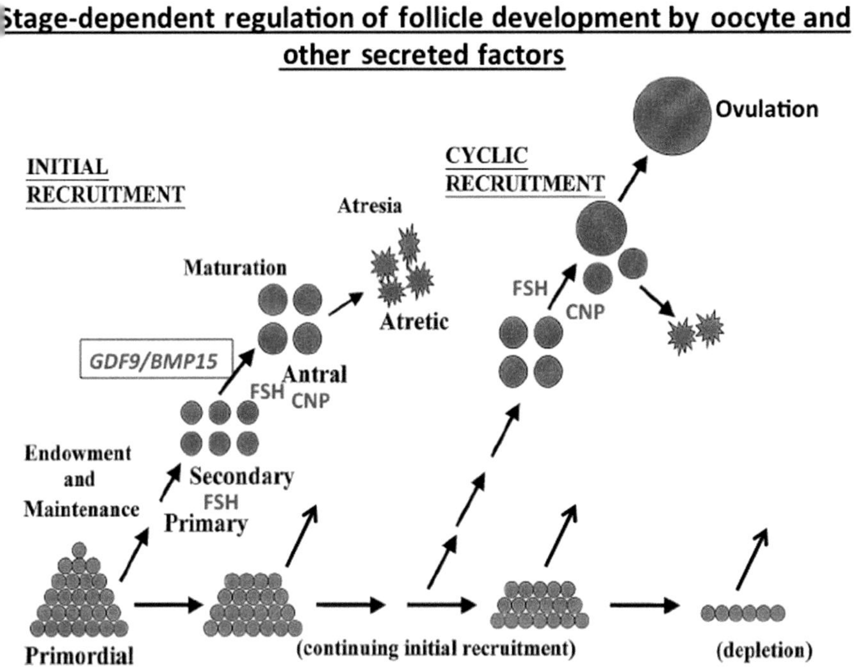

Figure 6.1 Stage-dependent regulation of follicle development by oocyte and other secreted hormonal factors. Ovarian follicles develop through primordial, primary, secondary, and antral stages before reaching the preovulatory follicles capable of releasing the mature oocyte. Although FSH is the major hormone regulating follicle development, several oocyte factors (GDF9, BMP15, and others) are important for the intraovarian regulation of follicle development. In addition, recent studies indicated that CNP produced by follicular somatic cells also promotes follicle development at different stages. BMP15, bone morphogenetic protein 15; CNP, C-type natriuretic peptide; FSH, follicle-stimulating hormone; GDF9, growth differentiation factor 9.

by secreting high levels of estrogens and inhibins to suppress pituitary FSH release. The result is a negative selection of the remaining cohort, leading to its ultimate demise [5]. Concomitantly, increases in local growth factors and vasculature allow a positive selection of the dominant follicle, thus ensuring its final growth and eventual ovulation and luteinization. After cyclic recruitment, it takes only 2 weeks for an antral follicle to become a dominant Graafian follicle in women. However, the overall development of human follicles from primordial to preovulatory stages requires more than 6 months.

In rodents, the duration of follicle development is much shorter than that needed for human follicles. The time required between the initial recruitment of a primordial follicle and its growth to the secondary stage is more than 30 days, whereas the time for a secondary follicle to reach the early antral stage is about 28 days [1]. Once reaching the early antral stage, these follicles are subjected to cyclic recruitment, and only 2–3 days are needed for them to grow into preovulatory follicles. For the first wave of follicle development in rodents, primordial and some primary follicles are formed soon after birth. After the breakdown of ovarian nests and the organization of oocytes and somatic cells into primordial follicles, newly formed follicles undergo a second differentiation process, in which the flattened pregranulosa cells surrounding each oocyte acquire a cuboidal morphology. The resulting primary follicles begin to grow via proliferation of these granulosa cells. These follicles progress to the early antral stage during the third week of life, when serum gonadotropin levels are elevated. After early antral follicles are formed, most of them undergo atresia whereas few of them are recruited into preovulatory follicles following cyclic changes in gonadotropins during each estrous cycle. The first wave of follicle development is accelerated by elevated gonadotropins in juvenile rodents. Around day 35 of age, cyclic ovarian function begins. The neonatal rodent model allows analysis of early follicle development in a synchronized population of growing follicles.

Although the "non-renewable follicle pool" concept is accepted by most ovarian researchers [6],

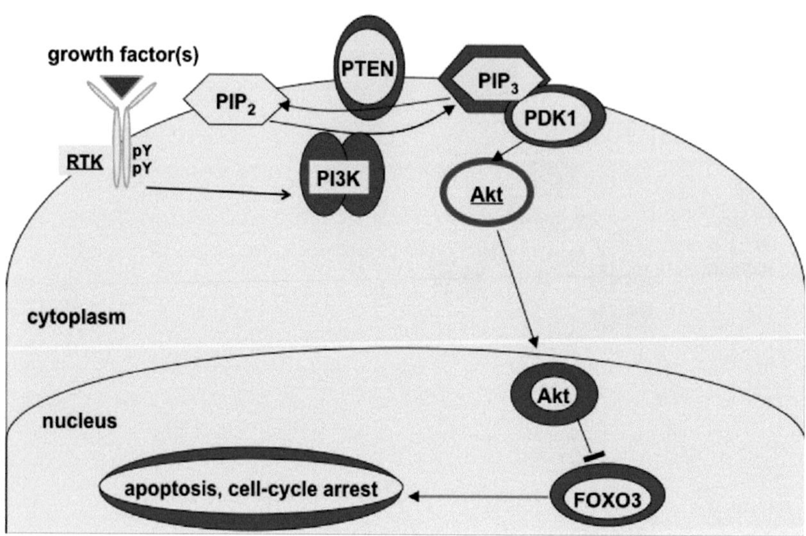

Figure 6.2 Oocyte genes important for the activation of dormant primordial follicles. The majority of ovarian follicles are arrested at the primordial stage for years in rodents and decades in women. The PTEN–PI3K–Akt–Foxo3 pathway in the oocyte is important in the regulation of the initiation of primordial follicle growth. Oocyte-specific deletion of the PTEN gene increased PIP_3 levels and activated the Akt enzyme, leading to the suppression of Foxo3 activity and follicle growth. Likewise, oocyte-specific deletion of the Foxo3 gene also promoted the development of primordial follicles.

several studies suggested postnatal derivation of new follicles from female germ stem cells of ovarian [7] and bone marrow origins [8]. However, these studies have been challenged based on elegant transplantation-parabiotic [9] and transgenic follicle tracing [10] studies.

Oocyte regulation of follicular dormancy

Although a large number of primordial follicles are formed early in life, only a limited number of these follicles initiate growth during a given time (Figure 6.1). Throughout reproductive life, the primordial follicle is gradually depleted and the near exhaustion of the follicle reserve marks the start of menopause or reproductive senescence. The mechanisms that regulate the gradual exit of ovarian follicles from the non-growing, primordial pool are poorly understood. Whether an individual follicle remains dormant or initiates growth likely depends on the balance of stimulatory and inhibitory factors. Blandau and colleagues performed organ culture of fetal mouse ovaries for 2–3 weeks and found increases in oocyte growth in some follicles [11]. Subsequent cultures of whole rodent ovaries from neonatal animals indicated that a small number of follicles leave the resting pool and begin to grow [12]. As in rodent ovaries, only a fraction of human primordial follicles initiate growth in culture [13]. Using in vitro cultures, mutant animals, specific inhibitors, and passive immuno-neutralization approaches, a number of factors have been found to be important for primordial follicle growth. These include Kit ligand [14, 15], platelet-derived growth factor (PDGF) [16], neurotrophins [17], vascular endothelial growth factor [18], bone morphogenetic protein (BMP)-4 [19], BMP-7 [20], basic fibroblast growth factor (FGF), keratinocyte growth factor [21], vascular endothelial growth factor (VEGF), and others. Although the exact intraovarian factor(s) underlying the initial recruitment of dormant primordial follicles to initiate growth is still unclear, many of the growth factors, including Kit ligand, PDGF, neurotrophins, and VEGF, found to activate the dormant primordial follicles in vitro are known to interact with receptors with tyrosine kinase activities. It is, thus, possible that diverse local paracrine hormones important for initial follicle recruitment could converge on the same intracellular signaling pathway downstream of receptors with tyrosine kinase activity (TrkR) (Figure 6.2).

Upon receptor activation by specific ligands, downstream phosphatidylinositol 3-kinase (PI3K) is activated, leading to the conversion of the lipid second messenger phosphatidylinositol-4, 5-bisphosphate (PIP_2) into phosphatidylinositol-3, 4, 5-triphosphate (PIP_3). PIP_3 then recruits and activates phosphatidylinositol-dependent kinase 1 (PDK1). PDK1, in turn, phosphorylates and activates PKB (protein kinase B, also known as Akt), which inhibits the activities of key forkhead (Foxo) transcription factors, resulting in cell proliferation and survival (Figure 6.2). Furthermore, other branches of the PI3K signaling pathway include SGK (serum- and glucocorticoid-induced kinase), TSC1/TSC2 (tuberous sclerosis complex 1 and 2), RHEB (Ras homolog enriched in brain), TOR (target of rapamycin), p70S6K (ribosomal protein, S6 kinase 70kD), and others.

In addition to the activation of Akt/PKB by PI3K, this important pathway is also regulated by an inhibitor. The tumor suppressor phosphatase with tensin homology (PTEN) protein negatively regulates PI3K signaling by dephosphorylating PIP_3, converting it back to PIP_2 (Figure 6.2). The *PTEN* gene is cloned as a candidate tumor suppressor gene from the chromosome 10q23 region, a locus frequently targeted for genetic loss in tumors. Studies using cKit ligand, which activate cKit (a TrkR), using mouse and rat oocytes demonstrated the stimulation of Akt/PKB activity and the suppression of a downstream transcriptional factor Foxo3 [22]. The important roles of the PI3K–PTEN–Akt–Foxo3 pathway were demonstrated by transgenic mouse studies. Deletion of the transcriptional factor Foxo3 in mice led to the activation of all dormant follicles during the neonatal stage, resulting in a premature ovarian failure phenotype during later life [23]. Subsequent studies using tissue-specific mutant mice indicated that oocyte-specific deletion of the *PTEN* gene promoted the growth of all primordial follicles in neonatal and adult animals [24]. Deletion of PTEN in the oocyte increases PKB/Akt phosphorylation and nuclear export of downstream Foxo3 proteins [25].

Earlier studies demonstrate that vanadate is a competitive reversible inhibitor for protein tyrosine phosphatases (PTPases). In particular, peroxovanadium (pV) compounds activate the insulin receptor kinase in hepatocytes and inhibit the dephosphorylation of insulin receptors in hepatic endosomes [26]. These vanadate derivatives, such as bisperoxovanadium (bpV), have been employed as PTPase inhibitors and insulin mimetics. Given that PTPases and PTEN share considerable homology in their active site, bpV compounds were found to inhibit the PI3K-phosphatase, PTEN [27]. These small-molecular-weight compounds, including bpV(pic), increased cellular PIP_3 levels, phosphorylation of Akt, and glucose uptake in adipocytes at nanomolar concentrations. We also checked for agents capable of activating PI3K through direct interactions. Binding of the SH2 domains of p85, the regulatory subunit of PI3K, to tyrosine auto-phosphorylation sites on activated TrkR receptors releases an autoinhibitory constraint that stimulates the catalytic domain (p110) of PI3K. Earlier studies designed a synthetic peptide (740Y) corresponding to a nine-amino-acid stretch of the PDGF receptor intracellular region fused to the protein transduction domain (16 aa) of a fly protein [28]. This cell-permeable peptide was phosphorylated at the key tyrosine residue to mimic the activated PDGF receptor and was shown to bind to the SH2 domain of p85 regulatory subunit of PI3K and activate enzyme activity.

We hypothesized that short-term treatment with PTEN inhibitors and PI3K activators could activate dormant follicles by synergistically stimulating the PKB/Akt signaling (Figure 6.2) in ovarian cells. Once activated, primordial follicles could grow into primary, secondary, and larger follicles through intrinsic follicular mechanisms. Our recent study indicated that treatment of neonatal mouse ovaries in vitro with a PTEN inhibitor and the PI3K-activating peptide activated dormant primordial follicles [29]. After in vitro activation, ovaries were transplanted into the kidney capsule of FSH-treated adult ovariectomized recipients to promote follicle growth. After transplantation, activated follicles reached the preovulatory stage in 2 weeks and mature oocytes were obtained for in vitro fertilization to generate blastocysts. These embryos were morphologically and epigenetically normal and developed to fetuses after embryo transfer to pseudopregnant mice. After normal term pregnancy, pups were delivered and grew to adults without abnormalities. These offspring were fertile and derived a normal second generation. Using human cortical fragments containing primordial follicles based on the same approach, human dormant follicles in ovarian cortical strips obtained from a 26-year-old patient with a benign ovarian tumor were also activated. After xenotransplantation into severe compromised immunodeficient (SCID) mice and treatment with FSH to stimulate activated follicle growth for 24 weeks, large numbers of mature oocytes were obtained after a single human chorionic gonadotropin (hCG) injection to induce oocyte maturation. These findings lay the foundation for future clinical applications to regulate follicle dynamics.

Oocyte factors regulate follicle development

Once reaching the primary stage, granulosa cells express FSH receptors and growth of these follicles can be facilitated by FSH (Figure 6.1). FSH receptors are found in neonatal ovaries, when primary and secondary follicles are present [30, 31]. This is followed closely by the formation of LH receptors in the thecal cells. In addition to the endocrine hormone FSH, GDF9 (growth differentiation factor 9) and BMP15 (bone morphogenetic factor-15) are local hormones produced by oocytes capable of modulating follicle development. Earlier studies using mutant mice demonstrated that GDF9 was an oocyte-derived paracrine factor important for growth of follicles beyond the primary stage [32]. GDF9 belongs to the transforming growth factor beta (TGFβ) superfamily having six or more cysteine residues which form a cysteine knot, characteristic for this family. Subsequent studies indicated that treatment with recombinant GDF9 enhanced growth and differentiation of early ovarian follicles in culture [33] and after in vivo treatment [34]. GDF9 was also found to be anti-apoptotic during follicular development by suppressing follicle atresia [35].

BMP15, also known as GDF9B, is a paralog gene for GDF9. Although both proteins belong to the TGFβ superfamily having six or more cysteine residues which form a cysteine knot, BMP15, similar to GDF9, lacks the cysteine residues for covalent dimer formation found in other members of this family. BMP15, like GDF9, is expressed in oocytes throughout folliculogenesis and is a potent stimulator of granulosa cell proliferation [36]. Similar to GDF9, a null mutation of BMP15 in sheep is associated with infertility [37]. However, there appear to be species differences in the role of BMP15, because BMP15-null mice only show a decrease in ovulation rate but not sterility [38]. Furthermore, natural mutations of BMP15 in sheep can cause both increased ovulation rate and infertility phenotypes in a dosage-sensitive manner. In the Inverdale (FecXI) sheep, a heterozygous mutant of BMP15 causes increased ovulation rate, and twin and triplet births, but primary ovarian failure in homozygotes [37, 39]. Individuals with mutations in both GDF9 and BMP15 have a greater ovulation rate than sheep with either of the mutations separately [40]. Although the exact cellular mechanism underlying the diametrically opposing actions of these oocyte factors in the regulation of fecundity is unclear, both oocyte factors are clearly involved in the control of proliferation and differentiation of somatic cells inside follicles. In addition to GDF9 and BMP15, BMP6 is also produced by the oocyte. However, the exact physiological role of this oocyte protein is still unclear [41].

Oocyte maturation arrest and re-initiation

During follicle growth, three populations of oocytes can be identified. In growing follicles before the antral stage, oocytes continue to grow and have not attained their full size. They are unable to resume maturation when released from follicles and cultured in vitro. For antral follicles, medium-sized oocytes arrested in metaphase I (MI) stage are present. Although these oocytes can resume maturation in vitro, they have not completed their maturation. For fully grown oocytes found in preovulatory follicles, they resume maturation in response to gonadotropins or when released from follicles and cultured in vitro. The meiotic progression is completed after oocytes reach metaphase II (MII) stage. This is the only stage when oocytes, in most mammals, can be successfully fertilized [42]. After oocytes begin to mature, their nuclei–germinal vesicles (GVs) break down and chromosomes condense (germinal vesicle breakdown, GVBD). Chromosomes are then arranged in MI stage which is followed by anaphase I to telophase I transition and oocytes are arrested in MII, ready for fertilization. Although oocytes acquire the ability to undergo meiotic maturation at the early antral follicle stage, meiotic progression is arrested until the preovulatory LH surge.

Depending on the animal species, meiotic arrest of oocytes starts from before or a short time after birth. The preovulatory surge of gonadotropins after puberty onset induces resumption of the meiotic division and the progression of the oocyte from the dictyate stage to the metaphase of the second meiotic division. Earlier studies have postulated the involvement of a follicular factor, oocyte maturation inhibitor (OMI), in meiotic arrest based on the following observations: (1) fully grown mammalian oocytes obtained from their follicles undergo meiotic maturation spontaneously, whereas follicle-enclosed ova remain immature until stimulated by LH; (2) co-culture of cumulus–oocyte complexes isolated from their follicles with follicular granulosa cells, granulosa cell extract, and follicular fluid inhibits the spontaneous maturation of oocytes; (3) the inhibition of oocyte maturation by OMI is reversible and can be removed by the addition of LH. Subsequent studies on OMI characterization and purification further suggested the involvement of a peptide of ~2000 dalton [43].

It took more than 20 years to demonstrate the chemical nature of this OMI. Natriuretic peptides comprise of atrial natriuretic peptide (ANP), brain natriuretic peptide (BNP), and C-type natriuretic peptide (CNP) encoded by the natriuretic peptide precursor type C (NPPC) gene. Unlike ANP and BNP, CNP does not have direct natriuretic activity and is a selective agonist for the B-type natriuretic receptor (NPRB, also known as NPR2). The precursor NPPC protein is cleaved to the 22-amino-acid peptide, CNP. A recent study indicated that mural granulosa cells of preovulatory follicles express NPPC mRNA whereas cumulus cells surrounding oocytes express mRNA of the NPPC receptor NPR2, a guanylate cyclase, in mice. Treatment with CNP increased cGMP levels in cumulus cells and oocytes and inhibited meiotic resumption of oocytes in vitro [44]. Meiotic arrest was not sustained in most Graafian follicles of NPPC or NPR2 mutant mice, and meiosis resumed precociously. The ligand CNP is secreted by granulosa cells and interacts with its receptor NPR2 in cumulus cells to prevent precocious meiotic maturation. This is critical for maturation and ovulation synchrony and for normal female fertility. These recent findings are consistent with the earlier identification of OMI in follicular fluid and granulosa cell extracts [43] as well as the identity of CNP as a small peptide hormone. Subsequent studies indicated that the ovulatory LH surge decreased CNP levels in murine ovaries and human follicular fluid [45] and further underscored the importance of decreasing CNP levels during the preovulatory period to allow the resumption of oocyte maturation for subsequent fertilization and early embryonic development.

In addition to the role of CNP as an OMI [44], our recent studies demonstrated the ability of CNP to promote preantral and antral follicle development [46]. The NPPC gene is expressed in somatic/granulosa cells of preantral and antral follicles and exogenous CNP is capable of promoting follicle growth by stimulating cGMP production mediated through the NPRB receptor. Furthermore, the paracrine hormone CNP, acting through the cGMP pathway, likely mediates some of the effects of the endocrine hormone FSH in the promotion of preantral follicle development, because FSH increased NPPC expression in cultured ovarian explants. In explants of juvenile ovaries, CNP treatment promoted the development of primary/early secondary follicles to the late secondary stage whereas treatment of cultured preantral follicles with CNP, like FSH, stimulated follicle growth. Similar to the known follicle-stimulating effects of FSH on preantral follicles in juvenile rats [47], in vivo CNP treatment of juvenile mice stimulated preantral follicle development to the early antral stage to allow subsequent stimulation by FSH and LH/hCG. Furthermore, CNP treatment of immature mice containing early antral follicles led to the formation of preovulatory follicles without the need for exogenous FSH. These follicles are capable of responding to the preovulatory LH/hCG stimulation, resulting in successful ovulation, fertilization, and pregnancy. These findings suggest that CNP can promote follicle development ranging from primary to antral stages and could substitute for FSH in the penultimate stage of follicle development to the preovulatory stage. These findings demonstrate that the regulation of oocyte maturation arrest and follicle growth is linked by the same intraovarian peptide CNP, underlying the importance of coordinated development of oocyte and somatic cells inside ovarian follicles (see Figure 6.3).

Meiotic errors in oocytes and aneuploidy

Aneuploidies, numerical chromosome errors, are common in human oocytes and embryos and are associated with increasing maternal age. Errors in chromosome segregation at first meiosis are the major cause for implantation failure, congenital abnormality, spontaneous abortion, and trisomy. Maternal age is the major etiological factor associated with chromosome non-disjunction at oocyte meiosis, possibly as a result of spindle aberrations [48]. Studies on male and female gametes have demonstrated that oogenesis is more error-prone compared with spermatogenesis and this

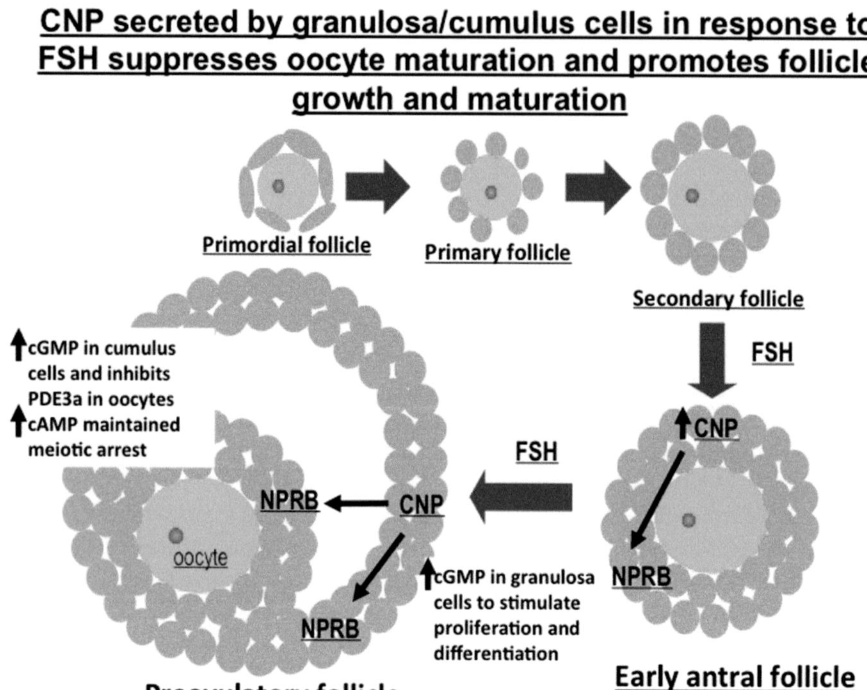

Figure 6.3 CNP as an intraovarian factor important for the suppression of oocyte maturation and for the stimulation of follicle growth and maturation. CNP is secreted by granulosa cells of secondary and early antral follicles in response to FSH stimulation. CNP acts through its receptor NPRB, expressed in granulosa cells, to increase cGMP production and to stimulate follicle development. In addition, CNP acts through its receptor NPRB, expressed in cumulus cells, to increase cGMP production. Cumulus cell cGMP, transported to the oocytes through the gap junctions, inhibits the activity of the PDE3 (phosphodiesterase 3) enzyme, leading to increased intra-oocyte cAMP levels, thus suppressing oocyte maturation. The preovulatory LH surge decreases CNP levels in the preovulatory follicles, thus allowing meiotic maturation of preovulatory oocytes.

is possibly a result of the prolonged arrest at the dictyotene stage in a process that begins during fetal life and becomes complete only after ovulation. During meiotic progression in oocytes, the first meiotic division involves homologous chromosome segregation rather than sister chromatids as in meiosis II.

Important information on oocyte aneuploidy has been provided by the preconceptional testing of polar bodies (PBs), in which fluorescence *in situ* hybridization (FISH) has confirmed that 70% of chromosomal abnormalities occur in meiosis I as reflected by an aneuploid first polar body (PB1). These findings supported the validity of proposing the analysis of PB1 to predict the chromosomal status of the oocyte, and to use the derived information as an additional tool for oocyte selection. Microtubules are the cytoskeletal components of meiotic spindles and are important for the alignment and segregation of chromosomes during meiosis and mitosis. Disruption and disorganization of spindles in oocytes are frequently manifested as a dispersal of chromosomes, resulting in chromosomal anomalies after fertilization, such as aneuploidy and polyploidy. The major technologies used to evaluate the integrity of spindles are immunofluorescent staining of microtubules and electron microscopy. Both provide only static, instead of kinetic, information since fixation of oocytes is essential in the procedures. Recent use of PolScope allows for non-invasive assessment and follow-up of changes in spindle dynamics and morphology, including non-disjunction in human oocytes [49]. This approach employs polarized light and can be used to view spindles in living oocytes, with electro-optical hardware and digital processing to image microtubules in cells on the basis of birefringence. Although the exact cellular mechanisms underlying the high incidence of aneuploidy in women is still unknown, potential roles of age-related decline in oocyte functions and gonadotropin-induced hyperstimulation of ovarian follicle maturation should be considered for future investigations.

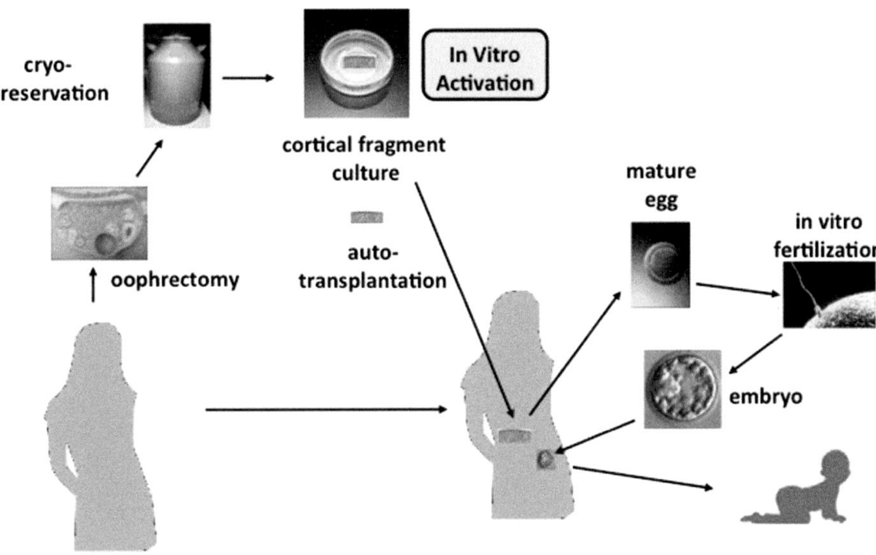

Figure 6.4 In vitro activation of dormant primordial follicles in patients with primary ovarian insufficiency. Patients with primary ovarian insufficiency are infertile at less than 40 years of age due to the lack of large follicles, but some patients still possess some primordial and primary follicles. One ovary was removed from these patients to obtain ovarian fragments for cryopreservation. After recovering from laparoscopic surgery, ovarian fragments were treated with PTEN inhibitors and PI3K-activating peptides to activate dormant ovarian follicles before auto-transplantation into the same patients. Some follicles started to grow inside the grafts and, after gonadotropin treatment and ultrasound monitoring, some mature oocytes could be retrieved. These oocytes could be fertilized in vitro for embryo transfer as a treatment option for infertility.

Pathophysiology and clinical implications

Studies on follicle and oocyte developmental dynamics provide new understanding of ovarian physiology. These findings also serve as the basis to elucidate ovarian pathophysiology and allow formulation of treatment options for infertility. The essential role of oocyte-derived GDF9 and BMP15 for optimal follicle development is underscored by genetic studies of patients with ovarian dysfunctions. In patients with primary ovarian insufficiency, different missense mutations in the BMP15 gene have been identified [50–52], but no clear mutation has been found for GDF9 [53]. It is, thus, becoming clear that mutations of these oocyte genes are only involved in rare cases of primary ovarian insufficiency. Similar to studies in sheep, heterozygous mutations of GDF9 were found in mothers of dizygotic twins [54] whereas a single nucleotide polymorphism in BMP15 is associated with high response to ovarian stimulation [55].

Ovarian functions decrease with age, characterized by the diminishing number of follicles and menstrual cycle cessation. Primary ovarian insufficiency, also known as premature ovarian failure, is diagnosed for women showing >1 year of no menstrual cycle before 40 years of age. They are infertile due to a lack of follicle growth and ovulation; oocyte donation is the only treatment option. For the general population, menopause occurs at ~51 years of age but many middle-aged women (40–50 years of age) suffer from infertility associated with profound psychological impacts, and sometimes societal repercussions. Infertile primary ovarian insufficiency patients and middle-aged women are minimally responsive to the traditional gonadotropin treatments, but a limited number of primordial follicles are still present [56]. For cancer patients with ovaries cryopreserved before chemo- or radiation therapy, auto-transplantation of human ovarian cortical strips has allowed the growth of preovulatory follicles, generation of mature oocytes, and more than a dozen successful pregnancies [57]. Based on prior success in activating human cortical fragments using compounds capable of activating the PI3K/Akt pathway in oocytes to initiate follicle growth, we are using this in vitro activation (IVA) approach to activate dormant residual follicles in patients with primary ovarian insufficiency. As shown in Figure 6.4, ovaries of primary ovarian insufficiency patients will be obtained by laparoscopic surgery. These ovaries will be fragmented for cryopreservation and stored until patients are ready to receive second laparoscopic surgery for auto-transplantation. Ovarian fragments will be thawed and treated with a PTEN enzyme inhibitor and the PI3K activator 740Y-P for 2 days before auto-transplantation. After surgery, ultrasound monitoring and serum sex steroid hormone measurements will be performed. It is anticipated that oocytes could be retrieved after injection of hCG and intracytoplasmic sperm injection (ICSI) will be performed for fertilization of oocytes. If successful, the present approach could also be useful for middle-aged (40–45 years of age) patients intending to become pregnant because these patients still contain residual follicles likely responding to the IVA treatment protocol if auto-transplanted. With the advances in biomedicine, women are living longer but the time of menopause has remained the same. Coupling with the options to use contraceptives and major delay in first pregnancy, the practical fertile window for modern women has narrowed substantially; future infertility treatment could involve the extension of this fertile window for middle-aged women.

References

1. McGee EA, Hsueh AJ. Initial and cyclic recruitment of ovarian follicles. *Endocr Rev* 2000; **21**(2): 200–14.
2. Macklon NS, Fauser BC. Aspects of ovarian follicle development throughout life. *Horm Res* 1999; **52**(4): 161–70.
3. Gougeon A. Regulation of ovarian follicular development in primates: facts and hypotheses. *Endocr Rev* 1996; **17**(2): 121–55.
4. Hsueh AJ, Billig H, Tsafriri A. Ovarian follicle atresia: a hormonally controlled apoptotic process. *Endocr Rev* 1994; **15**(6): 707–24.
5. Zeleznik AJ. Follicle selection in primates: "many are called but few are chosen". *Biol Reprod* 2001; **65**(3): 655–9.
6. Telfer EE, Gosden RG, Byskov AG, *et al.* On regenerating the ovary and generating controversy. *Cell* 2005; **122**(6): 821–2.
7. Johnson J, Canning J, Kaneko T, Pru JK, Tilly JL. Germline stem cells and follicular renewal in the postnatal mammalian ovary. *Nature* 2004; **428**(6979): 145–50.
8. Skaznik-Wikiel M, Lee HJ, Tschudy KS, *et al.* Oocyte generation in adult mammalian ovaries by putative germ cells in bone marrow and peripheral blood. *Cell* 2005; **122**: 303–15.
9. Eggan K, Jurga S, Gosden R, Min IM, Wagers AJ. Ovulated oocytes in adult mice derive from non-circulating germ cells. *Nature* 2006; **441**(7097): 1109–14.
10. Zhang H, Zheng W, Shen Y, *et al.* Experimental evidence showing that no mitotically active female germline progenitors exist in postnatal mouse ovaries. *Proc Natl Acad Sci USA* 2012; **109**(31): 12580–5.
11. Blandau R, Warrick E, Rumery RE. In vitro cultivation of fetal mouse ovaries. *Fertil Steril* 1965; **16**(6): 705–15.
12. Skinner MK. Regulation of primordial follicle assembly and development. *Hum Reprod Update* 2005; **11**(5): 461–71.
13. Carlsson IB, Laitinen MP, Scott JE, *et al.* Kit ligand and c-Kit are expressed during early human ovarian follicular development and their interaction is required for the survival of follicles in long-term culture. *Reproduction* 2006; **131**(4): 641–9.
14. Hutt KJ, McLaughlin EA, Holland MK. KIT/KIT ligand in mammalian oogenesis and folliculogenesis: roles in rabbit and murine ovarian follicle activation and oocyte growth. *Biol Reprod* 2006; **75**(3): 421–33.
15. Parrott JA, Skinner MK. Kit-ligand/stem cell factor induces primordial follicle development and initiates folliculogenesis. *Endocrinology* 1999; **140**(9): 4262–71.
16. Nilsson EE, Detzel C, Skinner MK. Platelet-derived growth factor modulates the primordial to primary follicle transition. *Reproduction* 2006; **131**(6): 1007–15. Epub 2006/06/01.
17. Ojeda SR, Romero C, Tapia V, Dissen GA. Neurotrophic and cell-cell dependent control of early follicular development. *Mol Cell Endocrinol* 2000; **163**(1–2): 67–71.
18. Roberts AE, Arbogast LK, Friedman CI, *et al.* Neutralization of endogenous vascular endothelial growth factor depletes primordial follicles in the mouse ovary. *Biol Reprod* 2007; **76**(2): 218–23.
19. Tanwar PS, O'Shea T, McFarlane JR. In vivo evidence of role of bone morphogenetic protein-4 in the mouse ovary. *Anim Reprod Sci* 2008; **106**(3–4): 232–40.
20. Lee WS, Otsuka F, Moore RK, Shimasaki S. Effect of bone morphogenetic protein-7 on folliculogenesis and ovulation in the rat. *Biol Reprod* 2001; **65**(4): 994–9.
21. Kezele P, Nilsson EE, Skinner MK. Keratinocyte growth factor acts as a mesenchymal factor that promotes ovarian primordial to primary follicle transition. *Biol Reprod* 2005; **73**(5): 967–73.

22. Reddy P, Shen L, Ren C, *et al.* Activation of Akt (PKB) and suppression of FKHRL1 in mouse and rat oocytes by stem cell factor during follicular activation and development. *Dev Biol* 2005; **281**(2): 160–70.

23. Castrillon DH, Miao L, Kollipara R, Horner JW, DePinho RA. Suppression of ovarian follicle activation in mice by the transcription factor Foxo3a. *Science* 2003; **301**(5630): 215–18.

24. Reddy P, Liu L, Adhikari D, *et al.* Oocyte-specific deletion of Pten causes premature activation of the primordial follicle pool. *Science* 2008; **319**(5863): 611–13.

25. John GB, Gallardo TD, Shirley LJ, Castrillon DH. Foxo3 is a PI3K-dependent molecular switch controlling the initiation of oocyte growth. *Dev Biol* 2008; **321**(1): 197–204.

26. Posner BI, Faure R, Burgess JW, *et al.* Peroxovanadium compounds. A new class of potent phosphotyrosine phosphatase inhibitors which are insulin mimetics. *J Biol Chem* 1994; **269**(6): 4596–604.

27. Rosivatz E, Matthews JG, McDonald NQ, *et al.* A small molecule inhibitor for phosphatase and tensin homologue deleted on chromosome 10 (PTEN). *ACS Chem Biol* 2006; **1**(12): 780–90.

28. Derossi D, Williams EJ, Green PJ, Dunican DJ, Doherty P. Stimulation of mitogenesis by a cell-permeable PI 3-kinase binding peptide. *Biochem Biophys Res Commun* 1998; **251**(1): 148–52.

29. Li J, Kawamura K, Cheng Y, *et al.* Activation of dormant ovarian follicles to generate mature eggs. *Proc Natl Acad Sci USA* 2010; **107**(22): 10280–4. Epub 2010/05/19.

30. White SS, Ojeda SR. Changes in ovarian luteinizing hormone and follicle-stimulating hormone receptor content and in gonadotropin-induced ornithine decarboxylase activity during prepubertal and pubertal development of the female rat. *Endocrinology* 1981; **109**(1): 152–61.

31. O'Shaughnessy PJ, McLelland D, McBride MW. Regulation of luteinizing hormone-receptor and follicle-stimulating hormone-receptor messenger ribonucleic acid levels during development in the neonatal mouse ovary. *Biol Reprod* 1997; **57**(3): 602–8.

32. Dong J, Albertini DF, Nishimori K, *et al.* Growth differentiation factor-9 is required during early ovarian folliculogenesis. *Nature* 1996; **383**(6600): 531–5.

33. Vitt UA, Hayashi M, Klein C, Hsueh AJ. Growth differentiation factor-9 stimulates proliferation but suppresses the follicle-stimulating hormone-induced differentiation of cultured granulosa cells from small antral and preovulatory rat follicles. *Biol Reprod* 2000; **62**(2): 370–7.

34. Vitt UA, McGee EA, Hayashi M, Hsueh AJ. In vivo treatment with GDF-9 stimulates primordial and primary follicle progression and theca cell marker CYP17 in ovaries of immature rats. *Endocrinology* 2000; **141**(10): 3814–20.

35. Orisaka M, Orisaka S, Jiang JY, *et al.* Growth differentiation factor 9 is antiapoptotic during follicular development from preantral to early antral stage. *Mol Endocrinol* 2006; **20**(10): 2456–68. Epub 2006/06/03.

36. Otsuka F, Yao Z, Lee T, *et al.* Bone morphogenetic protein-15. Identification of target cells and biological functions. *J Biol Chem* 2000; **275**(50): 39523–8. Epub 2000/09/22.

37. Galloway SM, McNatty KP, Cambridge LM, *et al.* Mutations in an oocyte-derived growth factor gene (BMP15) cause increased ovulation rate and infertility in a dosage-sensitive manner. *Nat Genet* 2000; **25**(3): 279–83. Epub 2000/07/11.

38. Yan C, Wang P, DeMayo J, *et al.* Synergistic roles of bone morphogenetic protein 15 and growth differentiation factor 9 in ovarian function. *Mol Endocrinol* 2001; **15**(6): 854–66. Epub 2001/05/29.

39. Davis GH, McEwan JC, Fennessy PF, *et al.* Infertility due to bilateral ovarian hypoplasia in sheep homozygous (FecXI FecXI) for the Inverdale prolificacy gene located on the X chromosome. *Biol Reprod* 1992; **46**(4): 636–40. Epub 1992/04/01.

40. Hanrahan JP, Gregan SM, Mulsant P, *et al.* Mutations in the genes for oocyte-derived growth factors GDF9 and BMP15 are associated with both increased ovulation rate and sterility in Cambridge and Belclare sheep (*Ovis aries*). *Biol Reprod* 2004; **70**(4): 900–9. Epub 2003/11/25.

41. Ebeling S, Topfer D, Weitzel JM, Meinecke B. Bone morphogenetic protein-6 (BMP-6): mRNA expression and effect on steroidogenesis during in vitro maturation of porcine cumulus oocyte complexes. *Reprod Fertil Dev* 2012; **23**(8): 1034–42. Epub 2011/12/01.

42. Eppig JJ. Coordination of nuclear and cytoplasmic oocyte maturation in eutherian mammals. *Reprod Fertil Dev* 1996; **8**(4): 485–9. Epub 1996/01/01.

43. Tsafriri A, Pomerantz SH. Oocyte maturation inhibitor. *Clin Endocrinol Metab* 1986; **15**(1): 157–70. Epub 1986/02/01.

44. Zhang M, Su YQ, Sugiura K, Xia G, Eppig JJ. Granulosa cell ligand NPPC and its receptor NPR2 maintain meiotic arrest in mouse oocytes. *Science* 2010; **330**(6002): 366–9. Epub 2010/10/16.

45. Kawamura K, Cheng Y, Kawamura N, *et al.* Pre-ovulatory LH/hCG surge decreases C-type natriuretic peptide secretion by ovarian granulosa cells

to promote meiotic resumption of pre-ovulatory oocytes. *Hum Reprod* 2011; **26**(11): 3094–101. Epub 2011/08/26.

46. Sato Y, Cheng Y, Kawamura K, Takae S, Hsueh AJ. C-type natriuretic peptide stimulates ovarian follicle development. *Mol Endocrinol* 2012; **26**(7): 1158–66.

47. McGee EA, Perlas E, LaPolt PS, Tsafriri A, Hsueh AJ. Follicle-stimulating hormone enhances the development of preantral follicles in juvenile rats. *Biol Reprod* 1997; **57**(5): 990–8.

48. Jones KT. Meiosis in oocytes: predisposition to aneuploidy and its increased incidence with age. *Hum Reprod Update* 2008; **14**(2): 143–58. Epub 2007/12/18.

49. Rienzi L, Martinez F, Ubaldi F, *et al.* Polscope analysis of meiotic spindle changes in living metaphase II human oocytes during the freezing and thawing procedures. *Hum Reprod* 2004; **19**(3): 655–9. Epub 2004/03/05.

50. Di Pasquale E, Beck-Peccoz P, Persani L. Hypergonadotropic ovarian failure associated with an inherited mutation of human bone morphogenetic protein-15 (BMP15) gene. *Am J Hum Genet* 2004; **75**(1): 106–11. Epub 2004/05/12.

51. Dixit H, Rao LK, Padmalatha VV, *et al.* Missense mutations in the BMP15 gene are associated with ovarian failure. *Hum Genet* 2006; **119**(4): 408–15. Epub 2006/03/02.

52. Tiotiu D, Alvaro Mercadal B, Imbert R, *et al.* Variants of the BMP15 gene in a cohort of patients with premature ovarian failure. *Hum Reprod* 2010; **25**(6): 1581–7. Epub 2010/04/07.

53. Laissue P, Christin-Maitre S, Touraine P, *et al.* Mutations and sequence variants in GDF9 and BMP15 in patients with premature ovarian failure. *Eur J Endocrinol* 2006; **154**(5): 739–44. Epub 2006/04/29.

54. Palmer JS, Zhao ZZ, Hoekstra C, *et al.* Novel variants in growth differentiation factor 9 in mothers of dizygotic twins. *J Clin Endocrinol Metab* 2006; **91**(11): 4713–16. Epub 2006/09/07.

55. Hanevik HI, Hilmarsen HT, Skjelbred CF, Tanbo T, Kahn JA. A single nucleotide polymorphism in BMP15 is associated with high response to ovarian stimulation. *Reprod Biomed Online* 2011; **23**(1): 97–104. Epub 2011/05/14.

56. Pal L, Santoro N. Premature ovarian failure (POF): discordance between somatic and reproductive aging. *Ageing Res Rev* 2002; **1**(3): 413–23.

57. Donnez J, Silber S, Andersen CY, *et al.* Children born after autotransplantation of cryopreserved ovarian tissue: a review of 13 live births. *Ann Med* 2011; **43**(6): 437–50. Epub 2011/01/14.

Chapter 7 Mouse models to identify genes throughout oogenesis

Jia Peng, Qinglei Li, and Martin M. Matzuk

Introduction

In mammals, oocytes initially develop from primordial germ cells (PGCs), which divide and migrate to the gonad to become oogonia during fetal development. At birth, a mammalian female contains about two million primary oocytes, which remain quiescent in the prophase of meiosis I (refer to Chapters 2 and 6). Eventually, a subset of these immature oocytes will be surrounded by granulosa cells to form the primordial follicle pool. Folliculogenesis begins with the activation of a primordial follicle and ends with either the release of a fertilizable oocyte or follicular atresia. The pathways involved in oogenesis and folliculogenesis have been extensively studied, with an attempt to better understand the molecular mechanisms underlying successful ovulation and fertilization. In this chapter, we highlight three major pathways critical for female germ cell development – transforming growth factor beta (TGFβ), phosphatidylinositol 3-kinase (PI3K), and small RNAs – and discuss mouse models used for dissecting the function of genes involved in these pathways.

TGFβ pathway

Overview of the TGFβ pathway

The TGFβ superfamily is the largest family of secreted proteins in mammals [1]. Members of the TGFβ family are involved in a variety of developmental and physiological processes. The canonical TGFβ signaling pathway begins with two dimeric ligands binding to type I and type II receptors to form an activated heterotetrameric receptor complex. The type II receptor within this activated complex phosphorylates the type I receptor, which in turn phosphorylates downstream SMAD proteins. These phosphorylated, receptor-regulated SMAD (R-SMAD) proteins can then bind to the common SMAD (co-SMAD; i.e., SMAD4), translocate into the nucleus, and interact with SMAD binding partners to regulate transcription of target genes (Figure 7.1).

Oocyte-secreted ligands: GDF9 and BMP15

Growth differentiation factor 9 (GDF9) and bone morphogenetic protein 15 (BMP15) are key oocyte-secreted members of the TGFβ superfamily involved in regulating female fertility in mammals [2, 3]. Although GDF9 and BMP15 are closely related paralogs, they signal via different SMAD pathways: SMAD2/3 for GDF9 and SMAD1/5 for BMP15. Mutations in these two ligands have been generated in mice [2, 4]. These mouse models along with relevant studies in human and other species have defined the critical roles of these two factors during oogenesis and folliculogenesis.

In 1996, our group showed that GDF9 is required for follicular development beyond the primary stage [2]. However, mice with null mutations in *Bmp15* only exhibit female subfertility with slightly decreased ovulation rate and litter sizes compared to wild-type mice [4]. In contrast, homozygous *BMP15* mutations in sheep ($FecX^I$ and $FecX^H$) are associated with complete infertility due to an arrest of folliculogenesis at the primary stage [3]. Interestingly, ewes heterozygous for these *BMP15* mutations have an increased rate of ovulation. A point mutation in sheep *GDF9* (FecG) results in a similar phenotype to the *BMP15* mutants in the homozygote state [5]. In humans, recent studies have also identified several point mutations in *BMP15* and *GDF9* that are associated with premature ovarian failure [6]. While the specific contributions of BMP15 and GDF9 appear to differ among species, the general importance of these oocyte-secreted paralogs in female reproduction is clearly evident.

Biology and Pathology of the Oocyte, 2nd edn., ed. Alan Trounson, Roger Gosden, and Ursula Eichenlaub-Ritter. Published by Cambridge University Press.

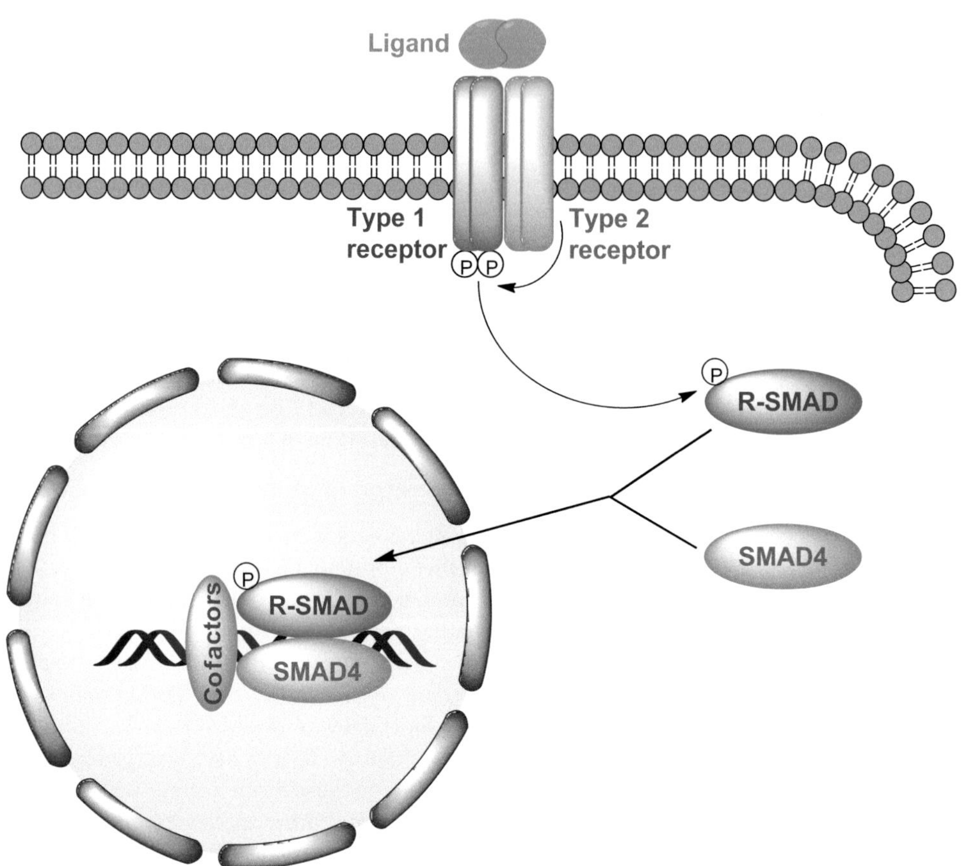

Figure 7.1 Overview of the canonical transforming growth factor beta (TGFβ) pathway. In the presence of dimeric ligands, the type II receptor phosphorylates the type I receptor and results in formation of an activated heterotetrameric receptor complex. The phosphorylated R-SMAD binds to SMAD4, then translocates into the nucleus to regulate target gene expression with other SMAD binding partners.

TGFβ superfamily ligands commonly form homodimers or heterodimers to bind their receptors and trigger downstream signaling pathways. Our previous studies found that *Gdf9*$^{+/-}$*Bmp15*$^{-/-}$ double mutant mice had more severe fertility defects compared to *Bmp15*$^{-/-}$ mice [4], suggesting these two genes may have synergistic functions during oogensis and folliculogenesis. Moreover, an in vitro study has detected GDF9:BMP15 protein heterodimer by immunoprecipitation [7]. However, the existence and functional roles of GDF9:BMP15 heterodimers in vivo still remain largely unknown.

Regulation of cumulus cell functions by GDF9 and BMP15

There are two major types of granulosa cells in a preovulatory ovarian follicle: mural cells and cumulus cells. Oocyte-secreted growth factors GDF9 and BMP15 play important roles in cumulus cell development and function before and after the luteinizing hormone (LH) surge [8]. In response to the ovulatory LH surge, cumulus cells become expanded and produce a complex extracellular matrix (ECM), which is indispensable for ovulation and therefore required for fertility. This highly coordinated process is called cumulus expansion. A number of key cumulus genes have been identified including hyaluronan synthase 2 (*Has2*), pentraxin 3 (*Ptx3*), prostaglandin-endoperoxide synthase 2 (*Ptgs2*), and tumor necrosis factor-α-induced protein 6 (*Tnfaip6*) [9–14]. Mouse knockout models of these cumulus genes have revealed effects on fertility through a range of mechanisms (Table 7.1).

Other genes in the TGFβ pathway involved in folliculogenesis

The crosstalk between the oocyte and surrounding granulosa cells is essential for successful

Table 7.1. Mouse models with defects in the TGFβ pathway or downstream genes

Gene name	Symbol	Targeting strategy	Reproductive phenotype	Reference
Activin/inhibin βB subunit	*Inhbb*	KO	Delivery and nursing defects	[20]
Activin/inhibin βA subunit	*Inhba*	cKO (*Amhr2-Cre*)	Increased corpora lutea	[21]
Activin receptor type 2A	*Acvr2*	KO	Antral follicle block	[22]
Bone morphogenetic protein	*Bmp15*	KO	Defects in cumulus–oocyte complex formation and ovulation	[4]
Bone morphogenetic protein receptor 1A	*Bmpr1a*	cKO (*Amhr2-Cre*)	Females are subfertile with reduced spontaneous ovulation	[23]
Growth differentiation factor 9	*Gdf9*	KO	Folliculogenesis arrest at the type 3b primary follicle stage	[2]
Inhibin α	*Inha*	KO	Granulosa/Sertoli tumors, gonadotropin hormone dependent	[24]
Pentraxin 3	*Ptx3*	KO	Impaired cumulus–oocyte complex structure and matrix stability; females are subfertile	[10, 11]
Prostaglandin-endoperoxide synthase 2	*Ptgs2*	KO	Defects in cumulus expansion, ovulation, fertilization, and embryo implantation; females are sterile	[12]
Sma/MAD homolog 1/5	*Smad1/5*	cKO (*Amhr2-Cre*)	Females are infertile and develop metastatic granulosa cell tumors	[25]
Sma/MAD homolog 2/3	*Smad2/3*	cKO (*Amhr2-Cre*)	Defective cumulus expansion and follicular development; impaired GDF9 signaling; females are subfertile	[26]
Sma/MAD homolog 4	*Smad4*	cKO (*Amhr2-Cre*)	Impaired cumulus–oocyte integrity; premature luteinization of follicles; females are subfertile	[27]
Tumor necrosis factor α-induced protein 6	*Tnfaip6*	KO	Defective cumulus expansion; females are sterile	[13, 14]

cKO, conditional knockout; KO, knockout.

folliculogenesis and ovulation. The oocyte-secreted proteins GDF9 and BMP15 are required for granulosa cell growth, proliferation, and differentiation, whilst other growth factors secreted by granulosa cells (e.g., activins, inhibins) also act on oocytes to regulate their development and function. Furthermore, mouse models with altered expression of other TGFβ pathway proteins, including receptors, R-SMADs, SMAD4, etc. have been created to identify functional roles of these factors in ovarian development (Table 7.1).

PI3K pathway

Overview of the PI3K pathway in the mammalian ovary

Recent studies have shown that the PI3K signaling pathway plays a key role in regulating ovarian follicle maturation [15]. Class IA PI3K consists of a regulatory subunit (p85) and a catalytic subunit (p110). In the presence of growth factors, receptor protein tyrosine kinase (RPTK) activates PI3K, which then phosphorylates phosphatidylinositol-4, 5-bisphosphate (PIP_2) to produce phosphatidylinositol-3, 4, 5-triphosphate (PIP_3). PIP_3 binds to kinase with pleckstrin homology (PH) domain (e.g., 3-phosphatidylinositol-dependent kinase-1 [PDK1] and AKT [protein kinase B]). PTEN (phosphatase and tensin homolog), known as a major negative regulator of PI3K signaling, converts PIP_3 back to PIP_2. AKT is fully activated after phosphorylation by both PDK1 and the mammalian target of rapamycin complex 2 (mTORC2) and subsequently inactivates a series of downstream targets including forkhead box transcription factors (i.e., FOXO1, FOXO3A, and FOXO4), BCL2-associated agonist of cell death (BAD), tuberous sclerosis complex 2 (TSC2), and p27 to regulate cell survival and proliferation (Figure 7.2).

Mouse models to study roles of the PI3K pathway in ovarian function

Over the past decade, the roles of PI3K signaling in the oocyte have been investigated using a variety of genetic mouse models (Table 7.2). PTEN has been found to

Table 7.2. Mouse models with defects in the PI3K pathway

Gene name	Symbol	Targeting strategies	Reproductive phenotype	Reference
Phosphatase and tensin homolog	*Pten*	cKO (*Gdf9-Cre*)	Premature primordial follicle activation, POF, in young adulthood	[16]
Phosphatase and tensin homolog	*Pten*	cKO (*Vasa-Cre^{ERT2}*)	Induced activation of primordial follicles, POF	[28]
Phosphatase and tensin homolog	*Pten*	cKO (*Amhr2-Cre*)	Accumulation of corpora lutea; ovarian stromal hyperplasia	[29]
Phosphatase and tensin homolog	*Pten*	cKO (*Cyp19-Cre*)	Accumulation of corpora lutea; increased granulosa cell proliferation and ovulation; decreased follicle atresia	[30]
3-phosphatidylinositol-dependent kinase-1	*Pdk1*	cKO (*Gdf9-Cre*)	Premature primordial follicle death, POF in young adulthood	[17]
Thymoma viral proto-oncogene 1	*Akt1*	KO	Retarded follicular development; enhanced oocyte apoptosis; reduced granulosa cell proliferation	[31]
Tuberous sclerosis complex 1	*Tsc1*	cKO (*Gdf9-Cre*)	Premature primordial follicle activation, POF in young adulthood	[32]
Tuberous sclerosis complex 2	*Tsc2*	cKO (*Gdf9-Cre*)	Premature primordial follicle activation, POF in young adulthood	[33]
Forkhead box O3	*Foxo3a*	KO	Premature primordial follicle activation, POF in young adulthood	[18]
Forkhead box O3	*Foxo3a*	cKO (*Vasa-Cre^{ERT2}*)	Induced activation of primordial follicles in postnatal and adult life	[28]

POF, premature ovarian failure.

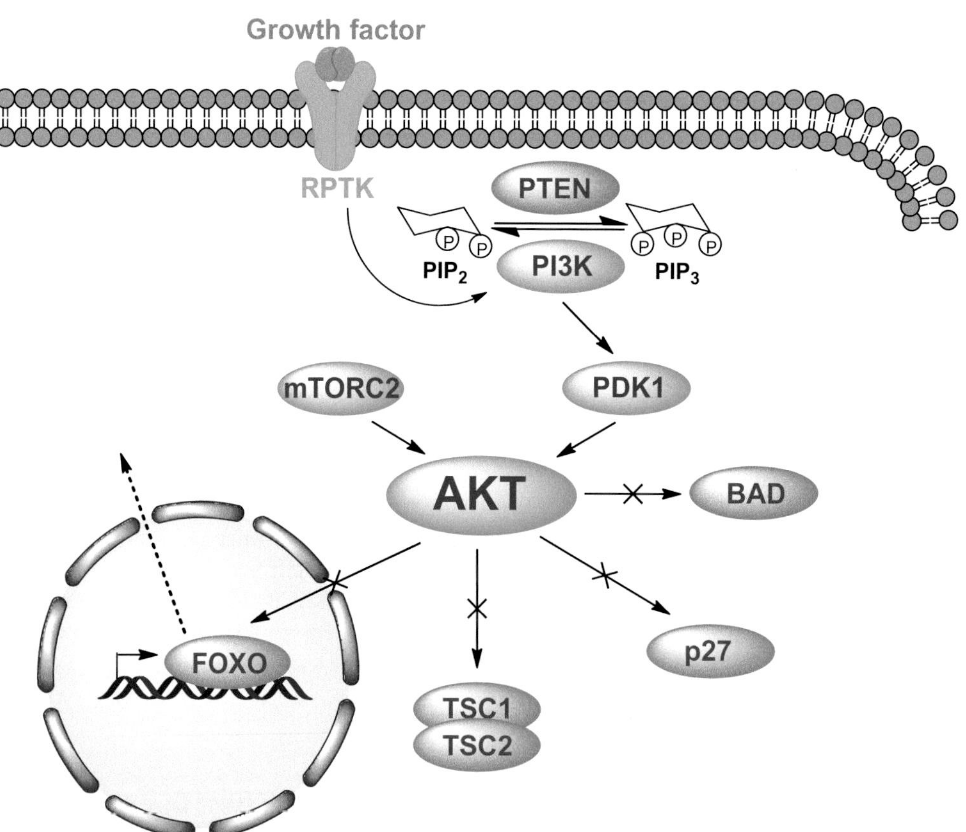

Figure 7.2 Overview of the PI3K pathway. Growth factors bind to RPTK to activate PI3K, which phosphorylates PIP_2 to produce PIP_3. PTEN, a key negative regulator in the PI3K signaling, converts PIP_3 back to PIP_2. PIP_3 then binds to PDK1. AKT is fully activated after phosphorylation by PDK1 and mTORC2 and in turn inactivates a series of downstream targets including FOXO, BAD, TSC2, and p27.

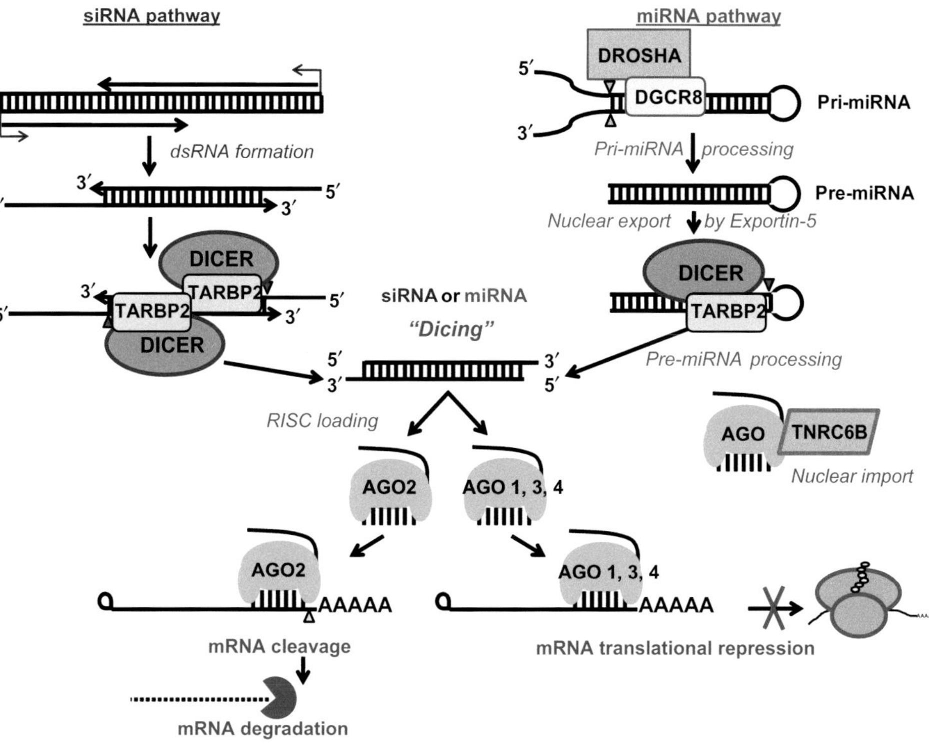

Figure 7.3 siRNA and miRNA biosynthesis. The initial siRNA transcript forms a long dsRNA, whereas miRNA transcripts fold into a hairpin-shaped pri-miRNA. Pri-miRNA is sequentially processed by Drosha and DGCR8 to produce pre-miRNA, and then exported to the cytoplasm where DICER and TARBP2 cleave the 5′-overhangs of the siRNA precursor or the loop of the pre-miRNA. The mature siRNA or miRNA is loaded onto RISC to accelerate degradation of target mRNAs or repress mRNA translation.

act as a key negative regulator of the PI3K pathway by dephosphorylating PIP_3. It is reported that mice lacking PTEN in the oocyte exhibited premature ovarian failure due to excessive activation and depletion of primordial follicles in early adulthood [16]. Female mice deficient in PDK1 also show female infertility due to primordial follicle loss during sexual maturity [17]. FOXO3A, one member of the FOXO subfamily, is another important downstream negative effector of the PI3K pathway in early folliculogenesis. After phosphorylation by AKT, FOXO3A is exported from the nucleus thus triggering primordial follicle activation (Figure 7.2). *Foxo3a* knockout female mice exhibited a similar ovarian phenotype to *Pten* oocyte-specific knockout mice, which also displayed premature ovarian failure [18]. Mouse models for a variety of other genes involved in PI3K signaling, including *Akt1*, *Tsc1*, and *Tsc2*, have further revealed their roles in ovarian function (Table 7.2).

Small RNA pathways

Overview of siRNAs and miRNAs

Current research indicates that non-coding small RNAs play significant roles in reproductive development in both males and females [19]. Generally, small RNAs can be divided into two major groups according to their length. Small RNAs greater than 24 nucleotides include the piRNAs (P-element-induced wimpy testis [PIWI]-interacting RNAs), whereas those RNAs less than 24 nucleotides include microRNAs (miRNAs) and small interfering RNAs (siRNAs). Since piRNAs are specifically required for male reproduction, here we highlight the functional roles of miRNAs and siRNAs in female germ cell development.

Although miRNAs and siRNAs are similar in length, their biosynthesis processes are largely different (Figure 7.3). The initial siRNA transcript forms a

Table 7.3. Mouse models created to study siRNA and miRNA function

Gene name	Symbol	Targeting strategies	Pathway altered	Phenotype	Reference
Argonaute 2	*Ago2*	KO	miRNA	E9.5 lethality; embryonic defects including neural tube and cardiac defects	[34]
Argonaute 2	*Ago2*	cKO (*Zp3-Cre*)	siRNA	Female sterility; oocyte meiosis I block	[35]
DICER	*Dicer1*	KO	miRNA (siRNA?)	E7.5 lethality; defects in embryonic stem cells	[36]
DICER	*Dicer1*	Hypomorphic allele	miRNA	Female sterility; defects in vasculature leading to ovarian corpus luteum defects	[37]
DICER	*Dicer1*	cKO (*Amhr2-Cre*)	miRNA	Female sterility; oviductal diverticuli and uterine implantation defects	[38–41]
DICER	*Dicer1*	cKO (*Zp3-Cre*)	siRNA	Sterile; disorganized spindles, defects in chromosome alignment, and a block at meiosis I	[34, 42]
DiGeorge syndrome critical region gene 8	*Dgcr8*	cKO (*Zp3-Cre*)	miRNA	Normal fertility; confirms that miRNAs are not required in oocytes	[43]

long double-stranded RNA (dsRNA), while a miRNA transcript folds into a hairpin structure known as a primary miRNA (pri-miRNA). Pri-miRNAs contain a dsRNA stem which undergoes sequential processing by the microprocessor complex (Drosha and DiGeorge syndrome region gene 8 protein [DGCR8] in mammals) to form precursor miRNA (pre-miRNA). Specifically, pre-miRNA intermediates arise via cleavage at the base of the pri-miRNA stem. Pre-miRNAs are then exported from the nucleus via Exportin-5. In the cytoplasm, the cytoplasmic type III RNA endonuclease DICER and cofactor TAR RNA-binding protein 2 (TARBP2) cleave the 5′-overhangs of the siRNA precursor and the loop of the pre-miRNA to yield a mature miRNA. Once formed, a mature siRNA or miRNA is loaded onto the Argonaute (AGO)-containing effector complex, RNA-induced silencing complex (RISC). Alternatively, miRNPs can accelerate degradation of target mRNAs or repress mRNA translation.

siRNA, but not miRNA, regulates oocyte meiosis

Initially, miRNAs were thought to be the major DICER-dependent small RNAs in mammals. However, recent studies have discovered functional roles for siRNAs in oogenesis. During small RNA biosynthesis, miRNAs are processed by Drosha and DGCR8 in the nucleus and DICER in the cytoplasm, while siRNAs only require DICER in cytoplasm. Since mice lacking DICER or AGO2 are embryonic lethal, several studies have used Cre-loxP-mediated recombination to conditionally knockout DICER or AGO2 specifically in oocytes (Table 7.3). Conditional deletion of *Dicer* in the oocyte using zona pellucida 3 (Zp3)-Cre results in oocyte arrest at metaphase of meiosis I. Similar oocyte phenotypes are observed in the *Ago2* oocyte-specific knockout mouse. Thus, DICER and AGO2 functions are required for normal oocyte meiosis and female fertility. Since DICER is required for miRNA and siRNA processing, the oocyte defects could be due to the ablation of miRNA, siRNA, or both. Surprisingly, absence of DGCR8 in oocytes has no major defect in oocyte maturation and fertilization. This indicates that DGCR8-independent, DICER-dependent production of siRNA is directly required for oogenesis whereas miRNAs are likely dispensable for oocyte function and thus fertility.

Conclusions

The major function of the ovary in female reproduction is to generate mature oocytes ready for successful fertilization. Proper development of the oocyte is crucial to ensure the integrity of the genome passed on to the next generation. In this chapter, we have discussed a number of mouse models created to study three major pathways involved in regulating ovarian development. The following important points can be gleaned from analysis of these genetic models: (1) oocyte-secreted GDF9 and BMP15 are crucial growth factors during oogenesis and folliculogenesis;

2) the major functional role of the PI3K pathway is to regulate primordial follicle survival and activation via two negative effectors, PTEN and FOXO3A; (3) siRNA, but not miRNA, is the key player in regulating oocyte meiosis. These updated findings lead us to a better understanding of intraovarian regulatory mechanisms, which provide potential improvements in treating human infertility in clinic.

Acknowledgments

Studies in the Matzuk laboratory on female fertility pathway have been supported by the Eunice Kennedy Shriver National Institute of Child Health and Human Development through R01 grants HD33438 and HD32067 and cooperative agreement U54 HD007495 as part of the Specialized Cooperative Centers Program in Reproduction and Infertility Research.

All authors contributed equally to this review.

References

1. Knight PG, Glister C. TGF-beta superfamily members and ovarian follicle development. *Reproduction* 2006; **132**(2): 191–206.
2. Dong J, Albertini DF, Nishimori K, *et al.* Growth differentiation factor-9 is required during early ovarian folliculogenesis. *Nature* 1996; **383**(6600): 531–5.
3. Galloway SM, McNatty KP, Cambridge LM, *et al.* Mutations in an oocyte-derived growth factor gene (BMP15) cause increased ovulation rate and infertility in a dosage-sensitive manner. *Nat Genet* 2000; **25**(3): 279–83.
4. Yan C, Wang P, DeMayo J, *et al.* Synergistic roles of bone morphogenetic protein 15 and growth differentiation factor 9 in ovarian function. *Mol Endocrinol* 2001; **15**(6): 854–66.
5. Hanrahan JP, Gregan SM, Mulsant P, *et al.* Mutations in the genes for oocyte-derived growth factors GDF9 and BMP15 are associated with both increased ovulation rate and sterility in Cambridge and Belclare sheep (*Ovis aries*). *Biol Reprod* 2004; **70**(4): 900–9.
6. Laissue P, Christin-Maitre S, Touraine P, *et al.* Mutations and sequence variants in GDF9 and BMP15 in patients with premature ovarian failure. *Eur J Endocrinol* 2006; **154**(5): 739–44.
7. Liao WX, Moore RK, Otsuka F, Shimasaki S. Effect of intracellular interactions on the processing and secretion of bone morphogenetic protein-15 (BMP-15) and growth and differentiation factor-9. Implication of the aberrant ovarian phenotype of BMP-15 mutant sheep. *J Biol Chem* 2003; **278**(6): 3713–19.
8. Su YQ, Sugiura K, Wigglesworth K, *et al.* Oocyte regulation of metabolic cooperativity between mouse cumulus cells and oocytes: BMP15 and GDF9 control cholesterol biosynthesis in cumulus cells. *Development* 2008; **135**(1): 111–21.
9. Chen L, Russell PT, Larsen WJ. Functional significance of cumulus expansion in the mouse: roles for the preovulatory synthesis of hyaluronic acid within the cumulus mass. *Mol Reprod Dev* 1993; **34**(1): 87–93.
10. Salustri A, Garlanda C, Hirsch E, *et al.* PTX3 plays a key role in the organization of the cumulus oophorus extracellular matrix and in in vivo fertilization. *Development* 2004; **131**(7): 1577–86.
11. Varani S, Elvin JA, Yan C, *et al.* Knockout of pentraxin 3, a downstream target of growth differentiation factor-9, causes female subfertility. *Mol Endocrinol* 2002; **16**(6): 1154–67.
12. Lim H, Paria BC, Das SK, *et al.* Multiple female reproductive failures in cyclooxygenase 2-deficient mice. *Cell* 1997; **91**(2): 197–208.
13. Fulop C, Szanto S, Mukhopadhyay D, *et al.* Impaired cumulus mucification and female sterility in tumor necrosis factor-induced protein-6 deficient mice. *Development* 2003; **130**(10): 2253–61.
14. Ochsner SA, Day AJ, Rugg MS, *et al.* Disrupted function of tumor necrosis factor-alpha-stimulated gene 6 blocks cumulus cell-oocyte complex expansion. *Endocrinology* 2003; **144**(10): 4376–84.
15. Zheng W, Nagaraju G, Liu Z, Liu K. Functional roles of the phosphatidylinositol 3-kinases (PI3Ks) signaling in the mammalian ovary. *Mol Cell Endocrinol.* 2012; **356**(1–2): 24–30.
16. Reddy P, Liu L, Adhikari D, *et al.* Oocyte-specific deletion of Pten causes premature activation of the primordial follicle pool. *Science* 2008; **319**(5863): 611–13.
17. Reddy P, Adhikari D, Zheng W, *et al.* PDK1 signaling in oocytes controls reproductive aging and lifespan by manipulating the survival of primordial follicles. *Hum Mol Genet* 2009; **18**(15): 2813–24.
18. Castrillon DH, Miao L, Kollipara R, Horner JW, DePinho RA. Suppression of ovarian follicle activation in mice by the transcription factor Foxo3a. *Science* 2003; **301**(5630): 215–18.
19. Hawkins SM, Buchold GM, Matzuk MM. Minireview: The roles of small RNA pathways in reproductive medicine. *Mol Endocrinol* 2011; **25**(8): 1257–79.
20. Vassalli A, Matzuk MM, Gardner HA, Lee KF, Jaenisch R. Activin/inhibin beta B subunit gene disruption leads to defects in eyelid development and female reproduction. *Genes Dev* 1994; **8**(4): 414–27.

21. Pangas SA, Jorgez CJ, Tran M, *et al.* Intraovarian activins are required for female fertility. *Mol Endocrinol* 2007; **21**(10): 2458–71.

22. Matzuk MM, Kumar TR, Bradley A. Different phenotypes for mice deficient in either activins or activin receptor type II. *Nature* 1995; **374**(6520): 356–60.

23. Edson MA, Nalam RL, Clementi C, *et al.* Granulosa cell-expressed BMPR1A and BMPR1B have unique functions in regulating fertility but act redundantly to suppress ovarian tumor development. *Mol Endocrinol* 2010; **24**(6): 1251–66.

24. Matzuk MM, Finegold MJ, Mather JP, *et al.* Development of cancer cachexia-like syndrome and adrenal tumors in inhibin-deficient mice. *Proc Natl Acad Sci USA* 1994; **91**(19): 8817–21.

25. Pangas SA, Li X, Umans L, *et al.* Conditional deletion of Smad1 and Smad5 in somatic cells of male and female gonads leads to metastatic tumor development in mice. *Mol Cell Biol* 2008; **28**(1): 248–57.

26. Li Q, Pangas SA, Jorgez CJ, *et al.* Redundant roles of SMAD2 and SMAD3 in ovarian granulosa cells in vivo. *Mol Cell Biol* 2008; **28**(23): 7001–11.

27. Pangas SA, Li X, Robertson EJ, Matzuk MM. Premature luteinization and cumulus cell defects in ovarian-specific Smad4 knockout mice. *Mol Endocrinol* 2006; **20**(6): 1406–22.

28. John GB, Gallardo TD, Shirley LJ, Castrillon DH. Foxo3 is a PI3K-dependent molecular switch controlling the initiation of oocyte growth. *Dev Biol* 2008; **321**(1): 197–204.

29. Fan HY, Liu Z, Paquet M, *et al.* Cell type-specific targeted mutations of Kras and Pten document proliferation arrest in granulosa cells versus oncogenic insult to ovarian surface epithelial cells. *Cancer Res* 2009; **69**(16): 6463–72.

30. Fan HY, Liu Z, Cahill N, Richards JS. Targeted disruption of Pten in ovarian granulosa cells enhances ovulation and extends the life span of luteal cells. *Mol Endocrinol* 2008; **22**(9): 2128–40.

31. Brown C, LaRocca J, Pietruska J, *et al.* Subfertility caused by altered follicular development and oocyte growth in female mice lacking PKB alpha/Akt1. *Biol Reprod* 2010; **82**(2): 246–56.

32. Adhikari D, Zheng W, Shen Y, *et al.* Tsc/mTORC1 signaling in oocytes governs the quiescence and activation of primordial follicles. *Hum Mol Genet* 2010; **19**(3): 397–410.

33. Adhikari D, Flohr G, Gorre N, *et al.* Disruption of Tsc2 in oocytes leads to overactivation of the entire pool of primordial follicles. *Mol Hum Reprod* 2009; **15**(12): 765–70.

34. Liu J, Carmell MA, Rivas FV, *et al.* Argonaute2 is the catalytic engine of mammalian RNAi. *Science* 2004; **305**(5689): 1437–41.

35. Kaneda M, Tang F, O'Carroll D, Lao K, Surani MA. Essential role for Argonaute2 protein in mouse oogenesis. *Epigenetics Chromatin* 2009; **2**(1): 9.

36. Bernstein E, Kim SY, Carmell MA, *et al.* Dicer is essential for mouse development. *Nat Genet* 2003; **35**(3): 215–17.

37. Otsuka M, Zheng M, Hayashi M, *et al.* Impaired microRNA processing causes corpus luteum insufficiency and infertility in mice. *J Clin Invest* 2008; **118**(5): 1944–54.

38. Nagaraja AK, Andreu-Vieyra C, Franco HL, *et al.* Deletion of Dicer in somatic cells of the female reproductive tract causes sterility. *Mol Endocrinol* 2008; **22**(10): 2336–52.

39. Hong X, Luense LJ, McGinnis LK, Nothnick WB, Christenson LK. Dicer1 is essential for female fertility and normal development of the female reproductive system. *Endocrinology* 2008; **149**(12): 6207–12.

40. Gonzalez G, Behringer RR. Dicer is required for female reproductive tract development and fertility in the mouse. *Mol Reprod Dev* 2009; **76**(7): 678–88.

41. Pastorelli LM, Wells S, Fray M, *et al.* Genetic analyses reveal a requirement for Dicer1 in the mouse urogenital tract. *Mamm Genome* 2009; **20**(3): 140–51.

42. Murchison EP, Stein P, Xuan Z, *et al.* Critical roles for Dicer in the female germline. *Genes Dev* 2007; **21**(6): 682–93.

43. Suh N, Baehner L, Moltzahn F, *et al.* MicroRNA function is globally suppressed in mouse oocytes and early embryos. *Curr Biol* 2010; **20**(3): 271–7.

Section 3 Developmental biology

Chapter 8

Structural basis for oocyte–granulosa cell interactions

Ursula Eichenlaub-Ritter and Carlos Plancha

Introduction

Cellular interactions are known to be essential not only in mammalian developing tissues and organs, but also during steady-state maintenance phases. In the mammalian ovary, cellular interactions are particularly important since follicle development is continuously initiated, during childhood and adulthood, until the follicle pool drops below a poorly understood threshold in menopause. In this context, the germ cell–soma interface is of major relevance since it is at this level that a fine tuning must take place to allow for correct ovarian follicle development and the full oocyte functionality, known as oocyte competence acquisition. This includes complex differentiation processes of the somatic cells, fine tuning in response to growth factors and hormones, and the regulation of meiotic arrest and metabolism to the demand of the growing and maturing oocyte.

Although the zona pellucida, an oocyte-specific extracellular layer, intercalates between oocytes and the innermost layer of cumulus granulosa cells (corona radiata), unique cellular structures are present at this level that emanate from the granulosa cell, extend across the zona pellucida, and reach direct contact with the oocyte's plasma membrane. These structures, known as the transzonal projections (TZPs), may contain cytoskeletal components, such as tubulin and/or actin, and possess membrane junctions such as gap and adhesion junctions, and cell organelles such as mitochondria. Between neighboring granulosa cells similar specialized junctions exist that allow direct cell–cell signaling but also permit nutrient access to the oocyte.

Oocyte–granulosa cell interactions imply that different levels of polarity must exist at both these cellular components of the ovarian follicle. The granulosa cumulus cell polarity is an example of tissue polarity, where most cells are morphologically homogeneous, but the innermost layer displays unique structures to account for this specific interaction. The oocyte polarity can be defined as a cellular polarity with microdomains, where the cortical region, including the subcortical cytoplasm and components accumulating in this region, like cortical vesicles and the "subcortical maternal complex," concentrates a series of structures and macromolecules that are of relevance in order to allow the correct oocyte functionality. Cellular processes know to be important for oocyte functionality include cortical spindle attachment and a markedly asymmetrical division during the process of oocyte maturation, and cortical accumulation of cell organelles ready for fertilization and activation by sperm after oocyte ovulation.

Oocyte quality is an attractive way of describing oocyte competence potential, and all assisted reproduction technologies (ARTs) aim at obtaining high quality oocytes, which would give rise to high quality embryos and consequently higher implantation rates and healthier live births. Unfortunately, reliable methods to predict the competence of particular oocytes are still not available. Furthermore, the growing need to rely on complex ovarian stimulation protocols, on long culture periods, and on different cryopreservation techniques is bound to interfere with the oocyte quality that we would like to optimize. We believe that a better understanding of oocyte physiology, a more rational design of culture environments, applying them to the in vivo situation, and the constant promotion of appropriate cell–cell signaling in all critical stage-specific transitions from oocyte growth, through maturation up to ovulation, will allow optimization of oocyte quality.

Biology and Pathology of the Oocyte, 2nd edn., ed. Alan Trounson, Roger Gosden, and Ursula Eichenlaub-Ritter.
Published by Cambridge University Press.

All these subjects will be discussed in this chapter that will end up with some simplified functional models to better clarify the current concepts at this stage of our understanding.

Defining the structure–function of germ cell–soma interface

Oocyte–granulosa cell interactions and the TZPs

Folliculogenesis and formation of a fully grown and developmentally competent oocyte are dependent on complex regulations involving endocrine, paracrine, and autocrine signaling pathways. The oocyte–granulosa cell dialog is essential for normal follicular development [1, 2]. It is a prerequisite for the acquisition of high maturational and developmental competence of the oocyte during the in vivo protracted folliculogenesis. In this dialog, several factors have been identified. For instance, the oocyte-secreted growth factors of the transforming growth factor beta (TGFβ) family, such as growth differentiation factor 9 (GDF9) and bone morphogenetic protein 15 (BMP15), absence of which causes sterility in mice [3, 4], as well as granulosa cell-secreted proteins such as cKIT being produced by preantral granulosa cells and their interactions with surface receptors on the oolemma promoting oocyte growth [5], are of particular relevance (see Chapter 10). Factors secreted by the oocyte regulate metabolism and exchange of nutrients between the two compartments (see Chapter 10) but also form a morphokinetic gradient that is involved in controlling gene expression and proliferation and differentiation of the granulosa cells (e.g., [6]), particularly in cumulus and corona radiata. This will not be reviewed here, and this chapter will focus on the cellular and structural differentiations that permit direct oocyte–cumulus/granulosa cell crosstalk and exchange, and that influence the stage- and hormone-dependent events particularly with respect to the organization of the cytoskeleton within the oocyte and its companion granulosa cells.

After the initial steps in oogenesis comprising meiotic S-phase, pairing, and meiotic exchange have taken place in the fetal ovary, clusters of oocytes surrounded by somatic cells exist (also termed cyst or nests, see Chapters 2 and 3). At this stage, oocytes are physically attached and communicate via cytoplasmic bridges containing microtubules and microtubule motor proteins like KIF23 for efficient interactions within the functional syncytium (for reference see Chapter 3). Primordial follicles are formed after cyst or nest breakdown shortly before or after birth (reviewed in Chapter 2) in which the surviving dictyate stage-arrested oocytes become surrounded by somatic cells resulting in follicle formation. Each primordial follicle consists of the meiotically arrested small oocyte and a few squamous granulosa cells surrounded by a basal membrane. That direct cell–cell signaling is required already at this early stage is implied by the fact that a gap junction blocker inhibits follicle formation as well as the expression of Par6 (partition-defective protein 6), a protein of the family of Par proteins involved in regulation of cell polarity, in the nuclei of oocytes of newly formed primordial follicles in the mouse [7].

Gonadotropin-independent recruitment of primordial follicles to the growing pool that is commencing throughout the female reproductive period is accompanied by prominent and characteristic changes in the granulosa cell architecture, from a flattened shape to a cuboidal, epithelial-like character. Recent studies have shown that this is not comparable with a classical mesenchymal–epithelial transition as granulosa cells initially lack all epithelial markers like E-cadherin, cytokeratin 8, and zonula occludens (ZO)-1alpha+ proteins that were tested so far [8]. At this early stage of folliculogenesis signaling and cohesion between oocyte and granulosa cells and among granulosa cells appears to involve adherens junctions, N-cadherin, and nectin 2 but not tight junctions as might have been expected from the epithelial-type shape of the granulosa cells [8]. The basal membrane may participate in regulation of cell shape at these early stages since rat granulosa cells plated on extracellular matrix coated surface maintain their epithelioid shape with fewer actin cables compared with granulosa cells that contain numerous stress fibers when they are placed on uncoated tissue culture dishes (reviewed by [9]). The cuboidal cells rather than the flatter granulosa cells rapidly radially divide, such that their density underneath the basal membrane increases, and they then divide perpendicularly to form a second and more granulosa cell layers [10]. Granulosa cells in the vicinity of the oocyte proliferate differentially from those of the outer layers such that in preantral and early antral stages of folliculogenesis frequently there are larger intercellular spaces between neighboring granulosa cells in the innermost layers but tightly

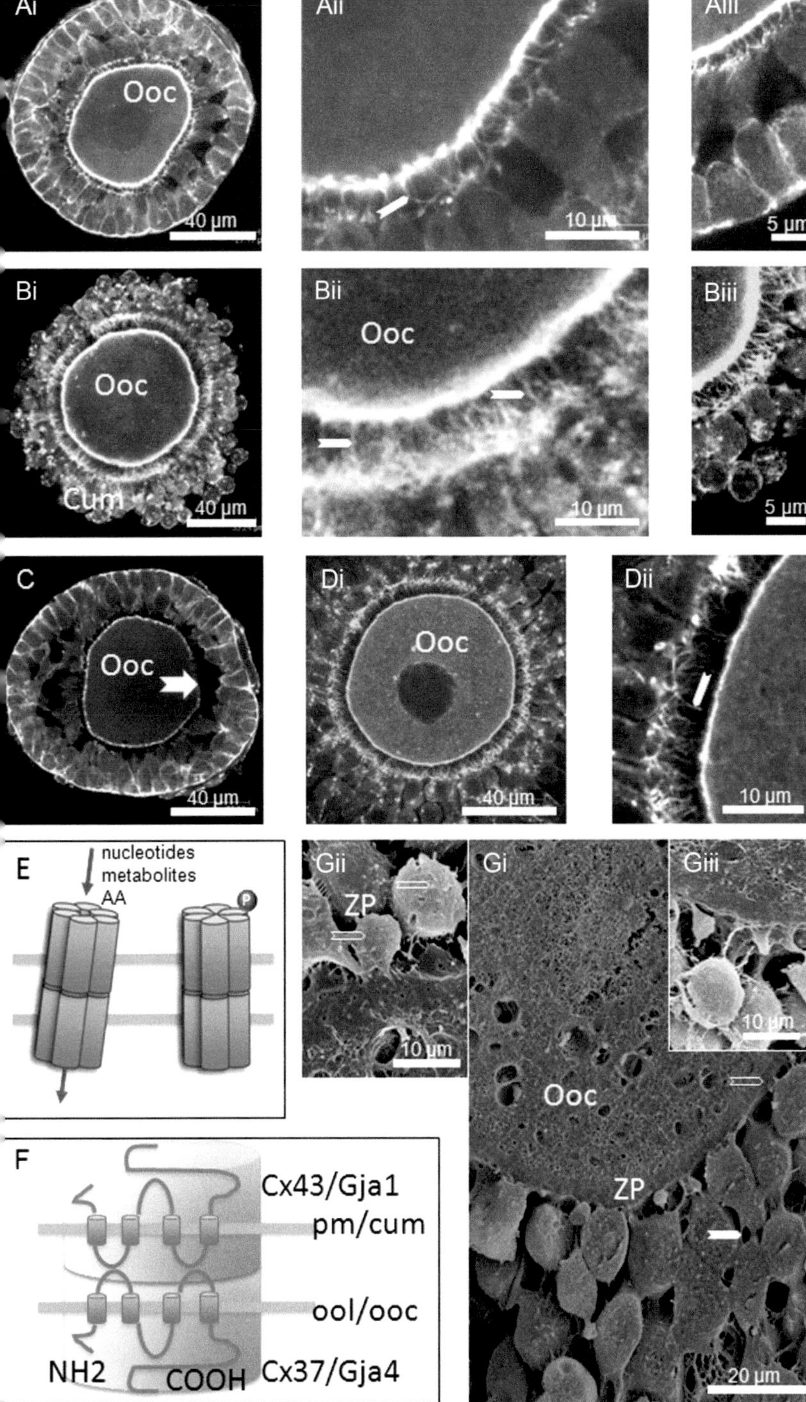

Figure 8.1 Presence of actin-rich TZPs (actTZPs) in preantral follicles of the mouse. Actin is enriched at the oolemma (Ai), in the actTZPs (arrow in Aii) and is present in the peripheral cytoplasm of granulosa cells that are located at the basal membrane (Aiii). Density and length of actTZPs becomes increased during preantral follicle culture as shown in the cumulus–oocyte complex (COC) isolated from follicle developed to large antral stage after 12 days of culture (Bi–Biii). Vitrification by Cryotop may transiently disrupt oocyte–granulosa cell apposition (large arrow in C) but actTZPs are restored after 12 days of culture to the antral stage (Di, Dii). Gap junctions consisting of two connexons on neighboring cells, each possessing six connexin molecules, so that in open conformation nucleotides, metabolites, and amino acids (AA) can be transmitted from one to the other cell (E). Heterologous gap junctions contain connexin 37 at oolemma (ool/ooc) and connexin 43 at the plasma membrane of the cumulus cell (pm/cum) in mouse and human oocytes in which extracellular domains can interact with each other (F). Scanning electron microscopy of fixed mouse follicles shows TZPs crossing the zona pellucida and extending from the granulosa cells towards the oocyte (Ooc) (open arrow) and long cell protrusions connecting adjacent granulosa cells (Gi–Giii). Ai–Dii: Confocal images of follicles/COCs from preantral follicle culture stained by phalloidin-TRITC. Gi–Giii: Mouse follicles processed for scanning electron microscopic analysis. Ai–Di and Gi–Giii. Courtesy of Tom Trapphoff, University of Bielefeld. For further explanation, see text.

packed cells in the more peripheral part of the follicle (see Figure 8.1). Granulosa cells have to be regarded as a functional syncytium at these stages as adjacent cells are connected by gap junctions (see below) while adherens junctions exist but do not block the diffusion of components through the extracellular space and towards the oocyte [8].

Throughout folliculogenesis and oocyte growth, oocytes secrete zona pellucida proteins, three in most mammals, four in the human (e.g., [11–13]), that form a dense three-dimensional, ordered network in the extracellular space as implicated by zona birefringence in polarizing microscopy (reviewed by [14]). Alterations in the density, order, and regular distribution of zona components as visible by analysis of birefringence by quantitative polarizing microscopy have been used in oocyte selection and quality assessment (e.g., [15]). Thin or extremely thick zonas, and those with irregularities presumably resulting from uncoordinated deposition of zona proteins and from loss of granulosa/cumulus–oocyte contacts and interactions have been shown to be indicators of reduced oocyte quality (reviewed by [14]). Thus, with the presence of a three-dimensional ordered structure of the extracellular matrix, the zona pellucida is reflecting the tight oocyte/somatic cell apposition and interactions although it basically spatially separates the two compartments and restricts the areas of direct contacts. Loss of apposition may for instance occur upon cryopreservation by osmotic stress and cell deformation (see [16, 17]) (Figure 8.1) and, when not restored, can contribute to oocyte death and follicular atresia, while restoration is a good indicator that integrity and cell–cell signaling has been retained (Figure 8.1). That somatic cell activities and presence are influencing the extracellular matrix can be deduced from the fact that the zona may harden and undergo rapid changes in organization and filament density/thickness during in vitro maturation, which may hinder fertilization, particularly of denuded oocytes, due to precocious release of cortical granules (e.g., [18]).

Throughout folliculogenesis granulosa cellular extensions, the TZPs, protrude from the apical side of the granulosa cells towards the oolemma, and terminate either at or within the zona matrix (Figures 8.1 and 8.2), thus anchoring the granulosa cell to this site, or cross the zona and terminate at the oocyte oolemma covered with microvilli at the oocyte periphery. There is also evidence that the TZPs extend deep into the ooplasm in a stage-specific fashion. Thus, morphology is continuously adapting to the stage-specific needs of the oocyte and cumulus cells and is dynamically regulated throughout folliculogenesis (e.g., [19, 20]). TZPs have been observed in all mammalian follicles analyzed so far, from human (e.g., [21]) to mouse, rat, hamster, bovine, pig, and marmoset (e.g., [22]/rat [23]/hamster, [24]/bovine, [25]/pig, [26]/marmoset]) (e.g., Figures 8.1 and 8.3).

Although these granulosa cumulus cellular extensions are collectively termed "TZPs" they can be distinguished not only by their localization, terminating in the zona or transversing and interacting with the oolemma, but also by their shape and intrinsic characteristic cytoskeletal organization into different functional units, either being rich in microtubules (Figure 8.3A) or in microfilaments/actin (Figures 8.1Ai–Di and 8.3B): mtTZPs and actTZPs, respectively. The actin and tubulin polymerized fibers can thus act not only in stabilizing the structure of the TZPs but also in promoting cargo-specific transport. For instance, microtubules and microfilaments can serve as tracks for promoting directional transport of mitochondria and secretory vesicles, for example, by microtubules and dynein/kinesin motor proteins and by microfilaments and myosin motor proteins as exemplified in axonal transport (for review, see [27]). Anchoring of cytoskeletal elements at the interface between the granulosa cell and the oocyte promotes and provides for cell organization, for example the organization of the granulosa cell's cytoskeleton (see below) or anchoring of the meiotic spindle eccentrically to provide for unequal division (as depicted in Figure 8.2). Particularly in early stages of folliculogenesis some TZPs appear to extend deeper into the oocyte. This facilitates local interactions between oolemma, cortical ooplasm, and its cellular components, and the exchange of signals of oocytes with granulosa cells and vice versa. Over time during development from the early preantral to the antral stage of folliculogenesis the density and length of actTZPs increases as visible from studies using polarizing microscopy and analyzing birefringence in three-dimensional in vitro follicle growth of the mouse [17, 28]. Long, thin cellular extensions exist also between neighboring granulosa cells, particularly in the innermost cumulus layer (corona radiata) of the follicle to mediate signaling between the somatic cells in the oocyte's vicinity and within granulosa cells from different layers (Figure 8.1Gi–Giii). Basically, the interactions between granulosa cells of the corona radiata,

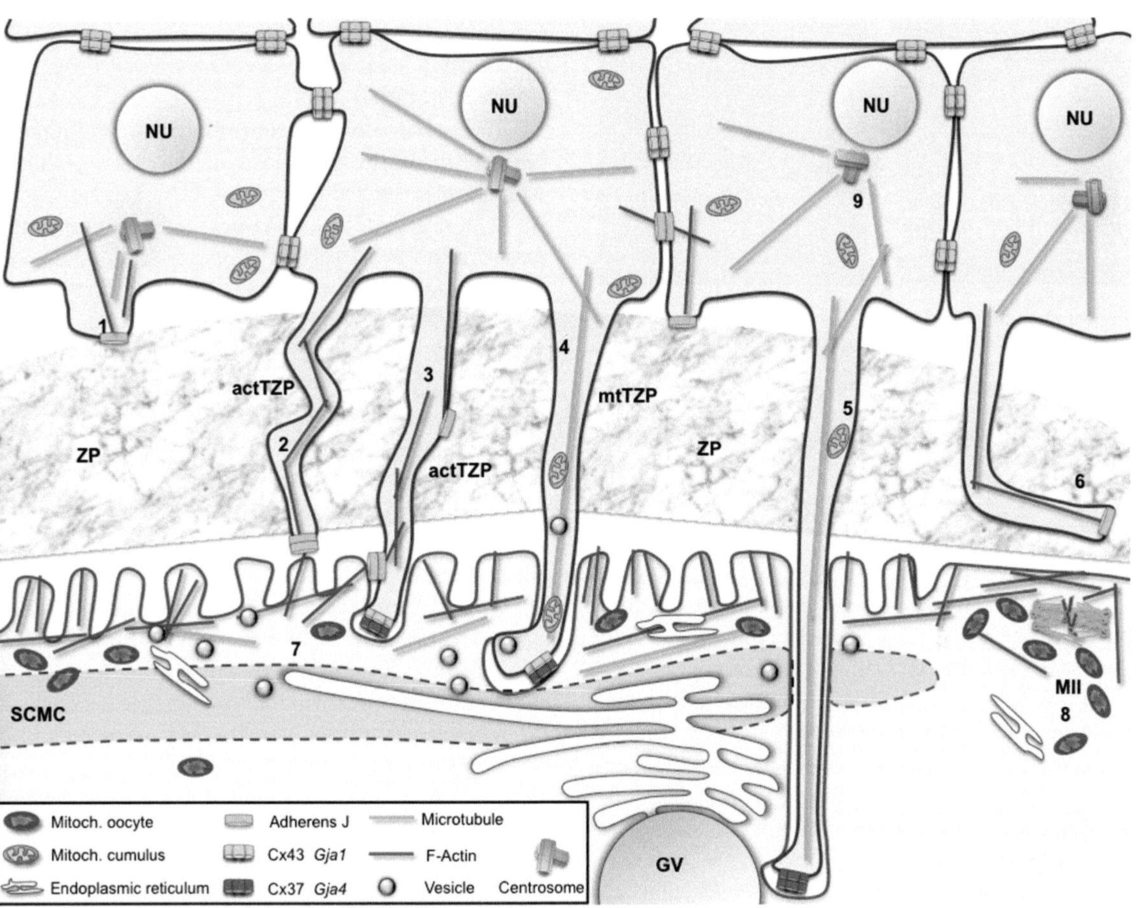

Figure 8.2 Different types of TZPs and the positioning of TZPs, cell organelles, cytoskeletal elements, junctional complexes of Cx37, Cx43, heterologous Cx37/Cx43, and adherens junctions and nuclei (NU in granulosa and GV in oocyte), and spindle during folliculogenesis and oogenesis. 1. Microvillar-like extensions of granulosa cells into the zona pellucida (ZP) containing adhesion junctions, connected to the cytoskeleton by actin fibers and in contact with the tubulin cytoskeleton that is organized by centrosomal microtubule-organizing centers (MTOCs) in the part of the granulosa/cumulus cell adjacent to the zona. 2. TZP rich in actin (actTZP) extending through the zona and anchored by adherens junction to the microvillar oolemma. 3. Straight actTZP anchored by adherens junction to ZP and microvillar oolemma, extending to bases or beyond bases of oolemmal microvilli and communicating with the oocyte via heterologous gap junctions. 4. Microtubule-rich TZP (mtTZP) extending with a bulbous end into the cortical ooplasm, containing typical cristae-rich mitochondria of the cumulus/granulosa cell and vesicles, and heterologous gap junctions. 5. mtTZP extending deep into ooplasm and terminating close to the GV, which is still centrally located as typical for early stages of folliculogenesis/oocyte growth, and not eccentrically positioned as characteristic for later antral stages in vivo. 6. actTZP anchored with perpendicular extensions within the ZP and stabilized by adherens junction. 7. Cortical cytoplasm of fully grown oocytes that is rich in actin, mitochondria with low inner membrane potential, endoplasmic reticulum, vesicles, and components of the subcortical maternal complex, and in contact with cytoskeletal fibers (actin cables, microtubules) that mediate eccentric position of GV and spindle at antral stages of folliculogenesis. 8. Spindle and chromosomes located eccentrically (here shown as characteristic for mouse oocytes aligned perpendicular to the oolemma in the subcortical cytoplasm underneath the actin cytoskeleton). 9. Centriolar MTOC with pair of centrioles in close vicinity of the "apical" part of the cumulus cell on the ZP facing portion of the cumulus cell and attached by microtubules to mtTZPs. For further explanation, see text.

the outermost cumulus, and the mural granulosa cells provide for efficient signaling and communication via gap junctions such that the compartment can act as a syncytium up to a certain degree.

TZPs appear most abundant in the human preantral stage. During the oocyte growth phase, some TZPs extend deep into the oocyte, reaching the germinal vesicle (GV), thus forming a large surface area along the sides between oolemma and granulosa cell membrane for interactions apart from the terminal small, more bulbous region. According to Motta *et al.* [19], observations in the human suggest that TZPs eventually retract and maintain fewer terminal connections with the oocyte at later antral stages of

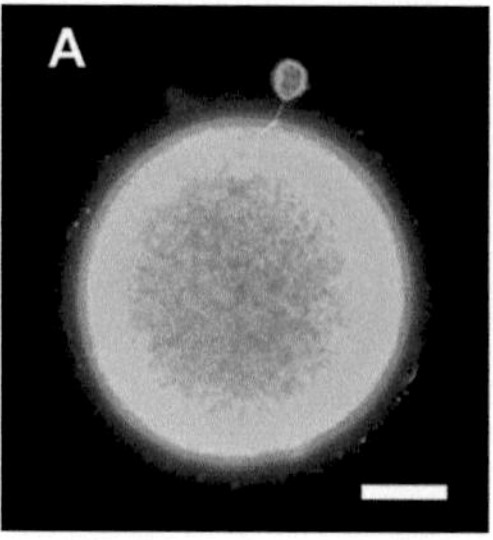

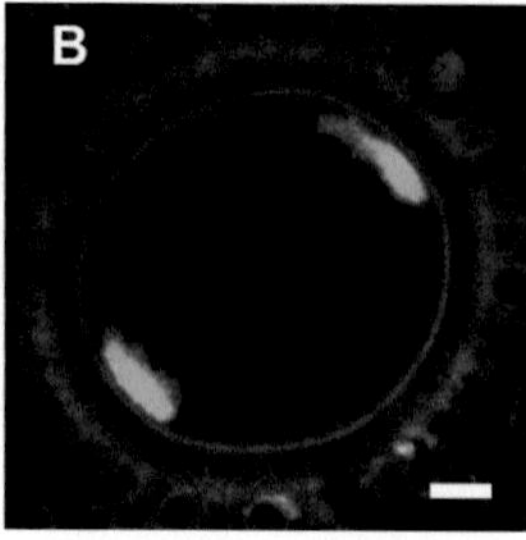

Figure 8.3 Mouse denuded oocyte (A) with just one cumulus granulosa cell and one mtTZP. Microtubules labeled in green and microfilaments in red (A). Hamster germinal vesicle (GV) oocyte inside a cumulus–oocyte complex (B) with the actin-containing TZPs and the actin-rich oocyte cortex and the innermost surface of the cumulus cells that attaches to the zona pellucida and is also an actin-rich domain. Microfilaments labeled in red and cytokeratin intermediate filaments in green (B). Bar: 20 μm.

folliculogenesis as compared to the early preantral stage. Finally, the electron microscopic analysis already suggested that at ovulation most TZPs were retracted in humans [19]. More recent analysis by transmission electron microscopy and high-resolution scanning microscopy fully confirmed and refined thosefindings, showing that in resting human oocytes, follicular cells project few and short cytoplasmic processes in the perioocytic space, and form bulbous terminals very close to the oolemma with fasciae adherens, maculae adherens, and gap junctions [29]. At this stage the oolemma possesses mostly few and short microvilli. In the resting stage the so-called "intra-ooplasmic processes" extend deep into the oocyte, nearly touching the GV but these become retracted upon oocyte growth. In antral follicles numerous long "curly hair-like microvilli" extend from the zona radiata through the zona to the oolemma. The corona cells themselves possess many short microvilli that may be involved in efficient nutrient interaction, receptor-mediated signaling, or removal of catabolites from the oocyte [29]. Interestingly, the dynamic and more stable microtubules within cells may be recognized by post-translational modifications. For instance, tyrosinated tubulin is commonly a hallmark of rapidly turning over microtubules [30, 31], for example in the metaphase spindle of oocytes [32], while acetylated tubulin more frequently is found in the less dynamic microtubules of interphase cells [31]. Human granulosa cells are rich in acetylated tubulin [33]. TZPs within the zona pellucida of human oocytes retrieved for in vitro fertilization also contain microtubules rich in acetylated tubulin [34], suggesting they present a fairly stable cytoskeletal support for TZP integrity throughout oocyte maturation.

TZPs observed in preantral follicles are anchored by F-actin at the periphery of the zona pellucida (Figure 8.1) and possess a few corkscrew-shaped mtTZPs deep into the zona pellucida [34]. That this organization is directed by oocyte-secreted factors can be deduced from the disturbed interactions in GDF9$^{-/-}$ murine oocytes. These oocytes lack anchoring, but instead possess organelle-rich TZPs that envelope the oocyte surface [35]. Influences of the hormonal homeostasis and stage-specific organization (Figure 8.4) are evident from FSHβ$^{-/-}$ mice. Folliculogenesis is blocked in these mutants at the late secondary preantral stage. In this model, granulosa cells persist to possess organelle-rich and anchoring TZPs [34].

Dramatic morphogenetic processes occur upon oocyte resumption of meiosis downstream from the gonadotropin surge as revealed in hamster folliculogenesis, showing that hormonal control drives cytoskeletal changes in both the somatic and germ cells [23]. Specifically, gonadotropins seem to modulate meiotic resumption by positive signal transmission through actin-containing cumulus processes. In fact, it was shown in that study that actTZPs persist during and after meiotic resumption until the prometaphase I stage, when retraction of actTZPs (or at least microfilament depolymerization from TZPs), accompanied by a marked increase of the actin microfilament polymerization cytoskeleton at the oocyte cortex, takes place, probably in preparation for first polar body emission [23].

In the bovine, similarly abundant, actTZPs were observed in mature GV-stage cumulus–oocyte complexes (COCs). At stages intermediate in the maturation process, the density of actTZPs decreased while more mtTZPs were present. At the end of maturation, numerous, long mtTZPs were still retained while only few actTZPs were apparent in this species [24]. In the pig, cumulus cells project numerous long and thin TZPs at resumption of meiosis, but these were largely disconnected when oocytes reached metaphase II, and decreased in numbers [25]. Concomitantly, a comparatively sparse distribution of short microvilli transformed into a dense distribution of well-developed microvilli on the oocyte oolemma. The proteasome inhibitor MG132, which blocks cell-cycle progression beyond metaphase I, not only prevented the

	actTZP	mtTZP	GJ coupling	Oo/GC coupling	GC cGMP/ cAMP	Ooc cGMP/ cAMP
Foxo3a ↑			↓	↓		
Cx43/*Gja1*$^{-/-}$			↓↓			
Cx37/*Gja4*$^{-/-}$				↓↓		
FSH				↑↓	↑	↑↑↑↓
Nrp/R	↑	↑	↑	↑↑	↑↑	↑↑
LH	↓	↑	↓↓		↓	↓
EGF-like	↓	↑	↓		↓	↓

igure 8.4 Overview of major alterations in actTZP, mtTZPs, gap junctional coupling (GJ coupling), oocyte–granulosa cell coupling (Oo/GC oupling), granulosa cell cAMP/cGMP (GC cAMP/cGMP), or oocyte cGMP/cAMP (Ooc cGMP/cAMP) in overexpressing or knockdown models Foxo3a overexpression; *Gja1*$^{-/-}$ or *Gja4*$^{-/-}$ knockout) or under influence of follicle-stimulating hormone (FSH), Nrp/R (natriuretic peptide ype C, NPPC, and natriuretic peptide receptor 2; NPR2) signaling, or luteinizing hormone (LH) and epidermal growth factor (EGF)-like growth actor. Increases and decreases are indicated by ↑ or ↓arrows, respectively. Transient increases followed by decreases are also depicted. Most tudies used COCs from a mouse model. For references and further explanation, see text.

xtrusion of the first polar body, but also the degralation of F-actin-rich TZPs interconnecting cumuus cells with the pig oocyte [36], demonstrating the ight cell-cycle control and coordination of morphogenetic processes with maturation kinetics involving TZP dynamics.

It was first shown in prepubertal mice that granlosa "apical" centrosome positioning occurs at sites f granulosa–zona contact and in close vicinity with TZPs(Figure 8.2) [37]. Dual labeling with antibodies to ubulin and pericentrin, a component of the pericenriolar material associated with centrosomal and acenrosomal microtubule-organizing centers (MTOCs) in granulosa cells, revealed a close relationship between granulosa cell centrosomes and the outer surface of he zona pellucida. Centrosomes often appeared at one nd of coiled or branching TZPs [34]. Centrosomes ppear thus to anchor microtubules from TZPs and nay presumably contribute to stabilize the somatic–germ cell interactions. The organization of the oocyte–granulosa cell junction is depicted in the scheme n Figure 8.2, reflecting the major characteristics in ocyte and granulosa cell interactions. They are at he oocyte interface: stage-specifically short or long nd abundant microvilli at the oolemma, containing ctin microfilaments and microtubules. In addition, he subcortical layer of ooplasm is also represented, haracterized by the presence of various vesicles and mitochondria with low inner membrane potential prior to maturation [38], endoplasmic reticulum, microfilaments, microtubules, and the subcortical maternal complex, which has been proposed to be enriched in maternal mRNA and protein [39]. All these elements, particularly the granulosa cell cytoskeletal fibers, may be ordered and polarized within a growing follicle, being dependent on hormones, growth factors, and gap junction signaling arising from the cumulus.

The membrane junctions

Gap junctions

Gap junctions are transmembrane channels with different conductance and permeability properties. Each gap junction consists of two hemi-channels, termed connexons, on the opposing membranes of adjacent cells. Every connexon consists of a hexamer of connexin (Cx) molecules. Connexins possess four transmembrane domains with cytoplasmic C- and N-termini, one cytoplasmic loop, and two extracellular loops (as indicated in Figure 8.1F). The C-terminal tails of connexins can interact with different protein partners and participate in gap junction conformation, interactions, and formations of plaques of gap junctions at the cell membrane or with partners that may modulate gene expression and signaling. Hemi-channels alone can also contribute to signaling when they are not docked on another hemi-channel or form a gap junction, thus allowing a multitude of signaling events.

The assembly of the six connexins occurs at the endoplasmic reticulum, and connexons can then be transferred by cytoskeletal-based routes to the cell periphery, where they become integrated into the membrane. The six connexins are subunits that form a cylinder with a central pore, depending on the conformation of the subunits. Docking of the connexon-son opposite cells requires rotation of one connexon by 30° to facilitate interdigitation of the extracellular domains (Figure 8.1E), forming in this way a dual concentric β-barrel configuration [40]. Under these conditions, the hydrophilic pore of the channel allows the transcellular flow of ions and small molecules of up to 1 kDa, such as cyclic nucleotides (cAMP and cGMP), inositol phosphates, amino acids, and calcium ions as well as other cell ions and small molecules. Adjacent cells become electrically and chemically coupled when apposed connexons dock, thereby facilitating passive diffusion. Ions and small molecules that have been shown to pass from granulosa cell to oocyte via gap junctions in mammals include Na^+, Cl^- [41], cAMP [42, 43], cGMP [44], ribonucleosides (e.g., [45]), certain amino acids [46], 2-deoxyglucose [47], choline (e.g., [45]), and inositol [48].

Paracrine signaling and autocrine regulatory events by hemi-channels or gap junctions depend on the type of connexin and on the specific cellular context, for example post-translational modifications like phosphorylation (e.g., [49]) and contact with the contractile cytoskeleton [50] that can influence the conformation and thus contribute to opening or closing of the pore. For instance, phosphorylation of tyrosine 247 appears as the key factor for the Cx43-channel closure. The ATP-dependent paracrine signaling by the Cx43-hemi-channel opening is also influenced by intracellular Ca^{2+}. The hemi-channel is opened by low and closed by high (<500 nM) concentration of Ca^{2+} and involves the RhoA GTPase activity and the actomyosin contractile network [51]. In autocrine activities, mitogen-activated protein kinase can phosphorylate Cx43, resulting in its interaction with cyclin E and in cyclin-dependent kinase 2 (CDK2) activity, thus influencing cell proliferation, for instance of smooth muscle cells [52]. Importantly, there is evidence from different cellular models that microtubule-dependent regulation of gap junctional communications, for example by Cx43, is involved in TGFβ signal transduction. Thus Cx43 positively regulates the TGFβ pathway by releasing sequestered SMADs from microtubules, increasing the level of phospho-SMAD2, its hetero-oligomerization, and activation as a transcription factor [53]. Whether and how such activities are important in feedback signaling from oocyte-secreted growth factors is currently unknown. Connexins can also modulate cell polarity and migration by control of microtubule dynamics [54]. Vice versa, intracellular interaction of Cx43 with microtubules facilitates transport and gap junction formation. Microtubules appear to enhance the assembly of gap junctions in the presence of cholesterol, and low density lipoprotein [55, 56]. Kinase activation can either effect an acute (within minutes) reduction of channel conductance and/or open probability. Prolonged activation may effect other cellular reactions including compromised connexin targeting/retention at gap junctions, and in some cases, altered gene expression. Many connexins undergo rapid synthesis/assembly and degradation, for example Cx43 has an unusually short half-life in cultured murine cells and tissues (reviewed by [57]). Gap junction channels formed of different connexins are differentially permeable to molecules based on size and molecular charge.

The connexin family comprises 21 isoforms in humans. Different connexins have been identified in porcine, ovine, bovine, mouse, and rat ovaries (reviewed by [58]). Connexins are expressed from the early stage of development in the mouse [59, 60]. Five connexin mRNAs were detected in human granulosa cells. Cx43 forms numerous gap junction-like plaques while Cx26, Cx30, Cx30.3, Cx32, and Cx40 appear to be restricted to the cytoplasm. This supports earlier findings that Cx43 is not the only gap junction protein present in granulosa cells of early preantral follicles, but it is the only one that makes a significant contribution to intercellular coupling (for reference, see [61]). Gap junctional conductance of human granulosa cells was significantly and positively correlated with Cx43 level and with embryo quality as judged by cleavage rate and morphology, and was significantly higher in patients who became pregnant than in those who did not [62], revealing the relevance of transcellular signaling in the somatic granulosa cell compartment for oocyte quality.

In fact, Cx43 is detectable in pregranulosa cells of primordial follicles, probably mediating the relationship between somatic cells [60]. The number of Cx43 gap junctions increases concomitantly with follicle development and, in particular, during the transition from the preantral to the antral stage. In the absence of Cx43 (termed gap junction protein 1, gene name in mouse is *gja1*), gap junctions between granulosa somatic cells do not form and folliculogenesis arrests at the unilaminar stage [59]. *Gja1*$^{-/-}$ mice die soon after birth whereas ovaries removed from prenatal Cx43 knockout mice placed under the kidney capsule of wild-type females can be sustained. However, follicles do not develop beyond the primary follicle stage and growth of oocytes is retarded [63, 64]. Oocytes recovered from these grafts failed to undergo meiotic maturation and fertilization. Since granulosa cell proliferation is arrested or impaired differentially in mice, depending on strain background, the cellular context and gene expression pattern may modulate activity [63, 65]. For instance, the homozygous *Gja1* null mutation causes arrest in the primary follicle stage on the C57BL/6 background [63], whereas some follicles can develop into antral stages when the same mutation is crossed into the CD1 background [65]. Targeted knockout of *gja1* in the oocyte by ZP3-promoter-driven Cre-Lox recombinanase expression caused ablation of Cx43 in the oocyte, but also a decrease in expression of this connexin in the surrounding somatic cells, with oogenesis appearing normal. However, the knockdown severely impaired implantation, suggesting that inefficient signaling between granulosa cells may have downstream effects on oocyte and embryo quality, and possibly maternal connexin may be involved in later events [58]. From analysis of the stage/age at which knockdown was functional in this model it appears that follicles that reached the primary stage are no longer dependent on Cx43 for their development [58]. Presence of Cx45 and Cx32 may be able to compensate for the loss of Cx43 (reviewed by [58]). From these and other studies, Cx43 has been proposed to represent the major mediator of granulosa–granulosa cell communication in vivo.

Cx43 turnover appears to be highly regulated by mitogen-activated protein kinase (MAPK)- and protein kinase C (PKC)-mediated phosphorylation in several cell types that are also implicated in keeping Cx43 hemi-channels closed and enhancing gap junction turnover [66]. It has been shown that MAPK phosphorylates Cx43 at serines 279 and 282 in granulosa cells of early follicles, and that this is involved in regulating follicle development [57]. Serines 255, 279, and 282 are phosphorylated directly by activated MAPK in epidermal growth factor (EGF)-treated cells with phosphorylation of one or both of the S279/S282 sites being sufficient to disrupt gap junctional communication (Figure 8.4) [67]. EGF treatment leads to internalization of Cx43 [66], potentially in a direct manner through phosphorylation of Cx43 at serines 279 and 282. In fact, Cx43 in primary and early secondary follicles appears predominately intracellular and relatively highly phosphorylated at serines 279 and 282. LH-induced gating mechanism of the gap junctions in rat ovarian follicles is in two steps, by a change in the phosphorylation state of the Cx43 protein, and a reduction of Cx43 protein level [68]. Analysis of transcription of six genes (*STAR*, *COX2*, *AREG*, *SCD1*, *CX43/GJA1*, and *SCD5*) in human cumulus from preovulatory follicles by real-time PCR showed that all excluding connexin 43 became increased at resumption of maturation [69], suggesting regulation of signaling between mural granulosa and cumulus granulosa cells by Cx43 is differentiation specific and occurs through different pathways. High levels of androgen reduce Cx43 expression and impair gap junction intercellular communication between human granulosa cells through the androgen receptors. This may play a role in polycystic ovary syndrome (PCOS) pathologies [70]. Furthermore, decreased Cx43 expression has been implicated in the increased granulosa cell apoptosis in acute hyperglycemia and chronic diabetes in mice [71] and apoptotic follicles in pig and bovine (for references, see [58]).

By contrast to Cx43 homotypic channels, Cx37 in oocytes forms gap junctions coupling the cumulus granulosa cells with the developing oocyte, thus linking the germline and somatic components of the follicle into a functional syncytium and allowing diffusional transfer of small molecules throughout folliculogenesis (reviewed by [61]) (Figure 8.4). In contrast to deficiency in Cx43, Cx37 (known as gap junction protein 4, gene *gja4*) deficiency in the mouse disrupts communication between the oocyte and the neighboring granulosa cells, leading to infertile females with ovaries devoid of Graafian follicles [72, 73]. Communication among the granulosa cells remained functional, as shown by fluorescently labeled neurobiotin transfer [72]. The oocyte is involved in inducing the formation of gap junctions containing Cx37 at the surface of granulosa cells such that heterotypic gap junctions composed of Cx37 and Cx43 can connect oocyte and granulosa cell (Figure 8.2) [74]. Thus Cx37 expression may be sufficient to establish gap junctional communication during folliculogenesis that allows for acquisition of oocyte meiotic competence and progression to metaphase II. This is supported by studies with chimeric ovaries in which follicle development and oocyte maturation were impaired when either wild-type oocytes and Cx43-deficient granulosa cells, or Cx37-deficient oocytes and wild-type granulosa cells were present, suggesting oocytes must express Cx37 that interacts with Cx43 for communication with granulosa cells [59]. In the human ovary, Cx37 is exclusively localized to oocytes of all follicle stages, and the estimated number of Cx37 gap junctions on the oolemma in follicles of stage 2 to stage 6 becomes increased in parallel to oocyte and follicle growth, reaching a maximum in the preantral stage. Acetylated α-tubulin and Cx37 double labeling revealed that the majority of Cx37 gap junctions, irrespective of follicle stage, were located on the outer surface of the oocyte cytoskeleton, demonstrating tight regulation in plaques and correlations to the intracytoplasmic cytoskeleton in the mouse oocyte [75]. Furthermore, communication via gap junctions between the oocyte and cumulus cells may also play a role in the regulation of chromatin remodeling and transcription during early stages of oocyte maturation, as for instance suggested by studies in bovine COCs [76]). When gap junctional functionality was experimentally interrupted, chromatin rapidly condensed, and RNA synthesis suddenly ceased in oocytes of COCs cultured in the presence of FSH [76]. Addition of a phosphodiesterase 3 inhibitor prevented chromatin changes, suggesting that gap junctional communication is essential to maintain a meiotic block (see below). Prolonging gap junctional coupling in COCs during oocyte culture before in vitro maturation enhanced the ability of early antral oocytes to undergo meiosis and early embryonic development [76]. In contrast, Cx37 protein (see below) was shown to be over 30% decreased in oocytes of a type 1 diabetic mouse model, pointing to the involvement of reduced gap junctional communication in decreased quality and impaired oocyte meiotic maturation in this pathology [77].

Presence of the cumulus and gap junctional communication is essential for maintenance of meiotic arrest. Thus, removal of the cumulus induces the spontaneous maturation of denuded oocytes [78]. Furthermore, gap junction inhibitors, such as carbenoxolone, induce resumption of meiosis in rat and mouse follicles [79, 80]. Initially it was believed that in vivo oocytes were kept in meiotic arrest by diffusion of cAMP from granulosa cells via gap junctions into the oocyte (e.g., [81]). This was suggested to render cAMP-dependent kinase active and prevent activation of maturation-promoting factor/Cdk1 (e.g., [82]). By now there is increasing evidence that cAMP originates mainly from Gs-coupled receptor GPR3 activation of adenylate cyclase within the oocyte ([83]; reviewed in Chapter 10) while cumulus-provided cGMP is essential to maintain phosphodiesterase PDE3A in oocytes in an inactive state and thereby prevents oocyte cAMP levels become critically lowered [80, 84]. Gap junctional communication is also essential for the initiation of resumption of maturation in response to gonadotropins, as shown in mice and cattle [73, 85]. Resumption of meiosis in oocytes in vivo has been found to coincide with a progressive interruption of cell-to-cell coupling following the gonadotropin surge [42]. In vitro oocyte–granulosa cell gap junctional coupling is abruptly decreased in a gonadotropin-dependent manner concurrent with the resumption of oocyte meiosis, as for instance demonstrated in porcine COC maturation (Figure 8.4) [86]. Cx43 became clustered to lipid rafts at the membrane concomitantly with GV breakdown (GVBD) in a gonadotropin-dependent manner. In this model and species it appears that the gonadotropin-dependent shutdown of junctional communication involves initially functional inactivation of Cx43 channels in lipid rafts, rather than removal of Cx43 from the cell surface [86]. At a later stage endocytosis might contribute to reduce gap junctional communication. Unfortunately, most in vitro models used to assess paracrine signaling in the COC do not fully retain and focus on preservation of physical interactions between the two cell types such that the relevance and role of TZPs and gap junctions in the oocyte–paracrine communication axis and gap junctional signaling feedback are still largely unknown [87]. However, undoubtedly the signaling is central to acquisition of maturational and high developmental potential of the oocyte. For instance, constitutively active Foxo3a in oocytes that is involved in regulation of primordial follicle arrest does not only dramatically reduce the expression of Bmp15, but also Cx37 and Cx43, and cell–cell coupling (Figure 8.4),

nd this causes retarded oocyte growth and follic-
ılar development, anovulation and infertility [88], onsistent with the mouse knockout models demon-strating the relevance of gap junctional signaling. njecting a fluorescent tracer into the oocyte has been ısed to assess junctional communication in response o LH [89]. Shortly after LH and epiregulin stim-ılation, relative fluorescence in mural/cumulus cells lecreased to 9% and 32% of the basal level, respec-ively. This suggests that epiregulin-induced signaling y the EGFR kinase contributes to the LH-induced neiotic resumption and is required for gap junction losure and decrease in follicle and oocyte cGMP (as ndicated in Figure 8.4). Since even 20 times higher piregulinand amphiregulin did not decrease fluores-ence levels as much as LH, there must be pathways part from the EGF-mediated ones that are involved n LH signaling [89]. For instance, a preovulatory lecrease in nitric oxide (NO) concentrations may also ontribute to the ovarian response to LH and to gap unction closure. NO interferes with LH-induced dis-uption of gap junctional communication as well as vith the decrease of the expression of Cx43 that may ıave a negative effect on MAPK activation and a posi-ive one on soluble guanylate cyclase [79]. NO appears lso involved in maintaining a physiologically inactive, quiescent" state in mitochondria in the subcortical ytoplasm of meiotically blocked oocytes retaining a ow inner membrane potential [38].

To conclude, the current status of research sug-gests that before the LH surge, cGMP is synthesized n the granulosa cells by the transmembrane guany-ate cyclase natriuretic peptide receptor 2 (NPR2) n response to the agonist C-type natriuretic pep-ide (CNP) (Figure 8.4). cGMP is transmitted from umulus to oocyte via gap junctions on TZPs and nvolved in meiotic arrest. The LH surge causes a lecrease in the amount of CNP, and in guanylate yclase activity of NPR2 [90] but also causes MAPK ctivation, phosphorylation of Cx43, and transient losure of gap junctions (Figure 8.4) [80]. Further-nore, alterations in the numbers and possibly activ-ty of actTZPs and mtTZPs contribute to modu-ation of oocyte–cumulus communication. Finally, umulus expansion physically decreases tight appo-ition and gap junctional communication within the OC. Thus several pathways contribute to resump-ion of meiosis, including phosphorylation of connex-ns and closure of gap junctions, while the kinetics and active retraction of mtTZPs may be a species-specific event.

Adherens junctions

The oocyte–granulosa cell interaction can also comprise adherens junctions, with transmembrane adhesion molecules binding to linker proteins that may anchor the adhesion complex to the cytoskeleton and mediate tight apposition (Figure 8.2). Cadherins and catenins form the adherens junctions between cells. Cadherins are connected to the actin cytoskeleton by αβ-catenins, and may act as foci for the transmission of cytoskeletal-mediated tension during cell motility and aggregation [91]. In many cell types, the cytoplasmic portion of E-cadherin interacts with catenins that mediate signaling events from the extracellular environment to the interior of the cell and from the attachment organization to the actin cytoskeleton. Thus, the cadherin family of transmembrane glycoproteins are particularly important for morphogenetic processes. N-cadherin exists in oocytes of primary follicles but later is exclusively found in granulosa cells particularly in growing follicles, possibly promoting proliferation and interactions among granulosa cells and interactions of granulosa cells with the oocyte. N-cadherin has been detected in rat granulosa cells in vivo [92] and in vitro [93, 94]. E-cadherin expression appears important for oocyte growth, and the acquisition of meiotic competence during gonad development in mice. Thus, E-cadherin appears stage-specifically expressed in folliculogenesis. In the hamster, E-cadherin expression was detected in oocytes of the neonatal ovary, but not in postnatal stages and in granulosa cells of preantral follicles or in later stages of follicle development. Alpha- and β-catenin are present in granulosa cells of all stages, but α-catenin becomes decreased at maturation and ovulation. Thus the catenins by interacting with the E-cadherin/N-cadherin may participate in the regulation of cytoskeletal structures and intracellular signaling between the oocyte and the granulosa cells, particularly in anchoring the granulosa cells to the zona pellucida and the oocyte in the early preantral stages of folliculogenesis [95]. Since apoptotic granulosa cells do not appear to express E-cadherin it is possible that expression of E-cadherin is important to maintain cell viability and thus to prevent apoptosis at the preantral stage [93, 95]. Beta-catenin is a prominent component of the WNT signaling pathway. WNT proteins comprise secreted, cysteine-rich glycoproteins involved in many processes in cell regulation. Studies in human cumulus suggest that WNT2 signals through its receptor FZD9 to regulate the β-catenin pathway in human cumulus cells, potentially recruiting the catenin into the plasma membrane and promoting the formation of adherens junctions. WNT2 stimulates proliferation in mouse granulosa cells, suggesting that it may universally act as a mitogen to promote follicle growth apart from roles in cell adhesion (reviewed by [96]). Gene expression microarray analysis of human cumulus suggests that the WNT–β-catenin pathway is differentially expressed in cumulus from lean controls and cumulus from lean PCOS patients, possibly contributing to the pathology [97]).

The cytoskeleton in interactions, and oocyte polarity and competence

Polymerization kinetics of microtubules can be regulated in numerous ways, for example by free α- and β-tubulin heterodimer concentration, presence of templates, Ran-GTP gradient, post-translational modifications of tubulin or of microtubule-associated proteins, including motor proteins as characteristic for spindle formation in mammalian oocytes (reviewed by [98]). Within the cellular context, the organization of microtubular networks by microtubule-organizing centers (MTOCs) is of relevance. Most somatic cells like the granulosa cells possess a major MTOC, the centrosome, consisting of a pair of centrioles surrounded by pericentriolar material [99]. The latter appears involved in anchoring and stabilization of microtubules. The oocyte does not contain pairs of centrioles as a major MTOC. Rather multiple MTOCs become recruited from the cytoplasm after GVBD and contribute to spindle formation (see Chapters 12 and 28). By contrast, the granulosa cells possess centriolar MTOCs and studies in mice suggest that they are involved in anchoring and stabilization of the TZP microtubules [34] and in polarization of the granulosa/cumulus cells that are next to and in direct contact with the oocytes [37].

Somatic cell contact appears to optimize oocyte quality during meiotic maturation by regulating the spatial organization and function of the meiotic spindle through actin-dependent mechanisms that enhance development [100]. In denuded oocytes the GV is centrally located in ooplasm and the meiosis I spindle, which is organized from a more centrally located ball of microtubular asters and chromosomes after the circular bivalent stage, has to move to the cortex for asymmetric cytokinesis and first polar body formation during in vitro maturation [98]. This and the anchoring of the metaphase II spindle at the cortex involves complex interactions between the chromatin-induced Ran-GTP gradient, the Arp2/3 complex, N-WASP, directional actin polymerization, and cytoplasmic streaming in murine oocytes (reviewed by [101]). Actin-driven chromosomal motility leads therefore to symmetry breaking in first and second meiotic division in mammalian meiotic oocytes [101]. Formin proteins nucleate actin and facilitate the elongation of actin filaments to generate long actin polymers. Formin-2 is expressed exclusively in oocytes and the nervous system in the mouse [102]. An actin meshwork exists throughout oogenesis but is absent in formin-2-null oocytes [103, 104]. Formin-2 also interacts with microtubules of the meiotic spindle and is required for spindle migration and polar body formation [105]. It is long known that spindle positioning and cortical cytoskeleton differ significantly between species such as human and mouse [106]. Both conserved and species-specific mechanisms of cellular organization in all mammals need to be explored further, but undoubtedly involve junctional signaling.

Cortical granule migration depends on the presence of microfilaments, while distribution of mitochondria involves the microtubules in in vitro maturing human oocytes [107]. Whether and how the microfilamentous and mitochondrial meshwork is influenced by the presence of TZPs and gap junction-associated organization of the oocyte cytoskeleton requires also further research. Confocal microscopic observations revealed that human oocytes obtained from PCOS patients and matured in vitro had a higher frequency of abnormal meiotic spindle and aberrant chromosomal alignment than in vivo matured oocytes [107]. Also, few immature oocytes from intracytoplasmic sperm injection (ICSI) cycles that are induced to mature in vivo without cumulus possess birefringent spindles [108] and a large percentage are aneuploid [109]. Aberrant up-regulation of mRNA of the human formin-2 (*FMN2*) and of another formin, *DIAPH2*, was detected in human oocytes of PCOS patients [110]. Apart from interactions between oocyte and cumulus that are mediated by oocyte-secreted factors and coordinate metabolism and gene expression in both compartments, absent signaling and organization of the cytoskeleton by gap junctions, cyclic ıucleotides, and TZPs may contribute to the inefficient n vitro maturation of immature oocytes and problems ·elated to certain pathologies such as PCOS.

Thus, in contrast to the in vitro situation, the GVs of in vivo grown oocytes in many species appear to be eccentrically localized [111]. In turn, spindle formaion occurs initially eccentrically in in vivo maturing nouse oocytes. This appears to rely on the organizaion of the cortical cytoskeleton and physical interacions between the oocyte and cumulus cells [100]. The organization of the cytoskeleton via elements that are anchored in the cortex and rely on contacts via TZPs and microtubular and actin cytoskeletal organization and organelle distribution appear therefore to conribute to efficient nuclear maturation, polar body fornation, and acquisition of high developmental potenial of the oocyte [100].

Optimizing ARTs and oocyte quality

Most bioassays for oocyte-secreted factors, and culures of isolated COCs in the presence of oocytesecreted factors such as GDF9, destroy or severely affect gap junctional communication [87]. Therefore, efforts have been established to prolong and retain oocyte–somatic cell dialog that is of significance for netabolic coupling, maintenance of polar organizaion, and for the regulation of stage-specific alterations in nucleotides controlling cell-cycle progresion/meiotic arrest. Unfortunately, roles of specific TZPs and junctions in the modulation of auto- and paracrine communication are still largely unknown. For instance, it is still unclear whether and which TZPs are enriched in the main receptors for oocyteecreted factors like BMPR-II, ALK4/5, and ALK6, and hereby may modulate communication stage specifically, although one can speculate from observations n different cell types that gap junctional communicaion and cytoskeletal organization contribute to mediate and amplify signaling.

An example that removal of the COC from its nornal environment during in vitro maturation dramatcally affects oocyte–granulosa cell dialog, maturation kinetics, and oocyte quality in a non-human primate, he marmoset, shows that the rate of nuclear maturaion is much faster for in vitro maturing oocytes in COCs compared with in vivo maturation. ActTZPs decreased after human chorionic gonadotropin (hCG) administration in the in vivo situation, and mtTZPs disappeared rapidly within the first three hours after the ovulatory stimulus. In contrast mtTZPs of oocytes in COCs decreased slowly during in vitro maturation. Embryo development was improved when maturation time was increased, implying that there may be correlations between turnover/stability of TZPs, nuclear maturation kinetics, and oocyte quality [29].

In conclusion, in order to obtain high quality oocytes, we must improve conditions to physically maintain intercellular signaling and communication. Specifically, special attention should be aimed at allowing temporally and spatially regulated alterations in cell polarization, cytoskeleton, TZPs, and gap junctional communication during follicle culture and oocyte maturation; in particular we should aim to maintain or even improve the regulation of junctional signaling required for normal development of the follicle, granulosa cell activity, and oocyte acquisition or maintenance of high developmental competence. This appears of particular relevance in cryopreservation of ovarian tissue, follicles, and oocytes when slow-cooling or vitrification protocols and handling may temporarily or terminally interfere with tight cell apposition, TZP integrity, and gap junction functionality, or in certain pathologies when there is no option for in vivo maturation due to risk of ovarian hyperstimulation syndrome (OHSS).

Conclusions

Despite the long-known critical role of granulosa cell/oocyte interactions in meiotic arrest, only in recent years some of the molecular players underlying bidirectional signaling, for instance oocytesecreted factors and cumulus-derived metabolites and nucleotides, have been identified, while the structural basis of the interactions is still only partially understood. In the future it will be of critical importance to develop methods to maintain and support follicular integrity for follicle and oocyte maturation in vitro. In particular, the integrity and spatial–temporal alterations in TZPs and junctional communication and the stage-specific cytoskeletal alterations ultimately optimizing the cell-to-cell dialog and supporting formation of a high quality oocyte in vivo as in vitro should be analyzed in efforts to improve fertility preservation and outcomes in ART, particularly in certain pathologies that relate to disturbed follicular and oocyte maturation. Furthermore, basic research on regulation of growth factor and receptor-mediated signaling, morphokinetic events in regulation of the cytoskeleton, and spatial distribution of cell components that influence ultimately embryo developmental capacity after fertilization will provide information that can be used in developing novel therapeutic strategies, improve counseling of patients, and design personalized treatments but will also be helpful in identifying non-invasive markers for oocyte quality, for instance in cumulus. Thus it is no surprise to find factors that are involved in signal transduction as well as in interactions with scaffolding proteins that may also bind and regulate components of the cytoskeleton and modulate calcium signaling as cumulus markers of high developmental capacity of human oocytes (for recent discussion, see [112]). Future work should focus on understanding the localized roles of modifications in subcellular structures in an effort to correlate the molecular composition and signaling networks with the stage-specific morphological alterations in oocytesand granulosa cells during folliculogenesis from the primordial to the large antral stage and oocyte maturation and ovulation that eventually will result in the production of a healthy oocyte and child.

References

1. Eppig JJ. Oocyte control of ovarian follicular development and function in mammals. *Reproduction* 2001; **122**: 829–38.
2. Gilchrist RB. Recent insights into oocyte-follicle cell interactions provide opportunities for the development of new approaches to *in vitro* maturation. *Reprod Fertil Dev* 2011; **23**: 23–31.
3. Dong J, Albertini DF, Nishimori K, *et al.* Growth differentiation factor-9 is required during early ovarian folliculogenesis. *Nature* 1996; **383**: 531–5.
4. Galloway SM, McNatty KP, Cambridge LM, *et al.* Mutations in an oocyte-derived growth factor gene (BMP15) cause increased ovulation rate and infertility in a dosage-sensitive manner. *Nat Genet* 2000; **25**: 279–83.
5. Packer AI, Hsu YC, Besmer P, Bachvarova RF. The ligand of the c-kit receptor promotes oocyte growth. *Dev Biol* 1994; **161**: 194–205.
6. Elvin JA, Yan C, Wang P, Nishimori K, Matzuk MM. Molecular characterization of the follicle defects in the growth differentiation factor 9-deficient ovary. *Mol Endocrinol* 1999; **13**: 1018–34.
7. Wen J, Zhang H, Li G, *et al.* PAR6, a potential marker for the germ cells selected to form primordial follicles in mouse ovary. *PLoS One* 2009; **4**: e7372.
8. Mora JM, Fenwick MA, Castle L, *et al.* Characterization and significance of adhesion and junction-related proteins in mouse ovarian follicles. *Biol Reprod* 2012; **86**: 1–14.
9. Berkholtz CB, Shea LD, Woodruff TK. Extracellular matrix functions in follicle maturation. *Semin Reprod Med* 2006; **24**: 262–9.
10. Da Silva-Buttkus P, Jayasooriya GS, Mora JM, *et al.* Effect of cell shape and packing density on granulosa cell proliferation and formation of multiple layers during early follicle development in the ovary. *J Cell Sci* 2008; **121**: 3890–900.
11. Bleil JD, Wassarman PM: Structure and function of the zona pellucida: identification and characterization of the proteins of the mouse oocyte's zona pellucida. *Dev Biol* 1980; **76**: 185–202.
12. Boja ES, Hoodbhoy T, Fales HM, Dean J: Structural characterization of native mouse zona pellucida proteins using mass spectrometry. *J Biol Chem* 2003; **278**: 34189–202.
13. Lefievre L, Conner SJ, Salpekar A, *et al.* Four zona pellucida glycoproteins are expressed in the human. *Hum Reprod* 2004; **19**: 1580–6.
14. Montag M, Köster M, van der Ven K, van der Ven H. Gamete competence assessment by polarizing optics in assisted reproduction. *Hum Reprod Update* 2011; **17**: 654–66.
15. Shen Y, Stalf T, Mehnert C, Eichenlaub-Ritter U, Tinneberg HR. High magnitude of light retardation by the zona pellucida is associated with conception cycles *Hum Reprod* 2005; **20**: 1596–606.
16. Navarro-Costa P, Correia SC, Gouveia-Oliveira A, *et al.* Effects of mouse ovarian tissue cryopreservation on granulosa cell-oocyte interaction. *Hum Reprod* 2005; **20**: 1607–14.
17. Trapphoff T, El Hajj N, Zechner U, Haaf T, Eichenlaub-Ritter U. DNA integrity, growth pattern, spindle formation, chromosomal constitution and imprinting patterns of mouse oocytes from vitrified pre-antral follicles. *Hum Reprod* 2010; **25**: 3025–42.
18. Schroeder AC, Schultz RM, Kopf GS, *et al.* Fetuin inhibits zona pellucida hardening and conversion of ZP2 to ZP2f during spontaneous mouse oocyte maturation *in vitro* in the absence of serum. *Biol Reprod* 1990; **43**: 891–7.
19. Motta PM, Makabe S, Naguro T, Correr S. Oocyte follicle cells association during development of human ovarian follicle. A study by high resolution scanning and transmission electron microscopy. *Arch Histol Cytol* 1994; **57**: 369 94.
20. Zuccotti M, Merico V, Cecconi S, Redi CA, Garagna S. What does it take to make a developmentally competent mammalian egg? *Hum Reprod Update* 2011; **17**: 525–40.

21. Hertig AT, Adams EC. Studies on the human oocyte and its follicle. I. Ultrastructural and histochemical observations on the primordial follicle stage. *J Cell Biol* 1967; **34**: 647–75.

22. Larsen WJ, Wert SE, Brunner GD. Differential modulation of rat follicle cell gap junction populations at ovulation. *Dev Biol* 1987; **122**: 61–71.

23. Plancha CE, Albertini DF. Hormonal regulation of meiotic maturation in the hamster oocyte involves a cytoskeleton-mediated process. *Biol Reprod* 1994; **51**: 852–64.

24. Allworth AE, Albertini DF. Meiotic maturation in cultured bovine oocytes is accompanied by remodelling of the cumulus cell cytoskeleton. *Dev Biol* 1993; **158**: 101–12.

25. Suzuki H, Jeong BS, Yang X. Dynamic changes of cumulus-oocyte cell communication during *in vitro* maturation of porcine oocytes. *Biol Reprod* 2000; **63**: 723–9.

26. de Prada JK, Hill DL, Chaffin CL, VandeVoort CA. Nuclear maturation and structural components of nonhuman primate cumulus-oocyte complexes during *in vivo* and *in vitro* maturation. *Fertil Steril* 2009; **91**: 2043–50.

27. Saxton WM, Hollenbeck PJ. The axonal transport of mitochondria. *J Cell Sci* 2012; **125**: 2095–104.

28. Barrett SL, Shea LD, Woodruff TK. Noninvasive index of cryorecovery and growth potential for human follicles *in vitro*. *Biol Reprod* 2010; **82**: 1180–9.

29. Makabe S, Naguro T, Stallone T. Oocyte–follicle cell interactions during ovarian follicle development, as seen by high resolution scanning and transmission electron microscopy in humans. *Microscopy Res Tech* 2006; **69**: 436–49.

30. Bulinski JC, Gundersen GG. Stabilization of post-translational modification of microtubules during cellular morphogenesis. *Bioessays* 1991; **13**: 285–93.

31. Janke C, Bulinski JC. Post-translational regulation of the microtubule cytoskeleton: mechanisms and functions. *Nat Rev Mol Cell Biol* 2011; **12**: 773–86.

32. de Pennart H, Houliston E, Maro B. Post-translational modifications of tubulin and the dynamics of microtubules in mouse oocytes and zygotes. *Biol Cell* 1988; **64**: 375–8.

33. Can A, Albertini DF. M-phase specific centrosome-microtubule alterations induced by the fungicide MBC in human granulosa cells. *Mutat Res* 1997; **373**: 139–51.

34. Albertini DF, Combelles CM, Benecchi E, Carabatsos MJ. Cellular basis for paracrine regulation of ovarian follicle development. *Reproduction* 2001; **121**: 647–53.

35. Carabatsos MJ, Elvin J, Matzuk MM, Albertini DF. Characterization of oocyte and follicle development in growth differentiation factor-9-deficient mice. *Dev Biol* 1998; **204**: 373–84.

36. Yi K, Li R. Actin cytoskeleton in cell polarity and asymmetric division during mouse oocyte maturation. *Cytoskeleton* 2012; **69**: 727–37, doi: 10.1002/cm.21048.

37. Combelles CM, Carabatsos MJ, Kumar TR, Matzuk MM, Albertini DF. Hormonal control of somatic cell oocyte interactions during ovarian follicle development. *Mol Reprod Dev* 2004; **69**: 347–55.

38. Van Blerkom J, Davis P, Thalhammer V. Regulation of mitochondrial polarity in mouse and human oocytes: the influence of cumulus derived nitric oxide. *Mol Hum Reprod* 2008; **14**: 431–44.

39. Li L, Baibakov B, Dean J. A subcortical maternal complex essential for preimplantation mouse embryogenesis. *Dev Cell* 2008; **15**: 416–25.

40. Perkins GA, Goodenough DA, Sosinsky GE. Formation of the gap junction intercellular channel requires a 30 degree rotation for interdigitating two apposing connexons. *J Mol Biol* 1997; **277**: 171–7.

41. Arellano RO, Martínez-Torres A, Garay E. Ionic currents activated via purinergic receptors in the cumulus cell-enclosed mouse oocyte. *Biol Reprod* 2002; **67**: 837–46.

42. Bornslaeger EA, Schultz RM. Regulation of mouse oocyte maturation: effect of elevating cumulus cell cAMP on oocyte cAMP levels. *Biol Reprod* 1985; **33**: 698–704.

43. Salustri A, Petrungaro S, De Felici M, Conti M, Siracusa G. Effect of follicle-stimulating hormone on cyclic adenosine monophosphate level and on meiotic maturation in mouse cumulus cell-enclosed oocytes cultured *in vitro*. *Biol Reprod* 1985; **33**: 797–802.

44. Norris RP, Ratzan WJ, Freudzon M, *et al.* Cyclic GMP from the surrounding somatic cells regulates cyclic AMP and meiosis in the mouse oocyte. *Development* 2009; **136**: 1869–78.

45. Heller DT, Cahill DM, Schultz RM. Biochemical studies of mammalian oogenesis: metabolic cooperativity between granulosa cells and growing mouse oocytes. *Dev Biol* 1981; **84**: 455–64.

46. Eppig JJ, Pendola FL, Wigglesworth K, Pendola JK. Mouse oocytes regulate metabolic cooperativity between granulosa cells and oocytes: amino acid transport. *Biol Reprod* 2005; **73**: 351–7.

47. Brower PT, Schultz RM. Intercellular communication between granulosa cells and mouse oocytes: existence and possible nutritional role during oocyte growth. *Dev Biol* 1982; **90**: 144–53.

48. Moor RM, Smith MW, Dawson RM. Measurement of intercellular coupling between oocytes and cumulus cells using intracellular markers. *Exp Cell Res* 1980; **126**: 15–29.

49. Solan JL, Lampe PD. Connexin43 phosphorylation: structural changes and biological effects. *Biochem J* 2009; **419**: 261–72.

50. Ponsaerts R, D'hondt C, Hertens F, *et al.* RhoA GTPase switch controls Cx43-hemichannel activity through the contractile system. *PLoS One* 2012; **7**: e42074.

51. Ponsaerts R, Wang N, Himpens B, Leybaert L, Bultynck G. The contractile system as a negative regulator of the connexin 43 hemichannel. *Biol Cell* 2012; **104**: 367–77.

52. Nakamoto RK, Koval M, Lo CW, *et al.* MAPK phosphorylation of connexin 43 promotes binding of cyclin E and smooth muscle cell proliferation. *Circ Res* 2012; **111**: 201–11.

53. Dai P, Nakagami T, Tanaka H, Hitomi T, Takamatsu T. Cx43 mediates TGF-β signaling through competitive Smads binding to microtubules. *Mol Biol Cell* 2007; **18**: 2264–73.

54. Francis R, Xu X, Park H, *et al.* Connexin43 modulates cell polarity and directional cell migration by regulating microtubule dynamics. *PLoS One* 2011; **6**: e26379.

55. Johnson RG, Meyer RA, Li XR, *et al.* Gap junctions assemble in the presence of cytoskeletal inhibitors, but enhanced assembly requires microtubules. *Exp Cell Res* 2002; **275**: 67–80.

56. Paulson AF, Lampe PD, Meyer RA, *et al.* Cyclic AMP and LDL trigger a rapid enhancement in gap junction assembly through a stimulation of connexin trafficking. *J Cell Sci* 2000; **113**: 3037–49.

57. Dyce PW, Norris RP, Lampe PD, Kidder GM. Phosphorylation of serine residues in the C-terminal cytoplasmic tail of connexin43 regulates proliferation of ovarian granulosa cells. *J Membr Biol* 2012; **245**: 291–301.

58. Gershon E, Plaks V, Dekel N. Gap junctions in the ovary: expression, localization and function. *Mol Cell Endocrinol* 2008; **282**: 18–25.

59. Gittens JE, Kidder GM. Differential contributions of connexin37 and connexin43 to oogenesis revealed in chimeric reaggregated mouse ovaries. *J Cell Sci* 2005; **118**: 5071–8.

60. Gittens JE, Barr KJ, Vanderhyden BC, Kidder GM. Interplay between paracrine signaling and gap junctional communication in ovarian follicles. *J Cell Sci* 2005; **118**: 113–22.

61. Kidder GM, Vanderhyden BC. Bidirectional communication between oocytes and follicle cells: ensuring oocyte developmental competence. *Can J Physiol Pharmacol* 2010; **88**: 399–413.

62. Wang HX, Tong D, El-Gehani F, Tekpetey FR, Kidder GM. Connexin expression and gap junctional coupling in human cumulus cells: contribution to embryo quality. *J Cell Mol Med* 2009; **13**: 972–84.

63. Ackert CL, Gittens JE, O'Brien MJ, Eppig JJ, Kidder GM. Intercellular communication via connexin43 gap junctions is required for ovarian folliculogenesis in the mouse. *Dev Biol* 2001; **233**: 258–70.

64. Juneja SC, Barr KJ, Enders GC, Kidder GM. Defects in the germ line and gonads of mice lacking connexin43. *Biol Reprod* 1999; **60**: 1263–70.

65. Tong D, Gittens JEI, Kidder GM, Bai D. Patch clamp study reveals that the importance of connexin43-mediated gap junctional communication for ovarian folliculogenesis is strain specific in the mouse. *Am J Physiol Cell Physiol* 2006; **290**: 290–7.

66. Leithe E, Rivedal E. Ubiquitination and down-regulation of gap junction protein connexin-43 in response to 12-O-tetradecanoylphorbol 13-acetate treatment. *J Biol Chem* 2004; **279**: 50089–96.

67. Warn-Cramer BJ, Cottrell GT, Burt JM, Lau AF. Regulation of connexin-43 gap junctional intercellular communication by mitogen-activated protein kinase. *J Biol Chem* 1998; **273**: 9188–96.

68. Granot I, Dekel N. Phosphorylation and expression of connexin-43 ovarian gap junction protein are regulated by luteinizing hormone. *J Biol Chem* 1994; **269**: 30502–9.

69. Feuerstein P, Cadoret V, Dalbies-Tran R, *et al.* Gene expression in human cumulus cells: one approach to oocyte competence. *Hum Reprod* 2007; **22**: 3069–77.

70. Wu CH, Yang JG, Yang JJ, *et al.* Androgen excess down-regulates connexin43 in a human granulosa cell line. *Fertil Steril* 2010; **94**: 2938–41.

71. Chang AS, Dale AN, Moley KH. Maternal diabetes adversely affects preovulatory oocyte maturation, development, and granulosa cell apoptosis. *Endocrinology* 2005; **146**: 2445–53.

72. Simon AM, Goodenough DA, Li E, Paul DL. Female infertility in mice lacking connexin 37. *Nature* 1997; **385**: 525–9.

73. Carabatsos MJ, Sellitto C, Goodenough DA, Albertini DF. Oocyte-granulosa cell heterologous gap junctions are required for the coordination of nuclear and cytoplasmic meiotic competence. *Dev Biol* 2000; **226**: 167–79.

74. Veitch GI, Gittens JE, Shao Q, Laird DW, Kidder GM. Selective assembly of connexin37 into heterocellular

gap junctions at the oocyte/granulosa cell interface. *J Cell Sci* 2004; **117**: 2699–707.

75. Teilmann SC. Differential expression and localisation of connexin-37 and connexin-43 in follicles of different stages in the 4-week-old mouse ovary. *Mol Cell Endocrinol* 2005; **234**: 27–35.

76. Luciano AM, Franciosi F, Modina SC, Lodde V. Gap junction-mediated communications regulate chromatin remodeling during bovine oocyte growth and differentiation through cAMP-dependent mechanism(s). *Biol Reprod* 2011; **85**: 1252–9.

77. Ratchford AM, Esguerra CR, Moley KH. Decreased oocyte-granulosa cell gap junction communication and connexin expression in a type 1 diabetic mouse model. *Mol Endocrinol* 2008; **22**: 2643–54.

78. Pincus G, Enzmann EV. The comparative behavior of mammalian eggs *in vivo* and *in vitro* : I. The activation of ovarian eggs. *J Exp Med* 1935; **62**: 665–75.

79. Sela-Abramovich S, Galiani D, Nevo N, Dekel N. Inhibition of rat oocyte maturation and ovulation by nitric oxide: mechanism of action. *Biol Reprod* 2008; **78**: 1111–18.

80. Norris RP, Freudzon M, Mehlmann LM, *et al.* Luteinizing hormone causes MAP kinase-dependent phosphorylation and closure of connexin 43 gap junctions in mouse ovarian follicles: one of two paths to meiotic resumption. *Development* 2008; **135**: 3229–38.

81. Sherizly I, Galiani D, Dekel N. Regulation of oocyte maturation: communication in the rat cumulus-oocyte complex. *Hum Reprod* 1988; **3**: 761–6.

82. Webb RJ, Marshall F, Swann K, Carroll J. Follicle-stimulating hormone induces a gap junction-dependent dynamic change in [cAMP] and protein kinase A in mammalian oocytes. *Dev Biol* 2002; **246**: 441–54.

83. DiLuigi A, Weitzman VN, Pace MC, *et al.* Meiotic arrest in human oocytes is maintained by a Gs signaling pathway. *Biol Reprod* 2008; **78**: 667–72.

84. Vaccari S, Weeks JL, II, Hsieh M, Menniti FS, Conti M. Cyclic GMP signaling is involved in the luteinizing hormone-dependent meiotic maturation of mouse oocytes. *Biol Reprod* 2009; **81**: 595–604.

85. Vozzi C, Formenton A, Chanson A, *et al.* Involvement of connexin 43 in meiotic maturation of bovine oocytes. *Reproduction* 2001; **122**: 619–28.

86. Sasseville' M, Gagnon MC, Guillemette C, *et al.* Regulation of gap junctions in porcine cumulus-oocyte complexes: contributions of granulosa cell contact, gonadotropins, and lipid rafts. *Mol Endocrinol* 2009; **23**: 700–10.

87. Gilchrist RB, Lane M, Thompson JG. Oocyte-secreted factors: regulators of cumulus cell function and oocyte quality. *Hum Reprod Update* 2008; **14**: 159–77.

88. Liu L, Rajareddy S, Reddy P, *et al.* Infertility caused by retardation of follicular development in mice with oocyte-specific expression of Foxo3a. *Development* 2007; **134**: 199–209.

89. Norris RP, Freudzon M, Nikolaev VO, Jaffe LA. Epidermal growth factor receptor kinase activity is required for gap junction closure and for part of the decrease in ovarian follicle cGMP in response to LH. *Reproduction* 2010; **140**: 655–62.

90. Robinson JW, Zhang M, Shuhaibar LC, *et al.* Luteinizing hormone reduces the activity of the NPR2 guanylyl cyclase in mouse ovarian follicles, contributing to the cyclic GMP decrease that promotes resumption of meiosis in oocytes. *Dev Biol* 2012; **366**: 308–16.

91. Dean DM, Morgan JR. Cytoskeletal-mediated tension modulates the directed self-assembly of microtissues. *Tissue Eng* 2008; **14**: 1989–97.

92. Farookhi R, Geng CH, MacCalman CD, Blaschuk OW. Hormonal regulation of N-cadherin mRNA levels in rat granulosa cells. *Ann NY Acad Science* 1997; **816**: 165–72.

93. Peluso JJ, Pappalardo A, Trolice MP. N-cadherin-mediated cell contact inhibits granulosa cell apoptosis in a progesterone-independent manner *Endocrinology* 1996; **137**: 1196–203.

94. Trolice MP, Pappalardo A, Peluso JJ. Basic fibroblast growth factor and N-cadherin maintain rat granulosa cell and ovarian surface epithelial cell viability by stimulating the tyrosine phosphorylation of the fibroblast growth factor receptors. *Endocrinology* 1997; **138**: 107–13.

95. Sundfeldt K, Piontkewitz Y, Billig H, Hedin L. E-cadherin–catenin complex in the rat ovary: cell-specific expression during folliculogenesis and luteal formation. *J Reprod Fertil* 2000; **118**: 375–85.

96. Wang HX, Li TY, Kidder GM. WNT2 regulates DNA synthesis in mouse granulosa cells through beta-catenin. *Biol Reprod* 2010; **82**: 865–75.

97. Kenigsberg S, Bentov Y, Chalifa-Caspi V, *et al.* Gene expression microarray profiles of cumulus cells in lean and overweight-obese polycystic ovary syndrome patients. *Mol Hum Reprod* 2009; **15**: 89–103.

98. Dumont J, Desai A. Acentrosomal spindle assembly and chromosome segregation during oocyte meiosis. *Trends Cell Biol* 2012; **22**: 241–9.

99. Nigg EA, Stearns T. The centrosome cycle: centriole biogenesis, duplication and inherent asymmetries. *Nat Cell Biol* 2011; **13**: 1154–60.

100. Barrett SL, Albertini DF. Cumulus cell contact during oocyte maturation in mice regulates meiotic spindle positioning and enhances developmental competence. *J Assist Reprod Genet* 2010; **27**: 29–39.

101. Verlhac MH. Spindle positioning: going against the actin flow. *Nat Cell Biol* 2011; **13**: 1183–5.

102. Dumont J, Million K, Sunderland K, *et al.* Formin-2 is required for spindle migration and for the late steps of cytokinesis in mouse oocytes. *Dev Biol* 2007; **301**: 254–65.

103. Schuh M, Ellenberg J. A new model for asymmetric spindle positioning in mouse oocytes. *Curr Biol* 2008; **18**: 1986–92.

104. Azoury J, Lee KW, Georget V, *et al.* Spindle positioning in mouse oocytes relies on a dynamic meshwork of actin filaments. *Curr Biol* 2008; **18**: 1514–19.

105. Kwon S, Shin H, Lim HJ. Dynamic interaction of formin proteins and cytoskeleton in mouse oocytes during meiotic maturation. *Mol Hum Reprod* 2011; **17**: 317–27.

106. Pickering SJ, Johnson MH, Braude PR, Houliston E. Cytoskeletal organization in fresh, aged and spontaneously activated human oocytes. *Hum Reprod* 1988; **3**: 978–89.

107. Liu S, Li Y, Feng HL, *et al.* Dynamic modulation of cytoskeleton during *in vitro* maturation in human oocytes. *Am J Obstet Gynecol* 2010; **203**: e1–7.

108. Shen Y, Betzendahl I, Tinneberg HR, Eichenlaub-Ritter U. Enhanced polarizing microscopy as a new tool in aneuploidy research in oocytes. *Mutat Res* 2008; **651**: 131–40.

109. Magli MC, Ferraretti AP, Crippa A, *et al.* First meiosis errors in immature oocytes generated by stimulated cycles. *Fertil Steril* 2006; **86**: 629–35.

110. Wood JR, Dumesic DA, Abbott DH, Strauss JF. Molecular abnormalities in oocytes from women with polycystic ovary syndrome revealed by microarray analysis. *J Clin Endocrinol Metab* 2007; **92**: 705–13.

111. Albertini DF, Barrett SL. The developmental origins of mammalian oocyte polarity. *Semin Cell Dev Biol* 2004; **15**: 599–606.

112. Feuerstein P, Puard V, Chevalier C, *et al.* Genomic assessment of human cumulus cell marker genes as predictors of oocyte developmental competence: impact of various experimental factors. *PLoS One* 2012; 7(7): e40449.

Chapter 9

Differential gene expression mediated by oocyte–granulosa cell communication

Saiichi Furukawa and Koji Sugiura

Introduction

The transition of preantral to antral follicles is accompanied by differentiation of preantral granulosa cells into two spatially and functionally distinct populations. Those located in close proximity to oocytes differentiate into cumulus cells and those lining the follicular wall differentiate into mural granulosa cells. Although many transcripts are expressed in common, there are subsets of differentially expressed transcripts that probably determine the different characteristics between cumulus and mural granulosa cells (summarized in Table 9.1). For example in mice, cumulus cells express higher levels of transcripts encoding amino acid transporters [1] and glycolytic enzymes when compared with mural granulosa cells [2]. This reflects the specialized role of cumulus cells in supporting oocyte development; cumulus cells provide oocytes with nutrients such as amino acids [3, 4] and substrates for energy production [5, 6]. In addition, reflecting their differences in steroidogenic capabilities, the expression levels of transcripts encoding steroidogenic enzymes are different between rat cumulus and mural granulosa cells [7, 8]. Likewise, mural granulosa cells exhibit a higher steady-state level of *Lhcgr* mRNA, which encodes luteinizing hormone (LH)/choriogonadotropin (CG) receptor, whereas it is barely detectable in cumulus cells [8–10]. This differential *Lhcgr* transcript expression may explain, at least in part, the differential responses to the LH surge between cumulus and mural granulosa cells. After the LH surge, while mural granulosa cells differentiate into luteal cells, cumulus cells undergo the cumulus expansion process which is required for normal ovulation [11]. Thus, cumulus and mural granulosa cells express many different transcripts, and proper coordination of the differential gene expression between the two granulosa cell populations is critical for normal follicular development and ovulation processes.

Emerging evidence shows the active role of oocytes in coordinating the differential gene expression between cumulus and mural granulosa cells. Oocyte-derived paracrine factors promote the expression of transcripts encoding amino acid transporters (Table 9.1) [1] and glycolytic enzymes in cumulus cells [2]. Therefore, the specialized role of cumulus cells in supporting oocyte development depends on the oocytes themselves. Likewise, oocytes suppress *Lhcgr* expression in cumulus cells before the LH surge [12]. This *Lhcgr* suppression is probably important in preventing cumulus cells from undergoing luteinization in response to LH. After the LH surge, oocyte-derived paracrine factors are required to enable cumulus cell-specific expression of the transcripts that are required for the normal cumulus expansion process [13]. Therefore, the ability of oocytes to coordinate differential gene expression within follicles appears essential for normal follicular development and ovulation processes. In fact, genetic models have revealed that some of the oocyte-derived paracrine factors have profound effects on follicular development and female fertility.

This chapter will review, firstly, the role of oocyte-derived paracrine factors in determining female fertility, and secondly, the current state of knowledge of the differential gene expression between cumulus and mural granulosa cells and the role of oocytes in coordinating the differential gene expression between these two granulosa cell populations. Although several animal models have been studied in this regard, we will mainly focus on the knowledge that has been acquired using rodent models.

Biology and Pathology of the Oocyte, 2nd edn., ed. Alan Trounson, Roger Gosden, and Ursula Eichenlaub-Ritter.
Published by Cambridge University Press.

Table 9.1. List of transcripts which are differentially expressed between cumulus and mural granulosa cells before the luteinizing hormone (LH) surge in mice

	Symbol	Name	Enriched in	Regulation by oocytes	References
	Lhcgr	Luteinizing hormone/choriogonadotropin receptor	MG	Yes	Eppig *et al.*, 1997 [12]
	Kitl	Kit ligand	MG	Yes	Joyce *et al.*, 1999 [76]
	Amh	Anti-Müllerian hormone	CC	Yes	Salmon *et al.*, 2004 [77]
	Ar	Androgen receptor	CC	Yes	Daiz *et al.*, 2007 [63]
	Cd34	CD34 antigen	MG	Yes	Daiz *et al.*, 2007 [63]
	Cyp11a1	Cytochrome P450, family 11, subfamily a, polypeptide 1	MG	Yes	Daiz *et al.*, 2007 [63]
Amino acid transporters					
	Slc38a3	Solute carrier family 38, member 3	CC	Yes	Eppig *et al.*, 2005 [1]
	Slc38a4	Solute carrier family 38, member 4	CC	Yes	Sugiura and Eppig, unpublished, 2005
	Slc38a5	Solute carrier family 38, member 5	CC	Yes	Sugiura and Eppig, unpublished, 2005
Glycolytic enzymes					Sugiura *et al.*, 2005 [2]
	Pfkp	Phosphofructokinase, platelet	CC	Yes	
	Ldha	Lactate dehydrogenase A	CC	Yes	
	Aldoa	Aldolase A, fructose-bisphosphate	CC	Yes	
	Eno1	Enolase 1, alpha non-neuron	CC	Yes	
	Pkm2	Pyruvate kinase, muscle	CC	Yes	
	Tpi	Triosephosphate isomerase 1	CC	Yes	
Cholesterol biosynthetic enzymes					Su *et al.*, 2008 [29]
	Mvk	Mevalonate kinase	CC	Yes	
	Pmvk	Phosphomevalonate kinase	CC	Yes	
	Fdps	Farnesyl diphosphate synthetase	CC	Yes	
	Sqle	Squalene epoxidase	CC	Yes	
	Cyp51	Cytochrome P450, family 51	CC	Yes	
	Sc4mol	Sterol-C4-methyl oxidase-like	CC	Yes	
	Ebp	Phenylalkylamine Ca antagonist (emopamil) binding protein	CC	Yes	
BMP antagonists					Sugiura *et al.*, 2009 [32]
	Grem2	Gremlin 2 homolog	MG	Yes*	
	Nog	Noggin	CC	Yes	
	Twsg1	Twisted gastrulation homolog 1	MG	No	
SMAD inhibitors					Sugiura *et al.*, 2009 [32]
	Smad7	MAD homolog 7	CC	No	
	Tob1	Transducer of ErbB-2.1	MG	No	
	Tob2	Transducer of ERBB2, 2	MG	No	
Receptor tyrosine kinase inhibitor					Sugiura *et al.*, 2009 [32]
	Spry2	Sprouty homolog 2	MG	Yes	
Co-regulator for nuclear receptors					Sugiura *et al.*, 2010 [48]
	Nrip1	Nuclear receptor interacting protein 1	MG	Yes	
Oocyte meiotic arrest (cGMP production in cumulus cells)					Zhang *et al.*, 2010 [41]
	Nppc	Natriuretic peptide type C	MG	ND	
	Npr2	Natriuretic peptide receptor 2	CC	Yes	

BMP, bone morphogenetic protein; CC, cumulus cells: MG, mural granulosa cells.
ND, not determined; *, expression was enriched in MG; however, it is promoted by oocytes in vitro.

Oocyte-derived paracrine factors

Mammalian oocytes produce two families of growth factors: the transforming growth factor beta (TGFβ) superfamily and fibroblast growth factors (FGFs). The functions of these growth factors in regulating female fertility are discussed briefly in the following section.

TGFβ superfamily

Growth differentiation factor 9 (GDF9), a member of the TGFβ superfamily, is the first oocyte-derived paracrine factor identified as indispensable for normal follicle growth and female fertility in mice [14]. While male mice deficient in *Gdf9* (*Gdf9*$^{-/-}$) exhibited a normal fertility phenotype, female *Gdf9*-null mice are completely infertile. In the *Gdf9*$^{-/-}$ ovary, folliculogenesis is blocked at the primary follicle stage, suggesting that GDF9 is required for the transition from primary to secondary follicles [14]. In fact, recombinant GDF9 promotes primary follicles to develop into early antral follicles in rat and human ovaries [15–17]. This indicates that the role of GDF9 in regulating follicular development is conserved among mammalian species. Interestingly, the follicular block in *Gdf9*-null mice appears to be attributable, at least in part, to the failure of *Gdf9*-deficient oocytes to suppress inhibin α expression in surrounding granulosa cells [18].

Since *Gdf9*-deficient follicles do not develop beyond the primary stage, the role of GDF9 in granulosa cell functions during antral follicle stage was examined using recombinant proteins. Recombinant GDF9 suppresses follicle-stimulating hormone (FSH)-stimulated expression of *Lhcgr* mRNA, promotes progesterone production by granulosa cells, and enables cumulus expansion in mice [19]. In addition, increasing the oocyte signals by supplying the medium with recombinant GDF9 during in vitro maturation culture enhances the developmental competence of mouse oocytes [20], whereas disrupting oocyte signals by a specific inhibitor of GDF9 signaling reduces developmental competence [21]. Therefore, the oocyte-derived paracrine factors are not only required for development of the follicles, but are critical for the oocytes to acquire their full developmental competence.

The first genetic evidence for the requirement of bone morphogenetic protein 15 (BMP15), another member of the oocyte-derived TGFβ superfamily, for female fertility was provided by studies of Inverdale and Hanna sheep, which carry naturally occurring point mutations in the *BMP15* gene [22]. Sheep homozygous for these mutations exhibit a blockage in folliculogenesis similar to that observed in the *Gdf9* knockout mice, and are infertile. Surprisingly, sheep heterozygous for these mutations exhibit increased ovulation rates and larger litter sizes than wild-type controls [22]. Therefore, a precise balancing of BMP15 signals appears to be critical for normal fertility in sheep. In mice, however, heterozygous or homozygous deletion of the *Bmp15* gene had minimal effects on female fertility [23]. This suggests that some other BMPs, such as BMP6, which is another oocyte-produced BMP member [24], may compensate for the loss of BMP15 in mice. However, female mice deficient in both *Bmp15* and *Bmp6* genes did not exhibit any fertility defects that were more severe than the defects in *Bmp6* or *Bmp15* single mutant mice [25]. Therefore, the requirement of BMP signals for female fertility appears to vary between mice and sheep. This species-specific difference in the requirement of BMP signals is implicated in the control of the different ovulation rates in different species [26]. Nonetheless, it is important to note that BMP signals are indeed required for female fertility in mice, as indicated by the impaired fertility phenotypes of female mice deficient in *Bmpr2b,* encoding one of the BMP receptors, or *Smad1/5/9* (formerly known as *Smad1/5/8*), encoding mediators of BMP signaling [27, 28]. In addition, a microarray study of the cumulus cell transcriptome of the *Bmp15*-deficient mice showed important functions of BMP15 during folliculogenesis in mice; there were more than 5000 transcripts whose levels were significantly different in wild-type and *Bmp15*$^{-/-}$ cumulus cells [29].

Interestingly, while *Bmp15*$^{-/-}$ female mice exhibit a relatively mild ovarian phenotype, female mice with an additional deletion of one allele of *Gdf9* (*Bmp15*$^{-/-}$/*Gdf9*$^{+/-}$) are infertile [23]. This indicates that synergistic interactions of BMP15 and GDF9 signals are critical for female fertility in mice. In fact, differential expression of more than 2600 transcripts was identified by a microarray analysis comparing cumulus cells of *Bmp15*$^{-/-}$ and *Bmp15*$^{-/-}$/*Gdf9*$^{+/-}$ mice [29]. The differentially expressed transcripts between cumulus cells of *Bmp15*$^{-/-}$ and *Bmp15*$^{-/-}$/*Gdf9*$^{+/-}$ mice are enriched in those related to metabolic processes, such as glycolysis and cholesterol biosynthesis [29]. Therefore, oocyte-derived TGFβ superfamily members act in concert to regulate granulosa cell metabolism (discussed further below).

Although the genetic models revealed the functions and interactions of the oocyte-derived TGFβ superfamily ligands [22, 23, 29], it is difficult to distinguish between acute and chronic effects of absence of these ligands throughout follicular development. Most studies in vitro, including the studies described below, however, used recombinant BMP15 of human sequence, since the mouse BMP15 ligand was not available. It needs to be noted that human BMP15 may not have the same effects on mouse cells as the mouse BMP15. Therefore, whether the human BMP15 reflects the actual functions of BMP15 in mice needs to be tested. Moreover, whether BMP15 and GDF9 act as monomers, homodimers, or BMP15/GDF9 heterodimers needs to be determined.

FGFs

Although expression of the *Fgf8* transcript by mouse oocytes was first reported more than a decade ago [30], the function of the oocyte-produced FGF8 during folliculogenesis was not reported until recently. As mentioned above, transcripts encoding glycolytic enzymes are differentially expressed between cumulus and mural granulosa cells (Table 9.1), and this is due to oocyte-derived factors [2]. Cumulus cells of *Bmp15*$^{-/-}$ mice express reduced levels of transcripts encoding glycolytic enzymes, suggesting that oocyte-derived BMP15 is required for greater expression of these transcripts in vivo. However, recombinant human BMP15 did not promote expression of these transcripts unless co-treated with recombinant FGF8 [31]. Thus, oocyte-derived BMP15 and FGF8 cooperate in promoting glycolysis in cumulus cells by promoting the expression of transcripts encoding glycolytic enzymes.

The mechanism of crosstalk between oocyte-derived BMP15 and FGF8 during folliculogenesis is yet to be determined; however, the involvement of sprouty homolog 2 (SPRY2), an antagonist of FGF signaling, has been implicated [32]. The *Spry2* transcript is differentially expressed between mouse cumulus and mural granulosa cells before the LH surge (Table 9.1). *Spry2* expression in cumulus cells is promoted by recombinant FGFs, whereas it is suppressed by recombinant BMP15, BMP6, or oocytes in culture. These results suggest that there may be a negative feedback mechanism of FGF signaling that involves SPRY2 within a follicle, and that this negative feedback mechanism may be suppressed by oocyte-derived BMP signals. It is possible that SPRY2 may act as a balancer of FGF and BMP signaling during folliculogenesis; however, future studies to test this possibility are necessary. In addition, since the recombinant human BMP15 was used in these studies [31, 32], it will be important to test whether the mouse BMP15 interacts with FGF signals in vivo.

Differential gene expression between cumulus and mural granulosa cells

The transcripts that are currently known to be differentially expressed between mouse cumulus and mural granulosa cells before the LH surge are summarized in Table 9.1. Oocytes play a critical role in determining the differential gene expression. In the following section, the roles of the proteins encoded by these transcripts in regulating follicle/oocyte development and ovulation are discussed.

Metabolic cooperativity between oocytes and cumulus cells

The presence of nutritional support from granulosa cells to oocytes was postulated more than a century ago [33], and the first physiological example was presented in the 1960s. Biggers and his co-workers reported that mouse oocytes did not resume meiosis in vitro in medium containing glucose as an energy substrate unless pyruvate or cumulus cells were also present [34]. Subsequent studies showed that cumulus cells produce pyruvate using glucose or lactate as substrates [5, 6]. Since pyruvate is the main energy substrate used by oocytes for their growth and the meiotic resumption [34, 35], it is likely that oocytes depend on the pyruvate provided by accompanying cumulus cells for their energy production. This phenomenon has long been known as an example of essential metabolic cooperativity between oocytes and cumulus cells [36, 37].

Amino acid uptake into oocytes is another example of the metabolic cooperativity between oocytes and cumulus cells. Colonna and Mangia [3] reported that certain amino acids, including alanine, were efficiently taken up into mouse oocytes enclosed within cumulus cells, whereas uptake into denuded oocytes was not efficient. This effect of cumulus cells on enhancing the uptake of amino acids into oocytes was blocked by an inhibitor of gap junctional communication [4]. This suggests that certain amino acids are first taken up by cumulus cells and are transported into oocytes through gap junctions.

As mentioned above, transcripts encoding glycolytic enzymes, including lactate dehydrogenase A (LDHA) and phosphofructokinase, platelet (PFKP), and amino acid transporters, including solute carrier family 38, member 3 (SLC38A3), are expressed at higher levels in cumulus cells than mural granulosa cells of Graafian follicles (Table 9.1) [1, 2]. These transcripts were barely detectable in oocytes by *in situ* hybridization [1, 2]. Removing oocytes from cumulus cell–oocyte complexes (COCs) resulted in reduced expression levels of these transcripts, whereas the reduction in transcript levels was prevented by co-culture with oocytes [1, 2]. Therefore, oocytes, by producing paracrine factors, promote expression of these transcripts in cumulus cells. The oocyte factors that promote expression of transcripts encoding glycolytic enzymes appear to be BMP15 and FGF8 [31]. The oocyte factors that promote *Slc38a3* expression are not yet identified.

Another example of the metabolic cooperativity between oocytes and cumulus cells has been reported recently. As mentioned above, cumulus cells of *Bmp15*$^{-/-}$/*Gdf9*$^{+/-}$ mice expressed lower levels of transcripts encoding cholesterol biosynthetic enzymes when compared with those of *Bmp15*$^{-/-}$ or wild-type mice [29]. This suggests that expression of these transcripts in vivo requires oocyte-derived BMP15 and/or GDF9. In fact, removal of oocytes from COCs resulted in reduced expression of these transcripts, whereas adding oocytes back into the cumulus cell culture prevented the reduction. Furthermore, cholesterol synthesis by mutant COCs or isolated cumulus cells cultured without oocytes was significantly lower than those of wild-type or cumulus cells cultured with oocytes. Co-culturing mutant COCs with wild-type oocytes promoted cholesterol synthesis in mutant cumulus cells, and increased cholesterol content in the mutant oocytes. Thus, cumulus cells synthesize cholesterol, not only for themselves, but also for the oocytes; the expression of transcripts encoding cholesterol biosynthetic enzymes depends on oocyte-derived BMP15 and/or GDF9. Therefore, the metabolic cooperativity between oocytes and cumulus cells is controlled by oocytes [36, 37].

Consistent with the fact that mammalian oocytes are deficient in carrying out glycolysis, cholesterol biosynthesis, and uptake of some amino acids [3, 29, 34], transcripts encoding proteins required for carrying out these metabolic processes are not expressed by oocytes [1, 2, 29]. Therefore, oocytes must obtain the amino acids, and the products of glycolysis and cholesterol biosynthesis, from companion cumulus cells for their own development. Accordingly, oocytes promote these metabolic processes in cumulus cells, at least in part, by inducing expression of these transcripts. Cumulus cells express higher levels of these transcripts than mural granulosa cells, which is because they are closer to the oocyte than mural granulosa cells and are exposed to higher concentrations of the oocyte-derived paracrine factors.

Meiotic arrest of oocytes

Fully grown oocytes in Graafian follicles are maintained in the diplotene stage of the first meiotic prophase. While the preovulatory LH surge triggers meiotic resumption and ovulation in vivo, simply releasing COCs from follicles results in gonadotropin-independent meiotic resumption in vitro [38, 39]. Thus, a factor(s), sometimes referred to as oocyte maturation inhibitor (OMI), produced by follicular somatic cells plays a critical role in maintaining the oocyte meiotic arrest. OMI appears to be a peptide of less than 2000 daltons, produced by mural granulosa cells, but not by the theca layer or ovarian bursa, and its action on the oocyte meiotic arrest is mediated by cumulus cells [40].

A recent study showed a critical role of natriuretic peptide type C (NPPC) and its receptor, natriuretic peptide receptor 2 (NPR2), in the meiotic arrest of mouse oocytes [41]. NPPC is a peptide of about 2000 daltons produced by mural granulosa cells of Graafian follicles. Supplying medium with NPPC prevented gonadotropin-independent meiotic resumption of oocytes enclosed within cumulus cells, but did not prevent that of denuded oocytes. Furthermore, oocytes in Graafian follicles of *Nppc* and *Npr2* mutant mice exhibited precocious resumption of meiosis [41]. In addition, levels of *Nppc* transcript and NPPC protein in ovaries decreased rapidly when equine chorionic gonadotropin (eCG)-primed mice were treated with human chorionic gonadotropin (hCG) [42], consistent with the releasing of oocytes from the meiotic arrest after the LH surge. The decrease in NPPC protein levels was also observed in human follicular fluids

[42]. Therefore, a similar mechanism of oocyte meiotic arrest that involves the NPPC/NPR2 system appears to exist in other mammals, including humans.

Interestingly, *Nppc* and *Npr2* are differentially expressed between cumulus and mural granulosa cells of Graafian follicles (Table 9.1). The previous report showed that *Npr2* was highly expressed in cumulus cells when compared with mural granulosa cells, whereas *Nppc* was specifically expressed by mural granulosa cells [41]. When cumulus cells were cultured alone, *Npr2* transcript levels decreased, but co-culturing with oocytes or supplying medium with recombinant human BMP15 and/or GDF9 prevented this decrease [41]. Moreover, cumulus cells of *Bmp15*$^{-/-}$/*Gdf9*$^{+/-}$ and *Bmp15*$^{-/-}$ mutant mice expressed lower levels of *Npr2* transcripts when compared to those of wild-type mice [29]. Therefore, the higher expression of *Npr2* transcript in cumulus cells when compared with mural granulosa cells requires oocyte-derived BMP15 and GDF9. Moreover, an estrogen signal was also critical for maintaining high *Npr2* expression in mouse cumulus cells [43], suggesting that oocyte and estrogen signals cooperate in regulating *Npr2* expression in cumulus cells.

Compared with *Npr2*, the regulation of *Nppc* expression in follicles is not well characterized. Since eCG-priming increased *Nppc* transcript levels in mouse mural granulosa cells [42], it is possible that FSH, which comes from outside of follicles, may be required for the greater *Nppc* expression in mural granulosa cells compared to that in cumulus cells. In addition, the lower expression of *Nppc* in cumulus cells compared to mural granulosa cells suggests that oocytes may suppress *Nppc* expression in cumulus cells. However, cumulus cells of *Bmp15*$^{-/-}$/*Gdf9*$^{+/-}$ and *Bmp15*$^{-/-}$ mutant mice did not exhibit increased levels of *Nppc* transcripts when compared with those of wild-type mice [29]. It is possible that the other oocyte factors such as BMP6 and FGF8 suppress *Nppc* expression in cumulus cells; however, there may be an unidentified mechanism that does not require oocyte signals for establishing the differential gene expression of *Nppc* mRNA between cumulus and mural granulosa cells. In addition, it will be interesting to assess the consequences on oocyte meiotic arrest and follicular development of disrupting the differential *Nppc* expression between cumulus and mural granulosa cells.

Cumulus expansion

During the transition of preantral to antral follicle granulosa cells associated with oocytes differentiate into cumulus cells and become competent to undergo expansion (mucification) [44]. Several intrafollicular signals, such as oocyte-derived BMP15 and GDF9, and estrogen, are required for cumulus cells to acquire the competence as demonstrated by the expansion-incompetent phenotypes of *Bmp15*$^{-/-}$/*Gdf9*$^{+/-}$ and estrogen receptor 2 mutant (*Esr2*$^{-/-}$) mice [23, 45–47].

A recent study showed a critical role of the interaction of oocyte and estrogen signals in maintaining cumulus cell competence to undergo expansion [48]. Isolated cumulus cells lost their competence to undergo expansion when they were kept in a prolonged culture, but the competence was maintained when medium was supplied with a combination of estrogen and either oocytes or recombinant human BMP15 and/or mouse GDF9. Therefore oocyte-derived BMP15 and GDF9 appear to cooperate with estrogen to maintain the competence of cumulus cells to undergo expansion [48]. Furthermore, in vitro-grown COCs developed without estrogen were less competent to undergo expansion when compared with those developed with estrogen [48]. This suggests that the interaction of oocyte and estrogen signals may also be critical for acquiring competence to undergo expansion.

Although the precise mechanism(s) of how oocyte-derived signals interact with estrogen signals in maintaining the competence is yet to be determined, a potential mechanism that involves nuclear receptor interacting protein 1 (NRIP1), whose encoding transcript is differentially expressed between cumulus and mural granulosa cells, has been proposed [48]. NRIP1, also known as receptor interacting protein 140 (RIP140), is one of the negative co-regulators of nuclear receptors including estrogen receptors [49, 50]. *Nrip1*-deficient female mice are infertile due to, at least in part, defective cumulus expansion [51, 52]. *Nrip1* transcript levels are significantly higher in mural granulosa cells than those in cumulus cells before the LH surge, and this is due to the suppression in cumulus cells by oocyte-derived BMP15 and/or GDF9 (Table 9.1) [48]. Therefore, oocytes may amplify the estrogen signal by suppressing cumulus cell expression of *Nrip1*, which encodes a potential negative regulator of estrogen signaling in cumulus cells.

Cumulus expansion in vivo is induced by the preovulatory LH surge, and it requires expression of transcripts encoding hyaluronan synthase 2 (HAS2), prostaglandin-endoperoxide synthase 2 (PTGS2), pentraxin-related gene (PTX3), and tumor necrosis factor alpha-induced protein 6 (TNFAIP6) in cumulus cells [53–57]. Since oocytes and cumulus cells do not express LH receptor (LHCGR) [8–10], the LH signal reaches COCs via epidermal growth factor (EGF)-like peptides [58]. EGF-like peptides produced by mural granulosa cells activate the EGF receptor (EGFR) signal in cumulus cells, and this EGFR signal, which is mediated by mitogen-activated protein kinase 3/1 (MAPK3/1, also known as ERK1/2), is required for cumulus expansion and ovulation processes [59, 60]. In addition to the EGFR signal, normal cumulus expansion in mice requires oocyte-produced enabling factors (cumulus expansion enabling factors: CEEFs) [13]. GDF9 appears to be one of the CEEFs [19, 61]. The intracellular signal of GDF9 is mediated by MAD homolog 2/3 (SMAD2/3) [62], and inhibiting the SMAD2/3 signal with a specific inhibitor or conditional deleting of *Smad2/3* genes prevented cumulus expansion in mice [63, 64].

The cumulus expansion-related transcripts are differentially expressed in spatially and temporally regulated manners during the ovulation period [54, 65–67]. These transcripts are barely detectable in any cell types of Graafian follicles. hCG treatment, which mimics the LH surge, transiently increases expression levels of the cumulus expansion-related transcripts in both cumulus and mural granulosa cells, but, subsequently, the levels are decreased in mural granulosa cells and become restricted/enriched in cumulus cells. The sustained expression of these transcripts in cumulus cells requires oocyte factors (i.e., CEEFs), and is probably critical for normal expansion [44, 68]. Oocytes probably sustain expression of these transcripts by maintaining the EGFR–MAPK3/1 cascade active in cumulus cells [69]. Oocytes promote EGFR signal-induced expression of *Spry2* mRNA in cumulus cells during the ovulation period [32]. Since SPRY proteins maintain activated EGFR signals by preventing degradation of EGFR [70–72], it is possible that oocytes sustain EGFR signals and expression of the cumulus expansion-related transcripts by promoting the expression of *Spry2* mRNA in cumulus cells.

Conclusions and future prospects

Although cumulus and mural granulosa cells are similar cell types, it has long been recognized that they play different roles in supporting follicular and oocyte development through their specialized abilities. The specialized abilities of cumulus and mural granulosa cells must be tightly coordinated for successful female reproduction. It is now apparent that oocytes play a critical role in coordinating the development and function of these cell types through the complex bidirectional communication between them [73]. Oocytes, at least in part, use their ability to affect gene expression in granulosa cells to coordinate the specialized functions of each granulosa cell compartment. Importantly, granulosa cell-derived factors also have a profound effect on transcript levels in oocytes as well as the quality of oocytes. For example, granulosa cell-derived KIT ligand, whose signal in oocytes is mediated by KIT, affects expression levels of oocyte-derived ligands: BMP15, GDF9, and FGF8 in rats [74, 75]. Thus, bidirectional communication is critical, not only for the development of granulosa cells, but also for that of oocytes. Since the oocyte-regulated transcripts tend to be differentially expressed between cumulus and mural granulosa cells in Graafian follicles, exploration of the differentially expressed transcripts has revealed significant new insights into our understanding of the mechanisms governing oocyte and follicular development. The current challenges are to discover other factors that are differentially expressed between cumulus and mural granulosa cells. This will lead to revelation of novel mechanisms that govern follicular and oocyte development, and provide new approaches in managing human fertility.

Acknowledgment

The authors thank Dr. John J. Eppig for helpful comments in preparing this manuscript.

References

1. Eppig JJ, Pendola FL, Wigglesworth K, Pendola JK. Mouse oocytes regulate metabolic cooperativity between granulosa cells and oocytes: amino acid transport. *Biol Reprod* 2005; **73**(2): 351–7.
2. Sugiura K, Pendola FL, Eppig JJ. Oocyte control of metabolic cooperativity between oocytes and

companion granulosa cells: energy metabolism. *Dev Biol* 2005; **279**(1): 20–30.

3. Colonna R, Mangia F. Mechanisms of amino acid uptake in cumulus-enclosed mouse oocytes. *Biol Reprod* 1983; **28**(4): 797–803.
4. Haghighat N, Van Winkle LJ. Developmental change in follicular cell-enhanced amino acid uptake into mouse oocytes that depends on intact gap junctions and transport system Gly. *J Exp Zool* 1990; **253**(1): 71–82.
5. Donahue RP, Stern S. Follicular cell support of oocyte maturation: production of pyruvate in vitro. *J Reprod Fertil* 1968; **17**(2): 395–8.
6. Leese HJ, Barton AM. Production of pyruvate by isolated mouse cumulus cells. *J Exp Zool* 1985; **234**(2): 231–6.
7. Zlotkin T, Farkash Y, Orly J. Cell-specific expression of immunoreactive cholesterol side-chain cleavage cytochrome P-450 during follicular development in the rat ovary. *Endocrinology* 1986; **119**(6): 2809–20.
8. Whitelaw PF, Smyth CD, Howles CM, Hillier SG. Cell-specific expression of aromatase and LH receptor mRNAs in rat ovary. *J Mol Endocrinol* 1992; **9**(3): 309–12.
9. Camp TA, Rahal JO, Mayo KE. Cellular localization and hormonal regulation of follicle-stimulating hormone and luteinizing hormone receptor messenger RNAs in the rat ovary. *Mol Endocrinol* 1991; **5**(10): 1405–17.
10. Peng XR, Hsueh AJ, LaPolt PS, Bjersing L, Ny T. Localization of luteinizing hormone receptor messenger ribonucleic acid expression in ovarian cell types during follicle development and ovulation. *Endocrinology* 1991; **129**(6): 3200–7.
11. Chen L, Russell PT, Larsen WJ. Functional significance of cumulus expansion in the mouse: roles for the preovulatory synthesis of hyaluronic acid within the cumulus mass. *Mol Reprod Dev* 1993; **34**(1): 87–93.
12. Eppig JJ, Wigglesworth K, Pendola F, Hirao Y. Murine oocytes suppress expression of luteinizing hormone receptor messenger ribonucleic acid by granulosa cells. *Biol Reprod* 1997; **56**(4): 976–84.
13. Buccione R, Vanderhyden BC, Caron PJ, Eppig JJ. FSH-induced expansion of the mouse cumulus oophorus in vitro is dependent upon a specific factor(s) secreted by the oocyte. *Dev Biol* 1990; **138**(1): 16–25.
14. Dong J, Albertini DF, Nishimori K, *et al.* Growth differentiation factor-9 is required during early ovarian folliculogenesis. *Nature* 1996; **383**(6600): 531–5.
15. Vitt UA, McGee EA, Hayashi M, Hsueh AJ. In vivo treatment with GDF-9 stimulates primordial and primary follicle progression and theca cell marker CYP17 in ovaries of immature rats. *Endocrinology* 2000; **141**(10): 3814–20.
16. Nilsson EE, Skinner MK. Growth and differentiation factor-9 stimulates progression of early primary but not primordial rat ovarian follicle development. *Biol Reprod* 2002; **67**(3): 1018–24.
17. Hreinsson JG, Scott JE, Rasmussen C, *et al.* Growth differentiation factor-9 promotes the growth, development, and survival of human ovarian follicles in organ culture. *J Clin Endocrinol Metab* 2002; **87**(1): 316–21.
18. Wu X, Chen L, Brown CA, Yan C, Matzuk MM. Interrelationship of growth differentiation factor 9 and inhibin in early folliculogenesis and ovarian tumorigenesis in mice. *Mol Endocrinol* 2004; **18**(6): 1509–19.
19. Elvin JA, Clark AT, Wang P, Wolfman NM, Matzuk MM. Paracrine actions of growth differentiation factor-9 in the mammalian ovary. *Mol Endocrinol* 1999; **13**(6): 1035–48.
20. Yeo CX, Gilchrist RB, Thompson JG, Lane M. Exogenous growth differentiation factor 9 in oocyte maturation media enhances subsequent embryo development and fetal viability in mice. *Hum Reprod* 2008; **23**(1): 67–73.
21. Yeo CX, Gilchrist RB, Lane M. Disruption of bidirectional oocyte-cumulus paracrine signaling during in vitro maturation reduces subsequent mouse oocyte developmental competence. *Biol Reprod* 2009; **80**(5): 1072–80.
22. Galloway SM, McNatty KP, Cambridge LM, *et al.* Mutations in an oocyte-derived growth factor gene (BMP15) cause increased ovulation rate and infertility in a dosage-sensitive manner. *Nat Genet* 2000; **25**(3): 279–83.
23. Yan C, Wang P, DeMayo J, *et al.* Synergistic roles of bone morphogenetic protein 15 and growth differentiation factor 9 in ovarian function. *Mol Endocrinol* 2001; **15**(6): 854–66.
24. Elvin JA, Yan C, Matzuk MM. Oocyte-expressed TGF-beta superfamily members in female fertility. *Mol Cell Endocrinol* 2000; **159**(1–2): 1–5.
25. Sugiura K, Su YQ, Eppig JJ. Does bone morphogenetic protein 6 (BMP6) affect female fertility in the mouse? *Biol Reprod* 2010; **83**: 997–1004.
26. Hashimoto O, Moore RK, Shimasaki S. Posttranslational processing of mouse and human BMP-15: potential implication in the determination of ovulation quota. *Proc Natl Acad Sci USA* 2005; **102**(15): 5426–31.

27. Yi SE, LaPolt PS, Yoon BS, *et al.* The type I BMP receptor BmprIB is essential for female reproductive function. *Proc Natl Acad Sci USA* 2001; **98**(14): 7994–9.

28. Pangas SA, Li X, Umans L, *et al.* Conditional deletion of Smad1 and Smad5 in somatic cells of male and female gonads leads to metastatic tumor development in mice. *Mol Cell Biol* 2008; **28**(1): 248–57.

29. Su YQ, Sugiura K, Wigglesworth K, *et al.* Oocyte regulation of metabolic cooperativity between mouse cumulus cells and oocytes: BMP15 and GDF9 control cholesterol biosynthesis in cumulus cells. *Development* 2008; **135**(1): 111–21.

30. Valve E, Penttila TL, Paranko J, Harkonen P. FGF-8 is expressed during specific phases of rodent oocyte and spermatogonium development. *Biochem Biophys Res Commun* 1997; **232**(1): 173–7.

31. Sugiura K, Su YQ, Diaz FJ, *et al.* Oocyte-derived BMP15 and FGFs cooperate to promote glycolysis in cumulus cells. *Development* 2007; **134**(14): 2593–603.

32. Sugiura K, Su YQ, Li Q, *et al.* Fibroblast growth factors and epidermal growth factor cooperate with oocyte-derived members of the TGFbeta superfamily to regulate Spry2 mRNA levels in mouse cumulus cells. *Biol Reprod* 2009; **81**(5): 833–41.

33. Paladino G. I ponti intercellulari fra l'uovo ovarico e le cellule follicolari, et la formazione della zona pellucida. *Anat Anz* 1890; **15**: 254–9.

34. Biggers JD, Whittingham DG, Donahue RP. The pattern of energy metabolism in the mouse oocyte and zygote. *Proc Natl Acad Sci USA* 1967; **58**(2): 560–7.

35. Eppig JJ. Analysis of mouse oogenesis in vitro. Oocyte isolation and the utilization of exogenous energy sources by growing oocytes. *J Exp Zool* 1976; **198**(3): 375–82.

36. Sugiura K, Eppig JJ. Society for Reproductive Biology Founders' Lecture 2005. Control of metabolic cooperativity between oocytes and their companion granulosa cells by mouse oocytes. *Reprod Fertil Dev* 2005; **17**(7): 667–74.

37. Su YQ, Sugiura K, Eppig JJ. Mouse oocyte control of granulosa cell development and function: paracrine regulation of cumulus cell metabolism. *Semin Reprod Med* 2009; **27**(1): 32–42.

38. Pincus G, Enzmann EV. The comparative behavior of mammalian eggs in vivo and in vitro: I. The activation of ovarian eggs. *J Exp Med* 1935; **62**(5): 665–75.

39. Edwards RG. Maturation in vitro of mouse, sheep, cow, pig, rhesus monkey and human ovarian oocytes. *Nature* 1965; **208**(5008): 349–51.

40. Tsafriri A, Pomerantz SH. Regulation of the development of meiotic competence and of the resumption of oocyte maturation in the rat. *Symp Soc Exp Biol* 1984; **38**: 25–43.

41. Zhang M, Su YQ, Sugiura K, Eppig JJ. Granulosa cell ligand NPPC and its receptor NPR2 maintain meiotic arrest in mouse oocytes. *Science* 2010; **330**: 366–9.

42. Kawamura K, Cheng Y, Kawamura N, *et al.* Pre-ovulatory LH/hCG surge decreases C-type natriuretic peptide secretion by ovarian granulosa cells to promote meiotic resumption of pre-ovulatory oocytes. *Hum Reprod* 2011; **26**(11): 3094–101.

43. Zhang M, Su YQ, Sugiura K, *et al.* Estradiol promotes and maintains cumulus cell expression of natriuretic peptide receptor 2 (NPR2) and meiotic arrest in mouse oocytes in vitro. *Endocrinology* 2011; **152**(11): 4377–85.

44. Diaz FJ, O'Brien MJ, Wigglesworth K, Eppig JJ. The preantral granulosa cell to cumulus cell transition in the mouse ovary: development of competence to undergo expansion. *Dev Biol* 2006; **299**(1): 91–104.

45. Emmen JM, Couse JF, Elmore SA, *et al.* In vitro growth and ovulation of follicles from ovaries of estrogen receptor (ER)α and ERβ null mice indicate a role for ERβ in follicular maturation. *Endocrinology* 2005; **146**(6): 2817–26.

46. Couse JF, Yates MM, Deroo BJ, Korach KS. Estrogen receptor-beta is critical to granulosa cell differentiation and the ovulatory response to gonadotropins. *Endocrinology* 2005; **146**(8): 3247–62.

47. Dupont S, Krust A, Gansmuller A, *et al.* Effect of single and compound knockouts of estrogen receptors alpha (ERalpha) and beta (ERbeta) on mouse reproductive phenotypes. *Development* 2000; **127**(19): 4277–91.

48. Sugiura K, Su YQ, Li Q, *et al.* Estrogen promotes the development of mouse cumulus cells in coordination with oocyte-derived GDF9 and BMP15. *Mol Endocrinol* 2010; **24**: 2303–14.

49. Augereau P, Badia E, Balaguer P, *et al.* Negative regulation of hormone signaling by RIP140. *J Steroid Biochem Mol Biol* 2006; **102**(1–5): 51–9.

50. Augereau P, Badia E, Carascossa S, *et al.* The nuclear receptor transcriptional coregulator RIP140. *Nucl Recept Signal* 2006; **4**: e024.

51. White R, Leonardsson G, Rosewell I, *et al.* The nuclear receptor co-repressor nrip1 (RIP140) is essential for female fertility. *Nat Med* 2000; **6**(12): 1368–74.

52. Tullet JM, Pocock V, Steel JH, *et al.* Multiple signaling defects in the absence of RIP140 impair both cumulus

expansion and follicle rupture. *Endocrinology* 2005; **146**(9): 4127–37.

53. Davis BJ, Lennard DE, Lee CA, *et al.* Anovulation in cyclooxygenase-2-deficient mice is restored by prostaglandin E2 and interleukin-1beta. *Endocrinology* 1999; **140**(6): 2685–95.

54. Varani S, Elvin JA, Yan C, *et al.* Knockout of pentraxin 3, a downstream target of growth differentiation factor-9, causes female subfertility. *Mol Endocrinol* 2002; **16**(6): 1154–67.

55. Ochsner SA, Day AJ, Rugg MS, *et al.* Disrupted function of tumor necrosis factor-alpha-stimulated gene 6 blocks cumulus cell-oocyte complex expansion. *Endocrinology* 2003; **144**(10): 4376–84.

56. Fulop C, Szanto S, Mukhopadhyay D, *et al.* Impaired cumulus mucification and female sterility in tumor necrosis factor-induced protein-6 deficient mice. *Development* 2003; **130**(10): 2253–61.

57. Sugiura K, Su YQ, Eppig JJ. Targeted suppression of Has2 mRNA in mouse cumulus cell-oocyte complexes by adenovirus-mediated short-hairpin RNA expression. *Mol Reprod Dev* 2009; **76**(6): 537–47.

58. Park JY, Su YQ, Ariga M, *et al.* EGF-like growth factors as mediators of LH action in the ovulatory follicle. *Science* 2004; **303**(5658): 682–4.

59. Su YQ, Wigglesworth K, Pendola FL, O'Brien MJ, Eppig JJ. Mitogen-activated protein kinase activity in cumulus cells is essential for gonadotropin-induced oocyte meiotic resumption and cumulus expansion in the mouse. *Endocrinology* 2002; **143**(6): 2221–32.

60. Fan HY, Liu Z, Shimada M, *et al.* MAPK3/1 (ERK1/2) in ovarian granulosa cells are essential for female fertility. *Science* 2009; **324**(5929): 938–41.

61. Gui LM, Joyce IM. RNA interference evidence that growth differentiation factor-9 mediates oocyte regulation of cumulus expansion in mice. *Biol Reprod* 2005; **72**(1): 195–9.

62. Roh JS, Bondestam J, Mazerbourg S, *et al.* Growth differentiation factor-9 stimulates inhibin production and activates Smad2 in cultured rat granulosa cells. *Endocrinology* 2003; **144**(1): 172–8.

63. Diaz FJ, Wigglesworth K, Eppig JJ. Oocytes determine cumulus cell lineage in mouse ovarian follicles. *J Cell Sci* 2007; **120**(Pt 8): 1330–40.

64. Li Q, Pangas SA, Jorgez CJ, *et al.* Redundant roles of SMAD2 and SMAD3 in ovarian granulosa cells in vivo. *Mol Cell Biol* 2008; **28**(23): 7001–11.

65. Elvin JA, Yan C, Wang P, Nishimori K, Matzuk MM. Molecular characterization of the follicle defects in the growth differentiation factor 9-deficient ovary. *Mol Endocrinol* 1999; **13**(6): 1018–34.

66. Joyce IM, Pendola FL, O'Brien M, Eppig JJ. Regulation of prostaglandin-endoperoxide synthase 2 messenger ribonucleic acid expression in mouse granulosa cells during ovulation. *Endocrinology* 2001; **142**(7): 3187–97.

67. Fulop C, Salustri A, Hascall VC. Coding sequence of a hyaluronan synthase homolog expressed during expansion of the mouse cumulus-oocyte complex. *Arch Biochem Biophys* 1997; **337**(2): 261–6.

68. Su YQ, Denegre JM, Wigglesworth K, *et al.* Oocyte-dependent activation of mitogen-activated protein kinase (ERK1/2) in cumulus cells is required for the maturation of the mouse oocyte-cumulus cell complex. *Dev Biol* 2003; **263**(1): 126–38.

69. Reizel Y, Elbaz J, Dekel N. Sustained activity of the EGF receptor is an absolute requisite for LH-induced oocyte maturation and cumulus expansion. *Mol Endocrinol* 2010; **24**(2): 402–11.

70. Wong ES, Fong CW, Lim J, *et al.* Sprouty2 attenuates epidermal growth factor receptor ubiquitylation and endocytosis, and consequently enhances Ras/ERK signalling. *EMBO J* 2002; **21**(18): 4796–808.

71. Egan JE, Hall AB, Yatsula BA, Bar-Sagi D. The bimoda regulation of epidermal growth factor signaling by human Sprouty proteins. *Proc Natl Acad Sci USA* 2002 **99**(9): 6041–6.

72. Rubin C, Litvak V, Medvedovsky H, *et al.* Sprouty fine-tunes EGF signaling through interlinked positive and negative feedback loops. *Curr Biol* 2003; **13**(4): 297–307.

73. Eppig JJ, Wigglesworth K, Pendola FL. The mammalian oocyte orchestrates the rate of ovarian follicular development. *Proc Natl Acad Sci USA* 2002; **99**(5): 2890–4.

74. Otsuka F, Shimasaki S. A negative feedback system between oocyte bone morphogenetic protein 15 and granulosa cell kit ligand: its role in regulating granulosa cell mitosis. *Proc Natl Acad Sci USA* 2002; **99**(12): 8060–5.

75. Miyoshi T, Otsuka F, Nakamura E, *et al.* Regulatory role of kit ligand-c-kit interaction and oocyte factors in steroidogenesis by rat granulosa cells. *Mol Cell Endocrinol* 2012; **358**(1): 18–26.

76. Joyce IM, Pendola FL, Wigglesworth K, Epping JJ. Oocyte regulation of kit ligand expression in mouse ovarian follicles. *Dev Biol* 1999; **214**(1): 342–53.

77. Salmon NA, Handyside AH, Joyce IM. Oocyte regulation of anti-Mullerian hormone expression in granulosa cells during ovarian follicle development in mice. *Dev Biol* 2004; **266**(1): 201–8.

Section 3 Developmental biology

Chapter 10 Hormones and growth factors in the regulation of oocyte maturation

Marco Conti

Introduction

Oocyte maturation is the process by which a fully grown oocyte completes the developmental program initiated during fetal life to become a fertilizable egg. It has long been known that this process is triggered by endocrine signals generated by the pituitary. However, only recently has it become clear that the extensive reprogramming of the oocyte and somatic cells associated with ovulation also requires local paracrine and autocrine signals. These local regulations functioning within the periovulatory follicle will be the focus of this chapter.

Oocyte development and the follicle environment

A unique property of the female germ cell is the specialized meiotic cell cycle. Female meiosis initiates in the fetal gonad but will be completed only at the time the follicle is preparing for ovulation [1]. Thus, completion of meiosis may take more than 40 years in a woman. Although recent data in mouse and human have challenged the dogma that meiosis initiation does not occur in the postnatal life [2], the most widely held view is that a neonatal ovary is endowed with a finite number of oocytes that have completed the meiotic prophase but are held in a suspended state of the cell cycle, termed the dictyate state or germinal vesicle (GV) stage.

In the fully grown follicle, the oocyte arrested in dictyate displays an easily identifiable nucleus with a prominent nucleolus, termed GV; a unique extracellular matrix, the zona pellucida, separates the oocyte from the several layers of epithelial somatic cells that compose the cumulus oophorus. Cumulus cells are in physical contact with the oocyte through an intricate network of projections that traverse the zona pellucida, with specialized points of contact stabilized by occluding and/or gap junctions; these intercellular communications are indispensable for the oocyte metabolism, for development, and final maturation [3]. Cumulus cells undergo profound morphological and functional changes at the time of ovulation but will continue to surround the oocyte even after it is expelled from the follicle and will be shed only after fertilization. Given their morphology after expulsion from the follicle, they are often referred to as *corona radiata*. In an antral preovulatory follicle, the cumulus–oocyte complex is attached to multiple layers of somatic epithelial cells that line the wall of the follicle termed mural granulosa cells. These cell layers are phenotypically different from cumulus cells: these are the cells responsive to gonadotropins and responsible for most of the secretory function in the follicle. The epithelial granulosa cells are surrounded by a basal lamina that separates them from stromal cells that form the theca layers of the follicle. Theca cells are also responsive to the gonadotropin luteinizing hormone (LH) and active in production of paracrine factors as well as steroid hormones, primarily androgens.

Oocyte meiotic arrest and meiotic re-entry

In mammals, oocytes acquire the competence to mature well before ovulation. Yet the meiotic cell cycle of an oocyte enclosed in a maturing follicle remains suspended in dictyate stage.

In the 1930s, Pincus and Enzmann [4] were the first to establish that rabbit oocytes, once removed from their follicular environment, resume meiosis without the need of gonadotropin stimulation, a phenomenon they termed spontaneous maturation. This finding,

Biology and Pathology of the Oocyte, 2nd edn., ed. Alan Trounson, Roger Gosden, and Ursula Eichenlaub-Ritter.
Published by Cambridge University Press.

later confirmed in human oocytes by Edwards [5], provided the foundation for the theory that the follicular environment controls the oocyte meiotic arrest. We now have a detailed understanding on how meiotic arrest is maintained in rodent oocytes as well as the somatic cell signals involved in the maintenance of this block.

The oocyte release from meiotic arrest and the re-entry into the meiotic cell cycle is triggered by the large, transient increase in circulating LH, which in women occurs in the middle of the menstrual cycle. LH acts by binding to a specific receptor that belongs to the family of seven transmembrane receptors or G protein-coupled receptors (GPCRs). Occupancy of the receptor by the LH ligand causes a GDP/GTP exchange in Gs protein, which in turn activates an adenylate cyclase and production of the second messenger cAMP [6]. In spite of the established dependence of oocyte maturation on LH, the general consensus is that receptors for this gonadotropin are not expressed by the oocyte [7]. Therefore, the induction of oocyte maturation is not a direct effect of the gonadotropin on the gamete; rather, it requires intermediate signals originating in the somatic cells once they are activated by LH. In support of this view, LH receptors are abundantly expressed on mural granulosa and theca cells but absent or expressed in minimal amount in cumulus cells. In some species, such as the mouse and rat, in vitro exposure of cumulus/oocyte complexes to LH produces little or no detectable effect, consistent with low or absent receptor expression. This restricted expression of LH receptors on the outer layers of somatic cells underscores that local regulations are required to transfer the gonadotropin signal from the periphery to the center of the follicle, to cumulus cells, and, ultimately, to the oocyte.

The gonadotropin surge induces cell-cycle re-entry and completion of meiosis I, followed by entry into meiosis II, collectively described as nuclear maturation of the oocyte. However, additional changes taking place in the cytoplasm of the oocyte are necessary to acquire competence for fertilization and to sustain embryo development; these changes are often defined as "cytoplasmic maturation." Although important in a clinical in vitro fertilization (IVF) setting, we have a very poor understanding of the biology underlying cytoplasmic maturation and the molecular basis of acquisition of developmental competence. Certainly, somatic–germ cell communications are necessary for this cytoplasmic component of oocyte

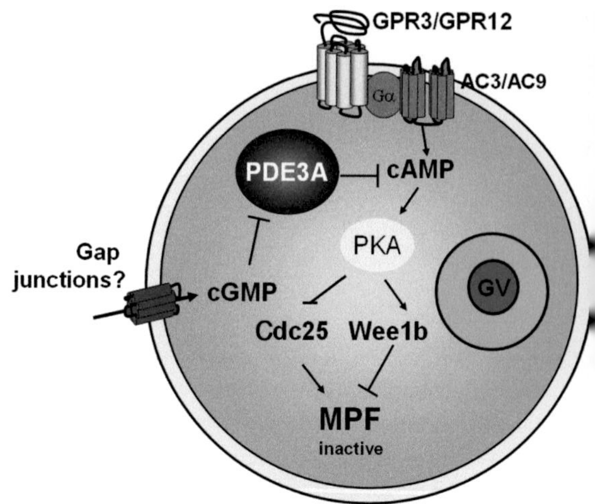

Figure 10.1 Intracellular cAMP pathway involved in oocyte meiotic arrest. In this scheme, the components involved in cAMP generation in the oocyte as well as the steps linking to MPF inactivation are reported. AC3, adenylate cyclase 3; AC9, adenylate cyclase 9; GPR3, G protein-coupled receptor 3; GPR12, G protein-coupled receptor 12; PDE3A, phosphodiesterase 3A; PKA, protein kinase A.

maturation, given the poor quality of denuded oocytes matured in the absence of cumulus cells.

The oocyte machinery maintaining meiotic arrest

As mentioned above, during follicle growth, oocytes are at a stage that corresponds to the prophase of mitosis. This state is maintained because the meiotic promoting factor (MPF) is inactive. This MPF activity was initially described in frog oocytes but was later identified as the master regulator of M-phase during both mitosis and meiosis and renamed M-phase factor [8]. MPF is a complex composed of a kinase, CDK1 (also termed Cdc2), and the cyclin B regulatory subunit. Cyclins are proteins that accumulate and degrade in synchrony with the different phases of the cell cycle. Their binding is an absolute requirement for the CDK1 kinase activity.

In the mouse, an oocyte derived from the antral follicle has accumulated a sufficient stockpile of cyclins to progress at least through the first part of metaphase, but in other species *de novo* synthesis of cyclins is necessary for meiotic re-entry. Thus, additional mechanisms are present to maintain MPF inactive (Figure 10.1). Indeed, an additional mode of regulation of MPF is through phosphorylation [9]. A family of dual specificity kinases termed Wee kinases, which include Wee1, Wee2, and Myt1, phosphorylate CDK1 at two residues (Thr14 and Tyr15) and these phosphorylations repress MPF activity. Wee2 is expressed exclusively in the oocyte, whereas the ortholog Wee1 is expressed in somatic cells [9]. The phosphatases that remove Wee phosphorylation on CDK1 belong to the family of CDC25 dual phosphatases (Figure 10.1). Thus, the regulation of meiotic arrest relies on concerted activity of MPF, the Wee kinases, and Cdc25 phosphatases as well as the control of cyclin synthesis and degradation (Figure 10.1) [9].

In species as diverse as frogs and humans, it has been conclusively established that the inactive state of MPF in oocytes is dependent on the accumulation of the second messenger cAMP [10]. Contrary to previous beliefs that the oocyte could not produce sufficient cAMP to maintain meiotic arrest and relied on its diffusion from somatic cells, it is now accepted that oocytes have all the components required for autonomous cAMP production. Human and mouse oocytes express the GPR3 receptor [11, 12], whereas rat oocytes express the cognate GPR12 receptor. These GPCRs, similar to lipid receptors, activate a Gs protein and cAMP production via activation of adenylate cyclases. When expressed in heterologous systems, the GPR3/12 receptors have substantial constitutive activity, underscoring the possibility that they function without a ligand. Some experimental evidence supports this possibility, and any definitive proof that an endogenous ligand is present in the follicle is lacking [7]. If present, this ligand could be used to suppress oocyte maturation and for pharmacological manipulation of fertility. In GV oocytes, cAMP is maintained at a steady state non-permissive for meiosis re-entry through balanced degradation catalyzed by phosphodiesterases (PDEs). PDE3A is the enzyme primarily responsible for cAMP degradation in the oocytes of frogs, mice, rats, and humans [7]. Its unique properties make this enzyme the central component required for meiotic arrest and meiotic maturation. It is now established that all the regulatory mechanisms involved in meiotic arrest and meiotic re-entry converge to regulate this enzyme. Inhibitors of this PDE are widely used to maintain meiotic arrest.

In the most commonly accepted view, cAMP, through activation of its target kinase PKA (protein kinase A), controls the activity of both Wee kinases (activation) and CDC25 phosphatases (repression), thus maintaining MPF in an inactivated state [9]. Most likely, more complex regulatory circuits are required to maintain MPF inactive but, at the same time, poised to become rapidly activated when meiosis resumes. For instance, additional regulatory mechanisms are necessary to control synthesis and degradation of cyclins [13].

Somatic cell signals maintaining meiotic arrest

Given the observations of Pincus and colleagues implying that somatic signals enforce the meiotic arrest, as well as the established oocyte signaling pathways required to maintain MPF inactive, regulation of cAMP levels in the oocyte is viewed as key for the control of meiotic arrest [10]. Although this decades-old hypothesis is essentially correct, it has taken more than 30 years to unravel the exact mechanisms involved. To account for the dependence of meiotic arrest on somatic cells, a long-held theory was that gap junctions connecting the oocyte and surrounding cells were essential to transfer cAMP produced by somatic cells [14]. However, several observations did not support this model. For instance, Tsafriri and collaborators had identified an activity in pig follicular fluid, termed oocyte maturation inhibitor (OMI), that prevented maturation of oocytes without the presence of somatic cells [15]. Both models were essentially correct and have been reconciled by three sets of observations made over the last 5 years. Firstly, it has been shown that genetic ablation of the PDE3A gene causes complete female infertility, with oocytes that cannot resume meiosis in vivo or in vitro, providing conclusive in vivo evidence that cAMP and PDE3A are critical components of the machinery that maintains meiotic arrest [16]. Secondly, it has been demonstrated that although cAMP is certainly required to maintain meiotic arrest, a pool of the cognate cyclic nucleotide cGMP is also required [17, 18]. Removal of cGMP by microinjection of the GV-arrested oocyte with a cGMP-specific PDE induced meiotic resumption. More importantly and to maintain the meiotic block, this pool of cGMP requires the activity of the oocyte PDE3A to signal meiotic arrest. PDE3A is a unique PDE that hydrolyzes both cAMP and cGMP, with the cGMP hydrolysis being very slow. Therefore, this enzyme behaves as a cAMP PDE that is inhibited by cGMP [19]. These and other experiments strongly indicated that meiotic arrest is maintained because

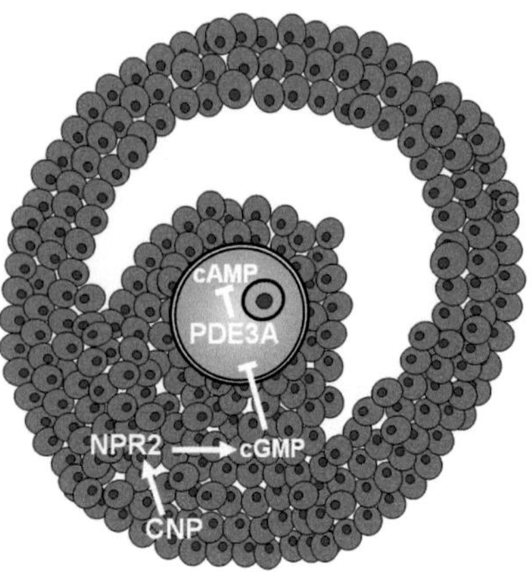

Figure 10.2 Signaling pathways controlling meiotic arrest. In this scheme, the paracrine signaling cassette controlling cGMP levels in granulosa and cumulus cells, as well as in the oocyte, is reported. The C natriuretic peptide (CNP) produced by mural granulosa cells binds and activates the natriuretic peptide receptor 2 (NPR2) with intrinsic guanylate cyclase activity to produce cGMP. Cyclic GMP diffuses to the oocyte to inhibit PDE3A, therefore blocking cAMP degradation. The resulting high cAMP levels do not permit meiotic progression.

a pool of cGMP maintains PDE3A sufficiently inactive to keep cAMP at levels non-permissive for meiotic re-entry. Thirdly, genetic analysis in the mouse follicle established that the natriuretic peptide receptor 2/C-type natriuretic peptide (NPR2/CNP) system is essential for cGMP production while the oocyte is arrested in GV [20], thus consolidating several previous reports of an important function of cGMP signaling in the follicle (reviewed in [7]). CNP is a member of the natriuretic peptide family that includes atrial natriuretic peptide (ANP) and B-type natriuretic peptide (BNP) and is synthesized as a precursor encoded by the NPPC (natriuretic peptide precursor C) gene. CNP binds and activates the membrane receptor guanylate cyclase NPR2 [21]. Mice with null mutations in *Nppc* and *Npr2* have similar phenotypes of defective meiotic arrest: all the oocytes in antral follicles resume meiosis in the absence of the gonadotropin surge [20]. It should be noted that the physicochemical properties of CNP are very similar to those described for OMI, as this was characterized as a small molecular weight protein. A largely overlooked publication also demonstrated that pig follicular fluid extracts stimulated cGMP production [22].

Taken together, these observations made in the mouse are consistent with the following paracrine loop controlling meiotic arrest within the antral follicle (Figure 10.2). Granulosa cells produce the CNP natriuretic peptide that in turn stimulates NPR2 receptors present on cumulus cells to produce cGMP. It is believed that cGMP diffuses through gap junctions to the oocyte, where it represses the activity of PDE3A. This inhibited state maintains a cAMP steady state in the mature oocyte sufficient to activate PKA and to maintain MPF in an inactive state.

It is most likely that this paracrine module and associated cell–cell communications function in species other than rodents, including primates and humans. The CNP peptide has been detected in human follicular fluid and NPR2 mRNA can be readily amplified from human granulosa cells retrieved during IVF [23]. In addition, regulation of this paracrine loop has been described in patients undergoing IVF (see below). Together with the facts that PDE3A is detected in human oocytes and PDE3A inhibitors prevent human oocyte maturation, it is most likely that this or very similar regulatory networks are also involved in the regulation of human oocyte meiotic arrest.

Paracrine regulation involved in meiotic maturation

The LH surge activates theca and mural granulosa cells, and perhaps cumulus cells in some species. This endocrine signal induces oocyte re-entry into meiosis within 3–4 hours in the mouse and 12 hours in humans. In terms of mechanism of action, LH induces accumulation of cAMP in the target cells; this is most likely the primary signal triggered by receptor activation. But it is now clear that cell signaling in the ovulatory follicle rapidly branches into both intracellular and extracellular pathways indispensable for orchestrating oocyte maturation and ovulation. In addition to PKA, activation of the downstream kinases MAPK (mitogen-activated protein kinase), AKT, and PKC are essential for ovulation, and these activations are mediated by paracrine loops functioning in the follicle [24].

LH functions through local activation of the epidermal growth factor (EGF) network

Although a possible involvement of growth factors in ovulation was suggested early on, the recent discovery that the LH surge causes activation of the EGF network has provided new insight into how the LH ction involves paracrine signals activated during ovuation. It has also provided important clues to undertand how the oocyte re-entry into the cell cycle is egulated. A large body of evidence supports a critial role for LH/human chorionic gonadotropin (hCG) ransactivation of the EGF receptor (EGFR) in the egulation of these processes and its involvement in the ontrol of cyclic nucleotide levels in the follicle and in he oocyte. Certainly, understanding the biochemical ircuits involved in this intrafollicular paracrine reglation will provide new tools to manipulate oocyte naturation and ovulation pharmacologically.

Work done in the 1970s and 1980s had explored ossible functions of EGF in follicle growth and matration but with conflicting results. Several reports ndicated that EGF represses the follicle-stimulating ormone (FSH)-induced differentiation of the follicle nd steroidogenesis, suggesting an inhibitory role on ranulosa cell differentiation [25]. On the other hand, t was convincingly demonstrated that EGF induces ocyte maturation at least in vitro [26, 27]. Given the ifficulty of detecting EGF accumulation in the folicular fluid of the periovulatory follicle [28, 29], a hysiological role of this growth factor for maturaion in vivo has remained elusive for decades. A beter understanding of the complexity of the ligands and eceptors of the EGF network has been key to elucilating the role of these growth factors in the ovaran follicle. In addition to EGF, it is now established hat several EGF-like growth factors are present in nammals, including amphiregulin (AREG), epireglin (EREG), betacellulin (BTC), heparin-binding GF (HB-EGF), epigen, and neuregulins [30]. These rowth factors act through at least four homodmeric or heteromeric tyrosine kinase receptors (see elow).

Rather than the long-sought EGF, recent work as demonstrated that AREG, EREG, and BTC are he growth factors rapidly and transiently accumuating in the follicle after LH/hCG stimulation [31, 2]. Induction of EGF-like growth factors is not estricted to rodent species, as similar regulations have een reported in primates, including humans, and in ther species [33–37]. These growth factors are bioogically active because human follicular fluid (hFF) rom hCG-stimulated follicles is capable of inducing umulus expansion and oocyte maturation in cultured nouse cumulus–oocyte complexes, and these biologcal activities are abolished when hFFs are immunoepleted of AREG [37].

These EGF-like growth factors are synthesized as membrane precursors where they may function as juxtacrine signals to activate adjacent cells. More often, they are released from the cell surface as mature, soluble peptides by proteolytic cleavage of the ectodomain and function as intermediate-range signals. Although the extracellular proteases in the follicle responsible for release of these growth factors are not well characterized, several metalloproteases potentially involved in this processing are induced by gonadotropin stimulation and may play a critical role in the release of these growth factors [38]. Indeed, inhibition of growth factor shedding by the matrix metalloprotease inhibitors GM6001 and TAPI-1 blocks the LH induction of maturation and cumulus expansion [39, 40]. This observation opens the possibility that targeting these ectoenzymes may be a novel strategy to prevent oocyte maturation and therefore fertility.

In humans, AREG is undetectable in FF prior to the LH surge but the concentration of this growth factor increases dramatically 36 hours after hCG treatment [37]. More detailed time courses with FF have been possible in primates, where an increase in AREG is detected 12 hours after hCG and remains elevated for at least 24 hours [41]. Surprisingly, it has been difficult to detect EREG in the human follicular fluid, even though a gonadotropin-dependent increase in Ereg mRNA is readily detectable. The fact that EREG does not accumulate in extracellular fluids may indicate a less prominent role for this EGF-like growth factor in humans or, perhaps, a function as a juxtacrine factor before it is shed from the surface of the granulosa cells. In an immature PMSG-primed mouse model of *Ereg* ablation, oocyte maturation is more affected than in the *Areg* knockout, underscoring both the physiological importance of this growth factor as well as the redundant nature of the EGF network.

Another property of the regulation of the EGF network underscores the transient and explosive accumulation of these growth factors at the time of ovulation. Shimada *et al.* have shown that prostaglandin E_2 (PGE_2) controls AREG production by cumulus cells [42]. A positive feedback loop whereby AREG controls expression of its own *Areg* mRNA has also been reported. All these positive regulatory loops point to a switch-like mechanism in the follicle leading to rapid and massive accumulation of these growth factors and activation of downstream pathways.

Studies using different genetic mouse models of disruption of the EGF network underscore a physiological role for this pathway in propagating the LH signal in the preovulatory follicle [43]. Mice null for either *Areg* or *Ereg* have a mild ovarian phenotype, likely due to compensation by the other EGF-like growth factors [44]. Conversely, mice null for *Areg* and homozygous for the hypomorphic *Egfrwa2* allele ($Areg^{-/-}/Egfr^{wa2/wa2}$) display a more severe dysfunction of the follicle [43]. Oocyte maturation, cumulus expansion, and ovulation are all impaired in these double mutant mice. It should be pointed out that the spatial propagation of the LH signal from the periphery to the center of the follicle is also compromised in these genetic mouse models. For instance in wild-type follicles, the activation of MAPK is initiated in mural granulosa cells and it then propagates to cumulus cells. Inactivation of the network in $Areg^{-/-}/Egfr^{wa2/wa2}$ mice causes a marked decrease or absence of MAPK activation in cumulus cells, confirming the view that the LH-dependent activation of the EGF network serves two purposes: it is required for amplification of the LH signal and for the transfer of the signal from the periphery to the cumulus [45].

In addition to EGFR, transcripts for the other members of the Egfr/Erbb1 family, including Erbb2, Erbb3, and Erbb4, have been detected in granulosa and cumulus cells of rodents and in human preovulatory follicles [37], opening the possibility that other receptors are involved in mediating the LH effects. Erbb2, which has no known ligand, becomes phosphorylated in mouse ovaries after hCG stimulation. Therefore, it is possible that upon ligand binding, EGFR forms not only homodimeric complexes, but also heterodimers with one or more of the other ERB receptors in the follicle. That different ligand–receptor complexes may form likely determines the specificity of the signals produced. Pharmacological inhibition of EGFR intrinsic kinase activity prevents these LH-induced events [31], demonstrating that the EGFR is involved. However, the physiological role for these other tyrosine kinase receptors in the ovary remains to be determined experimentally in vivo.

EGF signaling network regulation of cGMP

Given the role of cGMP in maintaining meiotic arrest, LH may signal oocyte maturation either by blocking cGMP production or by preventing cGMP diffusion from somatic cells to the oocyte. Although earlier observations had already implied an LH regulation of cGMP in granulosa cells, more recent data have unequivocally demonstrated that LH produces a profound decrease in cGMP concentration in the follicle [17, 18, 46]. More importantly, EGF-like growth factors share this property with LH, as follicle treatment with AREG or EREG causes a decrease in cGMP to almost undetectable levels [18, 46]. Since they are also known to modulate the permeability of gap junctions present in the follicle [45, 46], these growth factors likely regulate both cGMP synthesis and diffusion, confirming their critical intermediate role in the control of oocyte maturation (Figure 10.3).

The mechanism by which LH or the EGF-like growth factors regulate cGMP is unclear. However, recent observations suggest that the gonadotropin directly or indirectly inactivates the receptor guanylate cyclase [47] and/or induces a decrease in the Nppc mRNA and CNP protein as well [23]. Thus, it is likely that the LH signal for meiotic re-entry requires regulation of cGMP at different levels, possibly indirectly through EGF-like growth factor production.

Other paracrine regulations involved in oocyte maturation

One of the major downstream targets of LH in the follicle is prostaglandin-endoperoxide synthase 2 (PTGS2 or COX2), a rate limiting enzyme in the synthesis of prostaglandins. Induction of this enzyme is essential for ovulation, as documented by the phenotype of the *Ptgs2*-null mice. However, the possible involvement of PGEs in oocyte maturation is unclear. Notably, PGE stimulation causes accumulation of EGF-like growth factors [48], and *Ptgs2* gene ablation reduces *Areg* mRNA accumulation [42]. Interestingly, AREG itself induces *Ptgs2* in the cumulus–oocyte complex [42, 43]. These findings indicate an interplay between the EGF-like growth factor network and PGEs, suggesting complex positive feedback loops. Endothelin produced by granulosa cells is another paracrine signal that has been implicated in oocyte maturation [49].

It has been proposed that LH activation of theca cells may be also necessary for control of oocyte maturation. A report in cows suggested that theca cells may produce factors that inhibit maturation [50]. On the contrary in the mouse, it has been reported that insulin-like 3 (INSL3) produced by the theca may induce oocyte maturation. INSL 3, a ligand that belongs to the family of relaxin polypeptides,

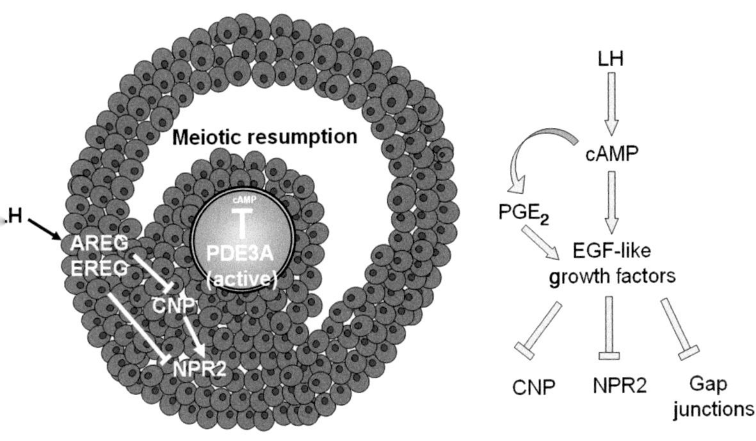

Figure 10.3 Signaling pathways controlling meiotic maturation. In this scheme, the paracrine signals controlling CNP and NPR2 activity are reported. Via stimulation of AREG and EREG secretion, LH represses NPR2 activity and inhibits CNP accumulation in the follicle. This inhibition causes a decrease in cGMP in granulosa cells, which is then translated into activation of PDE3A in the oocyte. On the right the signaling cascade involved in regulation of cGMP synthesis and diffusion through gap junctions is reported.

nduces meiotic resumption in the mouse via a perussis toxin-sensitive process, implying a Gi-mediated nechanism [51]. Others have shown that Gi signalng is not required for LH-mediated maturation in the nouse [52]; thus, it is presently unclear whether INSL3 ignal is indispensable for gonadotropin-induced naturation. Whether these observations are applicale to human is also unclear and requires further nvestigation. It should be pointed out that theca ells of growing and fully grown follicles respond to H, implying that LH induces these putative meioticnducing factors also in early antral follicles when ocytes remain arrested in GV. Thus, an involvement f theca cell-derived paracrine signals in oocyte matuation awaits better understanding of how these signals re synchronized with oocyte competence.

In the 1980s, Byskov and colleagues identified a terol moiety (follicular fluid meiosis-activating sterol, F-MAS) that induces maturation of denuded oocytes 53]. Although this compound may have an important ole in the granulosa/oocyte crosstalk, its function as a neiotic trigger has been challenged [54]. FF-MAS has n effect on oocyte cytoplasmic maturation [55].

Paracrine and autocrine signals nvolved in oocyte cytoplasmic naturation

Together with nuclear maturation, poorly defined ytoplasmic changes in the oocyte are necessary o acquire competence for fertilization and embryo levelopment. Interactions of the oocyte with cumuus cells are important [56], and denudation usually ompromises oocyte developmental competence. This is also true for human oocytes, as denuded oocytes are usually of poor quality. Early work by De La Fuente *et al.* [57] in the mouse, as well as data from other species, has indicated that EGF promotes oocyte developmental competence and is more potent than FSH in this role [57]. It is then likely that another function of the EGF network activation described above is to promote changes in the oocyte necessary to prepare it for fertilization and to sustain embryo development. Consistent with this view is the widespread use of EGF in the culture media for in vitro maturation (IVM) [58]. Since AREG and EREG activate signaling pathways slightly different from those activated by EGF, it is expected that these factors should be more effective in recreating a more physiological environment in IVM. Several other factors present in the follicle may play similar roles in promoting oocyte developmental competence even though the underlying mechanisms are largely unknown.

Neurotrophins are a family of peptide growth factors with a role in the crosstalk between glial cells and neurons that are also expressed and function outside the central nervous system. Brain-derived neurotrophic factor (BDNF) has been detected as mRNA in human granulosa cells, and BDNF protein accumulates in the follicular fluid of women undergoing IVF [59]. A function for this neurotrophin in oocyte maturation was first proposed by the observation that BDNF promotes polar body extrusion in an in vitro mouse model of maturation. This initial observation has been expanded and refined by studies investigating BDNF regulation by LH. BDNF mRNA increases two- to threefold after LH stimulation and the protein accumulation also increases twofold [60]. Via activation of the TrkB receptor expressed on the oocyte, BDNF promotes oocyte competence assessed as first polar body extrusion and improves oocyte ability to sustain embryo development to blastocyst. Data in humans also suggest that the levels of BDNF may be a predictor of human oocyte quality. Glial-derived neurotrophic factor (GDNF) is another neurotrophic factor potentially involved in promoting oocyte competence [61].

Conclusions

The data summarized above document that complex networks of paracrine regulation are necessary both to maintain meiotic arrest and to induce meiotic maturation. Thus, somatic cells of the preovulatory follicle provide continuous cues to the oocyte essential for its final maturation. This realization that these local paracrine circuits play critical roles in ovulation opens a number of opportunities for clinical intervention. Firstly, monitoring the accumulation of growth factors or local hormones in the follicular fluid may be useful to gauge the response of the antral follicle to gonadotropin stimulation and, therefore, provide new parameters to assess its function. Ultimately, biomarkers that predict the quality of the oocyte by probing the functions of the surrounding granulosa cells may be developed. Secondly, a better understanding of how these networks are activated at the time of ovulation will be invaluable to reproduce the appropriate environment for oocyte in vitro maturation. Supplementing the media with these bioactive molecules should improve the quality of the oocyte used for IVF or intracytoplasmic sperm injection (ICSI). Finally, one can envisage strategies to interrupt these paracrine signals in vivo, thus preventing oocyte maturation and ovulation. Thus, new windows of opportunity are opened by understanding the physiological role of these paracrine regulatory mechanisms, providing new ways to manipulate fertility, perhaps acting locally without disturbing the endocrine regulatory mechanisms affecting ovarian and uterine functions.

References

1. Gosden R, Lee B. Portrait of an oocyte: our obscure origin. *J Clin Invest* 2010; **120**: 973–83.
2. White YA, Woods DC, Takai Y, *et al.* Oocyte formation by mitotically active germ cells purified from ovaries of reproductive-age women. *Nat Med* 2012; **18**: 413–21.
3. Anderson E, Albertini DF. Gap junctions between the oocyte and companion follicle cells in the mammalian ovary. *J Cell Biol* 1976; **71**: 680–6.
4. Pincus G, Enzmann EV. The comparative behavior of mammalian eggs in vivo and in vitro: I. The activation of ovarian eggs. *J Exp Med* 1935; **62**: 665–75.
5. Edwards RG. Maturation in vitro of mouse, sheep, cow, pig, rhesus monkey and human ovarian oocytes. *Nature* 1965; **208**: 349–51.
6. Segaloff DL, Ascoli M. The lutropin/choriogonadotropin receptor…4 years later. *Endocr Rev* 1993; **14**: 324–47.
7. Conti M, Hsieh M, Zamah AM, Oh JS. Novel signaling mechanisms in the ovary during oocyte maturation and ovulation. *Mol Cell Endocrinol* 2012; **356**: 65–73.
8. Ferrell JE, Jr. *Xenopus* oocyte maturation: new lessons from a good egg. *Bioessays* 1999; **21**: 833–42.
9. Han SJ, Conti M. New pathways from PKA to the Cdc2/cyclin B complex in oocytes: Wee1B as a potential PKA substrate. *Cell Cycle* 2006; **5**: 227–31.
10. Conti M, Andersen CB, Richard F, *et al.* Role of cyclic nucleotide signaling in oocyte maturation. *Mol Cell Endocrinol* 2002; **187**: 153–9.
11. Mehlmann LM, Saeki Y, Tanaka S, *et al.* The Gs-linked receptor GPR3 maintains meiotic arrest in mammalian oocytes. *Science* 2004; **306**: 1947–50.
12. Hinckley M, Vaccari S, Horner K, Chen R, Conti M. The G-protein-coupled receptors GPR3 and GPR12 are involved in cAMP signaling and maintenance of meiotic arrest in rodent oocytes. *Dev Biol* 2005; **287**: 249–61.
13. Reis A, Madgwick S, Chang HY, *et al.* Prometaphase APCcdh1 activity prevents non-disjunction in mammalian oocytes. *Nat Cell Biol.* 2007; **9**(10): 1192–8.
14. Dekel N, Lawrence TS, Gilula NB, Beers WH. Modulation of cell-to-cell communication in the cumulus-oocyte complex and the regulation of oocyte maturation by LH. *Dev Biol* 1981; **86**: 356–62.
15. Tsafriri A, Pomerantz SH, Channing CP. Inhibition of oocyte maturation by porcine follicular fluid: partial characterization of the inhibitor. *Biol Reprod* 1976; **14**: 511–16.
16. Masciarelli S, Horner K, Liu C, *et al.* Cyclic nucleotide phosphodiesterase 3A-deficient mice as a model of female infertility. *J Clin Invest* 2004; **114**: 196–205.
17. Norris RP, Ratzan WJ, Freudzon M, *et al.* Cyclic GMP from the surrounding somatic cells regulates cyclic AMP and meiosis in the mouse oocyte. *Development* 2009; **136**: 1869–78.
18. Vaccari S, Weeks JL, 2nd, Hsieh M, Menniti FS, Conti M. Cyclic GMP signaling is involved in the luteinizing hormone-dependent meiotic maturation of mouse oocytes. *Biol Reprod* 2009; **81**: 595–604.

19. Manganiello VC, Smith CJ, Degerman E, Belfrage P. Cyclic GMP-inhibited cyclic nucleotide phosphodiesterase. In: Beavo JA, Houslay MD, eds. *Cyclic Nucleotide Phosphodiesterases: Structure, Regulation and Drug Action*. Chichester: John Wiley and Sons. 1990; 87–116.

20. Zhang M, Su YQ, Sugiura K, Xia G, Eppig JJ. Granulosa cell ligand NPPC and its receptor NPR2 maintain meiotic arrest in mouse oocytes. *Science* 2010; **330**: 366–9.

21. Schulz S. C-type natriuretic peptide and guanylyl cyclase B receptor. *Peptides* 2005; **26**: 1024–34.

22. Kolena J, Danisová A, Matulová L, Scsuková S. Stimulatory action of porcine follicular fluid on granulosa cell secretion of cyclic GMP. *Exp Clin Endocrinol* 1993; **101**(4): 262–4.

23. Kawamura K, Cheng Y, Kawamura N, *et al.* Pre-ovulatory LH/hCG surge decreases C-type natriuretic peptide secretion by ovarian granulosa cells to promote meiotic resumption of pre-ovulatory oocytes. *Hum Reprod* 2011; **26**: 3094–101.

24. Richards JS, Russell DL, Ochsner S, *et al.* Novel signaling pathways that control ovarian follicular development, ovulation, and luteinization. *Recent Prog Horm Res* 2002; **57**: 195–220.

25. May JV, Frost JP, Schomberg DW. Differential effects of epidermal growth factor, somatomedin-C/ insulin-like growth factor I, and transforming growth factor-beta on porcine granulosa cell deoxyribonucleic acid synthesis and cell proliferation. *Endocrinology* 1988; **123**: 168–79.

26. Dekel N, Sherizly I. Epidermal growth factor induces maturation of rat follicle-enclosed oocytes. *Endocrinology* 1985; **116**: 406–9.

27. Downs SM. Specificity of epidermal growth factor action on maturation of the murine oocyte and cumulus oophorus in vitro. *Biol Reprod* 1989; **41**: 371–9. Epub 2007 Sep 23.

28. Westergaard LG, Andersen CY. Epidermal growth factor (EGF) in human preovulatory follicles. *Hum Reprod* 1989; **4**: 257–60.

29. Reeka N, Berg FD, Brucker C. Presence of transforming growth factor alpha and epidermal growth factor in human ovarian tissue and follicular fluid. *Hum Reprod* 1998; **13**: 2199–205.

30. Bublil EM, Yarden Y. The EGF receptor family: spearheading a merger of signaling and therapeutics. *Curr Opin Cell Biol* 2007; **19**: 124–34.

31. Park JY, Su YQ, Ariga M, *et al.* EGF-like growth factors as mediators of LH action in the ovulatory follicle. *Science* 2004; **303**: 682–4.

32. Sekiguchi T, Mizutani T, Yamada K, *et al.* Expression of epiregulin and amphiregulin in the rat ovary. *J Mol Endocrinol* 2004; **33**: 281–91.

33. Fru KN, Cherian-Shaw M, Puttabyatappa M, VandeVoort CA, Chaffin CL. Regulation of granulosa cell proliferation and EGF-like ligands during the periovulatory interval in monkeys. *Hum Reprod* 2007; **22**: 1247–52.

34. Chen X, Zhou B, Yan J, *et al.* Epidermal growth factor receptor activation by protein kinase C is necessary for FSH-induced meiotic resumption in porcine cumulus-oocyte complexes. *J Endocrinol* 2008; **197**: 409–19.

35. Lindbloom SM, Farmerie TA, Clay CM, Seidel GE, Jr., Carnevale EM. Potential involvement of EGF-like growth factors and phosphodiesterases in initiation of equine oocyte maturation. *Anim Reprod Sci* 2008; **103**: 187–92.

36. Inoue Y, Miyamoto S, Fukami T, *et al.* Amphiregulin is much more abundantly expressed than transforming growth factor-alpha and epidermal growth factor in human follicular fluid obtained from patients undergoing in vitro fertilization-embryo transfer. *Fertil Steril* 2009; **91**: 1035–41.

37. Zamah AM, Hsieh M, Chen J, *et al.* Human oocyte maturation is dependent on LH-stimulated accumulation of the epidermal growth factor-like growth factor, amphiregulin. *Hum Reprod* 2010; **25**: 2569–78.

38. Curry TE, Jr., Osteen KG. The matrix metalloproteinase system: changes, regulation, and impact throughout the ovarian and uterine reproductive cycle. *Endocr Rev* 2003; **24**: 428–65.

39. Ashkenazi H, Cao X, Motola S, *et al.* Epidermal growth factor family members: endogenous mediators of the ovulatory response. *Endocrinology* 2005; **146**: 77–84.

40. Panigone S, Hsieh M, Fu M, Persani L, Conti M. Luteinizing hormone signaling in preovulatory follicles involves early activation of the epidermal growth factor receptor pathway. *Mol Endocrinol* 2008; **22**: 924–36.

41. Peluffo MC, Ting AY, Zamah AM, *et al.* Amphiregulin promotes the maturation of oocytes isolated from the small antral follicles of the rhesus macaque. *Hum Reprod*. 2012; **27**(8): 2430–7. doi: 10.1093/humrep/des158. Epub 2012 May 16.

42. Shimada M, Hernandez-Gonzalez I, Gonzalez-Robayna I, Richards JS. Paracrine and autocrine regulation of epidermal growth factor-like factors in cumulus oocyte complexes and granulosa cells: key roles for prostaglandin synthase 2 and

progesterone receptor. *Mol Endocrinol* 2006; **20**: 1352–65.

43. Hsieh M, Lee D, Panigone S, *et al.* Luteinizing hormone-dependent activation of the epidermal growth factor network is essential for ovulation. *Mol Cell Biol* 2007; **27**: 1914–24.

44. Kim K, Lee H, Threadgill DW, Lee D. Epiregulin-dependent amphiregulin expression and ERBB2 signaling are involved in luteinizing hormone-induced paracrine signaling pathways in mouse ovary. *Biochem Biophys Res Commun* 2011; **405**: 319–24.

45. Hsieh M, Thao K, Conti M. Genetic dissection of epidermal growth factor receptor signaling during luteinizing hormone-induced oocyte maturation. *PLoS One* 2011; **6**: e21574. doi: 10.1371/journal.pone.0021574. Epub 2011 Jun 30.

46. Norris RP, Freudzon M, Nikolaev VO, Jaffe LA. Epidermal growth factor receptor kinase activity is required for gap junction closure and for part of the decrease in ovarian follicle cGMP in response to LH. *Reproduction* 2010; **140**: 655–62.

47. Robinson JW, Zhang M, Shuhaibar LC, *et al.* Luteinizing hormone reduces the activity of the NPR2 guanylyl cyclase in mouse ovarian follicles, contributing to the cyclic GMP decrease that promotes resumption of meiosis in oocytes. *Dev Biol* 2012; **366**: 308–16.

48. Ben-Ami I, Freimann S, Armon L, *et al.* PGE2 up-regulates EGF-like growth factor biosynthesis in human granulosa cells: new insights into the coordination between PGE2 and LH in ovulation. *Mol Hum Reprod* 2006; **12**: 593–9.

49. Kawamura K, Ye Y, Liang CG, *et al.* Paracrine regulation of the resumption of oocyte meiosis by endothelin-1. *Dev Biol* 2009; **327**: 62–70.

50. Richard FJ, Sirard MA. Effects of follicular cells on oocyte maturation. II: Theca cell inhibition of bovine oocyte maturation in vitro. *Biol Reprod* 1996; **54**: 22–8.

51. Kawamura K, Kumagai J, Sudo S, *et al.* Paracrine regulation of mammalian oocyte maturation and male germ cell survival. *Proc Natl Acad Sci USA* 2004; **101**: 7323–8.

52. Mehlmann LM, Kalinowski RR, Ross LF, *et al.* Meiotic resumption in response to luteinizing hormone is independent of a Gi family G protein or calcium in the mouse oocyte. *Dev Biol* 2006; **299**: 345–55.

53. Byskov AG, Andersen CY, Nordholm L, *et al.* Chemical structure of sterols that activate oocyte meiosis. *Nature* 1995; **374**: 559–62.

54. Cao X, Pomerantz SH, Popliker M, Tsafriri A. Meiosis-activating sterol synthesis in rat preovulatory follicle: is it involved in resumption of meiosis? *Biol Reprod* 2004; **71**: 1807–12.

55. Marin Bivens CL, Grondahl C, Murray A, *et al.* Meiosis-activating sterol promotes the metaphase I to metaphase II transition and preimplantation developmental competence of mouse oocytes maturing in vitro. *Biol Reprod* 2004; **70**: 1458–64.

56. Luciano AM, Lodde V, Beretta MS, *et al.* Developmental capability of denuded bovine oocyte in a co-culture system with intact cumulus-oocyte complexes: role of cumulus cells, cyclic adenosine 3′,5′-monophosphate, and glutathione. *Mol Reprod Dev* 2005; **71**: 389–97.

57. De La Fuente R, O'Brien MJ, Eppig JJ. Epidermal growth factor enhances preimplantation developmental competence of maturing mouse oocytes. *Hum Reprod* 1999; **14**: 3060–8.

58. Richani D, Ritter LJ, Thompson JG, Gilchrist RB. Mode of oocyte maturation affects EGF-like peptide function and oocyte competence. *Mol Hum Reprod* 2013; **19**: 500–9.

59. Seifer DB, Feng B, Shelden RM, Chen S, Dreyfus CF. Neurotrophin-4/5 and neurotrophin-3 are present within the human ovarian follicle but appear to have different paracrine/autocrine functions. *J Clin Endocrinol Metab* 2002; **87**: 4569–71.

60. Kawamura K, Kawamura N, Mulders SM, Sollewijn Gelpke MD, Hsueh AJ. Ovarian brain-derived neurotrophic factor (BDNF) promotes the development of oocytes into preimplantation embryos. *Proc Natl Acad Sci USA* 2005; **102**: 9206–11.

61. Linher K, Wu D, Li J. Glial cell line-derived neurotrophic factor: an intraovarian factor that enhances oocyte developmental competence in vitro. *Endocrinology*. 2007; **148**(9): 4292–301. Epub 2007 May 31.

Chapter 11

Getting into and out of oocyte maturation

Hayden Homer

Introduction

The developmental journey from primordial germ cell to a mature oocyte (or egg) is unusually protracted, beginning during fetal life and concluding during postnatal life. In humans the entirety of this process can last a staggering four to five decades for those oocytes that are ovulated towards the end of a woman's reproductive lifetime. Two major components of this journey characteristic of most mammals, including humans, are firstly, an extended phase of oocyte growth leading to a 100- to 200-fold increase in oocyte volume and secondly, meiotic maturation which occurs after the fully grown oocyte re-awakens from a protracted arrest at prophase I (equivalent to G2-phase of the cell cycle).

Prophase I-arrested oocytes are characterized by the presence of an intact nucleus, the enlarged nucleus in oocytes with diffuse and weakly staining chromosomes being referred to as the germinal vesicle (GV). After prophase I arrest is lifted, oocytes re-enter and complete meiosis I (MI) before progressing uninterruptedly into meiosis II (MII) where a second arrest is imposed at metaphase II. Re-entry into MI is marked by GV breakdown (GVBD) after which the oocyte undergoes the first (or reductional) nuclear division when recombined homologous chromosomes (or bivalents) segregate followed shortly thereafter by exit from MI, evidenced by first polar body extrusion (PBE). The metaphase II arrest state that follows PBE is only broken if fertilization occurs or if oocytes are artificially activated by a parthenogenetic stimulus. Ultimately, this results in the completion of MII and, given the absence of DNA replication between MI and MII, the halving of the DNA complement, thereby allowing the diploid state to be restored in the zygote post-fertilization.

During maturation, mammalian oocytes are transcriptionally quiescent and rely exclusively on translational and post-translational mechanisms. Protein degradation constitutes a powerful post-translational means for ordering progression through the cell cycle [1]. Over the past decade, proteolysis orchestrated by the master regulon known as the anaphase-promoting complex/cyclosome (APC/C) has emerged as a key player in mammalian oocytes. This chapter will focus on the second phase of the oocyte's remarkable developmental journey, oocyte maturation, and particularly how the APC/C sustains the reservoir of oocytes and then steers them from immaturity through to fertilization-readiness.

Overview of APC/C-mediated control during M-phase

The APC/C is a multi-subunit E3 ubiquitin ligase that assembles polyubiquitin chains on lysine residues of substrates thereby earmarking them for destruction by the 26S proteasome [1]. APC/C substrate specificity is determined by the presence of conserved recognition motifs, two of the best known being the destruction box (D-box) and the KEN-box. The ability of the APC/C to target substrates in precise temporal order is conferred in part by substrate-specific co-activators, the two most extensively studied being Cdc20 (cell division cycle homolog 20) and Cdh1. The APC/C coupled with its Cdc20 co-activator (APC/C^{Cdc20}) engages substrates containing a D-box whereas Cdh1-activated APC/C (APC/C^{Cdh1}) can target either D-box- or KEN-box-containing substrates. Two of the most extensively characterized APC/C substrates are cyclin B1 (containing a D-box) and securin (containing both D- and KEN-boxes).

Biology and Pathology of the Oocyte, 2nd edn., ed. Alan Trounson, Roger Gosden, and Ursula Eichenlaub-Ritter. Published by Cambridge University Press.

Securin and cyclin B1 are well known for their roles during M-phase [1]. Cyclin B1 is the regulatory subunit of the master cell-cycle kinase known as cyclin-dependent kinase 1 (CDK1), otherwise known as maturation-promoting factor (MPF). In order to prevent chromosome mis-segregation cells must prevent unscheduled anaphase onset by keeping the protease, separase, in an inactive state. Once active, separase cleaves the molecular glue, cohesin, that tethers replicated chromosomes together, thereby allowing chromosomes to segregate. Securin is a molecular chaperone which, along with high CDK1 activity, maintains separase in an inactive state. Consequently, APC/C-mediated securin and cyclin B1 destruction culminate in separase activation and CDK1 inactivation thereby leading to anaphase onset and exit from M-phase.

Getting into meiosis

Prophase I arrest and re-entry into MI are critically dependent upon regulating CDK1 activity. The activity of the CDK1 heterodimer is controlled through competing stimulatory and inhibitory phosphorylation of the catalytic CDK1 subunit as well as by modulating the levels of its activating cyclin B subunit [2]. High levels of cyclic adenosine monophosphate (cAMP) acting via protein kinase A (PKA) favor CDK1 inhibition by promoting WEE1/MYT1 kinase family-mediated inhibitory phosphorylation of CDK1 on residues Thr14 and Tyr15 and by suppressing the dephosphorylation of these residues by stimulatory CDC25 phosphatases [2].

In addition to the CDK1 phosphorylation profile, sustaining the prophase I arrest state is also dependent upon cyclin B destruction mediated by the Cdh1-activated APC/C species. Notably, although three B-type cyclins (cyclin B1, cyclin B2, and cyclin B3) have been described in mammals [3], to date, the overwhelming majority of data pertaining to mammalian oocyte maturation involve cyclin B1 [2, 4].

APC/C^{Cdh1}-dependent maintenance of prophase I arrest

APC/C^{Cdh1}-mediated destruction of cyclin B1 is important for preventing CDK1 activation and for maintaining prophase I arrest [5–7]. Thus, the robust GV-stage arrest that ordinarily occurs when high cAMP levels are chemically induced – for instance, with 3-isobutyl-1-methylxanthine (IBMX) or milrinone, inhibitors of phosphodiesterase 3A (PDE3A) which hydrolyzes cAMP – is severely compromised in fully grown mouse oocytes which are depleted of Cdh1 using morpholino antisense [7]. It is important to note that even in the presence of high cAMP levels, and therefore an inhibitory CDK1 phosphorylation profile, reduced APC/C^{Cdh1} activity still leads to escape from GV arrest, underlining the indispensability of the cyclin B1 degradation pathway for maintaining prophase I arrest.

Studies involving mutant mice reinforce in vitro data and emphasize the importance of the APC/C for sustaining the oocyte reservoir through regulating prophase I arrest. By expressing Cre recombinase from the *ZP3* promoter, floxed alleles of either *FZR1* (encoding Cdh1) [8] or *APC2* (encoding the APC/C's APC2 subunit) [9] were deleted specifically in oocytes during the growing stage. $Fzr1^{\Delta/\Delta}$ oocytes exhibited reduced ability to sustain GV arrest both within the inhibitory follicular environment within the ovary and when cultured in vitro under conditions in which cAMP levels are artificially raised [8]. Furthermore, $Fzr1^{\Delta/\Delta}$ oocytes exhibited fivefold increased levels of cyclin B1, altogether supporting the notion that APC/C^{Cdh1}-mediated cyclin B1 degradation is important for sustaining the ovarian oocyte pool by maintaining prophase I arrest [8]. In keeping with findings from $Fzr1^{\Delta/\Delta}$ mice, ovaries from $APC2^{\Delta/\Delta}$ mice contained large numbers of oocytes which had undergone GVBD [9]. Altogether therefore, deregulation of the APC/C^{Cdh1}–cyclin B1 pathway within the ovary could be an important cause of premature depletion of oocytes and hence of premature ovarian failure.

Spatial regulation of GV-stage arrest

The breakdown of the nuclear envelope in both somatic cells and oocytes is preceded by a sudden increase in nuclear translocation of cyclin B1 [7, 10–12]. The significance of nuclear cyclin B1 accumulation for GVBD in oocytes was examined recently using a mutant form of cyclin B1 bearing a phenylalanine-to-alanine mutation (F146A) within its cytoplasmic retention signal (CRS). By virtue of impaired CRS-mediated nuclear export, F146A-cyclin B1 exhibits sixfold increased nuclear localization and ~8 minutes faster nuclear entry than wild-type cyclin B1 [11]. Compared with wild-type cyclin B1, overexpression of F146A-cyclin B1 induced greater GV escape during culture in milrinone-treated medium and accelerated GVBD after release into milrinone-free medium [11]. In contrast, another CRS-mutated cyclin B1, 5xA-cyclin B1, this time with poor nuclear localization properties because of resistance to the phosphorylation that enhances nuclear entry, did not augment GV escape and GVBD when compared with wild-type cyclin B1 [11].

Therefore, in order to maintain the prophase I arrest state, the oocyte must prohibit nuclear cyclin B1 accumulation. In keeping with this, CDK-cyclin B1 is itself primarily cytoplasmic at the GV stage [2], possibly because rapid export from the nucleus outstrips slower nuclear import. Another means for achieving this involves spatially enriching all of the components of the APC/C^{Cdh1}-mediated proteolytic machinery within the GV. Thus, oocytes do not express the cytoplasmic-localizing β-variant of *CDH1* and instead exclusively express the α-variant, which is nuclear because of a nuclear localization signal (NLS) [11]. Added to this, immunolocalization of Psmd11 (a 26S proteasomal subunit) and Cdc27 and Cdc16 (two APC/C subunits) points to enrichment of the APC/C and the proteasome within the GV [11]. This spatial bias is physiologically relevant as in spite of the 15-fold lower volume of the GV compared with the cytoplasm, nuclear-targeted F146A-cyclin B1 was degraded twofold faster than either wild-type cyclin B1 or 5xA-cyclin B1, both of which localize predominantly to the cytoplasm [11]. Furthermore, Cdh1 depletion significantly reduced the degradation of all cyclin B1 constructs. Altogether therefore, these data indicate that up-regulated APC/C^{Cdh1}-mediated cyclin B1 degradation within the GV is important for preventing nuclear cyclin B1 accumulation (Figure 11.1A).

It is noteworthy that cellular compartmentalization is also an important feature of other regulators of the prophase I arrest state. Thus, PKA-mediated phosphorylation on Ser 321 of CDC25B negatively regulates its activity by promoting complex formation with cytoplasmic 14–3–3 protein, thereby keeping it excluded from the nucleus [13]. Conversely, PKA increases the activity of inhibitory WEE1B which, due to its NLS, is sequestered in the GV in prophase I-arrested oocytes [13].

Overall therefore, CDK1-cyclin B1 activity is suppressed in the GV by locally reducing cyclin B1 levels through APC/C^{Cdh1}-dependent degradation and by nucleocytoplasmic cyclin B1 shuttling as well as by establishing an inhibitory CDK1 phosphorylation profile dependent upon nuclear and cytoplasmic localization respectively of WEE1B and CDC25B.

Positively regulating APC/C^{Cdh1} activity

Additional inputs serve to fine-tune APC/C^{Cdh1}-mediated degradation of cyclin B1 required for prophase I arrest. Unexpectedly, one of these turns out to be BubR1 (Bub-related 1), whose canonical role is to inhibit the Cdc20-activated APC/C species as a component of the spindle assembly checkpoint (SAC, see below). Depletion of BubR1 using morpholinos compromises IBMX-induced GV arrest as a result of Cdh1 instability [5]. Reduced APC/C^{Cdh1} activity following BubR1 depletion results in securin accumulation and escape from prophase I arrest [5] reminiscent of the effects produced by securin overexpression [14].

APC/C^{Cdh1} is inhibited by CDK1-mediated phosphorylation [1]. CDC14 is a dual specificity phosphatase that counteracts CDK1-mediated APC/C^{Cdh1} inhibition [3, 15]. CDC14B, one of two CDC14 homologs (the other being CDC14A) found in mammals, was recently shown to regulate prophase I arrest [16]. The efficiency of GV arrest in milrinone-treated medium was compromised when oocytes were depleted of endogenous CDC14B by means of double-stranded RNA (dsRNA)-mediated RNA interference (RNAi), whereas CDC14B overexpression had the opposite effect of delaying GVBD after transfer to milrinone-free medium [16]. Moreover, delayed GVBD after CDC14B overexpression was associated with reductions in both cyclin B1 levels and histone H1 kinase phosphorylation levels (a measure of CDK1 activity) and GVBD could be partially restored by co-depleting Cdh1 [16]. Unlike CDC14B, CDC14A does not appear to influence significantly APC/C^{Cdh1} activity at the G2–M boundary [17]. Altogether therefore, CDC14B is important for prophase I arrest by sustaining APC/C^{Cdh1}-mediated cyclin B1 degradation required for preventing CDK1 activation (Figure 11.1A).

APC/C^{Cdh1} regulation at the G2–M transition

In oocytes, securin, which ordinarily serves as an anaphase inhibitor during M-phase by preventing separase activation, is an important substrate of APC/C^{Cdh1} in GV-stage oocytes [14]. Experimentally increasing or decreasing securin levels in GV-stage mouse oocytes leads to parallel changes in cyclin B1 levels [14]. Significantly, depleting endogenous securin

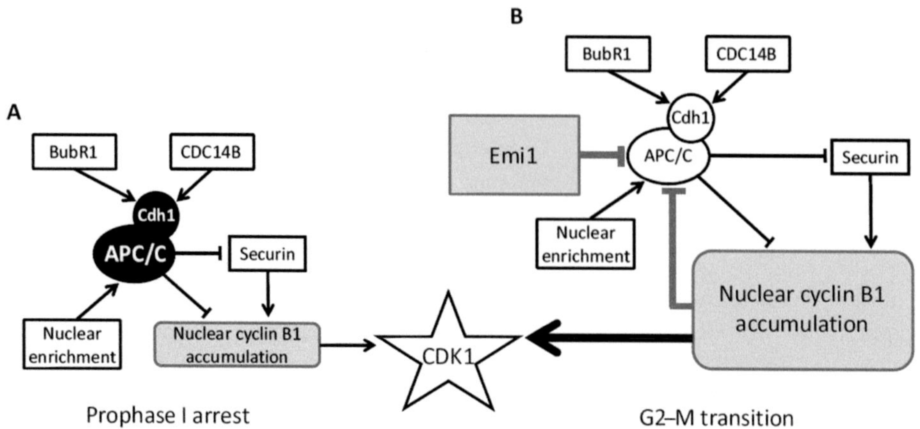

Figure 11.1 APC/C^{Cdh1} regulation during prophase I arrest (A) and at the G2–M transition (B). (A) In order to prevent nuclear cyclin B1 accumulation required for sustaining the prophase I arrest state, the APC/C^{Cdh1}-mediated proteolytic machinery is enriched within the GV and is positively regulated by BubR1 and CDC14B [5, 11, 16]. In GV oocytes, APC/C^{Cdh1} keeps securin levels low as its increase would lead to cyclin B1 accumulation and GVBD [14]. (B) Massive cyclin B1 influx into the GV around the time of GVBD [12] has been proposed to overwhelm nuclear APC/C^{Cdh1} [11]. Reinforced by early mitotic inhibitor 1 (Emi)1-mediated APC/C^{Cdh1} inhibition [6] this would then allow further cyclin B1 accumulation that would be further promoted by securin increases ultimately contributing to CDK1 activation and GVBD.

using morpholinos caused a 75% reduction in GVBD rates, which could be reversed by co-depleting Cdh1 [14]. Notably, the ability of securin to influence cyclin B1 is not shared by Aurora B, another APC/C substrate, and requires the presence of securin's D-box and KEN-box motifs [14]. Altogether these data indicate that securin and cyclin B1 act as specific co-competing APC/C^{Cdh1} substrates at the GV stage, which in turn enables securin to modulate cyclin B1 levels and hence the G2–M transition. Interestingly, unlike cyclin B1, which is largely excluded from the GV [11], immunolocalization studies reveal uniform securin distribution between the nuclear and cytoplasmic compartments in oocytes [14]. Therefore, it may be that following commitment to GVBD, nuclear securin reinforces nuclear cyclin B1 accumulation thereby promoting the G2–M transition (Figure 11.1B).

Another APC/C inhibitor active in prophase I oocytes is Emi1 (early mitotic inhibitor 1) [6]. Although Emi1 engages APC/C^{Cdh1} via a conserved D-box, it is resistant to ubiquitination and is therefore not a bona fide APC/C substrate [18]. Thus, unlike securin, which stabilizes cyclin B1 through co-competing as a substrate [14], Emi1 stabilizes cyclin B1 through pseudo-substrate inhibition [18], that is, binding of Emi1 to APC/C^{Cdh1} does not lead to its degradation but leads to its competion with other APC/C substrates for D-box binding. Depletion of endogenous Emi1 using morpholino antisense inhibited GVBD in vitro and was associated with delays in cyclin B1 accumulation and histone H1 phosphorylation [6], indicating that Emi1 is important for cyclin B1-dependent CDK1 activation at the G2–M transition. Furthermore, these defects in Emi1-depleted oocytes could be reversed by co-depleting Cdh1 such that double-depleted oocytes exhibited a similar tendency to escape from GV arrest whilst cultured in IBMX-treated medium as did Cdh1-depleted oocytes [6]. Altogether, these data show that Emi1 is required for GVBD by inhibiting APC/C^{Cdh1}-mediated cyclin B1 destruction and thereby facilitating CDK1 activation (Figure 11.1B).

The importance of Emi1-dependent APC/C^{Cdh1} inhibition for GVBD suggests that APC/C^{Cdh1} activity might decline at the G2–M transition to facilitate CDK1 activation. Such a decline has not been shown but if it did occur it would need to be transient to enable APC/C^{Cdh1} activity to rise again promptly post-GVBD to target its prometaphase I substrates (see below). Interestingly, temporal changes in Emi1 levels would support such an APC/C^{Cdh1} activity profile since Emi1 levels are maximal at the GV stage and decline markedly shortly after GVBD due to SCF (Skp1-Cul1-F-box)/βTrCP-mediated destruction [6].

Getting out of meiosis

Female mammalian MI has gained notoriety for its peculiar vulnerability to chromosome segregation errors with advancing female age, such oocyte-derived errors accounting for the overwhelming majority of human aneuploidy [19, 20]. One step beyond chromosome segregation at anaphase I is an intriguing but little understood property of all meiotic cells involving immediate entry into a second M-phase (MII) without any intervening DNA replication so as to obtain a haploid set of metaphase II chromosomes, each containing two sister chromatids. Having entered MII, oocytes then experience a unique cytostatic factor (CSF)-mediated arrest at metaphase II, which is broken by a fertilization-induced calcium signal. Therefore, understanding the regulation of these key transitions towards the end of meiosis in oocytes – metaphase I-to-anaphase I, MI-to-MII and egg-to-embryo, at the heart of all of which is the APC/C – will not only be key to unraveling the molecular basis for human reproductive catastrophe but will also provide important insight into how the cell cycle is adapted to meet the exacting requirements of meiosis.

Regulating APC/C during prometaphase I and at the metaphase I-to-anaphase I transition

APC/C^{Cdh1} during prometaphase I

One of the prominent features of meiotic maturation in mammalian oocytes is the very protracted nature of prometaphase I, lasting 7–11 hours in mouse oocytes and 24–36 hours in human oocytes. Earlier data showed that this timing is in part influenced by the rate of cyclin B1 synthesis, which in turn determines the tempo of CDK1 activation [21].

APC/C^{Cdh1}, which is important for maintaining prophase I arrest, remains active post-GVBD. It appears that in contrast to the rapid CDK1 activation following nuclear envelope breakdown (NEBD) in mitotic cells which immediately inhibits APC/C^{Cdh1}, the slow buildup of CDK1 activity in the first few hours after GVBD provides a permissive environment for APC/C^{Cdh1} activity [22]. More recently, we unexpectedly found that within this permissive CDK1 background during prometaphase I, APC/C^{Cdh1} continues to be positively regulated by BubR1 as it is during prophase I arrest [5] (Figure 11.2A). Importantly, reduced APC/C^{Cdh1} activity during early prometaphase I consequent upon BubR1 depletion culminated in an MI arrest [5]. Under these circumstances MI arrest was due to securin hyper-accumulation and could be partially rescued by suppressing securin synthesis. Intriguingly therefore, this indicated that key cell-cycle regulators such as securin are prone to become deregulated during the oocyte's unusually protracted M-phase and that an APC/C-dependent mechanism involving low-level proteolysis is important for maintaining forward progression (see Figure 11.2A).

APC/C^{Cdc20} brings about anaphase I in oocytes

Although CDK1 activity and cyclin B1 levels had long been known to decline on exit from MI in mouse oocytes [23, 24], it was initially unknown whether this was mediated by the APC/C. Indeed, data from *Xenopus* oocytes cast doubt on the role of APC/C^{Cdc20} at the MI-to-MII transition in vertebrate oocytes [25, 26]. This issue was subsequently addressed in mouse oocytes using time-lapse fluorescence imaging of green fluorescent protein (GFP)-tagged securin and cyclin B1 constructs [27]. In contrast to full-length constructs of both securin and cyclin B1 which were degraded on exit from MI, D-box mutated constructs were stable and inhibited homolog disjunction and PBE, pointing to a requirement for the APC/C [27]. Incontrovertible evidence of APC/C involvement subsequently arose when securin destruction, anaphase chromosome movements, and PBE were all found to be completely inhibited following Cre recombinase-mediated deletion of the APC/C's APC2 subunit [9].

Given that a D-box mutated securin mutant was resistant to degradation in spite of containing an intact KEN-box implicated APC/C^{Cdc20} and not APC/C^{Cdh1} in promoting anaphase I and MI exit [27]. These data were later corroborated when securin and cyclin B1 destruction and PBE were found to be inhibited or delayed in oocytes in which Cdc20 levels were reduced either by using *Cdc20*-targeting morpholinos in wild-type oocytes [22] or by generating mutant mice bearing hypomorphic *Cdc20* alleles [28]. Altogether these data showed that the APC/C, and specifically the Cdc20-activated species, underpins proteolysis-mediated anaphase I in mammalian oocytes as it does in mitosis.

Overall therefore, a striking feature of the APC/C in mammalian oocytes is that the sequence in which it engages co-activators is almost an exact reversal of the mitotic paradigm. Thus, during mitosis, APC/C^{Cdc20} activity predominates first during prometaphase and initiates securin and cyclin B1 degradation required for anaphase onset [1, 15]. As CDK1 activity falls, APC/C^{Cdh1} activity emerges to complete cyclin B1

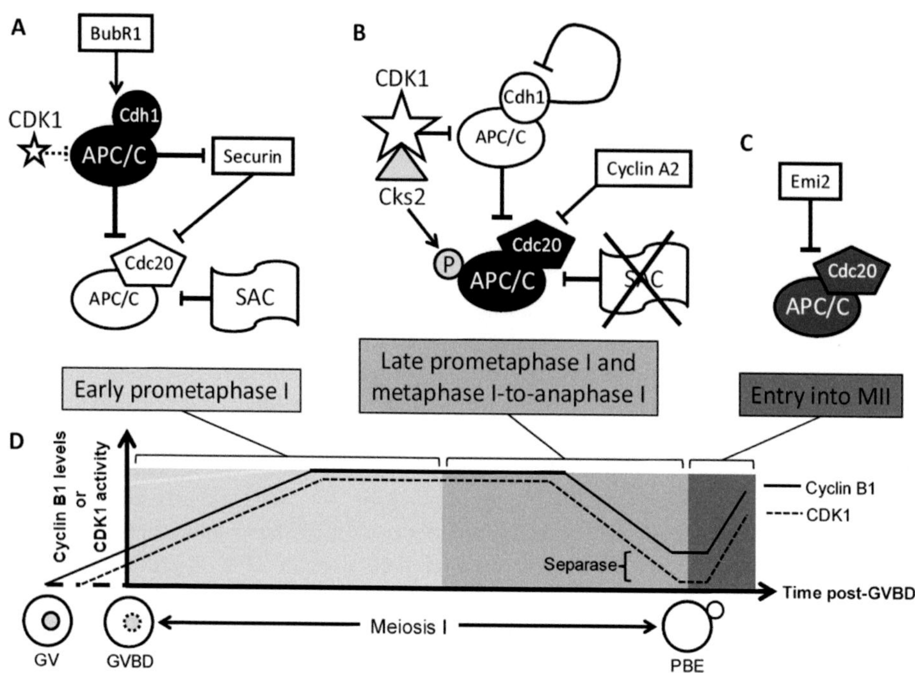

Figure 11.2 APC/C^{Cdh1} and APC/C^{Cdc20} regulation during MI (A–C) and accompanying changes in cyclin B1 levels and CDK1 activity (D). Active APC/C species are shown in black (A and B) whilst dark gray indicates partially active APC/C^{Cdc20} (C). The different shades indicated in the figure correspond with different stages of MI (D). (A) During early prometaphase I, APC/C^{Cdh1}-mediated Cdc20 degradation [22] and SAC inhibition [20] prevent APC/C^{Cdc20} activation. BubR1-dependent APC/C^{Cdh1} also prevents securin over-accumulation which would otherwise overwhelm later-acting APC/C^{Cdc20} [5]. The slow kinetics of CDK1 activation in early prometaphase I (D, lightly shaded area) allow APC/C^{Cdh1} to remain active [22]. (B) By late prometaphase I, APC/C^{Cdh1} is inhibited by maximally active CDK1 and possibly also by prior APC/C^{Cdh1}-mediated Cdh1 degradation [22, 67]. This allows Cdc20 accumulation which, along with silencing of the SAC at metaphase I and possibly CDK1-Cks2-mediated APC/C phosphorylation, enables APC/C^{Cdc20} activation. The resulting securin and cyclin B1 degradation and CDK1 inactivation lead to anaphase I and exit from MI (D, intermediately shaded area). Slow degradation kinetics could be related to the need to also degrade cyclin A2. Although cyclin B1 destruction is only partial [23, 24], separase may lead to a more complete inactivation of CDK1 (D, intermediately shaded area) [71]. (C) CDK1 reactivation required for entry into MII (D, darkly shaded area) is dependent upon Emi2-mediated suppression of APC/C^{Cdc20}-directed cyclin B1 destruction [70].

degradation and so drive mitotic exit [1, 15). In stark contrast, in oocytes, APC/C^{Cdh1} is the prominent species in prophase I-arrested oocytes and for much of prometaphase I and hands over to APC/C^{Cdc20} in late MI for executing anaphase I (see Figure 11.2). As I discuss next, a number of inputs contribute to regulating later-acting APC/C^{Cdc20}.

Modulating APC/C^{Cdc20} during early prometaphase I by regulating Cdc20 levels

An important substrate of prometaphase I APC/C^{Cdh1} is Cdc20; such APC/C^{Cdh1}-mediated Cdc20 destruction is crucial for preventing unscheduled accumulation of Cdc20 (Figure 11.2A) [22]. In wild-type oocytes, Cdc20 degradation is maximal during the first half of MI, about 1–2 hours ahead of the securin and cyclin B1 degradation that later brings about anaphase I [22]. Regulating Cdc20 levels is physiologically important since blunted Cdc20 destruction brought about by depleting Cdh1 leads to premature Cdc20 accumulation and APC/C^{Cdc20} activation, which accelerates anaphase I onset by ~1.5 hours and has disastrous consequences for chromosome segregation fidelity [22].

Intriguingly, chromosome segregation becomes uniquely error-prone in oocytes below a relatively sharply demarcated threshold level of Cdc20. This interesting discovery was made after generating mice which expressed graded reductions in Cdc20 [28]. Jin *et al.* [28] observed that mutant (*Cdc20*$^{-/H}$) female mice whose ovaries express 27% of wild-type levels of Cdc20 were severely infertile whereas mutants (*Cdc20*$^{H/H}$) with Cdc20 at 33% of wild-type levels exhibited essentially normal fertility. In stark contrast to females, *Cdc20*$^{-/H}$ and *Cdc20*$^{H/H}$ males exhibited similar fertility [28]. Remarkably, therefore, a change of <10% in Cdc20 expression levels led to a severely deleterious effect on fertility that was female specific. In an experimental tour de force, Jin *et al.* [28] then set out to determine exactly why this was. It was found that *Cdc20*$^{-/H}$ and *Cdc20*$^{+/+}$ females exhibited similar characteristics in terms of ovulatory capacity and numbers of embryos produced when mated with *Cdc20*$^{+/+}$ males but that ~90% fewer embryos derived from *Cdc20*$^{-/H}$ females reached the blastocyst stage of development, which in turn correlated closely with the reduced numbers of pups born to *Cdc20*$^{-/H}$ mothers. Strikingly, embryos of similar genotypes produced from *Cdc20*$^{+/-}$ and *Cdc20*$^{+/H}$ females showed normal survival rates. Altogether, these data indicated that the defect leading to impaired embryogenesis was not due to a defect at the embryonic stage but during oogenesis.

The poor developmental competence of embryos derived from *Cdc20*$^{-/H}$ mothers was associated with very high levels of embryonic aneuploidy suggesting that severe abnormalities in gene dosage underpinned embryonic lethality [28]. Whilst some of this aneuploidy stemmed from mis-segregation defects arising during the pre-meiotic mitotic divisions of Cdc20-deficient germ cells, the overwhelming majority reflected erroneous segregation that arose subsequently during MI in oocytes – 29% aneuploidy in primary oocytes soared to 90% in secondary oocytes. Significantly, male meiocytes did not exhibit this MI-specific vulnerability – 12% aneuploidy in primary spermatocytes increased modestly to 19% in secondary spermatocytes. Intriguingly, therefore, MI in oocytes was uniquely prone to deregulation when Cdc20 levels were reduced. The female-specific bias could reflect APC/C$^{\text{Cdh1}}$-mediated Cdc20 proteolysis in prometaphase I, which would exacerbate a preexisting Cdc20 defect in *Cdc20*$^{-/H}$ oocytes.

The authors sought to understand why MI in oocytes exhibited this striking vulnerability to reduced Cdc20 levels. They observed that securin and cyclin B1 degradation was far less efficient in hypomorphic oocytes compared with wild-type oocytes [28], consistent with APC/C$^{\text{Cdc20}}$ being the instigator of these events. Furthermore, live-cell imaging of fluorescently labeled chromosomes indicated that about half of *Cdc20*$^{-/H}$ oocytes exhibited three or more lagging chromosomes during anaphase I [28]. Although the reasons for this are unclear, destruction of cyclin A2 was also observed to be impaired even more than that of securin or cyclin B1 [28], raising the possibility that high cyclin A2 level could contribute to chromosome misalignment as it does during mitosis [29]. Importantly, apart from the female-specific fertility defect, *Cdc20*$^{-/H}$ mice are healthy with normal life expectancy, prompting speculation that reduced Cdc20 expression could be a cause of unexplained female infertility in otherwise healthy women [28].

SAC-mediated control of APC/C$^{\text{Cdc20}}$ activation

Overview of the SAC as a monitor of bi-orientation

The SAC is a quality control surveillance mechanism, which delays anaphase onset until chromosomes have all become properly bi-oriented on the bipolar spindle [30]. Key components of the SAC were first identified in yeast and include Mps1 and members of the Bub (budding uninhibited by benzimidazole) and Mad (mitotic arrest-deficient) family among others [30]. Two central players in SAC signaling, which can directly interact with and inhibit APC/C$^{\text{Cdc20}}$, are Mad2 and BubR1. Current models of SAC signaling emphasize the importance of Mad2 recruitment to improperly attached kinetochores for generating the downstream APC/C$^{\text{Cdc20}}$ inhibitor [31]. Although BubR1 is important for final APC/C$^{\text{Cdc20}}$ inhibition and indeed a more potent inhibitor than Mad2, the importance of a kinetochore activation step for BubR1 is less clear [32]. Ultimately, however, kinetochore recruitment of Mad2 transduces an inhibitory signal from improperly attached kinetochores to inhibit APC/C$^{\text{Cdc20}}$-directed securin and cyclin B1 destruction, thereby delaying anaphase.

Following bi-orientation, kinetochore pairs (sister kinetochores in mitosis and homologous kinetochores during MI) [33] have become attached in an end-on manner to microtubule bundles (termed K-fibers) emanating from opposite poles, thereby placing kinetochores under tension. It remains unclear which defect is monitored by the SAC prior to completion of bi-orientation, the lack of kinetochore occupancy or the lack of tension [34]. The "attachment versus tension" debate has been difficult to resolve due to the inter-dependency between the two entities – attachment is a prerequisite for tension and tension stabilizes attachment. Following bi-orientation, the resulting equilibrium between K-fiber-mediated forces acting in opposite directions and opposed by cohesion holding replicated chromosomes together culminates in chromosomes taking up a position at the equatorial region of the bipolar spindle; proper chromosome alignment is therefore one readout of bi-orientation whereas severe polar displacement reflects incomplete bi-orientation. Triggering anaphase when chromosomes are aligned and subjected to balanced forces promotes equitable chromosome partitioning. Conversely, inappropriately timed anaphase initiation prior to bi-orientation severely risks segregation errors for misaligned chromosomes subjected to unbalanced forces.

In order to prevent chromosome mis-segregation, therefore, it is crucial for the cell to be able to detect and respond to improper bi-orientation. During mitosis, kinetochore Mad2 recruitment plays a pivotal role in coupling the completion of bi-orientation to APC/C^{Cdc20} activation status. Thus, by virtue of submaximal tension/attachment, kinetochores of polar-displaced chromosomes recruit high levels of Mad2 thereby keeping APC/C^{Cdc20} in an inactive state, whereas following bi-orientation and equatorial chromosome alignment, kinetochores become devoid of Mad2 [35, 36]. Loss of Mad2 from kinetochores extinguishes the catalytic source of the SAC inhibitor, culminating in APC/C^{Cdc20} activation and anaphase initiation.

Bi-orientation in mammalian oocytes

Given the relationship between bi-orientation and SAC signaling, it is critically important to appreciate some of the unique features of MI in mammalian oocytes that directly impact the bi-orientation process. Spindle bipolarity – by providing two oppositely positioned spatial cues – is essential for bi-orientation, whilst kinetochore pairs that orient in opposite directions are favored over kinetochores facing in the same direction for acquiring attachments from opposite poles.

In mitosis, a pair of centrosomes predefine spindle bipolarity and kinetochore geometry inherently directs sister kinetochores in opposite directions. In stark contrast, in mouse oocytes spindle bipolarity is slowly acquired during an hours-long process in which over 80 microtubule-organizing centers (MTOCs) gradually coalesce to form two broad poles (Figure 11.3) [37, 38]. During this process, spindle morphology is progressively remodeled under the influence of microtubule motors from a spherical structure (completely lacking polarity) to its final barrel-shaped bipolar form (Figure 11.3) [37, 38].

Recent data provide new insight into unique facets of bi-orientation in oocytes. Bi-orientation in mammalian oocytes involves two major phases of chromosomal behavior, the resolution of chromosomes into individually discernible structures (termed individualization) followed by a striking reconfiguration of the morphology of individual chromosomes that occurs contemporaneously with bipolar spindle assembly [37–39]. High-resolution imaging of kinetochores in live and fixed oocytes reveals that kinetochore pairs initially orient to face in the same direction at the microtubule ball stage (Figure 11.4Ai and 11.4Aii) and gradually become re-oriented as bipolarization proceeds to eventually face in opposite directions (Figure 11.4Bi and 11.4Bii) [37, 39]. Kinetochore re-orientation is accompanied by a change in the shape of bivalents from an initially compact structure (referred to herein as a compact bivalent) (Figure 11.4Aii) to one with an extended morphology (referred to herein as an extended bivalent) (Figure 11.4Bii) [37]. Thus, in the absence of predefined bipolarity or inherently favorable kinetochore orientation, and bearing in mind that sister kinetochores must also be constrained to act as a single unit [33], bi-orientation in oocytes involves immense complexities not replicated in mitosis.

It is currently unclear exactly how these two phases of chromosome behavior come about. Spindle depolymerization prevents individualization [38], indicating that microtubules, likely through contacts with chromosomes, are required for individualization. Microtubules can engage chromosomes either through chromatin-based motor proteins (termed chromokinesins) or through kinetochore-based proteins. Interestingly, although the kinetics of chromosomal movement during individualization are consistent with this phase being chromokinesin-mediated, individualization in oocytes depleted of the major vertebrate chromokinesin, Kid, occurs completely normally [39]. This therefore raises the question of whether microtubules mediate individualization via the activity of an as-yet-unidentified mammalian chromokinesin or through interactions with kinetochores.

Regarding the second phase of chromosomal behavior, kinetochore re-orientation, interventions that impair Aurora kinase B or C such as small-molecule inhibitors [39] and dominant-negative mutants [40] lead to increased numbers of compact bivalents, pointing to a role for this kinase in re-orienting bivalents. The targets of Aurora kinase important for bringing about re-orientation are currently unknown. The plus-end-directed kinetochore motor, centromere protein E (CENP-E), is an important target of Aurora kinases A and B needed for bi-orientation in somatic cells [41]. Interestingly,

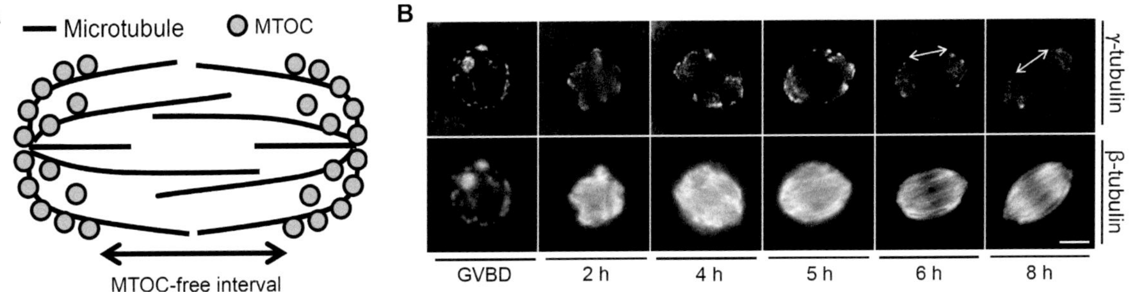

Figure 11.3 Acentrosomal spindle assembly in mouse oocytes of the MF-1 strain. (A) Schematic of criteria used for defining spindle bipolarity. For bipolarity, the spindle should be comprised of anti-parallel running longitudinal microtubule bundles and have two groups of microtubule-organizing centers (MTOCs) separated by an MTOC-free interval. (B) Confocal z-projections of fixed oocytes immunostained for γ-tubulin (for labeling MTOCs) and β-tubulin (for labeling microtubules) at the times shown post-GVBD. Note that based on the criteria set out in (A), bipolarity is established by ~6 h post-GVBD. White arrows highlight MTOC-free intervals at 6 h and 8 h post-GVBD. Scale bar = 10 μm. (Adapted with permission from [37]).

our recent data showed that re-orientation and chromosomal alignment were impaired in CENP-E-depleted oocytes, indicating that CENP-E-mediated re-orientation is required for bi-orientation in oocytes [37], raising the possibility that CENP-E could also be an important Aurora kinase target in oocytes.

SAC function in mammalian oocytes

A number of lines of evidence confirm that a SAC is functional in mammalian oocytes. Thus, PBE is delayed and securin and cyclin B1 are stabilized in wild-type oocytes in which kinetochore–microtubule attachments are experimentally perturbed using spindle poisons such as nocodazole and this delay could be overcome by disrupting Mad2 [42, 43]. Significantly, during an unperturbed MI, disrupting the function of a number of individual SAC components significantly accelerates MI progression and culminates in aneuploidy, showing that the SAC is indispensable for accurate homolog disjunction by delaying anaphase I onset in in vitro maturing oocytes [9, 20, 44, 45]. Therefore, exactly why female MI should remain so vulnerable to chromosome segregation errors when a functional SAC exists remains a perplexing question. Recent lines of investigation have focused on whether unique facets of SAC signaling in oocytes might be unusually permissive to chromosome mis-segregation.

On the face of it, SAC signaling in mammalian oocytes replicates the mitotic template in many key aspects. Thus, kinetochore recruitment of Mad2 is highest during early prometaphase I and declines to near-undetectable levels in late MI prior to anaphase onset when chromosome alignment and K-fiber formation are complete [37, 39, 43, 46, 47]. Moreover, the stage at which kinetochore Mad2 declines markedly is coincident with the onset of securin and cyclin B1 destruction [37, 45, 48] and delayed Mad2 loss from kinetochores arising following CENP-E depletion induces a concomitant delay in proteolysis that can be overridden by Mad2 co-depletion [37]. Overall, therefore, these data support a model in which kinetochore Mad2 levels directly influence APC/C^{Cdc20} activation entirely in keeping with the mitotic paradigm. This now raises the question of what other features of mammalian oocytes might predispose them to chromosome mis-segregation when core signaling pathways appear to remain conserved with somatic cells?

One possible explanation for the apparent leakiness of the female MI SAC is that the inhibitory signal generated from a minority of improperly attached kinetochores might be insufficient within the large oocyte volume – the volume of a mouse oocyte is ~270 pl versus ~6 pl for a PtK1 somatic cell. Thus, unlike mitotic cells in which a single unattached kinetochore can generate an SAC signal capable of inhibiting all of the cellular APC/C [49], propagating an inhibitory signal throughout a 40- to 50-fold greater cytosolic volume poses a far more challenging prospect.

Findings from *Mlh1* mutant mice in which recombination is severely compromised appeared to support such a model of sub-threshold inhibitory signal levels. Although loss of MLH1 on the C57BL/6J strain background induces a robust MI arrest [50], Nagaoka and colleagues found that transferring the *Mlh1* mutation to the C3H/HeJ strain enabled oocytes to eventually complete MI at levels comparable to wild-type oocytes [51]. Notably, however, they

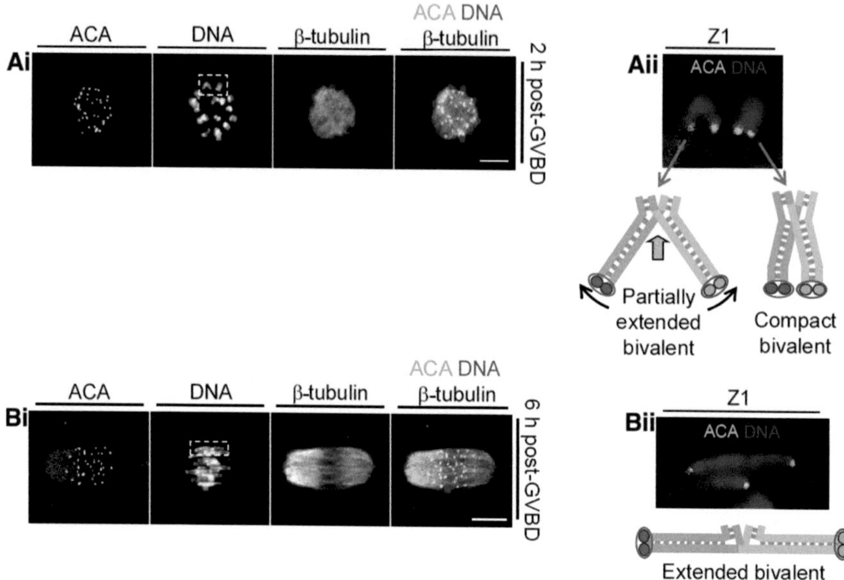

Figure 11.4 Kinetochore re-orientation during bi-orientation in mouse oocytes. Confocal z-projections of oocytes immunostained for microtubules, chromosomes, and kinetochores (using anticentromere antibodies, ACA) at the microtubule ball stage (Ai) and after completion of bipolarization (Bi). Shown are magnified single z-sections (Z1) of the white boxed areas, below which are accompanying schematics (Aii and Bii) to highlight bivalent morphology at different stages of MI. Note that kinetochore pairs initially face in the same direction in early MI (Aii) before re-orienting to face in opposite directions by late MI (Bii). Scale bar = 10 μm. (Adapted with permission from [37]).

observed that in both fixed specimens and live oocytes, severely polar-displaced chromosomes persisted right up until anaphase I onset. They then examined the bi-orientation status of chromosomes. Given that almost all chromosomes in these mutant oocytes were univalents (only ~1.9 bivalents per oocyte), it was important to adopt a method for determining the bi-orientation of the two sister kinetochores on univalent chromosomes, bearing in mind that sister kinetochores are usually constrained to act as a single unit during MI [33]. By analyzing the staining pattern of CENP-E, the authors observed that a "stretched" CENP-E signal was strongly correlated with equatorial chromosomal positioning [51]. They therefore used this stretched CENP-E signal as a measure of bi-orientation, the reasoning being that the stretched signal represented sister kinetochores that managed to attain bipolar attachments but became distorted because they could not separate into physically distinct kinetochore domains. Analyses of kinetochore appearance combined with cytogenetic analyses of chromosome composition in the resulting MII eggs indicated that four to five univalents failed to become bi-oriented prior to anaphase I [51]. On the basis of these data it was concluded that for satisfying the SAC and initiating anaphase I, a critical mass – but not all – of chromosomes need to become bi-oriented, suggesting that a minority of misaligned chromosomes could evade the SAC. It is important to note, however, that although bi-orientation status was evaluated, it is not known whether SAC protein recruitment differed between kinetochores of bi-oriented and misaligned chromosomes [51].

A subsequent study adopted oocyte bisection to produce "couplets" of two oocyte fragments each roughly half the volume of an oocyte [52]. The degradation of GFP-tagged cyclin B1 in fragments containing chromosomes (and hence kinetochores, termed karyoplasts) was observed to occur ~2 hours after that in fragments devoid of chromosomes (termed cytoplasts), altogether consistent with the notion that kinetochores generate an inhibitory SAC signal that sets the timing of APC/C activation [52]. Significantly, three couplets were produced in which one fragment contained a single bivalent and the other contained the remaining 19 bivalents. Interestingly, analysis of cyclin B1-GFP showed very similar degradation profiles for two of these couplets whilst for the third couplet the timing of cytokinesis (marked by PBE) was indistinguishable. Furthermore, in fragments with a single bivalent, cyclin B1-GFP degradation was comparable with that in whole oocytes and significantly delayed when compared with achromosomal fragments [52]. Altogether, these data indicate that a single bivalent (bearing four kinetochores) generates a sufficiently strong SAC signal to delay APC/C activation. Although it remains to be seen whether an intact oocyte can respond to a single unattached kinetochore as in mitosis, these findings indicate that relatively small inhibitory signals can be propagated throughout large cytosolic volumes (~135 pl). Significantly, these data indicate that four kinetochores within an oocyte-half (equivalent to eight kinetochores in a whole oocyte) emit a sufficiently strong inhibitory signal to delay APC/C activation [52]. This therefore argues against the notion that the failure of four to five polar-displaced univalents (that is, up to 10 improperly attached kinetochores) to prevent anaphase I onset in *Mlh1* mutant oocytes [51] reflects an inability to generate a signal capable of inhibiting cellular APC/C. If a minority of improperly attached polar kinetochores can inhibit the APC/C, why then do they fall below the SAC's radar in oocytes?

Examining the SAC's response to polar chromosomes in oocytes

Very recently, we and others have investigated polar-displaced chromosomes within the context of SAC signaling in oocytes. Given that the positional status of a bivalent – that is, polar-displaced or equatorially located – can only be assigned when two clearly defined poles are present and that spindle bipolarity is not predefined in oocytes, we first used stringent criteria to establish the phase of MI during which a bipolar spindle was present in oocytes from the strain of mice we worked with (see Figure 11.3A) [37]. We observed that establishment of bipolarity coincided with the completion of kinetochore re-orientation and alignment for the majority of bivalents and that during the bipolar stage, severely polar-displaced chromosomes were rare (see Figure 11.4Bi) [37]. Strikingly, quantification of kinetochore Mad2 levels revealed that Mad2 was not enriched at polar bivalents even when polar-displaced chromosomes occurred with markedly increased frequency in oocytes depleted of CENP-E [37]. Simultaneously with our paper, Lane *et al.* reported low-level Mad2 recruitment to kinetochores of polar chromosomes [48]. Notably, however, such polar kinetochores never recruit Mad2 to the levels normally observed in early prometaphase I [48] prior to APC/C^{Cdc20} activation, reaffirming that in oocytes, Mad2 recruitment is not enriched at severely misaligned chromosomes.

Independent data using a NuMA (nuclear mitotic apparatus) mutant mouse model have produced very similar findings regarding SAC signaling at polar chromosomes [53]. During mitosis, NuMA is important for anchoring microtubule minus-ends at the spindle poles. Examination of mutant mouse oocytes engineered to express a NuMA variant lacking a microtubule-binding domain revealed an important role for NuMA in organizing spindle poles during acentrosomal spindle assembly [53]. Although K-fibers form in mutant oocytes, polar-displaced chromosomes become frequent, perhaps because defective microtubule anchoring at poles leads to disordered force distribution along K-fibers and chromosomal dispersal [53]. Strikingly, in mutant oocytes, Mad2 is not preferentially retained at the increased numbers of polar-displaced chromosomes [53]. An important consequence of this is that mutant oocytes trigger anaphase I with many misaligned chromosomes, culminating in MI kinetics that are indistinguishable from wild-type oocytes but with high levels of aneuploidy and concomitant female sterility [53].

Thus, all three papers are broadly consistent insofar as polar chromosomes in mouse oocytes lack the ability to generate a robust SAC signal. Taken together, these data reconcile how mouse oocytes can possess a functional SAC with the capacity to respond to a small number of improperly attached kinetochores on the one hand [52] yet remain highly vulnerable to polar-displaced chromosomes on the other [51]. An important question arising from these findings is how kinetochores of polar chromosomes in mouse oocytes, which are not optimally placed to capture microtubules, nevertheless manage to become saturated.

Integrating kinetochore–microtubule attachment formation and SAC signaling

During mitosis, the SAC signal is only extinguished at kinetochore pairs that are attached to and placed under tension by K-fiber bundles emanating from opposite spindle poles [35]. As the polewards forces acting on chromosomes are balanced under such circumstances, the net result is that SAC silencing is coordinated with proper alignment. A prominent feature of mitosis important for promoting bi-orientation involves relocating chromosomes from the poles to the equator (termed congression) [54]; by moving chromosomes to the equator, congression establishes a positional bias where the likelihood of capturing microtubules from opposite spindle poles is maximal. A key player in mitotic bi-orientation is CENP-E, which is not only pivotal for actively congressing chromosomes but also for K-fiber formation [35, 41, 54]. Consequently, mitotic cells in which CENP-E function is compromised exhibit polar-displaced chromosomes that chronically recruit high levels of Mad2 [35]. Thus, the K-fiber mode in mitosis is important for ensuring that SAC signaling remains coupled with chromosomal alignment status.

In order to begin to understand why SAC monitoring of polar chromosomes in mammalian oocytes departs so markedly from the mitotic template, we recently examined the importance of K-fibers in oocytes. We observed that even when K-fiber formation was severely compromised by CENP-E-depletion, Mad2 eventually became completely depleted from kinetochores of all bivalents, including the most severely polar-displaced ones [37]. Displacement of Mad2 from polar chromosomes, even when K-fibers are lacking [37], shows that unstable kinetochore–microtubule contacts suffice for displacing all of Mad2 from kinetochores in oocytes even for polar chromosomes that are not optimally placed to capture microtubules. Our data suggest kinetochore–microtubule contacts form in oocytes with relative ease. A system that enables kinetochore–microtubule interactions to form as easily as occurs in mammalian oocytes could conceivably enable polar kinetochores to become saturated even when they lack a positional bias for accumulating attachments, thereby uncoupling chromosomal position and SAC activity.

Another issue relevant to SAC signaling at polar chromosomes involves the configuration of kinetochore–microtubule attachments that are formed in oocytes. A recent detailed analysis of kinetochore–microtubule attachment configurations in fixed specimens showed that a very high proportion (up to 61%) of the attachments that formed during the phase when tension was sub-maximal were merotelic [39] – a kinetochore–microtubule attachment configuration in which one kinetochore is attached to two different spindle poles [33]. In contrast with merotelic attachments, amphitelic attachments, the most advantageous attachment pattern for accurate chromosome segregation in which one kinetochore is attached exclusively to one pole and the other kinetochore is attached to the opposite pole [33], are associated with maximal interkinetochore tension [39]. Significantly, however, and in keeping with an increased ease of saturation of microtubule bindings sites in oocytes, kinetochore–microtubule attachments that generate sub-maximal interkinetochore tension still suffice for displacing the bulk of kinetochore Mad2 [48, 53]. Collectively, therefore, on the basis that many tensionless chromosomes that are displaced polewards must be merotelically attached [40, 48, 53], the propensity to form merotelic attachments could be a major determinant of aneuploidy in oocytes as although such attachments predispose to misalignment, they nevertheless efficiently evade the SAC.

Far greater investigation of the detailed mechanisms by which oocyte kinetochores engage microtubules will be required in order to better understand these unique features of SAC signaling.

Cks-dependent APC/C regulation at the metaphase I-to-anaphase I transition

In contrast to the negative regulation imposed by the SAC, anaphase I onset in oocytes appears to be positively regulated by Cks2 [55], one of two Cks (Cdc kinase subunit) homologs (the other being Cks1) found in mammals. Cks proteins are small accessory subunits of CDKs that are important for CDK1-dependent phosphorylation. Interestingly, unlike mitotic cells, which express both Cks1 and Cks2 [56], mammalian germ cells appear only to express Cks2 [55]. In mutant mouse oocytes lacking Cks2 (*CKS2*$^{-/-}$ oocytes), meiosis arrests at metaphase I [55], raising the possibility that Cks2 might promote APC/C^{Cdc20}-mediated anaphase I onset. Cks2 function in oocytes can be compensated for by Cks1 as expression of exogenous Cks1 restores meiotic progression in *Cks2*$^{-/-}$ oocytes [55] and mitosis is impaired when both Cks1 and Cks2 are co-depleted but not following Cks2 single depletion [56]. Notably, in contrast to wild-type Cks2, a mutant form of Cks2 defective in CDK1 interaction could not restore meiotic progression in *CKS2*$^{-/-}$ oocytes [55]. Added to this, immunoblot analyses of testes extracts from *CKS2*$^{-/-}$ mice suggested that the APC/C subunit, APC3 (or Cdc27), is hypophosphorylated when Cks2 is lacking [55]. Given that the *Xenopus* Cks2 homolog, Xe-p9 [57], and mammalian Cks1/2 [56, 58] are required for CDK-dependent APC/C phosphorylation which is in turn associated with APC/C activation, it is possible that Cks2 mediates phosphorylation-dependent APC/C^{Cdc20} activation in oocytes (Figure 11.2B) in the absence of which MI stalls at metaphase I. This remains to be tested, however, as phosphorylation-independent mechanisms of Cks1/2-induced enhancement of proteolysis might exist. For instance, Cks1/2 facilitates cyclin A destruction by acting as a targeting subunit that recruits cyclin A to the phosphorylated APC/C [56].

Cyclin A turnover and implications for Cks-versus SAC-mediated regulation in oocytes

Mammals possess two A-type cyclins, cyclin A1 and A2 [3]. Unlike cyclin A2 deficiency, which culminates in embryonic lethality around the peri-implantation stage [59], mutant mice lacking cyclin A1 are viable but exhibit a male-specific fertility defect reflecting an absolute requirement of cyclin A1 for MI progression in male germ cells. In contrast, it has been reported that cyclin A1 is not expressed in oocytes, in which the only A-type cyclin appears to be cyclin A2 [60]. Immunoblotting of mouse oocytes shows that cyclin A2 levels decrease between the GV stage and MII [61]. Time-lapse analysis of an exogenously expressed fluorescently tagged construct indicates that this decrease in cyclin A2 is a consequence of degradation that occurs concurrently with that of securin and cyclin B1 during late MI after SAC inactivation [9, 28]. In stark contrast, during mitosis, cyclin A is destroyed shortly after NEBD, well before the SAC is satisfied and therefore in advance of SAC-regulated securin and cyclin B1 destruction [29, 62]. The pattern of cyclin A turnover in mammalian oocytes therefore presents yet another striking contrast with mitosis and points to further unique mechanisms of APC/C regulation.

In mitosis, the N-terminus of cyclin A outcompetes the SAC for Cdc20 binding, which combined with Cks1/2-mediated cyclin A recruitment to the phosphorylated APC/C, results in cyclin A destruction during prometaphase even when the SAC is active [63]. In mitotic cells, consistent with the requirement of Cks for cyclin A destruction, co-depletion of Cks1 and Cks2 leads to cyclin A stabilization during prometaphase [56]. Intriguingly, and in contrast to mitosis, testes extracts lacking the only expressed Cks, Cks2, exhibit stabilization of cyclin B but not cyclin A [55]. This suggests that during mammalian MI, cyclin A destruction might not be promoted by Cks, thereby providing a possible explanation as to why cyclin A destruction does not occur during prometaphase I in oocytes but is delayed instead until late MI [9, 28]. This raises the intriguing possibility that, in oocytes, cyclin A falls under SAC control. We are currently addressing these and other important aspects of cyclin A and Cks-dependent regulation in oocytes.

Modulating the APC/C for MI exit and entry into MII

CDK1 inactivation during mitotic exit allows phosphatases to dephosphorylate mitotic substrates so promoting chromosome and spindle behavior required for anaphase, spindle disassembly, reformation of the nuclear envelope, and chromosome decondensation [15, 64]. CDK1 inactivation also allows pre-replicative complexes (PRCs) to be loaded onto DNA replication origins, thereby licensing DNA for replication when CDK activity rises again [15, 64].

The exacting demands of meiosis require that only anaphase and cytokinesis occur on exit from MI but not spindle disassembly, DNA replication, chromosome decondensation, or nuclear envelope reformation. Although increasing insight into how the delicate balance between kinase activity and protein dephosphorylation is fine-tuned to achieve this remarkable feat in yeast, far less is known about these processes in mammalian oocytes, in which the task is further complicated by the need for a highly asymmetric division.

Proteolysis during exit from MI in mammalian oocytes

A striking feature of mammalian oocytes is the extended (~2–3 hour-long) duration of proteolysis leading up to anaphase I and exit from MI [9, 22, 28, 45, 65], about 10 times longer than the equivalent phase of proteolysis during mitotic exit (~20–30 minutes) [66]. What might be the significance of such protracted proteolysis towards the end of MI within the context of the mammalian oocyte? Live-cell imaging has very recently shown that well after proteolysis is underway, bivalents that initially adopt an equatorial position not infrequently drift out to the poles [48]. Furthermore, in keeping with their stealth in evading the SAC, such polar chromosomes do not delay the kinetics of APC/C-mediated proteolysis so that anaphase I proceeds on schedule even in the 4% of cases in which polar chromosomes persist right up to the time of anaphase onset, culminating in aneuploidy [48]. Slow degradation kinetics could therefore furnish time for wayward chromosomes to find their way back to the equatorial fold ahead of the final anaphase I trigger, thereby limiting otherwise catastrophic mis-segregation.

It is not known what factors are involved in setting these slow proteolytic kinetics leading up to MI exit. It is possible that the oocyte requires this extended time simply because the absolute amount of substrate to be degraded within the large oocyte volume outstrips APC/C^{Cdc20} capacity. It is notable that although the onset of substrate degradation is advanced by 2–5 hours in oocytes lacking either Mad2 or Bub1, degradation still extends over 2–4 hours [9, 45] and the exponential fivefold increase in APC/C activity that occurs during this time is similar in SAC-compromised and wild-type oocytes [9]. Thus, even without SAC-induced inhibition, the rate of substrate degradation cannot be further augmented, supporting the notion that APC/C^{Cdc20} capacity might be rate-limiting in oocytes. During mitosis, the absolute amount of APC/C^{Cdc20} is in large excess of minimum requirements so that protein destruction is severely perturbed only when ~98% of Cdc20 is depleted [56]. Under such circumstances of APC/C^{Cdc20} excess in mitotic cells, Cdc20 only becomes rate-limiting for cyclin A destruction when ~90% of Cdc20 is depleted and cyclin A is overexpressed [56]. In contrast, protein destruction and MI exit are very sensitive to overexpression of securin, cyclin B1, or cyclin A2 even in wild-type oocytes fully replete with Cdc20 [28, 65], providing another indication of a less-than-favorable APC/C^{Cdc20}:substrate ratio in oocytes. It is possible that APC/C^{Cdc20} capacity might be limited in oocytes due to the APC/C^{Cdh1}-dependent Cdc20 destruction that occurs in prometaphase I [22].

Protracted substrate degradation may not only be a function of absolute APC/C^{Cdc20} capacity but may also be a consequence of the timing of substrate degradation. Thus, as discussed above, unlike mitosis in which cyclin A is degraded in early prometaphase prior to securin and cyclin B1 [29, 62], all three substrates appear to be destroyed in tandem in oocytes [9, 28], thereby increasing the APC/C^{Cdc20} substrate load at metaphase I (Figure 11.2B). In this regard it is of note that cyclin A stabilization in mitotic cells depleted of Cks1/2 is associated with protracted intervals between NEBD and anaphase onset and with markedly prolonged phases of securin and cyclin B1 degradation at metaphase [56, 58]. It is therefore interesting to speculate that unique Cks activity and cyclin A regulation in mammalian oocytes might contribute to their unusually protracted durations of prometaphase I and protein degradation.

Interestingly, inhibiting CDK1 with roscovitine accelerated the degradation phase in oocytes [48], suggesting that a CDK1-dependent process is in some way involved in prolonging destruction times. APC/C^{Cdh1} is known to be inhibited by CDK1 and to participate in mitotic exit [1, 15]. It is important to note that although Cdc20 depletion inhibits securin and cyclin B1 destruction required for PBE [22], clearly pointing to an important role for APC/C^{Cdc20} in meiotic exit, this does not preclude a role for APC/C^{Cdh1} very late during the exit pathway, for instance, after APC/C^{Cdc20} has induced sufficient cyclin B1 degradation (and hence CDK1 inactivation) to enable a very late rise in APC/C^{Cdh1}. With such a model, Cdc20 depletion by preventing the initial cyclin B1 decline would also prevent later APC/C^{Cdh1} activation. Added to this, although Cdh1 levels decline in mid-MI, perhaps due to earlier APC/C^{Cdh1}-mediated Cdh1 destruction [67], they rise again by very late MI [5]. One possibility therefore is that degradation kinetics on exit from MI reflect a composite of two APC/C species, firstly APC/C^{Cdc20}, which is later reinforced by APC/C^{Cdh1}. However, to test such a role for APC/C^{Cdh1} specifically during very late MI could be a challenging experimental prospect as it would involve modulating the function of distinct APC/C species with high temporal precision.

Regulating cyclin B1 destruction and CDK1 inactivation at the MI-to-MII transition

Meiotic cells must exert restraint during exit from MI in order to enable the meiotic cell cycle to sidestep interphase after cytokinesis and immediately catapult into a second M-phase. The APC/C comes to the fore again as a pivotal regulatory node during this unique cell-cycle transition. Partial CDK1 inactivation may allow anaphase I and cytokinesis whilst retaining sufficient CDK1 activity for promoting rapid MII spindle assembly with condensed chromosomes whilst preventing pre-replicative complex and nuclear envelope assembly. In keeping with this, in *Xenopus* oocytes [68] and fission yeast [69], restrained cyclin B destruction and CDK inactivation during MI exit is important for successful entry into MII.

In contrast to fission yeast and *Xenopus* oocytes, however, it is unclear to what extent restrained cyclin B1 destruction and CDK1 inactivation during exit from MI are absolutely required for the MI-to-MII transition in mammalian oocytes. An important APC/C inhibitor during meiotic divisions is early mitotic inhibitor 2 (Emi2)/Emi-related protein 1. Significant levels of Emi2 are detectable in mouse oocytes by the MII-arrested stage but not at the GV stage pointing to a restricted role late in meiosis [70]. Following Emi2 depletion using morpholinos, oocytes undergo PBE with normal kinetics but thereafter are incapable of assembling a bipolar spindle and maintaining condensed chromosomes, showing that Emi2 is important for establishing the MII-arrest state after MI exit [70]. Compromised spindle assembly and chromosome condensation following MI exit in Emi2-depleted oocytes appear to result from failure of CDK1 reactivation since Emi2-depleted oocytes are unable to re-establish elevated cyclin B1 levels following PBE [70]. The inability to re-establish cyclin B1 after MI exit was due to unrestrained APC/C^{Cdc20}-mediated proteolysis since spindle assembly and chromosome condensation could be rescued in Emi2-depleted oocytes by expressing either a non-destructible cyclin B1 construct or Mad2 after oocytes had undergone PBE [70].

Significantly, although Emi2 is important for restraining cyclin B1 destruction after exit from MI (Figures 11.2C and 11.2D), it does not appear to impact degradation during MI exit itself. In line with this, an exogenous fluorescently tagged cyclin B1 construct exhibited indistinguishable degradation kinetics during MI exit in Emi2-depleted and wild-type mouse oocytes [70]. Furthermore, exogenous cyclin B1 was degraded to the same degree in both Emi2-depleted and wild-type oocytes and either Mad2 or non-destructible cyclin B1 could rescue the MII state in Emi2-depleted oocytes when introduced after PBE had occurred [70]. Notably, these findings also indicate that Emi2-mediated APC/C inhibition does not contribute to the slow degradation profile (see above) and is not responsible for the incomplete cyclin B1 destruction [23, 24] that occurs in mouse oocytes during exit from MI. The significance of incomplete cyclin B1 degradation on exit from MI is uncertain since residual cyclin B1 might not sustain CDK1 activity as histone H1 phosphorylation has been reported to be inactivated down to basal levels during the MI-to-MII transition, perhaps via a separase-dependent mechanism (discussed below) [71]. Indeed, this has prompted suggestions that mammalian oocytes may require input from an auxiliary kinase akin to the CDK1-like kinase, Ime2, in budding yeast for sustaining the phosphorylation of key substrates required, for instance, for averting DNA replication during interkinesis [72]. Notably, however, a close mammalian relative of Ime2, Mak (male germ cell-associated kinase), does not appear to be expressed during the latter stages of oocyte development [73]. It remains to be seen whether other Ime2-like homologs such as Ick and Rage, transcripts for which are expressed in oocytes [74], modulate the phosphorylation status of important CDK1 substrates during interkinesis.

In addition to its more direct effect on CDK1 activity through mediating cyclin B1 destruction, the APC/C may also indirectly influence CDK1 during MI exit through its effects in bringing about separase activation by securin proteolysis. This is because separase fulfills a non-proteolytic function that is required for MI exit in mouse oocytes as evidenced by inhibition of PBE in separase-null oocytes, which can be restored by expressing a protease-dead form of separase [47]. It appears that separase influences MI exit at least in part through CDK1 inhibition mediated by separase–CDK1–cyclin B complex formation [75] as a highly specific antibody directed against the CDK1-binding determinants (anti-CBD antibody) in separase, which did not inhibit cohesin cleavage but counteracted separase–CDK1 complex formation, severely reduced PBE (~11%) compared with mock IgG injection (~63%) [71]. Furthermore, PBE could be rescued in anti-CBD-injected oocytes by the small-molecule CDK inhibitor, roscovitine, indicating that the cytokinesis defect with the anti-CBD antibody was consequent upon sustained CDK1 activity [71]. Although these data suggest that separase contributes to MI exit by binding to and inactivating CDK1 in vertebrate oocytes (Figure 11.2D), an important caveat is that CDK1 inactivation (measured using histone H1 kinase assays) occurred normally in separase-null oocytes [47].

The role of phosphatases in MI exit

In mitotic cells, CDK1 inactivation alone is not sufficient to drive mitotic exit, which also depends on phosphatase-mediated dephosphorylation of CDK substrates [15, 64]. In budding yeast, CDC14 is the key mitotic exit phosphatase, acting not only to dephosphorylate CDK1 (Cdc28 in budding yeast) substrates but also to complete CDK1 inactivation [15, 64]. As discussed earlier, in oocytes, CDC14B influences

GVBD whereas CDC14A has less impact at the G2–M boundary [16, 17]. Significantly however, both CDC14A and CDC14B are important for MI exit. Thus, overexpression of either CDC14A or CDC14B or injection of a polyclonal antibody directed against the C-terminal CDC14A region delayed MI progression [16, 17]. In both MII-arrested and GV-stage oocytes, histone H1 phosphorylation was found to be 1.5-fold greater after CDC14B depletion than after mock-depletion [16] suggesting that CDC14 impacts CDK1 substrates at multiple stages of meiosis. It therefore seems likely that CDC14 influences MI exit by dephosphorylating CDK1 substrates. Notably, CDC14A and CDC14B localize to the central spindle during late MI, suggesting that dephosphorylation of CDK1 substrates that reside here could be important for MI exit. In this regard it is noteworthy that in budding yeast, the midzone organizer, Ase1 (anaphase spindle elongation 1), is a CDK1 substrate whose CDC14-dependent dephosphorylation is required for proper interpolar microtubule sliding and anaphase spindle elongation [76]. It will therefore be interesting to determine whether CDC14B depletion impacts the activity and phosphorylation status of the mammalian Ase1 homolog, PRC1 (protein regulator of cytokinesis 1), which is expressed in oocytes [74] and is a CDK1 substrate important for cytokinesis in human somatic cells [77].

Although disrupting either CDC14A or CDC14B delays MI progression, PBE does eventually occur [16, 17]. Hence, CDC14 does not appear to be absolutely necessary for MI exit in oocytes but does contribute to the efficiency and integrity of the process. It will therefore also be important to determine whether other phosphatases might contribute to MI exit, such as those of the PP1 and PP2A families, which emerging evidence indicates are of greater significance than CDC14 for mitotic exit in animal cells [64].

CSF- and fertilization-mediated APC/C regulation during metaphase II arrest and egg activation

CSF and metaphase II arrest

After completing MI, oocytes enter MII where they arrest at metaphase II with elevated CDK1 activity. This unique metaphase II arrest state depends upon an activity known as CSF, which generates a suspended M-phase state by inhibiting APC/C-directed securin and cyclin B1 destruction. CSF-mediated arrest is broken at fertilization thereby ensuring that completion of MII and subsequent embryogenesis is coordinated with the introduction of a paternal genome.

This remarkable CSF arrest state is characterized by a fully formed bipolar spindle on which chromosomes, each consisting of two sister chromatids united by centromeric cohesion, are aligned at the equatorial region. Such a prolonged metaphase arrest goes counter to the mitotic paradigm in which metaphase is a fleeting state that, once achieved, triggers APC/C^{Cdc20}-mediated securin and cyclin B1 destruction shortly thereafter leading to anaphase and exit from M-phase.

Remarkably, however, although CSF suppresses APC/C activity to sustain metaphase II arrest, the APC/C does not become completely quiescent. Instead, APC/C-mediated cyclin B1 destruction perdures [78], giving cyclin B1 a half-life of around 1 hour in mouse eggs [79]. Sustained cyclin B1 levels during MII depend on continued protein synthesis as inhibiting protein synthesis using drugs such as puromycin culminates in net cyclin B1 destruction and exit from MII arrest [78].

The events surrounding MII arrest and the egg-to-embryo transition can be considered in terms of CSF establishment, CSF maintenance, and finally, the breaking of CSF at fertilization. As the mechanisms underpinning these events have been worked out in considerable detail in frogs, the ensuing discussion will frequently refer to the frog model as a template for dissecting the comparatively limited knowledge of mammalian CSF regulation. What has become clear is that in both mammalian and frog eggs, the oocyte-specific protein Emi2 constitutes a pivotal APC/C inhibitor and a cornerstone of CSF activity.

Establishing and maintaining CSF arrest

Many details that have been elucidated in frog eggs regarding CSF establishment and maintenance remain incompletely understood in mammalian oocytes. For instance, the precise role of the Mos–MAPK (mitogen-activated protein kinase) pathway in CSF arrest in mammals is unclear. Thus, although oocytes from Mos knockout mice fail to activate the MAPK pathway and do not sustain an MII arrest, they nevertheless often undergo a transient arrest lasting 2–4 hours [80–82]. Although one interpretation of this is that Mos–MAPK is involved in CSF maintenance but not in its establishment [70], such reasoning is not borne out by recent observations showing that Mos declines to undetectable levels amongst mouse eggs that remain arrested in MII [83]. Furthermore, exactly how the Mos–MAPK pathway might signal is unknown as Rsk (ribosomal S6 kinase), a crucial downstream Mos–MAPK effector in frogs [84], is dispensable in mammals as oocytes from triple Rsk [1–3] knockout mice establish and maintain MII arrest normally [85]. One role for Mos–MAPK in mammals appears to involve the maintenance of spindle integrity during MII, perhaps through the spindle regulators, MISS and DocR1, which are MAPK substrates [86, 87]. The involvement of the SAC in CSF arrest also witnesses a divergence between frogs and mammals as unlike frog eggs, in which the SAC is required for establishing and maintaining CSF arrest [88], in mouse oocytes expression of dominant negative versions of Mad2, Bub1, or BubR1 does not impair CSF arrest [89].

As mentioned previously, an integral CSF component that is conserved between frogs and mammals is Emi2. Consistent with a CSF role, endogenous Emi2 levels in mouse oocytes are low at the GV stage and increase by MII [70]. Furthermore, premature overexpression of Emi2 during oocyte maturation induces an MI arrest [70, 83]. Emi2 is required for establishing CSF arrest as preventing Emi2 accumulation using morpholino antisense during mouse oocyte maturation culminates in a failure to re-establish cyclin B1 and to assemble a MII spindle following PBE [70]. Moreover, small interfering RNA (siRNA)-induced Emi2 depletion in MII-arrested oocytes abrogates CSF arrest, underscoring Emi2's role in CSF maintenance [90]. The available evidence indicates that Emi2 mediates its effects through APC/C^{Cdc20} in mouse oocytes as Emi2 and Cdc20 interact in vitro, the establishment of MII arrest could be restored in maturing Emi2-depleted oocytes by co-depleting Cdc20, and the escape from MII arrest induced by Emi2 depletion is countered by co-depletion of Cdc20 [90]. Emi2 could also be linked with the observed requirement of Zn^{2+} for MII arrest in mouse eggs [91] as mutations within the putative Zn^{2+}-binding region (ZBR) in Emi2 compromised the MII-arresting ability of Emi2 overexpression [83].

In frog eggs, the Mos–MAPK pathway is intimately connected with Emi2-mediated MII arrest through Rsk-mediated Emi2 phosphorylation, which facilitates binding of protein phosphatase 2A (PP2A), in turn establishing an Emi2 phosphorylation profile that increases its stability and enhances APC/C binding and inhibition [84]. Although Rsk does not appear to be important in mice, it may be that the Mos–MAPK pathway still signals to mammalian Emi2 as mutating the T^{327} residue in mouse Emi2, thought to correspond to the Rsk target (T^{336}) in frogs, severely reduces the ability of Emi2 overexpression to induce an M-phase arrest in a functional assay [83]. Moreover, recent data indicate that PP2A is important for Emi2 stability as okadaic acid-induced PP2A inhibition in mouse eggs destabilized Emi2, leading to securin and cyclin B1 degradation, and could be reversed by preincubation with the PP2A-specific activator FTY720 [92]. Intriguingly, therefore, in mammals, Mos–MAPK might regulate Emi2 stability via PP2A through an as-yet-unidentified non-Rsk intermediary.

Breaking CSF arrest at fertilization

Fertilization induces a ~4–6-hour-long series of repetitive intracellular calcium oscillations that are both necessary and sufficient for inducing the events associated with egg activation, including lifting of MII arrest and cortical granule exocytosis, the latter being important for preventing polyspermy [93]. Based on the prevailing model, sperm–egg fusion delivers a soluble sperm factor, the leading candidate being the sperm-specific ζ isoform of phospholipase C (Plcζ), which, via increased inositol 1, 4, 5-trisphosphate (IP_3) levels acting through endoplasmic reticulum IP_3 receptors, leads to calcium release [94]. Recent evidence indicates that the mechanism by which calcium influx activates all of the downstream pathways leading to egg activation is not exclusively via its influence on bulk intracellular calcium oscillations and that calcium influx additionally mediates spatially restricted calcium signaling that is important for some aspects of activation such as spindle rotation and cortical granule exocytosis [95].

Increased intracellular calcium culminates in an approximately sixfold increase in APC/C-mediated proteolysis [79, 96]. Time-lapse imaging of fluorescently tagged securin and cyclin B1 constructs shows that their destruction commences approximately 12–13 minutes after the start of calcium spiking and that both undergo 80–90% degradation by the time of second PBE [96]. Although mouse eggs express both Cdc20 and Cdh1, the bulk of calcium-induced protein destruction is APC/C^{Cdc20}-mediated as a D-box mutated securin construct, which is resistant to APC/C^{Cdc20} but, by virtue of retaining a KEN-box still remains susceptible to APC/C^{Cdh1}, stayed stable until the time of second PBE [96]. APC/C^{Cdh1} is likely inhibited prior to second PBE due to high Cdh1-inhibitory

CDK1 activity, in keeping with which Cdh1 exhibits a mobility shift consistent with inhibitory phosphorylation [96]. Further in keeping with a prominent APC/C^{Cdc20} role, either siRNA-induced Cdc20 depletion or SAC activation (brought about either by spindle depolymerization or Mad2 overexpression) in MII mouse eggs prevents exit from MII [78, 79, 90, 97]. Taken together therefore, the primary mediator of calcium-induced proteolysis is APC/C^{Cdc20} whose principal substrates, as in MI and mitosis, are cyclin B1 and securin.

The steps linking calcium increase with APC/C^{Cdc20} activation in mammals are beginning to be deciphered but await full clarification. In frogs, fertilization-induced calcium signaling triggers sequential Emi2 phosphorylations by calmodulin kinase II (CaMKII) and polo-like kinase 1 (Plk1), leading to Emi2 degradation by the βTrCP-activated Skp-Cullin-Fbox ubiquitin ligase ($SCF^{\beta TrCP}$) [84]. In mouse eggs, in keeping with the notion that loss of Emi2 relieves APC/C^{Cdc20} inhibition, monitoring of a fluorescently tagged Emi2 construct indicated that Emi2 is stable in MII-arrested eggs until intracellular calcium levels rise, after which marked Emi2 destruction ensues [70]. Importantly, simultaneous time-lapse fluorescence imaging of Emi2 and cyclin B1 show that Emi2's destruction is temporally advanced compared with that of cyclin B1, consistent with the latter being a consequence of the former [70].

As in frogs, mammalian CaMKII is important for relaying the calcium signal. Thus, MII mouse oocytes express the γ3 and γJ isoforms of CaMKII in roughly equimolar amounts [83]. Furthermore, exit from MII arrest is promoted by expression of constitutively active CaMKII [97, 98] but impaired when CaMKIIγ levels are reduced either by morpholino antisense depletion of CaMKIIγ3 in oocytes [99] or by targeted deletion of the *CaMKIIγ* gene [100]. Unlike frogs, in which another important calcium-dependent enzyme important for transducing the calcium signal is the protein phosphatase calcineurin [101, 102], currently available evidence argues against a role for calcineurin in mammals as the calcineurin catalytic A subunit was undetectable in mouse oocytes and a cocktail of calcineurin inhibitors could not prevent MII exit [83]. The implication is that in mammals, CaMKIIγ is the primary mediator of calcium-induced Emi2 down-regulation. Notably, however, although CaMKIIγ transduces the calcium signal for initiating cell-cycle resumption, it is not required for cortical granule exocytosis [98–100].

Although the foregoing outline a broad framework whereby calcium oscillations trigger Emi2 destruction via CaMKII as intermediary, other details within this pathway remain unclear. In frogs, Emi2 is phosphorylated by CaMKII at a canonical RXST motif and by Plk1 at an N-terminally located DSGX$_3$S phoshodegron [84]. Notably, however, mouse Emi2 lacks the canonical CaMKII-targeted RXXT/S motif present in *Xenopus* Emi2 and in an in vitro assay, there was no detectable phosphorylation of either mouse or *Xenopus* Emi2 by CaMKIIγ [83]. These apparent anomalies could be reconciled if ^{173}KSST^{176} acts as an alternative CaMKII phosphorylation target in mouse Emi2, in support of which an Emi2 construct bearing a phosphorylation-resistant mutation within the ^{173}KSST^{176} sequence ($Emi2^{T176A}$) was resistant to calcium-induced destruction [83]. Also, it may be that lack of CaMKIIγ-mediated Emi2 phosphorylation in vitro could reflect the lack of an adaptor protein important for conferring in vivo phosphorylation [83]. Mammalian Emi2 sequences lack the N-terminally located DSGX$_3$S phoshodegron found in *Xenopus* [83, 103]. Instead, the corresponding phosphodegron in the mouse appears to be ^{274}DSGFCS^{279}, in keeping with which phosphorylation resistant mutations in this sequence, $Emi2^{D274A}$ and $Emi2^{S275N}$, were resistant to calcium-induced degradation [83].

Recently, it was shown that an independent requirement for exit from MII in mouse eggs is Wee1B kinase-mediated inhibitory CDK1 phosphorylation [104]. Thus, calcium-induced pronuclear formation was severely compromised in oocytes depleted of Wee1B using morpholinos. Interestingly, this work showed that Wee1B-dependent inactivation of CDK1 occurred ahead of cyclin B1–GFP proteolysis consistent with the notion that Wee1B is upstream of APC/C^{Cdc20}. Further in keeping with this, in Wee1B-depleted oocytes, Emi2 exhibited increased stability to calcium signaling as did securin and cyclin B1, altogether pointing to a model in which Wee1B not only made an indispensable contribution to CDK1 inactivation, but also initiated a cascade critical for fully activating APC/C^{Cdc20} through Emi2 destruction. It was also shown that the intermediary between calcium signaling and Wee1B was CaMKII, which activated Wee1B through S15 phosphorylation. Therefore, in addition to identifying an important role for inhibitory

CDK1 phosphorylation during MII exit, these data also point to another pathway between CaMKII and Emi2 involving Wee1B.

It is unclear what mediates Emi2's destruction in mammalian eggs. As yet there is no clear evidence that Emi2 destruction falls to $SCF^{\beta TrCP}$ as occurs in frogs as eggs from mice lacking one of the two mouse βTrCP isoforms, Trcpb1, degrade Emi2 normally in response to calcium increase [83]. Neither does responsibility fall on APC/C^{Cdc20} as Emi2 destruction is not sensitive to RNA interference (RNAi)-mediated Cdc20 depletion [83] and nocodazole-induced spindle depolymerization, which activates the SAC to inhibit APC/C^{Cdc20}, does not prevent Emi2 destruction [70]. It is possible that the other βTrCP isoform, Trcpb2, or an altogether different ubiquitin ligase confers degradation.

Conclusions

It is a little under a decade since the role of the APC/C in mammalian oocytes first became apparent. During this time it has become evident that the APC/C is instrumental in all of the key transitions during female mammalian meiotic maturation. Indeed, by straddling every phase of oocyte maturation from entry to exit, the APC/C holds a position of unrivaled importance with regard to female fertility.

Although the mechanisms by which the APC/C orchestrates these critical events in oocytes are beginning to be deciphered, many important questions remain to be elucidated. For instance, how does BubR1 regulate Cdh1 levels? Other key questions pertain to SAC signaling in oocytes, which in turn will require an in-depth understanding of how microtubules make contacts with kinetochores to enable SAC binding sites to become saturated with relative ease. Understanding how the APC/C targets cyclin A2 in oocytes could shed light on why prometaphase I and proteolysis during MI exit are unusually protracted. Clarification of cyclin B1 degradation and CDK1 inactivation and the role of auxiliary kinases and phosphatases during MI exit will be pivotal for understanding the regulation of the MI-to-MII transition. There is also a need for better understanding of Emi2 regulation during MII arrest and exit, such as the mechanism by which it might be influenced by the Mos–MAPK pathway, how Wee1B impacts its stability, and which ubiquitin ligase is responsible for executing its destruction. It will also be interesting to determine whether mammalian oocytes engage meiosis-specific APC/C activators similar to Cortex in *Drosophila* and Ama1 in yeast. Finally, whilst the APC/C is a pivotal node for regulating the levels of a number of proteins, it will be important to determine how the levels of APC/C components are themselves regulated. It is noteworthy in this regard that recent work indicates that all 12 core APC/C components are subject to finely tuned translational regulation during MI in mouse oocytes [105].

Undoubtedly, detailed understanding of the workings of the APC/C juggernaut will provide invaluable insight into the molecular underpinnings of medical conditions such as premature ovarian failure and of the female-specific age-related biological phenomenon that underlies high rates of embryonic aneuploidy, miscarriage and infertility for older women.

Acknowledgments

The author is supported by a Wellcome Trust Clinical Fellowship (082587/Z/07/Z).

References

1. Pines J. Cubism and the cell cycle: the many faces of the APC/C. *Nat Rev Mol Cell Biol* 2011; **12**(7): 427–38.
2. Solc P, Schultz RM, Motlik J. Prophase I arrest and progression to metaphase I in mouse oocytes: comparison of resumption of meiosis and recovery from G2-arrest in somatic cells. *Mol Hum Reprod* 2010; **16**(9): 654–64.
3. Satyanarayana A, Kaldis P. Mammalian cell-cycle regulation: several Cdks, numerous cyclins and diverse compensatory mechanisms. *Oncogene* 2009; **28**(33): 2925–39.
4. Polanski Z, Homer H, Kubiak JZ. Cyclin B in mouse oocytes and embryos: importance for human reproduction and aneuploidy. *Results Probl Cell Differ* 2012; **55**: 69–91.
5. Homer H, Gui L, Carroll J. A spindle assembly checkpoint protein functions in prophase I arrest and prometaphase progression. *Science* 2009; **326**(5955): 991–4.
6. Marangos P, Verschuren E, Chen R, Jackson P, Carroll J. Prophase I arrest and progression to metaphase I in mouse oocytes are controlled by Emi1-dependent regulation of APCCdh1. *J Cell Biol* 2007; **176**(1): 65–75.

7. Reis A, Chang H, Levasseur M, Jones K. APCcdh1 activity in mouse oocytes prevents entry into the first meiotic division. *Nat Cell Biol* 2006; **8**(5): 539–40.
8. Holt JE, Tran SM, Stewart JL, *et al.* The APC/C activator FZR1 coordinates the timing of meiotic resumption during prophase I arrest in mammalian oocytes. *Development* 2011; **138**(5): 905–13.
9. McGuinness BE, Anger M, Kouznetsova A, *et al.* Regulation of APC/C activity in oocytes by a Bub1-dependent spindle assembly checkpoint. *Curr Biol* 2009; **19**(5): 369–80.
10. Hagting A, Karlsson C, Clute P, Jackman M, Pines J. MPF localization is controlled by nuclear export. *EMBO J* 1998; **17**(14): 4127–38.
11. Holt JE, Weaver J, Jones KT. Spatial regulation of APCCdh1-induced cyclin B1 degradation maintains G2 arrest in mouse oocytes. *Development* 2010; **137**(8): 1297–304.
12. Marangos P, Carroll J. The dynamics of cyclin B1 distribution during meiosis I in mouse oocytes. *Reproduction* 2004; **128**(2): 153–62.
13. Oh JS, Han SJ, Conti M. Wee1B, Myt1, and Cdc25 function in distinct compartments of the mouse oocyte to control meiotic resumption. *J Cell Biol* 2010; **188**(2): 199–207.
14. Marangos P, Carroll J. Securin regulates entry into M-phase by modulating the stability of cyclin B. *Nat Cell Biol* 2008; **10**(4): 445–51.
15. Sullivan M, Morgan DO. Finishing mitosis, one step at a time. *Nat Rev Mol Cell Biol* 2007; **8**(11): 894–903.
16. Schindler K, Schultz RM. CDC14B acts through FZR1 (CDH1) to prevent meiotic maturation of mouse oocytes. *Biol Reprod* 2009; **80**(4): 795–803.
17. Schindler K, Schultz RM. The CDC14A phosphatase regulates oocyte maturation in mouse. *Cell Cycle* 2009; **8**(7): 1090–8.
18. Miller JJ, Summers MK, Hansen DV, *et al.* Emi1 stably binds and inhibits the anaphase-promoting complex/cyclosome as a pseudosubstrate inhibitor. *Genes Dev* 2006; **20**(17): 2410–20.
19. Hassold T, Hunt P. Maternal age and chromosomally abnormal pregnancies: what we know and what we wish we knew. *Curr Opin Pediatr* 2009; **21**(6): 703–8.
20. Homer H. New insights into the genetic regulation of homologue disjunction in mammalian oocytes. *Cytogenet Genome Res* 2011; **133**(2–4): 209–22.
21. Polanski Z, Ledan E, Brunet S, *et al.* Cyclin synthesis controls the progression of meiotic maturation in mouse oocytes. *Development* 1998; **125**: 4989–97.
22. Reis A, Madgwick S, Chang HY, *et al.* Prometaphase APCcdh1 activity prevents non-disjunction in mammalian oocytes. *Nat Cell Biol* 2007; **9**(10): 1192–8.
23. Hampl A, Eppig JJ. Analysis of the mechanism(s) of metaphase I arrest in maturing mouse oocytes. *Development* 1995; **121**: 925–33.
24. Winston NJ. Stability of cyclin B during meiotic maturation and the first meiotic cell division in mouse oocytes. *Biol Cell* 1997; **89**: 211–19.
25. Peter M, Castro A, Lorca T, *et al.* The APC is dispensable for first meiotic anaphase in *Xenopus* oocytes. *Nat Cell Biol* 2001; **3**: 83–7.
26. Taieb FE, Gross SD, Lewellyn AL, Maller JL. Activation of the anaphase-promoting complex and degradation of cyclin B is not required for progression from MI to II in *Xenopus* oocytes. *Curr Biol* 2001; **11**: 508–13.
27. Herbert M, Levasseur M, Homer H, *et al.* Homologue disjunction in mouse oocytes requires proteolysis of securin and cyclin B1. *Nat Cell Biol* 2003; **5**: 1023–5.
28. Jin F, Hamada M, Malureanu L, *et al.* Cdc20 is critical for meiosis I and fertility of female mice. *PLoS Genet* 2010; **6**(9): pii:e1001147.
29. den Elzen N, Pines J. Cyclin A is destroyed in prometaphase and can delay chromosome alignment and anaphase. *J Cell Biol* 2001; **153**: 121–36.
30. Musacchio A, Salmon ED. The spindle-assembly checkpoint in space and time. *Nat Rev Mol Cell Biol* 2007; **8**(5): 379–93.
31. Kulukian A, Han JS, Cleveland DW. Unattached kinetochores catalyze production of an anaphase inhibitor that requires a Mad2 template to prime Cdc20 for BubR1 binding. *Dev Cell* 2009; **16**(1): 105–17.
32. Malureanu LA, Jeganathan KB, Hamada M, *et al.* BubR1 N terminus acts as a soluble inhibitor of cyclin B degradation by APC/C(Cdc20) in interphase. *Dev Cell* 2009; **16**(1): 118–31.
33. Hauf S, Watanabe Y. Kinetochore orientation in mitosis and meiosis. *Cell* 2004; **119**(3): 317–27.
34. Pinsky BA, Biggins S. The spindle checkpoint: tension versus attachment. *Trends Cell Biol* 2005; **15**(9): 486–93.
35. Putkey F, Cramer T, Morphew M, *et al.* Unstable kinetochore-microtubule capture and chromosomal instability following deletion of CENP-E. *Dev Cell* 2002; **3**(3): 351–65.
36. Waters JC, Chen RH, Murray AW, Salmon ED. Localization of Mad2 to kinetochores depends on microtubule attachment, not tension. *J Cell Biol* 1998; **141**(5): 1181–91.
37. Gui L, Homer H. Spindle assembly checkpoint signalling is uncoupled from chromosomal position in mouse oocytes. *Development* 2012; **139**(11): 1941–6.

8. Schuh M, Ellenberg J. Self-organization of MTOCs replaces centrosome function during acentrosomal spindle assembly in live mouse oocytes. *Cell* 2007; **130**(3): 484–98.

9. Kitajima TS, Ohsugi M, Ellenberg J. Complete kinetochore tracking reveals error-prone homologous chromosome biorientation in mammalian oocytes. *Cell* 2011; **146**(4): 568–81.

0. Yang KT, Li SK, Chang CC, *et al.* Aurora-C kinase deficiency causes cytokinesis failure in meiosis I and production of large polyploid oocytes in mice. *Mol Biol Cell* 2010; **21**(14): 2371–83.

1. Kim Y, Holland AJ, Lan W, Cleveland DW. Aurora kinases and protein phosphatase 1 mediate chromosome congression through regulation of CENP-E. *Cell* 2010; **142**(3): 444–55.

2. Homer H, McDougall A, Levasseur M, Murdoch A, Herbert M. Mad2 is required for inhibiting securin and cyclin B degradation following spindle depolymerisation in meiosis I mouse oocytes. *Reproduction* 2005; **130**(6): 829–43.

3. Wassmann K, Niault T, Maro B. Metaphase I arrest upon activation of the MAD2-dependent spindle checkpoint in mouse oocytes. *Curr Biol* 2003; **13**: 1596–608.

4. Hached K, Xie SZ, Buffin E, *et al.* Mps1 at kinetochores is essential for female mouse meiosis I. *Development* 2011; **138**(11): 2261–71.

5. Homer H, McDougall A, Levasseur M, *et al.* Mad2 prevents aneuploidy and premature proteolysis of cyclin B and securin during meiosis I in mouse oocytes. *Genes Dev* 2005; **19**(2): 202–7.

6. Brunet S, Santa Maria A, Guillaud P, *et al.* Kinetochore fibers are not involved in the formation of the first meiotic spindle of mouse oocytes, but control the exit from the first meiotic M phase. *J Cell Biol* 1999; **146**: 1–12.

7. Kudo N, Wassmann K, Anger M, *et al.* Resolution of chiasmata in oocytes requires separase-mediated proteolysis. *Cell* 2006; **126**(1): 135–46.

8. Lane SI, Yun Y, Jones KT. Timing of anaphase-promoting complex activation in mouse oocytes is predicted by microtubule-kinetochore attachment but not by bivalent alignment or tension. *Development* 2012; **139**(11): 1947–55.

9. Rieder CL, Cole RW, Khodjakov A, Sluder G. The checkpoint delaying anaphase in response to chromosome monoorientation is mediated by an inhibitory signal produced by unattached kinetochores. *J Cell Biol* 1995; **130**(4): 941–8.

0. Woods L, Hodges C, Baart E, *et al.* Chromosomal influence on meiotic spindle assembly: abnormal meiosis I in female Mlh1 mutant mice. *J Cell Biol* 1999; **145**(7): 1395–406.

51. Nagaoka SI, Hodges CA, Albertini DF, Hunt PA. Oocyte-specific differences in cell-cycle control create an innate susceptibility to meiotic errors. *Curr Biol* 2011; **21**(8): 651–7.

52. Hoffmann S, Maro B, Kubiak JZ, Polanski Z. A single bivalent efficiently inhibits cyclin B1 degradation and polar body extrusion in mouse oocytes indicating robust SAC during female meiosis I. *PLoS One* 2011; **6**(11): e27143.

53. Kolano A, Brunet S, Silk AD, Cleveland DW, Verlhac MH. Error-prone mammalian female meiosis from silencing the spindle assembly checkpoint without normal interkinetochore tension. *Proc Natl Acad Sci USA* 2012; **109**(27): E1858–67.

54. Kapoor T, Lampson M, Hergert P, *et al.* Chromosomes can congress to the metaphase plate before biorientation. *Science* 2006; **311**(5759): 388–91.

55. Spruck CH, de Miguel MP, Smith AP, *et al.* Requirement of Cks2 for the first metaphase/anaphase transition of mammalian meiosis. *Science* 2003; **300**(5619): 647–50.

56. Wolthuis R, Clay-Farrace L, van Zon W, *et al.* Cdc20 and Cks direct the spindle checkpoint-independent destruction of cyclin A. *Mol Cell* 2008; **30**(3): 290–302.

57. Patra D, Dunphy WG. Xe-p9, a *Xenopus* Suc1/Cks protein, is essential for the Cdc2-dependent phosphorylation of the anaphase-promoting complex at mitosis. *Genes Dev* 1998; **12**(16): 2549–59.

58. van ZW, Ogink J, ter Riet B, Medema RH, *et al.* The APC/C recruits cyclin B1-Cdk1-Cks in prometaphase before D box recognition to control mitotic exit. *J Cell Biol* 2010; **190**(4): 587–602.

59. Murphy M, Stinnakre MG, Senamaud-Beaufort C, *et al.* Delayed early embryonic lethality following disruption of the murine cyclin A2 gene. *Nat Genet* 1997; **15**(1): 83–6.

60. Persson JL, Zhang Q, Wang XY, *et al.* Distinct roles for the mammalian A-type cyclins during oogenesis. *Reproduction* 2005; **130**(4): 411–22.

61. Winston N, Bourgain-Guglielmetti F, Ciemerych MA, *et al.* Early development of mouse embryos null mutant for the cyclin A2 gene occurs in the absence of maternally derived cyclin A2 gene products. *Dev Biol* 2000; **223**(1): 139–53.

62. Geley S, Kramer E, Gieffers C, *et al.* APC/C-dependent proteolysis of human cyclin A starts at the beginning of mitosis and is not subject to the spindle assembly checkpoint. *J Cell Biol* 2001; **153**: 137–48.

63. Di Fiore, Pines J. How cyclin A destruction escapes the spindle assembly checkpoint. *J Cell Biol* 2010; **190**(4): 501–9.

64. Wurzenberger C, Gerlich DW. Phosphatases: providing safe passage through mitotic exit. *Nat Rev Mol Cell Biol* 2011; **12**(8): 469–82.

65. Ledan E, Polanski Z, Terret M-E, Maro B. Meiotic maturation of the mouse oocyte requires an equilibrium between cyclin B synthesis and degradation. *Dev Biol* 2001; **232**: 400–13.

66. Clute P, Pines J. Temporal and spatial control of cyclin B1 destruction in metaphase. *Nat Cell Biol* 1999; **1**: 82–7.

67. Listovsky T, Oren YS, Yudkovsky Y, *et al.* Mammalian Cdh1/Fzr mediates its own degradation. *EMBO J* 2004; **23**(7): 1619–26.

68. Iwabuchi M, Ohsumi K, Yamamoto TM, Sawada W, Kishimoto T. Residual Cdc2 activity remaining at meiosis I exit is essential for meiotic M-M transition in *Xenopus* oocyte extracts. *EMBO J* 2000; **19**(17): 4513–23.

69. Izawa D, Goto M, Yamashita A, Yamano H, Yamamoto M. Fission yeast Mes1p ensures the onset of meiosis II by blocking degradation of cyclin Cdc13p. *Nature* 2005; **434**(7032): 529–33.

70. Madgwick S, Hansen D, Levasseur M, Jackson P, Jones K. Mouse Emi2 is required to enter meiosis II by reestablishing cyclin B1 during interkinesis. *J Cell Biol* 2006; **174**(6): 791–801.

71. Gorr IH, Reis A, Boos D, *et al.* Essential CDK1-inhibitory role for separase during meiosis I in vertebrate oocytes. *Nat Cell Biol* 2006; **8**(9): 1035–7.

72. Holt LJ, Hutti JE, Cantley LC, Morgan DO. Evolution of Ime2 phosphorylation sites on Cdk1 substrates provides a mechanism to limit the effects of the phosphatase Cdc14 in meiosis. *Mol Cell* 2007; **25**(5): 689–702.

73. Matsushime H, Jinno A, Takagi N, Shibuya M. A novel mammalian protein kinase gene (mak) is highly expressed in testicular germ cells at and after meiosis. *Mol Cell Biol* 1990; **10**(5): 2261–8.

74. Pan H, O'Brien MJ, Wigglesworth K, Eppig JJ, Schultz RM. Transcript profiling during mouse oocyte development and the effect of gonadotropin priming and development in vitro. *Dev Biol* 2005; **286**(2): 493–506.

75. Gorr IH, Boos D, Stemmann O. Mutual inhibition of separase and Cdk1 by two-step complex formation. *Mol Cell* 2005; **19**(1): 135–41.

76. Khmelinskii A, Roostalu J, Roque H, Antony C, Schiebel E. Phosphorylation-dependent protein interactions at the spindle midzone mediate cell cycle regulation of spindle elongation. *Dev Cell* 2009; **17**(2): 244–56.

77. Jiang W, Jimenez G, Wells NJ, *et al.* PRC1: a human mitotic spindle-associated CDK substrate protein required for cytokinesis. *Mol Cell* 1998; **2**(6): 877–85.

78. Kubiak J, Weber M, de Pennart H, Winston N, Maro B. The metaphase II arrest in mouse oocytes is controlled through microtubule-dependent destruction of cyclin B in the presence of CSF. *EMBO J* 1993; **12**(10): 3773–8.

79. Nixon VL, Levasseur M, McDougall A, Jones KT. Ca^{2+} oscillations promote APC/C-dependent cyclin B1 degradation during metaphase arrest and completion of meiosis in fertilizing mouse eggs. *Curr Biol* 2002; **12**: 746–50.

80. Colledge PM, Carlton MBL, Udy GB, Evans MJ. Disruption of c-mos causes partenogenetic development of unfertilized mouse eggs. *Nature* 1994; **370**: 65–8.

81. Hashimoto N, Watanabe N, Furuta Y, *et al.* Parthenogenetic activation of oocytes in c-mos-deficient mice. *Nature* 1994; **370**(6484): 68–71.

82. Verlhac MH, Kubiak JZ, Weber M, *et al.* Mos is required for MAP kinase activation and is involved in microtubule organization during meiotic maturation in the mouse. *Development* 1996; **122**(3): 815–22.

83. Suzuki T, Suzuki E, Yoshida N, *et al.* Mouse Emi2 as a distinctive regulatory hub in second meiotic metaphase. *Development* 2010; **137**(19): 3281–91.

84. Wu JQ, Kornbluth S. Across the meiotic divide – CSF activity in the post-Emi2/XErp1 era. *J Cell Sci* 2008; **121**(Pt 21): 3509–14.

85. Dumont J, Umbhauer M, Rassinier P, Hanauer A, Verlhac MH. p90Rsk is not involved in cytostatic factor arrest in mouse oocytes. *J Cell Biol* 2005; **169**(2): 227–31.

86. Lefebvre C, Terret ME, Djiane A, *et al.* Meiotic spindle stability depends on MAPK-interacting and spindle-stabilizing (MISS), a new MAPK substrate. *J Cell Biol* 2002; **157**(4): 603–13.

87. Terret ME, Lefebvre C, Djiane A, *et al.* DOC1R: a MAP kinase substrate that controls microtubule organization of metaphase II mouse oocytes. *Development* 2003; **130**(21): 5169–77.

88. Tunquist B, Eyers P, Chen L, Lewellyn A, Maller J. Spindle checkpoint proteins Mad1 and Mad2 are required for cytostatic factor-mediated metaphase arrest. *J Cell Biol* 2003; **163**(6): 1231–42.

89. Tsurumi C, Hoffmann S, Geley S, Graeser R, Polanski Z. The spindle assembly checkpoint is not essential for

CSF arrest of mouse oocytes. *J Cell Biol* 2004; **167**(6): 1037–50.

90. Shoji S, Yoshida N, Amanai M, *et al.* Mammalian Emi2 mediates cytostatic arrest and transduces the signal for meiotic exit via Cdc20. *EMBO J* 2006; **25**(4): 834–45.

91. Suzuki T, Yoshida N, Suzuki E, Okuda E, Perry AC. Full-term mouse development by abolishing Zn^{2+}-dependent metaphase II arrest without Ca^{2+} release. *Development* 2010; **137**(16): 2659–69.

92. Chang HY, Jennings PC, Stewart J, Verrills NM, Jones KT. Essential role of protein phosphatase 2A in metaphase II arrest and activation of mouse eggs shown by okadaic acid, dominant negative protein phosphatase 2A, and FTY720. *J Biol Chem* 2011; **286**(16): 14705–12.

93. Jones KT. Intracellular calcium in the fertilization and development of mammalian eggs. *Clin Exp Pharmacol Physiol* 2007; **34**(10): 1084–9.

94. Kashir J, Jones C, Coward K. Calcium oscillations, oocyte activation, and phospholipase C zeta. *Adv Exp Med Biol* 2012; **740**: 1095–121.

95. Miao YL, Stein P, Jefferson WN, Padilla-Banks E, Williams CJ. Calcium influx-mediated signaling is required for complete mouse egg activation. *Proc Natl Acad Sci USA* 2012; **109**(11): 4169–74.

96. Chang H, Levasseur M, Jones K. Degradation of APCcdc20 and APCcdh1 substrates during the second meiotic division in mouse eggs. *J Cell Sci* 2004; **117**(Pt 26): 6289–96.

97. Madgwick S, Levasseur M, Jones KT. Calmodulin-dependent protein kinase II, and not protein kinase C, is sufficient for triggering cell-cycle resumption in mammalian eggs. *J Cell Sci* 2005; **118**(Pt 17): 3849–59.

98. Knott JG, Gardner AJ, Madgwick S, *et al.* Calmodulin-dependent protein kinase II triggers mouse egg activation and embryo development in the absence of Ca^{2+} oscillations. *Dev Biol* 2006; **296**(2): 388–95.

99. Chang HY, Minahan K, Merriman JA, Jones KT. Calmodulin-dependent protein kinase gamma 3 (CamKIIgamma3) mediates the cell cycle resumption of metaphase II eggs in mouse. *Development* 2009; **136**(24): 4077–81.

100. Backs J, Stein P, Backs T, *et al.* The gamma isoform of CaM kinase II controls mouse egg activation by regulating cell cycle resumption. *Proc Natl Acad Sci USA* 2010; **107**(1): 81–6.

101. Mochida S, Hunt T. Calcineurin is required to release *Xenopus* egg extracts from meiotic M phase. *Nature* 2007; **449**(7160): 336–40.

102. Nishiyama T, Yoshizaki N, Kishimoto T, Ohsumi K. Transient activation of calcineurin is essential to initiate embryonic development in *Xenopus laevis*. *Nature* 2007; **449**(7160): 341–5.

103. Perry AC, Verlhac MH. Second meiotic arrest and exit in frogs and mice. *EMBO Rep* 2008; **9**(3): 246–51.

104. Oh JS, Susor A, Conti M. Protein tyrosine kinase Wee1B is essential for metaphase II exit in mouse oocytes. *Science* 2011; **332**(6028): 462–5.

105. Chen J, Melton C, Suh N, *et al.* Genome-wide analysis of translation reveals a critical role for deleted in azoospermia-like (Dazl) at the oocyte-to-zygote transition. *Genes Dev* 2011; **25**(7): 755–66.

Chapter 12

Chromosome behavior and spindle formation in mammalian oocytes

Heide Schatten and Qing-Yuan Sun

Abstract

The formation of the meiotic spindle is a critical process to assure accurate chromosome segregation and subsequent embryo development. Coordinated formation and organization of microtubules, centrosomes, and chromosomes is important for meiotic spindle formation at the oocyte's center after germinal vesicle breakdown (GVBD), for the formation of the MI (meiosis I) spindle to segregate homologous chromosomes, and for the formation of the MII (meiosis II) spindle to segregate chromatids, resulting in oocyte haploidy. The human oocyte is particularly susceptible to errors in chromosome segregation which may be related to defective centrosome and microtubule organization and to defective chromosome attachment to kinetochore microtubules and loss of molecular surveillance factors. The present chapter is focused on (1) formation of central, MI and MII spindle, with focus on microtubules and centrosomes; (2) chromosome dynamics and segregation during MI and MII, with focus on molecular aspects and surveillance mechanisms; and (3) spindle abnormalities, environmental influences, and possible treatments to restore spindle integrity with implications for assisted reproductive technologies (ART).

Introduction

The formation of the meiotic spindle is a critical step during oocyte maturation and begins when the germinal vesicle breaks down (GVBD) as a result of stimulation by luteinizing hormone (LH). Spindle formation in most mammalian oocytes takes place at the oocyte's center and involves significant restructuring of the cytoskeleton that will impact subsequent cellular and molecular functions that are also important for later development [1]. Coordinated formation and organization of microtubules, centrosomes, and chromosomes begins directly after GVBD with remodeling of these major spindle components in the oocyte's center to form the meiotic spindle.

The entire process of spindle formation and meiosis is complex and is critical for the production of haploid cells from diploid progenitors. After DNA duplication and centralized spindle formation two chromosomal divisions take place to first segregate homologous chromosomes (meiosis I; MI) followed by separation of sister chromatids (meiosis II; MII).

The program of oocyte maturation and spindle formation is precisely regulated when successful but the efficiency of these processes during oocyte maturation is remarkably low in humans compared to other animal species and results in maturation failures associated with female factor infertility problems. It has been estimated that in humans about 15–20% of oocytes undergo chromosomal segregation errors [2] and that 5% of all pregnancies are aneuploid [3]. The number of maturation failures is still higher when considering that many of the aneuploid oocytes deteriorate during maturation and may not reach oocyte quality required for fertilization, which typically takes place at the MII stage. When all these factors are included the maturation efficiency is low and aneuploidy may be as high as 40–60% [4–6]. A new study testing over 20 000 oocytes for aneuploidies revealed that almost every second oocyte (46.8%) is abnormal in human in vitro fertilization (IVF) clinics, involving chromosomes 13, 16, 18, 21, and 22 [7]. Several factors have been identified to play a role in aneuploidy and these are most frequently associated with oocyte aging and when oocytes are exposed to toxic environments affecting oocyte quality. Loss of surveillance, and destabilization of

Biology and Pathology of the Oocyte, 2nd edn., ed. Alan Trounson, Roger Gosden, and Ursula Eichenlaub-Ritter.
Published by Cambridge University Press.

centrosomes and the microtubule network, which affects microtubule organization, microtubule attachment to chromosomes, and subsequent chromosomal segregation, are factors that primarily affect women past age 35 [8–10] and are the topic of investigations in several laboratories worldwide.

Compared to mitosis, meiosis includes specific adaptations of DNA-damage and meiosis-specific spindle checkpoint mechanisms in which a specific surveillance program regulates meiotic targets, as will be detailed in the sections below. While only a few meiotic checkpoint substrates have been reported so far, this area of research has accelerated in recent years in part because of the advances in assisted reproductive technologies (ART) for which oocyte quality and accurate meiosis progression are important criteria for success [11–13]. The need to obtain oocytes with an error-free machinery to allow proper embryo development has been well recognized and excellent recent basic and applied research investigations have contributed significantly to study of the molecular program of meiosis [14–16]. The present chapter is focused on (1) formation of the centrally located and peripheral MI and MII spindle, with focus on microtubules and centrosomes; (2) chromosome dynamics and segregation during MI and MII, with focus on molecular aspects and surveillance mechanisms; and (3) spindle abnormalities, environmental influences, and possible treatments to restore spindle integrity with implications for ART.

Formation of the centrally located and peripheral MI and MII spindles, with focus on microtubules and centrosomes

The accurate formation of the central meiotic spindle requires several steps of regulation and includes phosphorylation and dephosphorylation cascades that play a role in remodeling the cytoskeleton. Cytoskeletal reorganization is a major requirement for accurate formation of the meiotic spindles formed at the oocyte's center followed by cytoskeleton-mediated spindle migration to the oocyte cortex and subsequent cytoskeletal reorganization during MI and MII [17–20]. Microtubules, centrosomes, and chromosomes are the main components of meiotic spindles that are precisely synchronized to participate synergistically in the process required for meiotic spindle formation and separation of homologous chromosomes during MI and separation of chromatids during MII that follows fertilization of the MII oocyte. Two successive highly asymmetric cell divisions take place during this process [21], with the first being completed after MI and the second after fertilization during MII, resulting in small polar bodies and a large polarized oocyte. Errors during formation of the central meiotic spindle will result in errors leading to chromosome mis-segregation during MI and MII.

While the majority of previous studies on meiosis had been focused on chromosomes and chromosome–microtubule interactions, in this section we will highlight the role of centrosomes, as relatively few studies have focused on centrosomes although these complex organelles play critical roles in the meiotic process and in precise microtubule organization and chromosome segregation.

Centrosomes (oftentimes also referred to as microtubule-organizing centers; MTOCs) are important for the organization of microtubules into a functional meiotic spindle in which the centrosomal proteins γ-tubulin, pericentrin, and the centrosome-associated protein NuMA (nuclear mitotic apparatus protein) serve major functions. γ-Tubulin is a component of the γ-tubulin ring complex (γ-TuRC) and is part of the centrosome core structure with a major role in microtubule nucleation [22, 23]. In the unfertilized oocyte, centrosomal material is localized throughout the ooplasm and it is concentrated at the meiotic spindle poles that start to assemble after GVBD and form the central, MI, and MII meiotic spindles. Pericentrin is an important centrosomal protein that along with γ-tubulin plays a role in assembling microtubules during spindle formation [24, 25, 26]. NuMA is a multifunctional protein that in the nucleus serves specific functions as nuclear matrix protein and becomes a critical component of the spindle during mitosis and meiosis, serving as centrosome-associated protein to tether microtubules into the well-known spindle formations. NuMA is localized to the GV before spindle formation [27, 28, 29]. Both pericentrin and NuMA depend on the microtubule motor protein dynein for their recruitment and assembly onto centrosomes [27, 30, 31].

The terminology used for oocyte centrosomes has oftentimes been inconsistent and at times inaccurate, which we have recently addressed in detail in a review paper on oocyte maturation [12]. In the present chapter we will only briefly address this topic. Briefly, oocyte centrosomes do not contain centrioles, as centrioles have been lost during oogenesis, which is reflected in the term "acentriolar centrosomes" most frequently used to describe oocyte centrosomes, referring to centrosomes that do not contain centrioles. The term "acentrosomal" has also been used by some investigators but this term may be misleading and does not reflect the fact that centrosomes are present in the oocyte and contain the well-known centrosome proteins that fulfill all functions known for somatic cell centrosomes and contain centrosomal proteins that undergo regulation as known for somatic cell centrosomes (in which centrioles are present). The term "pericentriolar material" has also been used at times to describe centrosomes, which is incorrect when used for oocytes that do not contain centrioles. We use the term centrosomes throughout the chapter for oocytes and meiotic spindle formation and will explain details in the specific subsections of this chapter. In all cases centrosomes are composed of a proteinaceous not yet clearly defined substance containing numerous centrosomal proteins with cell cycle-specific functions and further contain centrosome-associated proteins during specific cell-cycle phases. Centrosomes are multifunctional organelles. Signal transduction molecules, proteolytic enzymes, and several cell cycle-regulatory proteins are also associated with centrosomes, as centrosomes serve as gathering and distribution centers, using their microtubule organizing capabilities for cellular communication, and therefore play a central role in cellular metabolism, cell-cycle regulation, and several other cellular functions (for detailed reviews on cell cycle-specific centrosome functions in embryos, stem cells, and embryo development, please see Schatten [30] and Schatten and Sun [11–13, 31]).

Many of the previous studies on meiotic centrosomes have been performed in the mouse but it is important to emphasize that by now we know for absolute certain that the cytoskeletal and centrosome mechanisms and dynamics during oocyte maturation and meiotic spindle formation differ significantly and critically in the mouse compared to all other non-rodent mammalian systems studied so far, including humans. To highlight briefly the major and most significant differences in the mouse compared to non-rodent mammalian systems we will use the MII oocyte, which is the stage at which oocytes are arrested before fertilization takes place, as an example. The most prominent feature of the MII mouse oocyte is the presence of cytoplasmic asters [32–35] that contain γ-tubulin foci, which is different from MII oocytes of pig [36], sheep [37], cow [38], and human [28], [29], which do not contain cytoplasmic asters (Figure 12.1). Furthermore, the MII spindle in the mouse is characterized by foci of dense centrosomal aggregates that contain γ-tubulin as the major component, while centrosome organization at the meiotic poles in non-rodent mammalian species, including humans, displays a more continuous band of centrosomal components which are clearly distinguished from the meiotic spindle poles in the mouse. These differences reflect the different mechanism by which they are assembled. The formation of mouse oocyte spindle poles has been studied by several investigators [33–35] and it has been revealed that mouse MII spindle poles are formed by assembly of the cytoplasmic asters containing centrosomal material that has clearly been detected with the 5051 autoantibody [33, 34] and with γ-tubulin [39]. Schuh and Ellenberg [35] built on these earlier studies, using live-cell imaging to show the assembly of the mouse cytoplasmic asters into the mouse MII spindle poles. Different from the mouse, the porcine MII spindle is primarily formed by NuMA that bundles microtubules and by γ-tubulin while the mouse meiotic spindle is formed by incorporating the pre-existing smaller cytoplasmic MTOCs, resulting in a spindle pole primarily containing γ-tubulin.

Differences in the MII spindle of mouse and non-rodent species also include different drug sensitivities [32, 33, 40]. Lee *et al.* [40] showed that the microtubule inhibitor nocodazole at 10 μg/ml resulted in disappearance of NuMA staining at the porcine MII spindle while mouse meiotic spindle poles were resistant to this concentration of nocodazole treatment. These studies are also relevant when using the mouse model for toxicity studies as the effects may be different in the mouse and may not reflect the effects on human oocytes. One morphological distinction of MII oocytes in the mouse and non-rodent species is the orientation of the MII spindle; this is parallel in mouse oocytes while it is perpendicular in non-rodent MII oocytes, including those of humans, which may reflect different mechanisms for spindle anchorage and may also influence the described different drug sensitivities in these different systems. Although not addressed in the present chapter, one of the most significant differences between the mouse and non-rodent mammalian systems is the mode of

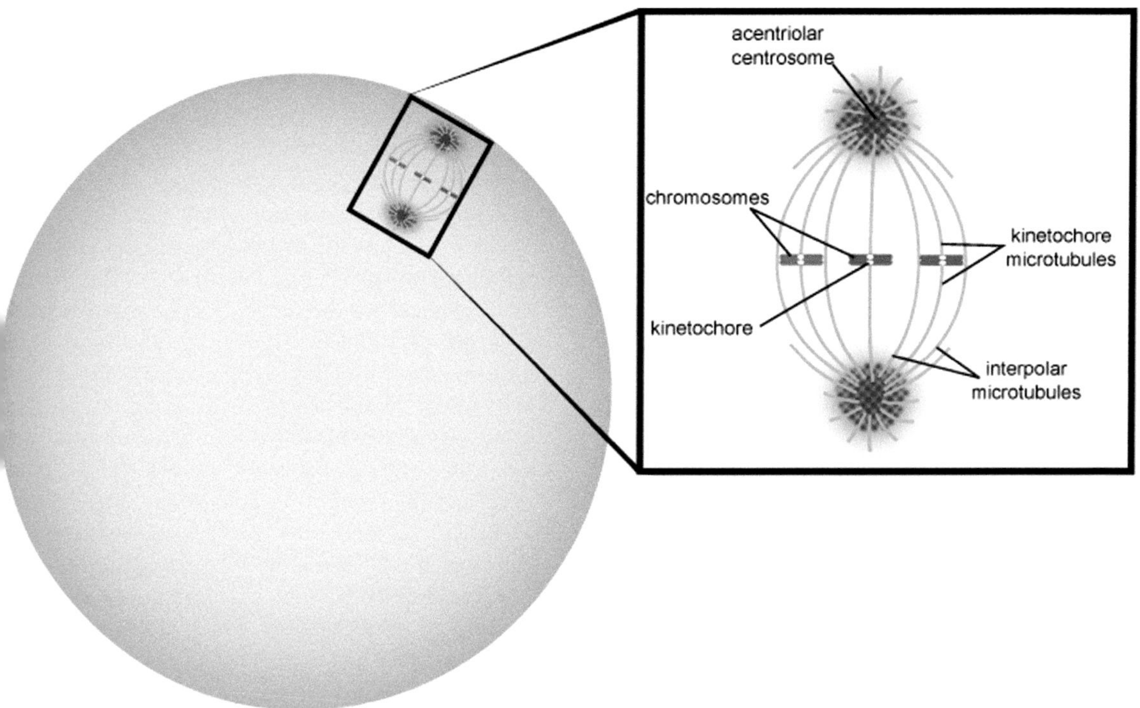

igure 12.1 Schematic diagram of MII spindle in oocytes before fertilization. The MII spindle is organized by acentriolar centrosomes that ucleate kinetochore and pole-to-pole microtubules for separation of chromosomes.

ertilization. The mouse ooplasm does not tolerate cenrioles while all other non-rodent systems studied so ar depend on sperm-derived centrioles for successful ertilization, sperm aster formation, and subsequent mbryo development [11, 13, 31, 41, 42]. These signifcant differences had not been recognized in early ferilization studies but they are well recognized now, as eterologous fertilization to assess human sperm qualty is now recommended to be performed in porcine r bovine oocytes because of the incompatibilities etween mouse oocytes and non-rodent sperm.

With these differences between the mouse and on-rodent mammalian species in mind we will turn o specific mechanisms that have been reported for pindle formation. Because the mouse has been the hoice model representing mammalian species for nany years most of the early studies on centrosomes ad been performed in the mouse and continued to e performed in the mouse for years, as it was difficult to overcome the previously held notion that the nouse is a most suitable model for mammals, which is ertainly true for numerous other studies but not for entrosome- or cytoskeleton-related maturation and ertilization studies. The porcine and bovine animal models are now being used for studying centrosomes as adequate representatives for mammalian systems, including humans.

Compared to studies on chromosomes, research on meiotic centrosomes has lagged behind studies on chromosome–microtubule interactions and we do not yet have sufficient information on mechanisms underlying regulation of centrosomes during meiosis. The formation of the centrally located spindle has been explored with immunofluorescence for the mouse [43, 44], the pig [45–47], and several other animal systems [18] and spindle migration and anchorage to the oocyte cortex has been reported for various invertebrate and mammalian oocytes in which microfilaments and/or microtubules play a role, with some differences in different species. Spindle migration and anchorage to the oocyte cortex involve proteins of the Rho family, formins, the Arp2/3 complex, myosins, microtubule motor proteins such as dynein, MOS/MEK/MAPK pathway proteins, PAR proteins, and others that have been reported for the mouse as has been reviewed in detail by Ai *et al.* [18].

Only sparse and fragmented knowledge is available to date on the roles of γ-tubulin, pericentrin, and

NuMA that are essential for the establishment of functional central, MI, and MII spindles; the specific role of centrosomal proteins in this process is still incompletely understood on molecular levels. Cytoskeletal remodeling for central, MI, and MII spindle formation includes microtubule and centrosome reorganization and restructuring [32, 48–50] that is driven in part by cell-cycle kinases as known for cell-cycle regulation in mitotic cells. The molecular cascades involving phosphorylation/dephosphorylation during oocyte maturation and spindle movement have been reviewed in detail by Fan *et al.* [19, 47] and Swain and Pool [17]; they have been addressed for meiosis in several original and review papers [14, 19, 20, 44, 51–56] and will not be addressed in the present chapter, while the formation of the centrosome–microtubule complex will be highlighted.

Early studies by Szollosi *et al.* [57] used transmission electron microscopy (TEM), describing compacted electron-dense foci around the GVs of fully grown G2-arrested mouse oocytes. These electron-dense foci were associated with microtubule asters and they were later identified as centrosomal material by using the 5051 centrosomal autoimmune serum [48] that had first been used for detection of centrosomal material in the mouse by Calarco-Gillam *et al.* [58]. We now know that chromosomes and centrosomes both play a role in microtubule organization during central spindle formation [12]; while chromosomes are not essential for initiating spindle assembly they are important for directing centrosome aggregation. Several studies proposed that the chromatin-bound Ran-GEF, RCC1, is able to catalyze the Ran-GDP/Ran-GTP transition and generate high local concentration of Ran-GTP around chromosomes that may be involved in microtubule growth. In a more recent study, Dumont *et al.* [59] reported a Ran-GTP-independent spindle assembly pathway for MI mouse oocytes, while MII spindle assembly required Ran-GTP. These studies indicate that different molecular mechanisms may be used for central, MI, and MII spindle formations and, as mentioned above, different species may employ different mechanisms. Clearly, more studies are needed to determine the precise mechanisms for MI and MII spindle formation and more studies are needed in systems other than the mouse to determine similarities or differences compared to the mouse system. By using *Drosophila* [60] and *Xenopus* egg extracts [61], in vitro experiments determined that γ-tubulin is the microtubule-nucleating component of meiotic spindle formation, aided by Ran-GTP that is localized in the vicinity of chromosomes during early stages of spindle formation.

Lee *et al.* [40] described amorphous staining of γ-tubulin around condensed chromosomes after GVBD that was associated with microtubule formation. The formation of a central assembly of microtubules and lateral attachment of chromosomes as detected by confocal microscopy is discussed in more detail by Kitajima *et al.* [62] and in Chapter 29. At this stage of central spindle formation NuMA comes into play and moves out of the nucleus to associate with the central spindle. It later participates as a centrosome-associated protein by forming a crescent around the centrosomal area facing chromosomes in MI and MII spindles [28, 29, 40]. As mentioned above, there are clear differences in NuMA and γ-tubulin participation in meiotic spindle formation between the mouse and non-rodent mammalian systems which have been elaborated by Lee *et al.* [40] by comparing immunolocalization of α-tubulin, γ-tubulin, and NuMA in mouse and pig oocytes starting at late G2. These studies showed that, in the pig, during MI spindle formation NuMA became strongly associated with both spindle poles at metaphase I while γ-tubulin was localized along the spindle microtubules. In the mouse, spindle poles contained several γ-tubulin foci but NuMA was not a major component. This study proposed that in porcine MI spindle poles NuMA is a major component while in mouse MI spindle poles γ-tubulin is a major component. Recent reports on human oocytes confirmed that the human MI and MII spindles are more similar to the pig model than the mouse model and showed clearly that NuMA is a major component of MI and MII spindles [28]. These studies also showed that translocation of NuMA from the nucleoplasm in GV-stage oocytes required dynein for translocation to the spindle poles, which had previously been shown for NuMA translocation in somatic cells. These studies further revealed that NuMA abnormalities are associated with female factor infertility and with failures in oocyte maturation, although the precise mechanisms underlying NuMA abnormalities are not yet known at the present time and further more detailed functional studies will be necessary to assess the regulation of NuMA during oocyte maturation and its misregulation associated with fertility problems [28], [29]. In somatic cells, cyclin B has been identified as a major regulator for NuMA [27] but data on regulation of NuMA by cyclin

3 in oocytes have not yet been obtained. It is also not yet known whether different factors in maturation medium play a role in cytoskeletal and nuclear maturation but this is likely, as a number of studies have shown that in vitro maturation yields fewer high-quality oocytes compared to in vivo maturation 20, 63], which may in part be related to different pH or calcium conditions, as microtubule and centrosome dynamics depend on regulation by calcium and pH [64]. The differences in cytoskeletal dynamics observed in vivo and in vitro [50] may be the result of lack of nuclear and cytoplasmic maturation factors n vitro that are supplied under physiological conditions [50, 65–68] and may affect cytoskeletal dynamics and cell-cycle progression during meiotic spindle formation, as has been reported for the mouse [50].

The MII spindle is formed following completion of MI and first meiotic division without undergoing a G2 nterphase stage between MI and MII. We do not yet have accurate knowledge about the transition stages from MI to MII and details on the mechanisms for centrosomal reorganization into the MII spindle are still sparse. More studies are available for the completely formed MII spindle which has to be maintained by several active mechanisms during MII cell-cycle arrest until fertilization takes place. These active mechanisms are important, as they are in place to prevent spindle deterioration; they are defective in aged MII [10]. As will be addressed in the section on spindle abnormalities, below, spindle deterioration is associated with loss of tension between centrosomes, microtubules, and chromosome attachment at the kinetochores. Spindle abnormalities are clearly detected with immunofluorescence methods revealing disintegration of centrosomal material at the spindle poles, chromosome scattering, and microtubule formation abnormalities.

Chromosome dynamics and segregation during MI and MII, with focus on molecular aspects and surveillance mechanisms

The purpose of MI and MII spindle formation is the separation of homologous chromosomes during MI and of chromatids during MII to produce a haploid gamete with oocyte quality that supports subsequent embryo development. As mentioned in the introduction, in humans, significant errors in chromosome segregation exist especially during the MI phase that follows after oocytes have been kept in the GV stage for a very long time (for months in mice and for years in humans); defects in the homologous chromosome pairs (homologs) may have accumulated during this time perhaps as a result of environmental factors or other influences that may have affected GV-stage oocyte quality. While checkpoint controls and surveillance mechanisms do exist during MI and MII [14–16] defects may not be repairable during MI and MII if they are excessive. The need for proper maturation from the GV stage through the meiotic stages to achieve optimal oocyte quality has been reviewed in previous papers [12, 13] and will not be addressed in detail here. This section is focused on molecular aspects of chromosome separation during MI and MII.

Much of our knowledge regarding chromosome condensation, alignment at the metaphase plate, segregation, and migration to the spindle poles comes from mitosis. This includes molecular mechanisms of chromosome attachment to kinetochore microtubules and cellular surveillance mechanisms to assure proper alignment and attachment for each individual chromosome before mitotic cell-cycle progression can proceed. Chromosome organization after GVBD in mammalian oocytes, and mechanisms involved in chromosome alignment and separation during MI and MII, has primarily been obtained from studies in the mouse system and may differ for other mammalian species. New studies on molecular mechanisms important for meiosis are now being pursued and while the newly generated data show some similarities of meiosis with mitosis, they also show significant differences [14–16].

The complex regulation of meiotic prophase and associated checkpoint controls have recently been reviewed in excellent detail [15, 69] and include responses to errors, coordinated progression of meiotic double-strand break (DSB) repair, chromosome dynamics, and homologous synapsis. Physical association of a chromosome pair is important during this process to assure equal and accurate orientation and separation. During MI in the fetal oocytes chromosomes undergo crossover recombination and establish physical links between homologous chromosomes for accurate MI chromosome segregation. The intimate association between homologous chromosomes includes a well-structured protein lattice termed synaptonemal complex (SC) [70, 71]. During prophase of MI components of the DNA-damage checkpoint machinery play a role as key regulators for prophase chromosomal events [69].

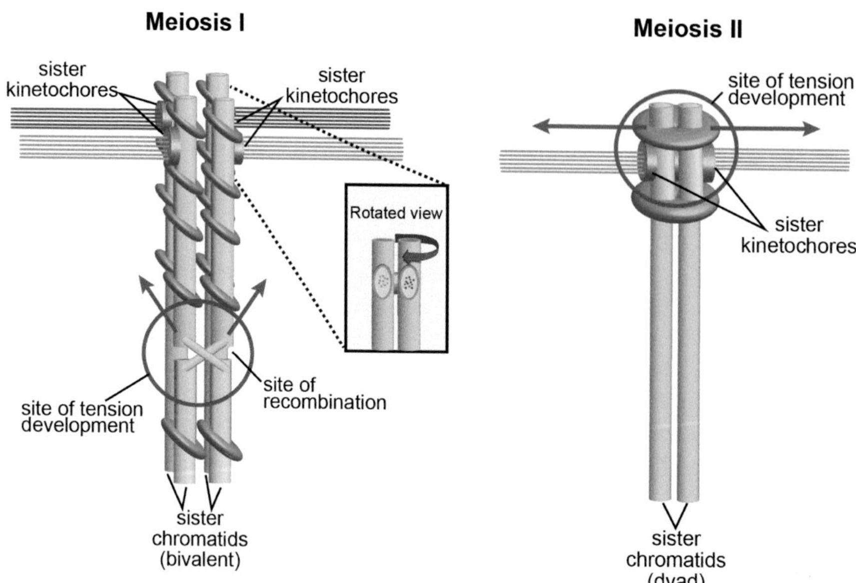

Figure 12.2 Segregation of chromosomes (MI) and chromatids (MII). In meiosis I crossovers between homologs and cohesin bonds between sister chromatid arms ensure maintenance of a bivalent structure, with tension arising from crossover sites once microtubules attach to kinetochores. Sister kinetochores are attached in a "side-by-side" conformation to the same spindle pole, so that each homolog of the pair is attached to opposite poles. Sister chromatids remain physically linked by centromeric cohesin, which is protected from degradation during meiosis I, until meiosis II. In meiosis II, the sister kinetochores resume a "back-to-back" conformation and attach to opposite poles, with tension arising from centromeric cohesion bonds, similar to mitosis. Red = kinetochore; yellow = cohesins; green = microtubules; blue = chromatin

In MI crossover of homologous chromosomes takes place and results in the presence of chiasmata at sites of recombination as shown in the schematic diagram in Figure 12.2. Up to anaphase II sister chromatids remain attached at their centromeres; final separation of sister chromatids takes place in MII. In MI and MII microtubules become attached to the kinetochores and exert pulling forces, which signals that proper microtubule–kinetochore attachment has occurred. The cohesin complex that holds chromosomes (MI) and chromatids (MII) together needs to be destructed for chromosome or chromatid separation to occur and proceed with cell cycle-specific anaphase movement. To assure that sister chromatid separation does not occur during MI and sister chromatids of the same chromosome will move to the same spindle pole the cohesin complex at centromeres is protected from degradation during MI.

Several molecular mechanisms have been uncovered in recent years that are important for accurate MI and MII cell-cycle progression. The main components that will be addressed below are cohesin components, the spindle assembly checkpoint (SAC) and its target, the anaphase-promoting complex/cyclosome (APC/C), and the shugoshins that are critical for ensuring segregation of homologs in MI and of sister chromatids in MII.

Cohesins are a family of proteins whose function includes holding chromosomes or sister chromatids together. They are placed onto chromosomes before recombination and are thought to be involved in recruiting synaptonemal complex protein (SYCP) members onto the SC. The cohesin complex contains the meiosis-specific subunits REC8, STAGE3, SMC1, and SMC3 [72, 73, 74]. Cohesins are localized along chromosome arms and at the centromere region. In meiosis, sister chromatids retain cohesin along their arms until the beginning of anaphase I when REC8 degradation by separase activity occurs [75, 76]. Cohesin remains at the sister centromeres, allowing sister chromatids to move to the same spindle pole. Centromeric REC8 is cleaved in anaphase II to allow sister chromatid segregation for the formation of haploid cells.

The spindle assembly checkpoint (*SAC*) monitors attachment and tension on kinetochores by spindle microtubules; it has recently been reviewed by Sun and Kim [77] for meiosis. SAC controls the timing of cohesin loss on chromosomes and transition into anaphase. SAC monitors unattached chromosomes and the accurate chromosomal bipolar orientation. SAC responds to various signals, including dynein that plays a role in chromosome movement. Recent studies have shown that differential regulation by phosphorylation/dephosphorylation of centromeric proteins is involved in SAC, and MCAK (mitotic centromere-associated kinesin) has been identified to be present specifically in centromeres, midspindle, and chiasmata and in silencing SAC [78].

The anaphase-promoting complex/cyclosome (APC/C) is a key regulator for controlling degradation of cohesion between chromosomes. Ubiquitin E3 ligase activity of the APC/C assures degradation of securin whose function before metaphase includes keeping the protease separase inactive. As key regulator during meiosis the APC/C is also responsible for the degradation of cyclin B. Cleavage of securin by release of active separase results in degradation of the RAD21/REC8 component of cohesin and by doing so allows chromosome separation in MI and exit from MI. The shugoshin family of proteins (shugoshin 1 and shugoshin 2) is localized to the centromeric region and plays a role in protecting REC8 at centromeres from cleavage during MI by recruiting protein phosphatase 2A (PP2A) to the centromere. During MII the pole to kinetochore microtubule attachment exerts tension across the centromere and induces relocation of SGO2/PPA apart from the centromeric cohesin resulting in separase-induced cleavage of REC8 [14–16].

As discussed in the section on the formation of MI and MII spindles, above, the main components involved in spindle formation are centrosomes and microtubules that are formed to separate chromosomes (MI) or sister chromatids (MII). Kinetochore microtubules attach to kinetochores while interpolar microtubules overlap at the center of the spindle and aid in force generation during chromosome/chromatid separation. Kinetochores are formed over centromeric regions as tripartite structures that are clearly seen in electron micrographs. Kinetochores are composed of a chromatin-containing inner plate, a protein-rich outer plate, and an outer fibrous corona layer. More than 60 kinetochore proteins have been identified in yeast but not yet in mammalian cells because of greater experimental challenges. Kinetochores are formed at the GV stage and connect to the plus ends of the polarized microtubule fibers that connect with their opposite ends (minus ends) to centrosomes. The plus ends indicate the fast growing side of microtubule polymerization. Regulators of kinetochore assembly include polo-like kinase I (Plk1). SAC checkpoint proteins include BUB1, BUBR1, BUB3, MAD1, MAD2, MPS1, and perhaps other not yet identified components. Motor proteins and SAC components play a role in kinetochore dynamics [79]. It is generally accepted that a "search and capture" process allows microtubule attachment to kinetochores which is probably directed by precise centrosomal microtubule nucleation, perhaps even aided by the formation of interpolar microtubules, although detailed information on this aspect of mechanisms employed for meiosis is not yet available.

Microtubule attachment errors are detected by surveillance mechanisms through members of the SAC and chromosomal passenger complex systems. Components of the chromosomal passenger complex include INCENP, Aurora B, Survivin, and Borealin/Dasra. Components of the SAC system play a role in intracellular signaling and prevent APC/C activity when chromosomes are not attached. MAD and BUB proteins accumulate at kinetochores that lack proper attachment to microtubules. Whether and by which mechanisms tension plays a role in SAC signaling in meiosis I, where sister chromatids in a bivalent attach to the same pole, is not yet clear [80]. A waiting phase is observed during which lagging chromosomes may still be aligned at the equatorial spindle region but errors are encountered when the surveillance mechanisms fail.

Spindle abnormalities, environmental influences and possible treatments to restore spindle integrity with implications for ART

The study of MII spindles in aged oocytes has become of increasing interest in recent years, as it is well known that aged oocytes display spindle abnormalities and aneuploidies that are associated with developmental abnormalities. Frequently, aneuploidies result in spontaneous abortions that have been reported to be the case for 75% of women over 40 years of age and about 12% in women younger than 20 years of age [8–10, 81, 82].

Aneuploidy is the result of chromosome missegregation that may be associated with loss of meiotic spindle integrity [10, 16]. Several failures in mechanisms responsible for accurate chromosome segregation have been implicated in the causes underlying

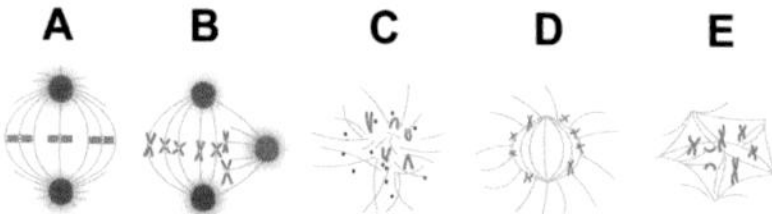

Figure 12.3 Representative examples of MII spindles of fresh and aged oocytes: (A) Fresh oocyte with bipolar spindle. (B–E) Aged oocytes with abnormal spindles. (B) Tripolar spindle with microtubules emanating from three poles and irregular chromosome attachments. (C) Highly disorganized spindle with scattered centrosomes and chromosomes. (D) Large irregular spindle with a dense microtubule network and attachment to chromosomes localized to the outer edges of the spindle in a rosette formation. (E) Multipolar spindle.

aneuploidy and include loss of centrosome integrity [10], loss of microtubule integrity, and loss of chromosome integrity, or loss of surveillance mechanism as has been reviewed by Wang *et al.* [16]. The loss of cohesins with maternal aging has been identified as one of the causes in mouse oocytes. Other causes have been identified in mouse oocytes, including loss of the SAC proteins Mad1 and Mad2 during MI and Bub1 in MII as well as others involved in SAC functions [16]. While results from human and mouse oocytes show a clear increase in the frequency of aneuploidy with advanced maternal age, recent results by Hornak *et al.* [83] reported no increase in the frequency of age-related aneuploidy in pig oocytes that were analyzed using comparative genomic hybridization (CGH). Our own studies in pig oocytes [84] and mice [10] revealed several patterns of deteriorated meiotic spindles as shown in the schematic diagram in Figure 12.3. In pig oocytes, decrease in Mad2 protein was shown to be associated with oocyte aging, but this does not necessarily lead to increased aneuploidy (see Chapter 29).

Aside from oocyte aging several environmental toxic components have been associated with meiotic spindle abnormalities. One of the best known environmental molecules resulting in spindle abnormalities is exposure of oocytes to bisphenol A (BPA), an endocrine disruptor found in several plastic components that are used in daily consumption. Details on specific effects have been addressed in several recent original and review papers [16, 41, 85] and are not addressed here.

While only briefly mentioned in this chapter because of space limitations, several other lines of investigation are in progress to determine specific spindle abnormalities and several treatments have been proposed to correct spindle deterioration. These approaches are especially important for ART, for which oocyte quality is a major factor for success. As reviewed by Miao *et al.* [10] caffeine has been used to restore abnormal spindles although practical applications have not yet been pursued. Identifying the cause for defects will allow specific repair and will benefit an increasing percentage of the worldwide population that choses to postpone having children until later in life and past the optimal reproductive age. In specific cases (e.g., risks for ovarian hyperstimulation syndrome) ART requires in vitro maturation that in addition to the challenge of maturing sometimes older oocytes or oocytes of patients suffering from pathologies like polycystic ovary syndrome (PCOS) also uses culture conditions that may not be optimal and produce abnormalities that may be corrected if the underlying causes are identified.

Conclusions and future perspectives

Taken together, significant progress has been made in recent years in analyzing components of the central MI and MII meiotic spindles to determine factors that play a role in the regulation of centrosomes, microtubules, chromosomes, and their interactions leading to spindle integrity. Several molecular factors have been identified that play a role in spindle abnormalities which are increased in aged oocytes and in oocytes exposed to environmental toxicants. Studies on aged and environmentally affected oocytes are particularly important to correct specific abnormalities that will allow molecular repair to improve the success rate for ART.

References

1. Sirard MA, Richard F, Blondin P, Robert C. Contribution of the oocyte to embryo quality. *Theriogenology* 2006; **65**: 126–36.
2. Pellestor F, Anahory T, Hamamah S. Effect of maternal age on the frequency of cytogenetic abnormalities in human oocytes. *Cytogenet Genome Res* 2005; **111**: 206–12.
3. Hassold T, Hunt, P. To err (meiotically) is human: the genesis of human aneuploidy. *Nat Rev Genet* 2001; **2**: 280–91.
4. Kuliev A, Cieslak J, Verlinsky Y. Frequency and distribution of chromosome abnormalities in human oocytes. *Cytogenet Genome Res* 2005; **111**: 193–8.
5. Rosenbusch BE, Schneider M. Cytogenetic analysis of human oocytes remaining unfertilized after intracytoplasmic sperm injection. *Fertil Steril* 2006; **85**: 302–7.

6. Pacchierotti F, Ranaldi R, Eichenlaub-Ritter U, Attia S, Adler ID. Evaluation of aneugenic effects of bisphenol A in somatic and germ cells of the mouse. *Mutat Res* 2008; **651**(1–2): 64–70.

7. Kuliev A, Zlatopolsky Z, Kirillova I, Spivakova J, Cieslak Janzen J. Meiosis errors in over 20,000 oocytes studied in the practice of preimplantation aneuploidy testing. *Reprod Biomed Online* 2011; **22**(1): 2–8.

8. Eichenlaub-Ritter U, Stahl A, Luciani J M. The microtubular cytoskeleton and chromosomes of unfertilized human oocytes aged in vitro. *Hum Genet* 1988; **80**: 259–64.

9. Eichenlaub-Ritter U. Genetics of oocyte aging. *Maturitas* 1998; **30**: 143–69.

10. Miao Y-L, Kikuchi K, Sun Q-Y, Schatten H. Oocyte aging: cellular and molecular changes, developmental potential and reversal possibility. *Hum Reprod Update* 2009; **15**(5): 573–85.

11. Schatten H, Sun QY. The role of centrosomes in mammalian fertilization and its significance for ICSI. *Mol Hum Reprod* 2009; **15**(9): 531–8.

12. Schatten H, Sun Q-Y. Centrosome dynamics during meiotic spindle formation in oocyte maturation. *Mol. Reprod. Develop* 2011; **78**: 757–68.

13. Schatten H, Sun Q-Y. New insights into the role of centrosomes in mammalian fertilisation and implications for ART. *Reproduction* 2011; **142**: 793–801.

14. Jones KT. Meiosis in oocytes: predisposition to aneuploidy and its increased incidence with age. *Hum Reprod Update* 2008; **14**(2): 143–58.

15. Holt JE, Jones KT. Control of homologous chromosome division in the mammalian oocyte. *Mol Hum Reprod* 2009; **15**(3): 139–47.

16. Wang Z-B, Schatten H, Sun Q-Y. Why is chromosome segregation error in oocytes increased with maternal aging? *Physiology* 2011; **26**(5): 314–25.

17. Swain JE, Pool TB. ART failure: oocyte contributions to unsuccessful fertilization. *Hum Reprod Update* 2008; **14**(5): 431–46.

18. Ai J-S, Li M, Schatten H, Sun Q-Y. Regulatory mechanism of spindle movements during oocyte meiotic division. *Asian Aust J Anim Sci* 2009; **22**: 1447–86.

19. Fan H-Y, Liu Z, Shimada M, *et al.* MAPK3/1 (ERK1/2) in ovarian granulosa cells are essential for female fertility. *Science* 2009; **324**: 938–41.

20. Gosden R, Lee B. Portrait of an oocyte: our obscure origin. *J Clin Invest* 2010; **120**(4): 973–83.

21. Brunet S, Verlhac MH. Positioning to get out of meiosis: the asymmetry of division. *Hum Reprod Update* 2011; **17**(1): 68–75.

22. Stearns T. The tubulin superfamily. In: Nigg E, ed. *Centrosomes in Development and Disease.* Weinheim: Wiley-VCA Verlag GmbH & CoKGaG. 2004; 17–25.

23. Moritz M, Rice LM, Agard DA. Microtubule nucleation. In: Nigg E, ed. *Centrosomes in Development and Disease.* Weinheim: Wiley-VCA Verlag GmbH & CoKGaG. 2004; 27–41.

24. Doxsey SJ, Stein P, Evans L, Calarco P, Kirschner M. Pericentrin, a highly conserved protein of centrosomes involved in microtubule organization. *Cell* 1994; **76**: 639–50.

25. Dictenberg J, Zimmerman W, Sparks C, *et al.* Pericentrin and gamma-tubulin form a protein complex and are organized into a novel lattice at the centrosome. *J Cell Biol* 1998; **141**: 163–74.

26. Young A, Dictenberg JB, Purohit A, Tuft R, Doxsey SJ Cytoplasmic dynein-mediated assembly of pericentrin and γ-tubulin onto centrosomes. *Mol Biol Cell* 2000; **11**: 2047–56

27. Sun QY, Schatten H. Multiple roles of NuMA in vertebrate cells: review of an intriguing multi-functional protein. *Front Biosci* 2006; **11**: 1137–46.

28. Alvarez Sedó CA, Schatten H, Combelles C, Rawe VY. The nuclear mitotic apparatus protein NuMA: localization and dynamics in human oocytes, fertilization and early embryos. *Mol Hum Reprod* 2011; **17**(6): 392–8.

29. Schatten H, Rawe VY, Sun QY. Cytoskeletal architecture of human oocytes with focus on centrosomes and their significant role in fertilization. In: Nagy ZP, Varghese A, Agarwal A, eds. *Practical Manual of In Vitro Fertilization: Advanced Methods and Novel Devices.* New York: Springer. 2012; 667–76.

30. Schatten H. The mammalian centrosome and its functional significance. *Histochem Cell Biol* 2008; **129**: 667–86.

31. Schatten H, Sun QY. The role of centrosomes in fertilization, cell division and establishment of asymmetry during embryo development. *Semin Cell Dev Biol* 2010; **21**: 174–84.

32. Schatten G, Simerly C, Schatten H. Microtubule configurations during fertilization, mitosis and early development in the mouse and the requirement for egg microtubule-mediated motility during mammalian fertilization. *Proc Natl Acad Sci USA* 1985; **82**: 4152–6.

33. Schatten H, Schatten G, Mazia D, Balczon R, Simerly C. Behavior of centrosomes during fertilization and cell division in mouse oocytes and in sea urchin eggs. *Proc Natl Acad Sci USA* 1986; **83**: 105–9.

34. Maro B, Howlett SK, Webb M. Non-spindle microtubule organizing centers in metaphase

II-arrested mouse oocytes. *J Cell Biol* 1985; **101**: 1665–72.

35. Schuh M, Ellenberg J. Self-organization of MTOCs replaces centrosome function during acentrosomal spindle assembly in live mouse oocytes. *Cell* 2007; **130**: 484–98.

36. Kim N-H, Funahashi H, Prather RS, Schatten G, Day BN. Microtubule and microfilament dynamics in porcine oocytes during meiotic maturation. *Mol Reprod Dev* 1996; **43**: 248–55.

37. Le Guen P, Crozet N. Microtubule and centrosome distribution during sheep fertilization. *Eur J Cell Biol* 1989; **48**: 239–49.

38. Long CR, Pinto-Correia C, Duby RT, *et al.* Chromatin and microtubule morphology during the first cell cycle in bovine zygotes. *Mol Reprod Dev* 1993; **36**: 23–32.

39. Gueth-Hallonet C, Antony C, Aghion J, *et al.* γ-Tubulin is present in acentriolar MTOCs during early mouse development. *J Cell Sci* 1993; **105**: 157–66.

40. Lee J, Miyano T, Moor RM. Spindle formation and dynamics of γ-tubulin and nuclear mitotic apparatus protein distribution during meiosis in pig and mouse oocytes. *Biol Reprod* 2000; **62**: 1184–92.

41. Schatten H, Sun QY. The functional significance of centrosomes in mammalian meiosis, fertilization, development, nuclear transfer, and stem cell differentiation. *Environ Mol Mutagen* 2009; **50**(8): 620–36.

42. Schatten H, Sun Q-Y. The significant role of centrosomes in stem cell division and differentiation. *Microsc Microanal* 2011; **17**(4): 506–12.

43. Can A, Semiz O, Çinar O. Centrosome and microtubule dynamics during early stages of meiosis in mouse oocytes. *Mol Hum Reprod* 2003; **9**(12): 749–56.

44. Brunet S, Maro B. Cytoskeleton and cell cycle control during meiotic maturation of the mouse oocyte: integrating time and space. *Reproduction* 2005; **130**: 801–11.

45. Ai J-S, Wang Q, Li M, *et al.* Roles of microtubules and microfilaments in spindle movements during rat oocyte meiosis. *J Reprod Dev* 2008; **54**: 391–6.

46. Ai J-S, Wang Q, Yin S, *et al.* Regulation of peripheral spindle movement and spindle rotation during mouse oocyte meiosis: new perspectives. *Microsc Microanal* 2008; **14**(4): 349–56.

47. Fan HY, Huo LJ, Meng XQ, *et al.* Involvement of calcium/calmodulin-dependent protein kinase II (CaMKII) in meiotic maturation and activation of pig oocytes. *Biol Reprod* 2003; **69**: 1552–64.

48. Messinger SM, Albertini DF. Centrosome and microtubule dynamics during meiotic progression in the mouse oocyte. *J Cell Sci* 1991; **100**: 289–98.

49. Combelles CM, Albertini DF. Microtubule patterning during meiotic maturation in mouse oocytes is determined by cell cycle-specific sorting and redistribution of gamma-tubulin. *Dev Biol* 2001; **239**: 281–94.

50. Sanfins A, Plancha CE, Overstrom, EW, Albertini DF. Meiotic spindle morphogenesis in *in vivo* and *in vitro* matured mouse oocytes: insights into the relationship between nuclear and cytoplasmic quality. *Hum Reprod* 2004; **19**(12): 2889–99.

51. Fan HY, Sun QY. Involvement of mitogen-activated protein kinase cascade during oocyte maturation and fertilization in mammals. *Biol Reprod* 2004; **70**: 535–47.

52. Yu LZ, Xiong B, Gao WX, *et al.* MEK1/2 regulates microtubule organization, spindle pole tethering and asymmetric division during mouse oocyte meiotic maturation. *Cell Cycle* 2007; **6**: 330–8.

53. Kubiak JZ, Weber M, Geraud G, Maro B. Cell cycle modification during the transitions between meiotic M-phases in mouse oocytes. *J Cell Sci* 1992; **102**: 457–67.

54. Hampl A, Eppig JJ. Analysis of the mechanism(s) of metaphase I arrest in maturing mouse oocytes. *Development* 1995; **121**: 925–33.

55. Sun QY, Lai L, Wu G, *et al.* Regulation of mitogen-activated protein kinase phosphorylation, microtubule organization, chromatin behavior, and cell cycle progression are regulated by protein phosphatases during pig oocyte maturation and fertilization *in vitro*. *Biol Reprod* 2002; **66**(3): 580–8.

56. Yin S, Sun X-F, Schatten H, Sun Q-Y. Molecular insights into mechanisms regulating faithful chromosome separation in female meiosis. *Cell Cycle* 2008; **7**(19): 2997–3005.

57. Szollosi D, Calarco P, Donahue RP. Absence of centrioles in the first and second meiotic spindles of mouse oocytes. *J Cell Sci* 1972; **11**: 521–41.

58. Calarco-Gillam PC, Siebert MC, Hubble R, Mitchison T, Kirschner M. Centrosome development in early mouse embryos as defined by an autoantibody against pericentriolar material. *Cell* 1983; **35**(3 Pt 2): 621–9.

59. Dumont J, Petri S, Pellegrin F, *et al.* A centriole- and RanGTP-independent spindle assembly pathway in meiosis I of vertebrate oocytes. *J Cell Biol* 2007; **176**: 295–305.

60. Moritz M, Braunfeld MB, Sedat JW, Alberts B, Agard DA. Microtubule nucleation by gamma-tubulin-containing rings in the centrosome. *Nature* 1995; **378**: 638–40.

61. Zheng Y, Wong ML, Alberts B, Mitchison T. Nucleation of microtubule assembly by a

gamma-tubulin-containing ring complex. *Nature* 1995; **378**: 578–83.

62. Kitajima TS, Ohsugi M, Ellenberg J. Complete kinetochore tracking reveals error-prone homologous chromosome biorientation in mammalian oocytes. *Cell* 2011; **146**(4): 568–81.

63. Zhang Q-H, Wei L, Tong J-S, *et al.* Localization and function of Spindly during mouse oocyte meiotic maturation. *Cell Cycle* 2010; **9**(11): 2230–6.

64. Schatten H, Walter M, Biessmann H, Schatten G. Activation of maternal centrosomes in unfertilized sea urchin eggs. *Cell Motil Cytoskel* 1992; **23**: 61–70.

65. Leibfried-Rutledge ML, Critser ES, Eyestone WH, Northey DL, First NL. Development potential of bovine oocytes matured in vitro and in vivo. *Biol Reprod* 1987; **36**: 376–83.

66. Liu H, Krey LC, Zhang J, Grifo JA. Ooplasmic influence on nuclear function during the metaphase II-interphase transition in mouse oocytes. *Biol Reprod* 2001; **65**: 1794–9.

67. Trounson A, Anderiesz C, Jones G. Maturation of human oocytes in vitro and their developmental competence. *Reproduction* 2001; **121**: 51–75.

68. Combelles CM, Cekleniak NA, Racowsky C, Albertini DF. Assessment of nuclear and cytoplasmic maturation in *in vitro* matured human oocytes. *Hum Reprod* 2002; **17**: 1006–16.

69. MacQueen AJ, Hochwagen A. Checkpoint mechanisms: the puppet masters of meiotic prophase. *Trends Cell Biol* 2011; **21**: 393–400.

70. Zickler D. From early homologue recognition to synaptonemal complex formation. *Chromosoma* 2006; **115**: 158–74.

71. Battaglia DE, Goodwin P, Klein NA, Soules MR. Influence of maternal age on meiotic spindle assembly in oocytes from naturally cycling women. *Hum Reprod* 1996; **11**: 2217–22.

72. Garcia-Cruz R, Brieno MA, Roig I, *et al.* Dynamics of cohesin proteins REC8, STAG3, SMC1 beta and SMC3 are consistent with a role in sister chromatid cohesion during meiosis in human oocytes. *Hum Reprod* 2010; **25**: 2316–27.

73. Prieto I, Tease C, Pezzi N, *et al.* Cohesin component dynamics during meiotic prophase I in mammalian oocytes. *Chromosome Res* 2004; **12**: 197–213.

74. Revenkova E, Jessberger R. Keeping sister chromatids together: cohesins in meiosis. *Reproduction* 2005; **130**: 783–90.

75. Terret ME, Wassmann K, Waizenegger I, *et al.* The meiosis I-to-meiosis II transition in mouse oocytes requires separase activity. *Curr Biol* 2003; **13**: 1797–802.

76. Kudo NR, Wassmann K, Anger M, *et al.* Resolution of chiasmata in oocytes requires separase-mediated proteolysis. *Cell* 2006; **126**: 135–46.

77. Sun SC, Kim NH. Spindle assembly checkpoint and its regulators in meiosis. *Hum Reprod Update* 2012; **18**(1): 60–72.

78. Vogt E, Sanhaji M, Klein W, *et al.* MCAK is present at centromeres, midspindle and chiasmata and involved in silencing of the spindle assembly checkpoint in mammalian oocytes. *Mol Hum Reprod* 2010; **16**(9): 665–84.

79. Maiato H, DeLuca J, Salmon ED, Earnshaw WC. The dynamic kinetochore-microtubule interface. *J Cell Sci* 2004; **117**: 5461–77.

80. Kolano A, Brunet S, Silk AD, Cleveland DW, Verlhac MH. Error-prone mammalian female meiosis from silencing the spindle assembly checkpoint without normal interkinetochore tension. *Proc Natl Acad Sci USA* 2012; **109**(27): E1858–67.

81. Speroff L. The effect of aging on fertility. *Curr Opin Obstet Gynecol* 1994; **6**: 115–20.

82. Eichenlaub-Ritter U, Chandley AC, Gosden RG. Alterations to the microtubular cytoskeleton and increased disorder of chromosome alignment in spontaneously ovulated mouse oocytes aged in vivo: an immunofluorescence study. *Chromosoma* 1986; **94**: 337–45.

83. Hornak M, Jeseta M, Musilova P, *et al.* Frequency of aneuploidy related to age in porcine oocytes. *PLoS One* 2011; **6**(4): e18892.

84. Miao Y-L, Sun Q-Y, Zhang X, *et al.* Centrosome abnormalities during porcine oocyte aging. *Environ Mol Mutagen* 2009; **50**(8): 666–71.

85. Eichenlaub-Ritter U, Vogt E, Cukurcam S, *et al.* Exposure of mouse oocytes to bisphenol A causes meiotic arrest but not aneuploidy. *Mutat Res* 2008; **651**: 82–92.

Chapter 13

Transcription, accumulation, storage, recruitment, and degradation of maternal mRNA in mammalian oocytes

Santhi Potireddy, Dasari Amarnath, and Keith E. Latham

Introduction

The mammalian oocyte is a remarkable cell, providing for a diverse range of essential functions to initiate each new life. Unique demands at the start of embryogenesis are met by equally unique capacities in the oocyte. These include the ability to undergo early oocyte activation and blocks to polyspermy upon fertilization, suppressing cell death after successful fertilization, supporting early nuclear reprogramming and remodeling events that enable production of a totipotent genome (a capacity that underlies cloning by somatic cell nuclear transfer), temporal regulation of the cell cycle, continuous provision of macromolecules required for cellular physiology and organization, and eventually transcriptional activation of the embryonic genome with the correct array of genes being activated. The reservoir of stored maternal mRNAs deposited in the oocyte provides the driving force behind these processes, as temporally regulated recruitment and translation of stored mRNAs provides for the dynamic production of different proteins at the correct times when they are needed. This chapter reviews the dynamic regulation of gene transcription, genome silencing, and maternal mRNA storage during oogenesis, and the subsequent mechanisms that enable regulated use of these mRNAs during oocyte maturation and after fertilization.

Gene transcription

The transition of primordial follicles to antral follicles and subsequent ovulation of high quality oocytes that are capable of undergoing successful fertilization and development to term are accompanied by stage-specific changes in mRNA expression [1]. Oocytes obtained from mouse primordial follicles display a pattern distinct from oocytes obtained from other stages. Of the 11 660 mRNAs detected in these oocytes, 5020 genes display a twofold change in relative abundance, with 50% of genes up- or down-regulated in their level of expression at the transition from primordial to primary follicles. This phenomenal change in the oocyte transcriptome coincides with a dramatic reorganization of follicle structure and initiation of development of growth in primary follicles. The second biggest change in the oocyte transcriptome is observed between the secondary and small antral follicle stages, and noticeably affects genes involved in microtubule-based processes. The overall transition from secondary to large antral follicles coincides with acquisition of oocyte meiotic and developmental competence, including the ability to form a meiotic spindle [2, 3].

Acquisition of meiotic and development competence is also marked by large-scale genomic changes. Oocytes remodel their genomes from less to more condensed forms, signified by non-surrounded nucleoli (NSN) in primordial follicles transitioning to surrounded nucleoli (SN) type by completion of oocyte growth. This coincides with global transcriptional silencing. NSN type oocytes are transcriptionally active and produce all classes of RNA, whereas SN oocytes are transcriptionally inactive. Transcriptional silencing is mediated by changes in chromatin structure, and eventually chromosomes condense to allow congression on the spindle [4]. Fully grown NSN and SN type oocytes are both meiotically competent and can reach metaphase II (MII) in vitro, but NSN oocytes are less competent to mature, and embryos derived from them arrest at the 2-cell stage [5].

The changes in chromatin structure lead to global changes in transcription activity. Global repression

Biology and Pathology of the Oocyte, 2nd edn., ed. Alan Trounson, Roger Gosden, and Ursula Eichenlaub-Ritter. Published by Cambridge University Press.

of transcription occurs just before the resumption of meiosis and is maintained until embryonic genomic activation during early cleavage. Global repression of transcription is essential for the heterochromatin formation, proper segregation of chromosomes at meiosis, and acquisition of developmental competence in oocytes. Transcriptional silencing is usually marked by global deacetylation. Deacetylation of pericentric heterochromatin is essential for the recruitment of heterochromatin protein 1 to centromeres and binding of the chromatin remodeling protein, ATRX, to centromeric heterochromatin in condensed chromosomes [6]. ATRX, a member of the SNF2 family, is required for chromosome alignment and meiotic spindle organization in metaphase II stage mouse oocytes. Disruption of ATRX binding using a histone deacetylase inhibitor such as trichostatin A results in abnormal chromosome alignment at the meiotic spindle. Global histone deacetylation is an important mechanism responsible for erasure of epigenetic memory of differentiated cells, and may likewise help erase oocyte epigenetic memory, so that the newly formed embryonic genome can initiate the developmental program. While the precise mechanism responsible for transcriptional silencing in oocytes remains to be fully elucidated, changes in the expression of key transcription factors, modification of RNA polymerase II, or changes in their access to the oocyte genome may contribute to transcriptional silencing. Additionally, MLL2, a histone 3 lysine 4 (H3K4) methyltransferase, is required for trimethylation at H3K4 and transcriptional silencing [7].

A complex network of interactions between granulosa cells, cumulus cells, and oocytes maintains meiotic arrest of oocytes. Fully grown oocytes competent to re-enter meiosis remain meiotically arrested until the preovulatory surge of luteinizing hormone (LH). A high level of cAMP (cyclic adenosine 3′, 5′-monophosphate) produced within the oocyte prevents the oocyte from resuming meiosis. A high cAMP concentration inside the oocyte is sustained by cGMP (cyclic guanosine 3′, 5′-monophosphate), a potent inhibitor of the oocyte-specific phosphodiesterase enzyme (PDE3A) responsible for hydrolysis of cAMP. Before the LH surge, cGMP produced in the cumulus cells diffuses through the gap junctions and inhibits activity of PDE3A inside the oocyte [8, 9]. LH causes a decrease in cGMP production by somatic cells and/or closure of somatic cell gap junctions, activation of oocyte PDE3A, and hydrolysis of cAMP, leading to meiotic maturation. Natriuretic precursor type C (NPPC) and its receptor guanylate cyclase, NPR2, which are expressed in mural granulosa and cumulus cells, respectively, also play critical roles in meiotic arrest. Binding of NPPC to its receptor stimulates synthesis of cGMP by cumulus cells. Interestingly, expression of *Npr2* mRNA by cumulus cells is regulated by the oocyte-derived paracrine factors growth differentiation factor 9 (GDF9), bone morphogenetic protein 15 (BMP15), and fibroblast growth factor 8B (FGF8B) [10]. Microsurgical extirpation of oocytes from the cumulus–oocyte complex significantly reduces the *Npr2* mRNA expression in cumulus cells. NPPC prevents spontaneous resumption of meiosis in cumulus-enclosed oocytes but not in denuded oocytes. The oocyte thus serves as a master regulator of meiotic arrest.

Genomic imprinting is an epigenetic mechanism responsible for parental origin-specific monoallelic expression of some genes, and typically involves differential DNA methylation. Methylation imprints are erased in primordial germ cells and then sex-appropriate imprints imposed anew during gametogenesis. The need to erase and re-establish imprints creates a window of opportunity for biallelic expression, which may affect oocyte phenotype. Fully grown mouse oocytes (75–80 μm) can support term development, whereas growing oocytes (60–65 μm) cannot. Nuclear transfer studies reveal progressive acquisition of imprints that enable extended parthenogenesis, and moreover reveal that early stage nuclei lacking complete maternal imprints can complement fully imprinted oocyte genomes in supporting parthenogenesis in conjunction with genetic modifications in the H19 differentially methylated region (DMR) and *Dlk1-Dio3* [11]. In vitro fertilization of reconstructed oocytes with incomplete imprints results in pups with phenotypic abnormalities [12]. Imprinted genes acquire imprinting methylation marks asynchronously in growing oocytes. The parental alleles retain their epigenetic memory of their origin even in the absence of DNA methylation, as maternal alleles acquire methylation signals first in growing oocytes [13]. Altered expression of imprinted genes with in vitro maturation seen in rhesus monkey oocytes [14] raises the possibility that maternal imprints are either incomplete or remain sensitive to environmental effects until just before maturation is completed, which may affect the outcome of in vitro manipulations.

Maternal mRNA storage

Maternal mRNAs drive early development of embryos prior to transcriptional activation. Oocytes have developed unique ways to store and regulate mRNAs, and mammalian oocytes differ from oocytes of other species in key respects. Maternal mRNAs are stored in an inactive form in the oocyte and activated for translation in a temporally complex manner throughout maturation, fertilization, and early cleavage.

RNA-binding proteins sequester the maternal mRNAs to messenger ribonucleoprotein (mRNP) particles. These proteins inhibit mRNA translation by subjecting mRNAs to degradation or by localizing mRNAs away from the translation apparatus in mRNP particles. Much of our knowledge of maternal mRNA regulation has come from studies in amphibian and invertebrate species, where biochemical or genetic studies have often been more facile. These data provide an invaluable basis for conceptualizing mechanisms that operate across species; however, species differences exist. In amphibian oocytes, Y-box proteins such as FRGY2 and MRNP3 are major RNP components [15–17]. Many other mRNA-binding proteins comprise a diverse range of proteins that regulate translation initiation and elongation. Some of these will be discussed in later sections.

A conserved core of proteins found in processing bodies (P bodies) from yeast to mammals may be involved in translation repression at some stages, and consists of the mRNA decapping enzyme DCP1P/DCP2P, activators of decapping DHH1P/RCK/p54, PAT1P, SCD6P/RAP55, EDC3P, the LSM1P-7P complex, and the 5′ to 3′ exonuclease, XRN1P [18]. P bodies are RNP aggregates in the cytoplasm that are involved in mRNA repression by sequestration from the translation apparatus. P bodies accumulate translationally repressed mRNAs and associated repressor proteins. Protein components of P bodies include XRN1, TNRC6A, LSM14A, EDC4, CPEB1, DDX6, EIF4E, EIF4ENIF1, EIF2C, and decapping enzymes [19]. *Drosophila* CUP (mammalian EIF4ENIF1) blocks EIF4G (eukaryotic translation initiation factor 4 gamma) recruitment and inhibits translation [20]. Sequestration of EIF4E in conjunction with CUP/EIF4ENIF1 to P bodies prevents mRNA from undergoing decapping and degradation and thereby promotes storage [18].

The mammalian oocyte cortex contains a storage form of granules related to P bodies [21, 22]. Maternal mRNA storage in mammals appears to differ from other species in key respects, with maternal mRNA localized to subcortical RNP particle domain (SCRD) [22]. P bodies are involved in mRNA storage in meiotically incompetent oocytes. As the oocyte develops, P bodies disappear and subcortical aggregates (SCA) appear. These SCAs contain RNA and RNA-binding proteins, forming SCRDs in the cortex of growing oocytes, which serve as a storage compartment for maternal mRNAs. Subcortical localization of DDX6 [23] and YBX2 [24] has been detected in oocytes and early embryos. Another structure termed the subcortical maternal complex (SCMC) has been described in mouse oocytes, and contains MATER, FLOPED, TLE6, and FILIA [25]. The SCMC is essential for embryonic developmental progression but does not appear to be related to maternal mRNA localization [22].

MATER also associates with the cytoplasmic lattices (CPLs), which require the oocyte-restricted peptidylarginine deiminase 6 (PADI6). In PADI6-null oocytes, acetylated tubulin is depleted, indicating the key role played by PADI6/CPLs. Additionally, the CPL may function in ribosome storage, and PADI6-null mouse oocyte protein synthesis can be incorrectly regulated, indicating an indirect role for the CPL in maternal mRNA translation [26].

Another key protein for mRNA storage in mammalian oocytes is the germ cell-specific RNA-binding protein YBX2 (also known as MSY2). This protein is essential for mRNA storage. Deficiency disrupts oocyte growth and maturation in mice [27].

Regulation of translation initiation and elongation

Proper development and differentiation of the oocyte and development of fertilized cell embryos to the 2-cell stage and beyond are dependent on the correct temporal recruitment and translation of the maternal mRNAs. Correct regulation during oogenesis and oocyte maturation establishes a high quality oocyte, whereas correct regulation after fertilization enables proper execution of key developmental processes during early embryogenesis, and sets the stage for continued development.

Maternal mRNAs recruited for translation before and after fertilization differ in the mechanism by which they are recruited for translation and vary in the sets of biological functions performed

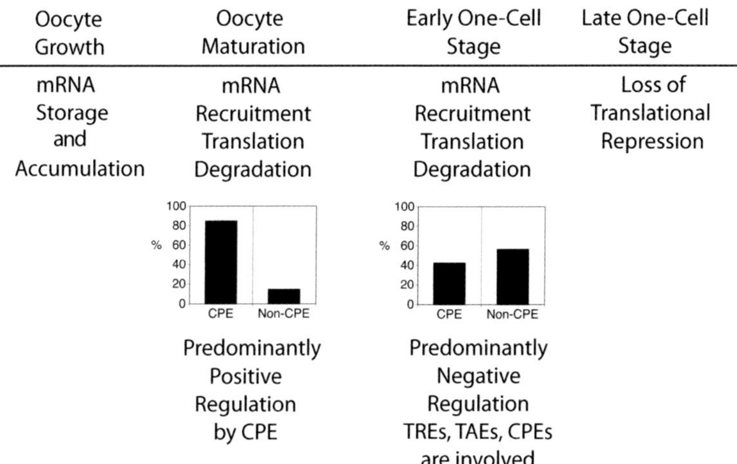

Figure 13.1 Changes in translational control during mouse oogenesis and early embryogenesis. During oocyte growth a large store of maternal mRNA accumulates in specialized storage forms. Upon oocyte maturation a large portion of this stored mRNA is recruited for translation by polyadenylation controlled predominantly by the cytoplasmic polyadenylation element (CPE) and other cis-regulatory motifs in the 3′ untranslated region. During this period, translational control is dominated by positive events driving translational recruitment via unmasking of mRNAs. After fertilization, the class of maternal mRNAs recruited onto polysomes changes dramatically, and this is regulated by a combination of non-CPE translation activator and translation repressor elements (TAEs and TREs). During this period, translation control is mediated by repressive mechanisms that suppress precocious recruitment of many mRNAs. By the late 1-cell stage these translation repression mechanisms disappear, as indicated by prompt recruitment of injected reporter mRNAs regardless of the cis-regulatory elements that they contain. This allows final recruitment, translation, and degradation of the bulk of the remaining maternal mRNA in preparation for the transition to embryonic control of development at the 2-cell stage as the newly created embryonic genome is reprogrammed and activated to produce the required array of stage-appropriate embryonic transcripts.

(Figure 13.1). The dormant maternal mRNAs are activated by reversible polyadenylation that is controlled by cytoplasmic polyadenylation elements (CPEs). These elements are sequence specific and present in the 3′ untranslated region (UTR) of mRNAs. The CPE-binding protein (CPEB) binds to the CPE, and then further interacts with and recruits other proteins for polyadenylation and ultimately translation [28]. Analysis of maternal mRNAs that undergo translation at the MII stage in mice (before fertilization) and at the 1-cell stage (after fertilization) for the presence of CPE motifs revealed that over 80% of maternal mRNAs translated at the MII stage contained known CPEs but fewer than half of maternal mRNAs translated at the 1-cell stage had CPEs [29]. This indicated that motifs other than CPE must regulate translation of many maternal mRNAs after fertilization. A novel motif that plays a major role in translation of the *Bag4* maternal mRNA at the 1-cell stage was identified [30]. This motif is distinct from classical CPE type motifs, and is not AU rich.

Analysis of the polysomal mRNA populations from the MII and 1-cell stages led to identification of mRNAs that undergo stage-specific translation [29]. Approximately 495 transcripts were translated at the MII stage with threefold or greater enrichment over the 1-cell stage and a large population of 1816 maternal mRNAs was translated preferentially at the late 1-cell stage. This shows that maternal mRNAs are highly regulated after fertilization as well as during oocyte maturation. Proteins synthesized at the MII stage are mostly involved in homeostasis and those recruited at the 1-cell stage are more related to macromolecular biosynthesis. Thus, subsets of maternal mRNAs are recruited in a temporally complex manner to suit the changing needs of the maturing oocyte and the early embryo.

Proteins such as EIF4E, EIF4G, and EIF4A bind to the 5′ cap of mRNAs and initiate translation. These proteins together form the EIF4F complex, which recruits the ribosomal subunits onto the mRNA. The MASKIN protein binds to the CPEB protein on the CPE. MASKIN interacts with EIF4E, which is bound on the 5′ end of the mRNA, thus preventing its interaction with the EIF4G. When CPEB is phosphorylated during oocyte maturation, the interaction between MASKIN and EIF4E is disrupted and CPEB interacts with cleavage and polyadenylation specific factor (CPSF), which recruits poly(A) polymerase to add a poly(A) tail. Poly(A)-binding protein (PABP) protects the newly formed poly(A) tail from degradation and interacts with the 40S ribosome to recruit other translation initiation factors [31]. Translation repression is also mediated by EIF4EBP (EIF4E-binding protein). Hypophosphorylated EIF4EBP has a high affinity for EIF4E and prevents the formation of the EIF4F complex required for translation initiation. Phosphorylation of EIF4EBP, for example by mTOR, causes the release of EIF4E during germinal vesicle breakdown (GVBD) in frog oocytes. The EIF4ET/mouse homolog CLAST4 also regulates EIF4E by transporting EIF4E from the cytoplasm to the nucleus [32]. Translation repression is also achieved by association with the cytoplasmic deadenylation complex, which includes CCR4 and CAF1. CAF1 represses translation in a deadenylation-independent manner and dependent on the 5′ cap of the mRNA [33].

Another mechanism of regulated translation initiation was reported for the *Xenopus* system. Translation initiation of the *Nanos* mRNA (*Nanos* is itself a translational regulator) is regulated by a secondary structural element located downstream of the initiator codon, which affects ribosome loading [34].

Translational regulation is also possible at the level of translation elongation. In *Drosophila*, the *Oscar* mRNA is repressed at the level of elongation until the mRNA is localized [35]. Translation elongation can modulate production of cell cycle-related proteins via conserved mechanisms, and can be integrated with signaling pathways, for example calcium signaling [36]. Regulation at the level of translation employs a different set of regulatory molecules than those employed in the control of initiation, and thus provides another means of achieving regulatory flexibility.

Cytoplasmic activation of maternal mRNAs requires the coordinated action of various motifs. Two important cis-regulatory motifs with well-defined roles are the CPE and the polyadenylation hexanucleotide (AAUAAA). In *Xenopus* the CPE activates and represses mRNA translation by interaction with MASKIN via the CPEB. The reason behind certain mRNAs with CPE being activated while others are repressed at the same time lies in the interplay between motifs. The differential regulation of mRNA translation is attributed to the number of CPEs, the CPE sequence, position of CPE and distance between CPEs [37, 38], and the interactions with other motifs [39]. CPE-mediated repression of mRNA translation is directed by the presence of at least two CPE elements, and a minimum distance of 10–12 nt defines maximum repression [39]. mRNAs with single CPE or a distance of more than 10–12 nt between CPE motifs do not undergo repression. Repression by the CPE is enhanced by the presence of a PUMILIO binding element (PBE) along with two or more CPE motifs [39, 40]. An optimal distance of 25 nt between the CPE and the hexanucleotide provides maximal and early translation, but an mRNA with two CPEs and one of them overlapping the hexanucelotide undergoes late translation. This is due to the masking of the hexanucelotide by CPEB and prevention of the interaction with CPSF. Upon activation of maturation-promoting factor/cyclin-dependent kinase 1(CDK1), CPEB is phosphorylated and a small amount degraded to allow CPSF to interact with the hexanucleotide [41]. The presence of a PBE with a single CPE enhances translation by twofold [39], stabilizing CPEB binding to the CPE, although in the case of mRNAs with two CPEs stabilization by the PBE is not necessary. Along with the CPE and PBE motifs, the MUSASHI binding motif is present in the 3′ UTRs of most mRNAs that undergo early or late translation [27]. MUSASHI displays interesting species specificity in its functions [42].

CPEB plays a vital role in germ cell development. In CPEB knockout mice, both male and female germ cell development is blocked at pachytene, a consequence of inhibition of translation of CPE-containing mRNAs encoding synaptonemal complex proteins – SCP1 and SCP3 [43]. The MASKIN protein, which binds to the CPEB in *Xenopus*, is homologous to mammalian transforming acidic coiled coil (TACC) proteins. TACC proteins in mammals regulate spindle formation [44]. Interestingly, the mammalian TACC proteins do not appear to bind EIF4E, indicating that the paradigm of MASKIN regulation of translational-controlling EIF4E interactions likely does not apply to mammals.

SMAUG response elements (SREs) and NANOS response elements (NREs) regulate both maternal mRNA translation and stability in *Drosophila*. SMAUG functions by either recruiting EIF4EBP to the mRNA 5′ end or by subjecting mRNAs to rapid deadenylation and instability [45, 46]. The human SMAUG homolog SAMD4A plays a role in translational control and mRNA storage in particles in neurons [47].

Stringent temporal regulation of maternal mRNAs is needed to avoid simultaneous translation of all mRNAs. This regulation is achieved by a variety of different regulatory motifs, and is influenced y the spacing between those motifs. For example, the relative CPE and hexanucleotide (AAUAAA) ositions affect the timing of polyadenylation. A horter distance between the CPE and hexanucleotide dvances the timing of polyadenylation [48]. The PBE vorks in conjunction with the CPE for temporal egulation of translation [39]. Splice variation of CPE-earing mRNAs affects timing of translation in mamnalian oocytes and embryos [49].

Translational control in mouse embryos requires nultiple elements other than the CPE [30]. The prinary mode of regulation after fertilization is one of epression rather than activation, distinguishing post-ertilization control from oocyte maturation control, vith four translation repression elements (TREs) and hree translation activating elements (TAEs) being mployed in the control of the model *Bag4* maternal mRNA. Removal of the TREs permits early transational recruitment. The major TRE identified coinides with a region of maternal mRNA secondary tructure. At a population level, bioinformatics analsis indicated a rich diversity of multiple motifs residng within the 3′ UTRs of over 40% of the maternal nRNAs analyzed. The number of putative motifs could e quite high for a single mRNA, one reaching as high s 95 occurrences.

Maternal mRNA degradation

Translational recruitment and mRNA polyadenylaion are often coupled to mRNA degradation. Hence, ecruitment of maternal mRNAs during maturation lso reduces availability of those mRNAs for later se. Additionally, degradation of maternal transcripts s necessary to establish embryonic control of develpment after fertilization. Maternal mRNAs must be liminated in coordination with transcriptional actiation of the genome, in order to avoid crippling leficiencies in mRNA and protein availability, and vidence indicates that transcriptional activity in the mbryo regulates maternal mRNA degradation. The nechanisms regulating mRNA adenylation, deadenyation, translation, and small RNA-mediated destrucion are components of this overall process.

The CPE regulates a choice between default leadenylation and storage versus degradation pathvays during *Xenopus* oocyte maturation. Deadenylaion is independent of translation, as some mRNAs ndergo immediate deadenylation and degradation, ome undergo deadenylation and storage, and some mRNAs undergo mRNA degradation after translation. The CPE and hexanucleotide motifs regulate the timing of degradation of specific mRNAs. mRNAs with no CPEs undergo default deadenylation, are less stable, and are subjected to degradation earlier than mRNAs with long poly(A) tails [50]. Microarray studies of wild-type and *Smaug* mutant *Drosophila* oocytes indicate that 55% of the proteins synthesized are maternally expressed and, upon egg activation, 20% of the mRNAs (~1600 mRNAs) are destabilized [51]. SMAUG plays a major role in the elimination of 76% of the destabilized mRNAs.

In mouse oocytes, the CPE is required for deadenylation and polyadenylation, hence the initial coining of the word adenylation control element (ACE). mRNAs with CPEs either undergo immediate translation or are deadenylated and stored as dormant transcripts during oogenesis. Transcripts that are degraded or stable were identified using expression microarrays, focusing on transcript changes between GV and MII mouse oocytes. A large population of 3002 probe sets was down-regulated during maturation to the MII stage and 9260 were unchanged. Biofunction analysis of the transcripts degraded during maturation reveals diverse biological functions such as protein synthesis, DNA replication, recombination and repair, energy production, and molecular transport. Biofunction analysis of transcripts that are stable at the MII stage indicates many are involved in signaling pathways [52]. In humans, there is also a dramatic reduction in numbers of mRNAs upon oocyte maturation [53].

YBX2 (also known as MSY2) is an abundant protein found in oocytes, with a role in mRNA stability. Deletion of YBX2 leads to sterile female mice. The major role of YBX2 is confirmed by the microarray analysis of wild-type and YBX2-deficient oocytes. The stability and abundance of a large number of transcripts is diminished in the YBX2-deficient oocytes. A total of 6940 and 6497 transcripts representing ~70% of transcripts detected are either increased or decreased, respectively [27]. The decapping enzyme DCP2 and other proteins involved in decapping are specifically localized to P bodies. mRNA decay and decapping can occur even within polysomes and in the absence of P bodies, illustrating the connection between translation and degradation [54].

Small RNAs (piRNAs, miRNAs, siRNAs) contribute to the control of mRNA stability. The complex regulation of mRNA degradation by piRNAs involving Argonaute (AGO) proteins targets the *Nanos* maternal mRNA in *Drosophila* embryos by recruiting or stabilizing the CCR4–NOT deadenylation complex together with SMAUG [55]. AGO proteins in *Drosophila* oocytes persist throughout early development. miRNAs (e.g., miR-430) regulate the stability of hundreds of mRNAs in zebrafish [56]. In *Xenopus*, AGO2 activity is regulated during early stages of development but its role is unclear. Expression of exogenous AGO2 does not have any deleterious effects, but expression of siRNA for AGO proteins causes developmental defects. Thus, depletion of AGO proteins results in inhibition of release of cleavage products from DICER during miRNA biogenesis and formation of RNA-induced silencing complexes (RISCs). Exogenous siRNAs in *Xenopus* can bind and inactivate AGO, and can block the production of miR-427 to support miRNA-mediated deadenylation of maternal mRNAs until AGO proteins are up-regulated at the mid-blastula transition [57].

In the mouse, hundreds of transcripts undergo degradation at meiosis I or II during oogenesis, revealing the transcript-dependent nature of mRNA degradation. Along with degradation, mRNA translocation and storage also play vital roles in regulation of transcripts that are stable during maturation but then eliminated from the polysomal fraction [58]. This maternal mRNA regulation process is controlled in part by CPEB and DAZL proteins, and without DAZL, oocytes display meiotic spindle defects as proteins essential for spindle formation and function are not produced as needed.

AGO2 is expressed during mouse preimplantation development and depletion of its mRNA leads to developmental arrest at the 2-cell stage. However, mammalian oocytes and embryos differ markedly from invertebrates with respect to miRNA and siRNA functions. Endogenous siRNAs are essential for mouse oocyte meiosis, and miRNAs are not essential during preimplantation development. miRNAs are abundant in oocytes, but miRNA function is suppressed in fully grown oocytes even though miRNA targets are present [59]. After fertilization, distinct populations of siRNAs and miRNAs likely control stage-specific mRNA degradation and possibly lineage restriction [60].

Interestingly, the mechanisms that suppress maternal mRNA translation appear to disappear by the late 1-cell stage in the mouse, as injected reporter mRNAs are efficiently recruited for translation even when lacking TAEs [30]. By relieving translational repression and permitting translation-coupled degradation, this transition may contribute to the dramatic elimination of maternal mRNAs between the late 1-cell and late 2-cell stages in mouse embryos.

As indicated above, mechanisms to coordinate transcriptional activation with mRNA degradation must exist. It is well known that transcriptional blockade, with RNA polymerase inhibitors, in 2-cell embryos can stabilize a large number of maternal transcripts, leading to increased relative abundance. Embryos produced by somatic cell nuclear transfer display altered patterns of maternal mRNA degradation and stabilization, indicating that the gene expression pattern of the nucleus affects maternal mRNA degradation [61].

Relationship of maternal mRNAs to oocyte and embryo quality

The degradation of maternal mRNAs is tightly regulated and it is transcript dependent. The differential recruitment of biologically distinct classes of maternal mRNAs onto polysomes before and after fertilization [29] indicates that the overall process is highly regulated. Array-based gene expression profiling revealed dramatic changes in maternal mRNA populations in mouse oocytes during oogenesis [1]. Likewise, dramatic changes in protein synthesis patterns after fertilization as well as array-based transcript profiling reveal dynamic changes in the spectrum of maternal mRNAs being recruited, translated, and degraded at different times. The correct disposition of maternal mRNAs contributes to the elaboration of overall oocyte quality. In vitro maturation in mice leads to reduced oocyte quality and defects in maternal mRNA regulation, particularly with mRNAs related to gene transcription [1]. Correct translation of maternal mRNAs during oogenesis is critical for proper spindle formation [1]. However, in the rhesus monkey only a small number of maternal mRNAs were affected by in vitro maturation [14]. Studies of human oocytes indicate that in vitro maturation of oocytes that fail to mature in vivo following gonadotropin stimulation is associated with abnormal maternal mRNA regulation and reduced oocyte quality [62]. Incorrect handling of maternal mRNAs could reflect poor initial quality of the oocyte rather than an effect of in vitro maturation, but illustrates the correlation of incorrect maternal mRNA regulation and poor oocyte quality.

Perspectives

The study of maternal mRNA in mammalian oocytes and embryos has revealed a complex and dynamic mode of developmental control about which much remains to be learned. Comparisons between mammalian and non-mammalian maternal mRNA regulation reveal many common features, but also many differences. Hence, it is imperative to continue unravelling the specific modes of regulation that operate in mammalian oocytes and early embryos. One interesting facet of maternal mRNA control is how it is coordinated with other ongoing processes, such as cell-cycle progression and nuclear events. Great strides have been made in deciphering how cell-cycle regulators control the phosphorylation and activities of RNA-binding proteins; however, no insight has yet been gained concerning the connection between transcription and maternal mRNA degradation. Additionally, while several intriguing papers recently suggested roles for localized mRNAs in mammalian oocytes, differences in interpretation persist on this point, and the extent to which this occurs or is required for normal embryogenesis has not yet been established.

Acknowledgments

Work in the authors' laboratory has been supported by grants from the National Institutes of Health, National Institute of Child Health and Development (RO1-HD43092, RC1-HD06337), and The National Center for Research Resources and the Office of Research Infrastructure Programs (ORIP) RO1-RR018907 and R24-RR015253/R24 OD012221) to KEL.

References

1. Pan H, O'Brien MJ, Wigglesworth K, *et al.* Transcript profiling during mouse oocyte development and the effect of gonadotropin priming and development in vitro. *Dev Biol* 2005; **286**: 493–506.
2. Wickramasinghe D, Albertini DF. Centrosome phosphorylation and the developmental expression of meiotic competence in mouse oocytes. *Dev Biol* 1992; **152**: 62–74.
3. Matzuk MM, Burns KH, Viveiros MM, *et al.* Intercellular communication in the mammalian ovary: oocytes carry the conversation. *Science* 2002; **296**: 2178–80.
4. De La Fuente R, Viveiros MM, Burns KH, *et al.* Major chromatin remodeling in the germinal vesicle (GV) of mammalian oocytes is dispensable for global transcriptional silencing but required for centromeric heterochromatin function. *Dev Biol* 2004; **275**: 447–58.
5. Inoue A, Nakajima R, Nagata M, *et al.* Contribution of the oocyte nucleus and cytoplasm to the determination of meiotic and developmental competence in mice. *Hum Reprod* 2008; **23**: 1377–84.
6. De La Fuente R, Viveiros MM, Wigglesworth K, *et al.* ATRX, a member of the SNF2 family of helicase/ATPases, is required for chromosome alignment and meiotic spindle organization in metaphase II stage mouse oocytes. *Dev Biol* 2004; **272**: 1–14.
7. Andreu-Vieyra CV, Chen R, Agno JE, *et al.* MLL2 is required in oocytes for bulk histone 3 lysine 4 trimethylation and transcriptional silencing. *PLoS Biol* 2010; **8**: pii: e100453.
8. Norris RP, Ratzan WJ, Freudzon M, *et al.* Cyclic GMP from the surrounding somatic cells regulates cyclic AMP and meiosis in the mouse oocyte. *Development* 2009; **136**: 1869–78.
9. Vaccari S, Weeks JL, 2nd, Hsieh M, *et al.* Cyclic GMP signaling is involved in the luteinizing hormone-dependent meiotic maturation of mouse oocytes. *Biol Reprod* 2009; **81**: 595–604.
10. Zhang M, Su YQ, Sugiura K, *et al.* Granulosa cell ligand NPPC and its receptor NPR2 maintain meiotic arrest in mouse oocytes. *Science* 2010; **330**: 366–9.
11. Kawahara M, Wu Q, Takahashi N, *et al.* High-frequency generation of viable mice from engineered bi-maternal embryos. *Nat Biotechnol* 2007; **25**: 1045–50.
12. Obata Y, Hiura H, Fukuda A, *et al.* Epigenetically immature oocytes lead to loss of imprinting during embryogenesis. *J Reprod Dev* 2011; **57**: 327–34.
13. Lucifero D, Mann MR, Bartolomei MS, *et al.* Gene-specific timing and epigenetic memory in oocyte imprinting. *Hum Mol Genet* 2004; **13**: 839–49.
14. Lee YS, Latham KE, Vandevoort CA. Effects of in vitro maturation on gene expression in rhesus monkey oocytes. *Physiol Genomics* 2008; **35**: 145–58.
15. Tafuri SR, Wolffe AP. *Xenopus* Y-box transcription factors: molecular cloning, functional analysis and developmental regulation. *Proc Natl Acad Sci USA* 1990; **87**: 9028–32.
16. Matsumoto K, Tanaka KJ, Aoki K, *et al.* Visualization of the reconstituted FRGY2-mRNA complexes by electron microscopy. *Biochem Biophys Res Commun* 2003; **306**: 53–8.
17. Skabkin MA, Kiselyova OI, Chernov KG, *et al.* Structural organization of mRNA complexes with

major core mRNP protein YB-1. *Nucleic Acids Res* 2004; **32**: 5621–35.

18. Parker R, Sheth U. P bodies and the control of mRNA translation and degradation. *Mol Cell* 2007; **25**: 635–46.
19. Eulalio A, Behm-Ansmant I, Izaurralde E. P bodies: at the crossroads of post-transcriptional pathways. *Nat Rev Mol Cell Biol* 2007; **8**: 9–22.
20. Richter JD, Sonenberg N. Regulation of cap-dependent translation by eIF4E inhibitory proteins. *Nature* 2005; **433**: 477–80.
21. Buchet-Poyau K, Courchet J, Le Hir H, *et al.* Identification and characterization of human Mex-3 proteins, a novel family of evolutionarily conserved RNA-binding proteins differentially localized to processing bodies. *Nucleic Acids Res* 2007; **35**: 1289–300.
22. Flemr M, Ma J, Schultz RM, *et al.* P-body loss is concomitant with formation of a messenger RNA storage domain in mouse oocytes. *Biol Reprod* 2010; **82**: 1008–17.
23. Swetloff A, Conne B, Huarte J, *et al.* Dcp1-bodies in mouse oocytes. *Mol Biol Cell* 2009; **20**: 4951–61.
24. Yu J, Hecht NB, Schultz RM. Expression of MSY2 in mouse oocytes and preimplantation embryos. *Biol Reprod* 2001; **65**: 1260–70.
25. Li L, Baibakov B, Dean J. A subcortical maternal complex essential for preimplantation mouse embryogenesis. *Dev Cell* 2008; **15**: 416–25.
26. Yurttas P, Vitale AM, Fitzhenry RJ, *et al.* Role for PADI6 and the cytoplasmic lattices in ribosomal storage in oocytes and translational control in the early mouse embryo. *Development* 2008; **135**: 2627–36.
27. Medvedev S, Pan H, Schultz RM. Absence of MSY2 in mouse oocytes perturbs oocyte growth and maturation, RNA stability, and the transcriptome. *Biol Reprod* 2011; **85**: 575–83.
28. Richter JD. CPEB: a life in translation. *Trends Biochem Sci* 2007; **32**: 279–85.
29. Potireddy S, Vassena R, Patel BG, *et al.* Analysis of polysomal mRNA populations of mouse oocytes and zygotes: dynamic changes in maternal mRNA utilization and function. *Dev Biol* 2006; **298**: 155–66.
30. Potireddy S, Midic U, Liang CG, *et al.* Positive and negative cis-regulatory elements directing postfertilization maternal mRNA translational control in mouse embryos. *Am J Physiol Cell Physiol* 2010; **299**: C818–27.
31. Barnard DC, Cao Q, Richter JD. Differential phosphorylation controls Maskin association with eukaryotic translation initiation factor 4E and localization on the mitotic apparatus. *Mol Cell Biol* 2005; **25**: 7605–15.
32. Dostie J, Ferraiuolo M, Pause A, *et al.* A novel shuttling protein, 4E-T, mediates the nuclear import o the mRNA 5′ cap-binding protein, eIF4E. *EMBO J* 2000; **19**: 3142–56.
33. Cooke A, Prigge A, Wickens M. Translational repression by deadenylases. *J Biol Chem* 2010; **285**: 28506–13.
34. Luo X, Nerlick S, An W, *et al.* *Xenopus* germline nanos1 is translationally repressed by a novel structure-based mechanism. *Development* 2011; **138**: 589–98.
35. Braat AK, Yan N, Arn E, *et al.* Localization-dependent oskar protein accumulation; control after the initiatior of translation. *Dev Cell* 2004; **7**: 125–31.
36. Pigott CR, Mikolajek H, Moore CE, *et al.* Insights into the regulation of eukaryotic elongation factor 2 kinase and the interplay between its domains. *Biochem J* 2012 **442**: 105–18.
37. de Moor CH, Richter JD. The Mos pathway regulates cytoplasmic polyadenylation in *Xenopus* oocytes. *Mol Cell Biol* 1997; **17**: 6419–26.
38. Mendez R, Barnard D, Richter JD. Differential mRNA translation and meiotic progression require Cdc2-mediated CPEB destruction. *EMBO J* 2002; **21**: 1833–44.
39. Pique M, Lopez JM, Foissac S, *et al.* A combinatorial code for CPE-mediated translational control. *Cell* 2008; **132**: 434–48.
40. Nakahata S, Kotani T, Mita K, *et al.* Involvement of *Xenopus* Pumilio in the translational regulation that is specific to cyclin B1 mRNA during oocyte maturation. *Mech Dev* 2003; **120**: 865–80.
41. Richter JD. Breaking the code of polyadenylation-induced translation. *Cell* 2008; **132**: 335–7.
42. MacNicol MC, Cragle CE, MacNicol AM. Context-dependent regulation of Musashi-mediated mRNA translation and cell cycle regulation. *Cell Cycle* 2011; **10**: 39–44.
43. Tay J, Richter JD. Germ cell differentiation and synaptonemal complex formation are disrupted in CPEB knockout mice. *Dev Cell* 2001; **1**: 201–13.
44. Peset I, Vernos I. The TACC proteins: TACC-ling microtubule dynamics and centrosome function. *Trends Cell Biol* 2008; **18**: 379–88.
45. Nelson MR, Leidal AM, Smibert CA. *Drosophila* Cup is an eIF4E-binding protein that functions in Smaug-mediated translational repression. *EMBO J* 2004; **23**: 150–9.
46. Jeske M, Meyer S, Temme C, *et al.* Rapid ATP-dependent deadenylation of nanos mRNA in a cell-free system from *Drosophila* embryos. *J Biol Chem* 2006; **281**: 25124–33.

7. Baez MV, Boccaccio GL. Mammalian Smaug is a translational repressor that forms cytoplasmic foci similar to stress granules. *J Biol Chem* 2005; **280**: 43131–40.

8. Simon R, Richter JD. Further analysis of cytoplasmic polyadenylation in *Xenopus* embryos and identification of embryonic cytoplasmic polyadenylation element-binding proteins. *Mol Cell Biol* 1994; **14**: 7867–75.

9. Oh B, Hwang S, McLaughlin J, *et al.* Timely translation during the mouse oocyte-to-embryo transition. *Development* 2000; **127**: 3795–803.

0. Varnum SM, Wormington WM. Deadenylation of maternal mRNAs during *Xenopus* oocyte maturation does not require specific cis-sequences: a default mechanism for translational control. *Genes Dev* 1990; **4**: 2278–86.

1. Tadros W, Goldman AL, Babak T, *et al.* SMAUG is a major regulator of maternal mRNA destabilization in *Drosophila* and its translation is activated by the PAN GU kinase. *Dev Cell* 2007; **12**: 143–55.

2. Su YQ, Sugiura K, Woo Y, *et al.* Selective degradation of transcripts during meiotic maturation of mouse oocytes. *Dev Biol* 2007; **302**: 104–17.

3. Wells D, Patrizio P. Gene expression profiling of human oocytes at different maturational stages and after in vitro maturation. *Am J Obstet Gynecol* 2008; **198**: 455.e1–9; discussion 55.e9–11.

4. Hu W, Sweet TJ, Chamnongpol S, *et al.* Co-translational mRNA decay in *Saccharomyces cerevisiae*. *Nature* 2009; **461**: 225–9.

55. Rouget C, Papin C, Boureux A, *et al.* Maternal mRNA deadenylation and decay by the piRNA pathway in the early *Drosophila* embryo. *Nature* 2010; **467**: 1128–32.

56. Giraldez AJ, Mishima Y, Rihel J, *et al.* Zebrafish MiR-430 promotes deadenylation and clearance of maternal mRNAs. *Science* 2006; **312**: 75–9.

57. Lund E, Sheets MD, Imboden SB, *et al.* Limiting Ago protein restricts RNAi and microRNA biogenesis during early development in *Xenopus laevis*. *Genes Dev* 2011; **25**: 1121–31.

58. Chen J, Melton C, Suh N, *et al.* Genome-wide analysis of translation reveals a critical role for deleted in azoospermia-like (Dazl) at the oocyte-to-zygote transition. *Genes Dev* 2011; **25**: 755–66.

59. Svoboda P. Why mouse oocytes and early embryos ignore miRNAs? *RNA Biol* 2010; **7**: 559–63.

60. Ohnishi Y, Totoki Y, Toyoda A, *et al.* Small RNA class transition from siRNA/piRNA to miRNA during pre-implantation mouse development. *Nucleic Acids Res* 2010; **38**: 5141–51.

61. Vassena R, Han Z, Gao S, *et al.* Tough beginnings: alterations in the transcriptome of cloned embryos during the first two cell cycles. *Dev Biol* 2007; **304**: 75–89.

62. Jones GM, Cram DS, Song B, *et al.* Gene expression profiling of human oocytes following in vivo or in vitro maturation. *Hum Reprod* 2008; **23**: 1138–44.

Chapter 14

Setting the stage for fertilization: transcriptome and maternal factors

Boram Kim and Scott A. Coonrod

Introduction

Toward the end of oocyte growth, an oocyte matures so that it can be fertilized by a sperm and develop into an early embryo. Oocyte maturation encompasses two main interrelated developmental programs, nuclear maturation and cytoplasmic maturation [1]. Nuclear maturation involves the progression from prophase I of meiosis to metaphase II and can be visualized microscopically as germinal vesicle breakdown (GVBD), spindle formation, chromosomal condensation/segregation, and polar body extrusion. Cytoplasmic maturation prepares the oocyte for activation and early development and is characterized structurally by the dramatic redistribution of endoplasmic reticulum (ER) and mitochondria from a relatively diffuse localization in germinal vesicle (GV) stage oocytes to a much more polarized distribution pattern in mature eggs. The targeting of mitochondria around the spindle apparatus is thought to provide energy, in the form of ATP, to drive processes such as chromosome segregation, while the targeting of the ER to distinct cortical clusters underneath the microvillar cortex is believed to be required for the generation of repetitive Ca^{2+} transients that are necessary for activation of development [2, 3]. At the molecular level, cytoplasmic maturation involves the accumulation and processing of mRNA and proteins that are also required for successful activation and early development [4]. Microtubules (MTs) play a central role in orchestrating the events of nuclear maturation and are also thought to be important mediators of organelle redistribution during cytoplasmic maturation [5]. Once mature, the oocyte is then competent for fertilization. Sperm–egg interaction is a sequential process whereby sperm first passes through the cumulus cell extracellular matrix, binds to and penetrates the zona pellucida (ZP), and then binds to and fuses with the oocyte plasma membrane (oolemma) [6]. The molecular mechanisms behind each of these interactions are now coming to light, thus greatly increasing our understanding of the fertilization process in mammals. Due, in part, to the transcriptional arrest that occurs upon resumption of meiotic maturation and prior to activation of the embryonic genome (EGA), the embryo must rely on stores of maternal transcripts and proteins to provide the material necessary to make the oocyte-to-embryo transition (OET) [4]. These stored factors are encoded by maternal-effect genes (MEG), which can be defined as genes encoded by the maternal genome that are essential for early embryogenesis. In light of advanced genomic and proteomics technologies, and with assistance from studies in non-mammalian organisms, over the last 10 years or so, there has been considerable progress in the identification and functional analysis of the role of MEG in mammalian development [7]. This chapter will focus on reviewing several aspects of oocyte and early embryo biology during the OET including cytoplasmic maturation, the mechanisms of sperm–egg binding and fusion, and the role of stored maternal factors in mediating early development. Most of the insights into early development that will be highlighted here arose from studies using mouse models.

Cytoplasmic maturation

Cytoplasmic organelles

Cytoplasmic maturation is characterized at the organelle level, in part, by the dramatic coalescence of ER and mitochondria around the spindle apparatus and microvillar cortex, thus providing localized pools of calcium and ATP for subsequent activation and early development (Figure 14.1). (We note here that

Biology and Pathology of the Oocyte, 2nd edn., ed. Alan Trounson, Roger Gosden, and Ursula Eichenlaub-Ritter.

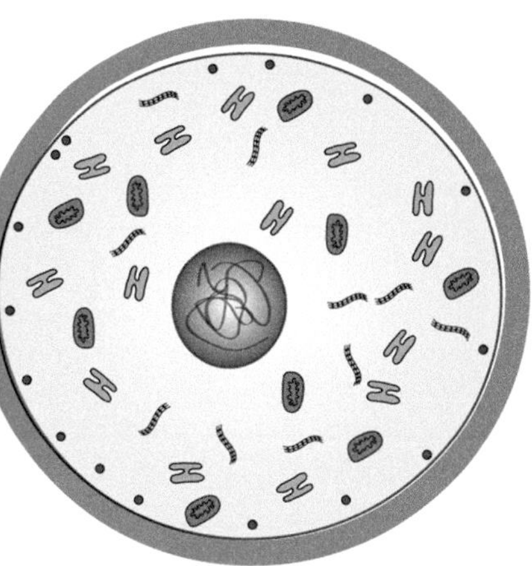

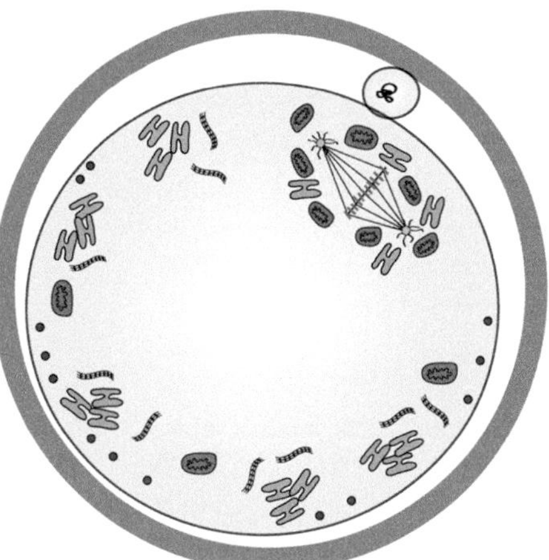

igure 14.1 Organelle redistribution during oocyte maturation. In the fully grown prophase I-arrested GV stage oocyte, the ER (blue) and nitochondria (orange) are diffusely distributed throughout the cytoplasm while cortical granules (red) localize to the subcortex. The GV ucleus is shown in gray and oocyte lattices are shown as black fibers. In the mature metaphase II-arrested oocyte, the ER is targeted to lusters opposite to that of the spindle apparatus while mitochondria are found to be clustered around the spindle, with some yperpolarized mitochondria being found at the subcortex. Microtubule organization centers (MTOCs) are shown in green.

s opposed to human oocytes where microvilli are nore evenly distributed, mouse oocytes contain a nicrovillus-free region which overlies the spindle pparatus.) Below, we will first discuss what is known bout mitochondrial, and then ER redistribution luring maturation. We will not discuss the redistri-ution of other organelles due, in part, to the fact hat very little is known about their dynamics at this levelopmental time point.

Mitochondria

Oocytes become uncoupled from cumulus cells ollowing ovulation and must sustain their own netabolism through the generation of ATP by nitochondria via oxidative phosphorylation [8]. Mitochondria are one of the most abundant organelles n oocytes and embryos must rely exclusively upon naternally inherited mitochondria until the peri-mplantation stage, at which point they begin to make heir own mitochondrial stores [9]. During matu-ation, mitochondria undergo a highly conserved, out poorly understood reorganization process; with nitiation of mitochondrial redistribution coinciding vith, and requiring, the resumption of meiosis. In he immature oocyte, mitochondria are more-or-less venly distributed throughout the cytoplasm and, as he oocyte begins to mature, they coalesce around he GV nucleus at GVBD and then become polarized around the spindle during the metaphase II (MII) stage [2, 10]. This redistribution event seems to be critical for the production of functional mitochondria and also for the oocyte to reach its full developmental potential. This prediction is based on findings from a range of species which show that a successful mito-chondrial redistribution in mature oocytes correlates with increased ATP activity and/or with a higher developmental potential [11–15]. Not too surprisingly perhaps, an oocyte's developmental potential is appar-ently not determined by its total amount of ATP, but instead it is determined by where these ATP pools localize within the oocyte. In other words, to meet the increasing local ATP demands, toward the end of oocyte maturation, subsets of mitochondria at the cortex are thought to become hyperpolarized ($\Delta\Psi_m$). Interestingly, localization of these high potential mitochondria at the subplasmalemma has been corre-lated with fertilization competency [16]. Importantly, mitochondria can be visualized in oocytes, using non-invasive light microscopy [14]; thus the non-polarized mitochondrial phenotype in poor quality oocytes may, one day, prove to be an invaluable tool for clinician embryologists to select embryos with high developmental potential for implantation. Regarding the mechanisms mediating maturation-induced mito-chondrial redistribution, a key driver of this process is thought to be the fraction of MTs that are not directly associated with the meiotic spindle apparatus

[5, 15, 17]. The methods by which mitochondria are trafficked along MTs in somatic cells are well documented and involve MT motors such as the ATPases, kinesin, and dynein [18, 19]. However, much work remains to be done before similar conclusions can be drawn in oocytes. In addition to MTs, microfilaments have also been found to play a role in mitochondrial transport in oocytes. Recently, for example, Yu *et al.* found that mitochondrial redistribution closely coincided with changes in mitochondrial ATP synthase activity during maturation. Surprisingly, while nocodazole-mediated MT depolymerization was found to inhibit the perinuclear accumulation of mitochondria during GVBD, this drug did not affect ATP production. However, cytochalasin B (which interferes with actin polymerization) both suppressed the formation of mitochondrial clusters and also suppressed ATP production [20]. These strong correlative findings suggest that microfilaments are important for the positioning of functional mitochondria in mature eggs and that mitochondrial clustering may be prompted by increasing energy demands at specific subcellular locations during oocyte maturation.

Endoplasmic reticulum

Mammalian development is initiated when a sperm delivers the oocyte-activating factor, phospholipase Cζ (PLCζ), into the egg cytoplasm at fertilization. PLCζ then cleaves phosphatidylinositol 4, 5-bisphosphate (PIP_2) to inositol trisphosphate (IP_3) and IP_3 binds to the IP_3R on the ER, which induces the opening of ER Ca^{2+} channels and subsequent release of Ca^{2+} into the cytosol. The resulting $[Ca^{2+}]_i$ oscillations are required for the activation of development, a process which includes: meiotic resumption, cortical granule exocytosis, and the initiation of embryonic development [21]. Prior to fertilization, the capacity for IP_3-induced Ca^{2+} release increases throughout oocyte maturation, with oocytes finally acquiring the ability to initiate fertilization-like oscillations late in maturation [22]. This up-regulation of the Ca^{2+}-releasing machinery likely depends upon a number of factors including changes in Ca^{2+} stores, changes in Ca^{2+} homeostasis, IP_3R functionality, and/or the distribution of ER [23]. Regarding the last point, the dramatic redistribution of ER during maturation is seen in a range of vertebrate species and the close correlation between ER positioning and functional $[Ca^{2+}]_i$ oscillations is well documented [24]. For example, a spatiotemporal correlation was found between the release of Ca^{2+} and the appearance of IP_3R-rich ER clusters at the cortex in mature MII stage oocytes [3, 25]. These clusters form at the vegetal cortex, which is the initiating site for $[Ca^{2+}]_i$ oscillations. Thus, the appearance of ER clusters at this site is likely the cause of increased IP_3 sensitivity [26]. As with mitochondria, MTs and microfilaments appear to be responsible for ER redistribution during maturation. Additionally, similar to mitochondria, the ER undergoes two major rearrangements during maturation, with the ER first congregating around the nucleus prior to GVBD followed by the targeting of ER to the microvillar cortex in the mature egg. Based on inhibitor studies, the targeting of ER to the perinuclear region at GVBD appears to require MTs and the MT motor, dynein, while targeting of ER to the cortex in the mature egg appears to be mediated primarily by microfilaments [27].

ER and mitochondrial clustering

Electron microscopic and confocal analysis of oocytes finds that mitochondria appear to undergo an ordered clustering during maturation and also come into close proximity with ER during this time [9]. In somatic cells, a number of studies have found that close physical interactions between ER and mitochondria facilitate organelle crosstalk via coordinated signaling events. For example, mitochondrial-derived ATP was found to activate ER membrane Ca^{2+} pumps, which in turn, propagated Ca^{2+} signals to mitochondria, thus altering their metabolic rate. Additionally, mitochondria can act as a Ca^{2+} buffer by regulating both local Ca^{2+} concentrations and the rate of Ca^{2+} signaling events [28]. Based on these (and other) observations, it seems likely that a functional interplay exists between ER and mitochondria in oocytes and that this relationship modulates both Ca^{2+} homeostasis and ATP supply [29, 30]. Additionally, the coordinated crosstalk between these two organelles in oocytes may prove to be the key determinate of successful developmental outcomes in early embryos [31].

Molecular inventory

Fate of transcripts

In light of our extended discussion on organelle redistribution during maturation above, here we will discuss the molecular aspects of cytoplasmic maturation. During their extended growth phase, mouse oocytes increase in size from ~20 to ~80 μm, and, during this time, RNA is synthesized and stored at relatively high rates [32]. Toward the end of oocyte growth, the rate of transcript synthesis slows and mRNA degradation then commences upon oocyte maturation. Degradation of the majority of mRNAs is accomplished during maturation and is almost complete in 2-cell embryos [33]. The fate of mRNA is often correlated with the length of the transcript's poly(A) tail, with some polyadenylated mRNAs being immediately translated into proteins, which may then be stored for later use by the oocyte during or following maturation and fertilization. Interestingly, it appears that a good many mammalian MEG products fall into this category. For example, proteins encoded by most of the MEG discussed below are actually first expressed during the early stages of oocyte growth. Additionally, proteomic studies have found that the mass and isoelectric point of a number of maternal proteins are altered at this time, suggesting that some of these stored proteins are activated during meiotic maturation by post-translational modifications such as phosphorylation [34]. Transcripts that are not immediately translated are often deadenylated and subsequently either are degraded during maturation or are masked from degradation and then stored in ribonucleoprotein particles. These dormant transcripts can then be readenylated and recruited for translation at later time points [35]. Regulation of these activities is mediated, in part, by the transcript's 5′ and 3′ untranslated regions, which can associate with different regulatory factors such as cytoplasmic polyadenylation element-binding protein (CPEB) [36]. Additionally, a role for small non-coding RNAs in regulating this activity is now coming to light with, for example, siRNAs being found to modulate maternal mRNA degradation [37].

Role of PADI6/cytoplasmic lattices in organelle redistribution

While the redistribution of organelles during oocyte maturation has been reported in diverse arrays of species, the mechanisms by which the cytoskeleton mediates this dynamic event remain poorly defined. As noted, most studies in this area treat oocytes with drugs (such as taxol or cytochalasin B) that alter MT or microfilament dynamics and then observe the effects of these drugs on organelle distribution [20, 27]. Few studies have actually directly observed the proximate relationship between organelles and the cytoskeleton during maturation, nor have many studies investigated the molecular mechanisms involved in tethering organelles to MTs or microfilaments. Given that the dynamic redistribution of organelles during oocyte maturation is occurring within an exceedingly large volume (relative to somatic cells), it stands to reason that the oocyte and early embryo may have evolved a specific structure to help facilitate organelle positioning and distribution. Recent studies suggest that the oocyte cytoplasmic lattices may represent just such a structure. The cytoplasmic lattices (also called cytoskeletal sheets, plaques, lamellae, and fibrillar arrays) are absent from non-growing oocytes but increase in number dramatically throughout oocyte growth, eventually becoming a dominant feature of the fully grown mouse oocyte [38]. Electron microscopic analysis of the oocyte lattices finds that these structures are composed of five to seven ~20 nm filaments lying side by side with the filaments appearing to be held in place by cross-bridges spaced every 23–25 nm [39]. Regarding the molecular composition of the lattices, previous studies suggested that the lattices represented a storage site for yolk, ribosomes, or possibly intermediate filaments [40–42]. More recently, immunoelectron microscopy analysis found that peptidylarginine deiminase 6 (PADI6), a highly abundant oocyte and embryo-restricted maternal protein, localizes to the lattices [43]. Regarding expression, PADI6 protein is observed in the oocyte cytoplasm as soon as oocytes enter their growth phase and the protein persists in embryos up to the blastocyst stage of development, which is similar to that of the lattices. Analysis of *Padi6*-null oocytes found that lattices are not observed in mutant oocytes at any point in oocyte growth or in early embryos, suggesting that PADI6 is a component of the lattice complex and that in the absence of PADI6, the lattices do not form [44]. In addition to PADI6, two other maternal factors, MATER and FLOPED, have also been found to localize to, and be required for, lattice formation [45, 46]. MATER is a member of the NLRP gene family and contains five tandem hydrophilic repeats at its N-terminus, a NACHT-NTPase domain within its core region, and a leucine-rich repeat (LRR) domain at its C-terminus [47]. The functional significance of these domains within MATER has yet to be explored. FLOPED encodes an atypical KH-domain RNA-binding domain [48]. The expression patterns for both MATER and FLOPED in oocytes and early embryos are similar to PADI6 [43, 49, 50]. Regarding a role for the lattices in early development, a recent study has found that α-tubulin interacts with PADI6 at the oocyte lattices and that tubulin solubility is greatly increased in *PADI6*-null oocytes [17]. These and other findings raise the possibility that the lattices may play a direct role in MT-mediated organelle distribution during oocyte maturation. This prediction was supported by the observation that both mitochondria and ER fail to undergo maturation-induced redistribution in *PADI6*-null oocytes. Further, the diffuse organelle distribution pattern observed in mature *Padi6*-null oocytes was not affected by taxol-mediated MT hyperpolymerization, suggesting that loss of *Padi6* results in an uncoupling of organelles from MTs. Additionally, levels of acetylated tubulin, a marker for stable MTs, were strongly suppressed in *Padi6*-null oocytes, suggesting that the lattices either contain, or are associated with, stable MTs [17]. Interestingly, a recent publication examined whether mitochondrial distribution or function was altered in mutant *Mater* oocytes during maturation. Indeed, mitochondria were found to be distributed in a non-polarized fashion and mitochondrial activity was also disrupted in mutant metaphase II-arrested oocytes [51]. Taken together, these findings raise the possibility that the lattices represent a novel form of stable MTs that have evolved within the oocyte cytoplasm to facilitate organelle positioning and redistribution in oocytes and possibly early embryos.

Fertilization: the role of egg proteins in sperm–egg binding and fusion

Mammalian fertilization occurs in a stepwise fashion and initiates when sperm come into contact with, and then penetrate, the oocyte's vestments; the cumulus mass and the ZP. Sperm then enter the perivitelline space and the sperm's plasma membrane then binds to, and fuses with, the microvillar region of the oocyte's plasma membrane. Following fusion, in addition to releasing PLCζ, sperm also release their highly condensed paternal genome into the oocyte cytoplasm whereby the sperm chromatin deconsenses and the male and female pronuclei form. These nuclei then fuse and the two parental genomes unite, thus completing the fertilization process.

Interaction of sperm with the egg vestment

The cumulus–oocyte complex (COC) consists of the ZP-encased oocyte and the surrounding layers of cumulus oophorus cells. Cumulus cells secrete a robust extracelluar matrix and it is this matrix that sperm must first traverse to reach the ZP. While cumulus-free oocytes can be fertilized in vitro, a number of genetic studies have found that deletion of genes that are involved in stabilizing the cumulus cell matrix, such as *Ambp*, *Tnfip6*, and *Ptx3*, can affect COC integrity and also suppresses female fertility [52]. Therefore, the passage of sperm through the cumulus matrix appears to facilitate the fertilization process in vivo. While the precise role that cumulus cells play in fertilization remains unclear, several reports suggest that the cumulus matrix may promote the acrosome reaction [52]. Following penetration of the cumulus cell matrix sperm then interact with, and pass through, the ZP. In mice, the ZP is composed of three glycosylated proteins, ZP1, ZP2, and ZP3, while human oocytes contain a fourth zona protein, ZP4. Numerous older reports indicated that *O*-glycan carbohydrate moieties on ZP3 appear to function as the primary sperm receptor and also to induce the acrosome reaction [53]. These models also suggested that, following the acrosome reaction, the exposed inner acrosomal membrane of sperm then binds to ZP2 in a secondary reaction that allows for the penetration of sperm through the ZP [54]. This long-standing model may now have to be significantly revised as more recent genetic ablation studies in mice suggest that ZP3 is not the primary sperm receptor, but instead the receptor appears likely to be ZP2 [55]. This finding could potentially simplify the mechanism of sperm penetration through the zona, with the new model suggesting that sperm–zona binding and penetration are mediated by interactions between sperm and the N-terminus of ZP2 throughout the zona matrix. Additionally, the model posits that, following fertilization, cortical granules exocytose their contents into the perivitelline space and these enzymes then cleave ZP2, thus destroying the zona's sperm receptor, thereby preventing polyspermy. Recently one of the proteolytic factors responsible for ZP2 cleavage has been identified as ovastacin (*Astl*), an oocyte-specific metalloendoprotease [56].

Sperm–oolemma interaction

SAS1B

Having penetrated the ZP, the acrosome reacted sperm enters the perivitelline space and then binds to, and fuses with, the oolemma at the microvillar region of the plasma membrane. A number of earlier studies uggested that the initial binding events may be medi-ted by interactions between integrins on the oolem-nal surface and their cognate ligands, the ADAMs (A)isintegrin And Metalloprotease domain), on sperm. Iowever, analysis of knockout oocytes which lacked he various integrin subunits thought to mediate gamete binding found that these molecules do not ppear to play a role in this process [57]. Recently, a perm-specific acrosomal membrane protein, SLLP1, vas found to bind specifically to the oocyte plasma nembrane and its binding partner on the oolemma vas then identified through a panning screen as the ocyte microvillar membrane-restricted metallopro-einase, SAS1B (sperm acrosomal SLLP1 binding) [58, 9]. In vitro studies then found that SLLP1 and SAS1B lirectly interact and that anti-SAS1B antibodies block ertilization. Lastly, analysis of *Sas1b*-null mice found hat these females were subfertile. These new stud-es provide the first defined pair of molecules (i.e., perm membrane SLLP1 and oolemmal SAS1B) that ppear to specifically mediate sperm–oolemmal bind-ng, but do not appear to play a role in subsequent usion events.

etraspanins

n addition to SAS1B, tetraspanins and glycosyl-hosphatidylinositol-anchored proteins (GPI-AP) on he oolemma have also been found to play impor-ant roles in sperm–egg binding and fusion (Figure 4.2). Tetraspanins are known to function as "molec-ılar facilitators" by bringing together and stabiliz-ng molecular complexes called tetraspanin webs, vhich form between tetraspanins and other trans-nembrane proteins and also associate with signal-ng pathways and cytoskeletal elements [60]. The irst clues that tetraspanins may play an impor-ant role in sperm–oocyte membrane binding and usion came from a study in the late 1990s that ound a function blocking antibody to the tetraspanin CD9 strongly suppressed sperm–oocyte binding and usion in a dose-dependent manner [61]. A number of subsequent studies in *Cd9*-null mice found that, lespite its nearly ubiquitous expression pattern, the nly discernible phenotype in mutant mice was that emale mice were severely subfertile and that, while perm could bind to *Cd9*-null oocytes, fusion was ılmost completely blocked [62–64]. Results from these nutant mouse studies suggested that CD9 is primarily nvolved in membrane fusion; however, more recent tudies have found that CD9 may also play a role in sperm–oocyte binding, thus supporting the initial anti-CD9 function-blocking antibody study [65]. In addition to CD9, genetic and molecular analysis of another tetraspanin, CD81, have found that this protein also appears to play an important role in sperm–egg interaction; however, the defects observed in *Cd81* mutant oocytes are less severe [66]. It is possible that these tetraspanins are directly involved in mediating sperm–oocyte interaction by, for example, functioning as a receptor for a sperm ligand. However, complementary sperm ligands for CD9 have not yet been identified.

The potential mechanism by which CD9 regulates sperm–egg interaction

While CD9's putative sperm ligand remains unknown, the best candidate ligand for mediating sperm–oolemmal interaction on the sperm side is the sperm-specific protein IZUMO1. Analysis of *Izumo1* mutant mice finds that males are infertile and that while *Izumo1*-null sperm can penetrate the ZP, they cannot bind or fuse with the oocyte plasma membrane [57]. In an ideal world, CD9 would be found to be the receptor for IZUMO1; however, an interaction between these two proteins has not been demonstrated and the receptor for IZUMO1 remains to be determined. An alternate indirect mechanism by which CD9 could facilitate sperm–oolemma interaction is by regulating the structural landscape of the oolemma in *cis*. For example, CD9 may interact with other molecules in the oocyte plasma membrane to form tetraspanin-enriched microdomains that are required for sperm–egg interaction. In support of this prediction, previous studies found that preincubation of eggs, but not sperm, with the large extracellular loop of CD9, which tetraspanin-associated proteins normally bind, hampered gamete fusion [67]. Another indirect mechanism by which CD9 may regulate sperm–egg interaction is by mediating the microvillar architecture. A recent electron microscopy study found that CD9 localizes to oocyte microvilli and that the microvillar morphology of *Cd9*-deficient oocytes is altered in length, density, and thickness [68]. Lastly, other studies have found that oocytes appear to release CD9-containing exosomes that can bind to sperm and thus facilitate sperm–egg fusion by allowing for direct interactions between sperm-localized CD9 and oocyte-localized CD9 [69].

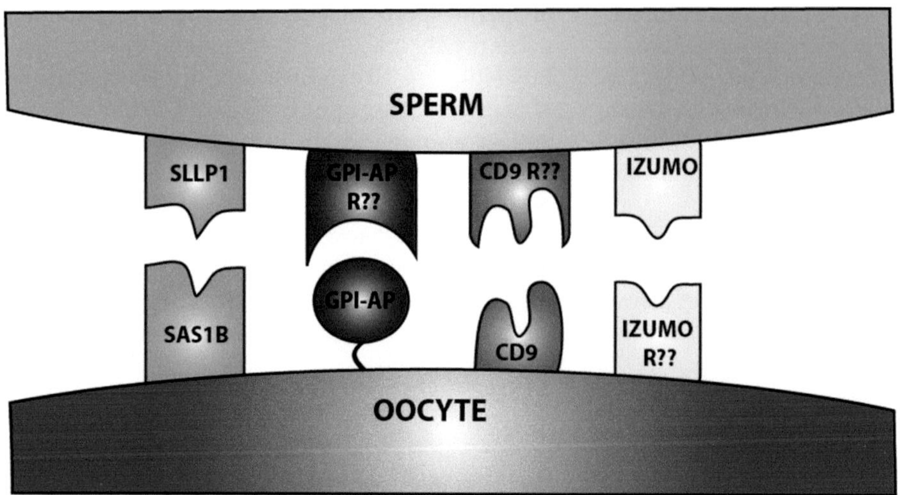

Figure 14.2 Molecular "players" involved in sperm–oocyte binding and fusion. Sperm SLLP1 has recently been shown to interact directly with oocyte-restricted SAS1B, thus defining the first pair of molecules known to mediate sperm–oolemma binding. On the sperm side, IZUMO has been shown to be required for sperm–oocyte binding and fusion; however, its cognate receptor on the oolemma is not known. On the oocyte side, GPI-anchored proteins (GPI-AP) and CD9 have been found to be required for sperm–oocyte binding and fusion; however, their putative cognate receptors on sperm have not been identified.

Glycosyl-phosphatidylinositol-anchored proteins

GPI-APs on the oolemma have also been found to be required for sperm–egg binding and fusion. A role for GPI-APs in sperm–egg interaction was identified when investigators found that treatment of mouse oocytes with phosphatidylinositol-specific phospholipase C (PI-PLC), an enzyme that cleaves the lipid tether in GPI-APs, significantly diminished the ability of the egg to bind to, and fuse with, sperm. This effect appeared to be limited to oocytes as PI-PLC-treated sperm could fertilize oocytes at a normal rate [70]. This study was supported by another report which asked a similar question using a mouse genetic model system. These investigators generated an oocyte-specific knockout mouse lacking the *Pig-a* (phosphatidylinositol glycan class-A) gene, which encodes the enzyme that catalyzes the first steps of GPI-AP biosynthesis. Results showed that oocytes which lacked the *Pig-a* gene matured normally, yet possessed a significantly reduced ability to fuse with sperm [71]. To date, the molecular identity of the GPI-anchored protein mediating these events remains unknown.

Maternal-effect genes (MEG)

In the final section, we will briefly discuss a panel of maternal factors stored within the oocyte that facilitate the OET. These genes fit well within the category of MEG because, while their gene products are synthesized by the oocyte, these factors are essential for early development. In this summary, we will focus on germ cell-specific MEG, as it seems likely that factors that have evolved specifically to mediate effects in the egg and early embryo are likely to be fundamentally important for early development (Figure 14.3).

Chromatin remodeling

NPM2

Maternal and paternal chromatin undergoes remodeling upon fertilization to ensure proper formation of the diploid genome. Following entry into the oocyte cytoplasm, decondensation of paternal chromatin occurs over a 30-minute to 1-hour time period [72]. In *Xenopus*, this process is thought to be largely mediated by histone chaperones such as nucleoplasmin (NPM) and nucleosome assembly protein 1 (NAP1) [73, 74]. In mammals, NPM2 protein expression initiates in growing oocytes and persists until the blastocyst stage. NPM2 predominantly localizes to the nucleus of GV stage oocytes, is dispersed throughout the cytoplasm following GVBD, and then translocates back to the nucleus upon pronuclear formation; with nucleocytoplasmic shuttling potentially being mediated by phosphorylation [34]. *Npm2*-null females are subfertile, with ~60% of embryos arresting around

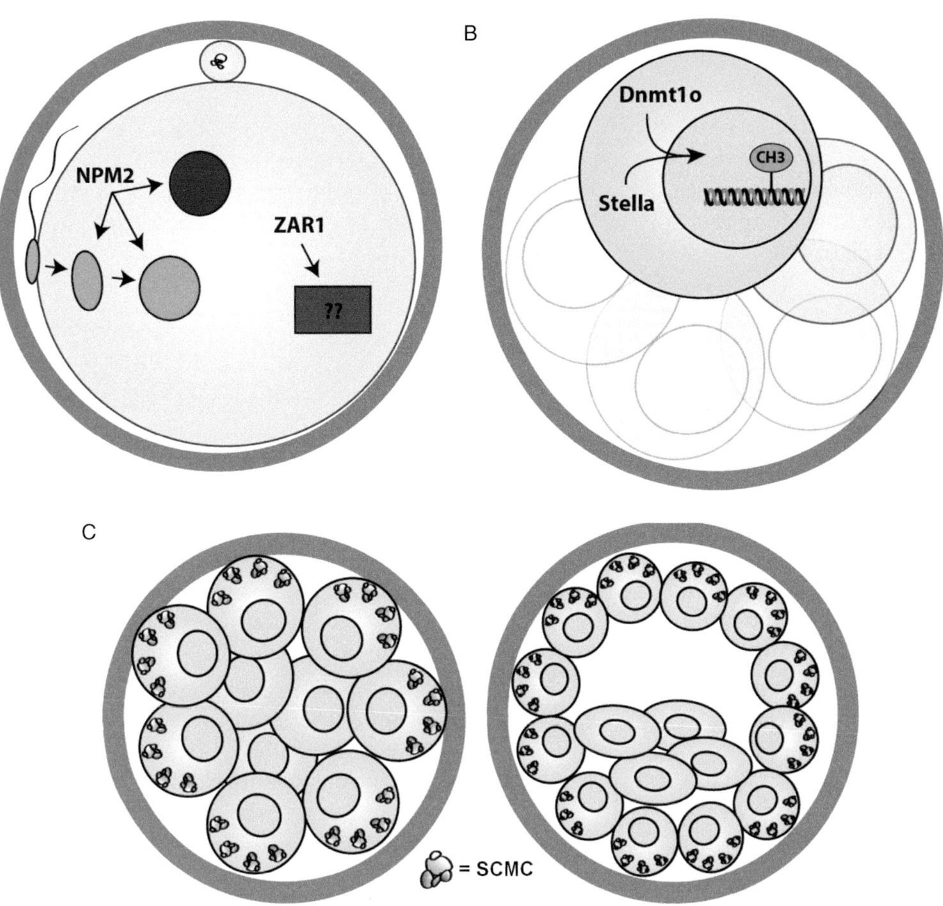

igure 14.3 Potential role for maternal-effect genes in early development. (A) Nucleoplasmin 2 (NPM2) is targeted to chromatin of econdensing sperm and to male and female pronuclei where, as a histone chaperone, it is believed to play a role in chromatin remodeling. AR1 is essential for female fertility; however, a role for this maternal factor has yet to be defined. (B) Dnmt1o and Stella are both believed to lay a role in the maintenance of DNA methylation at imprinted loci. (C) The subcortical maternal complex (SCMC) is thought to localize to ne non-apposed cytocortex of outer blastomeres and excluded from inner cells, thus potentially playing a role in cell fate determination in ne early embryo.

he 2-cell stage of development. In mammals, defects n decondensation of the sperm nucleus were not bserved in zygotes derived from *Npm2*-null females, hus NPM2 was originally thought not to play a role n sperm decondensation. However, a recent report ound that removal of the nucleolus-like body from GV stage oocytes slowed sperm decondensation and hat microinjection of NPM2 mRNA partially resued this defect [75]. A potential role for NPM2 in perm decondensation was further supported by the bservations that sperm decondensation was retarded n zygotes derived from *Npm2*-null females and that ecombinant NPM2 could induce sperm decondenation in vitro. In addition to sperm decondensaion defects, nuclear and nucleolar abnormalities were detected in null zygotes as were defects in histone deacetylation and heterochromatin formation, thus further supporting a role for NPM2 as a histone chaperone [76].

ZAR1

Zar1 (zygote arrest 1) is conserved across various vertebrate species, including zebrafish, frog, mice, and humans. In mice, ZAR1 protein expression initiates in growing oocytes and persists until the 2-cell stage of development. *Zar1*-deficient females are sterile, with embryonic arrest occurring either at the pronuclear stage (due to the zygote's inability to form a diploid genome) or at the 2-cell stage (due to a suppression of embryonic transcription) [77]. ZAR1 contains an atypical plant homeobox domain (PHD) that is found in many transcription factors, thus suggesting that this maternal protein may play a role in gene regulation [78]. Additionally, ZAR1 was recently found to interact with its homolog ZAR1-like, which colocalizes with mRNA processing factors, suggesting that ZAR1 may also regulate RNA metabolism [79].

DNA methylation in preimplantation embryos

DNMT1o

Following fertilization, a small subset of imprinted paternal and maternal genes are spared from global DNA demethylation during remodeling of the genome in order to preserve parent-specific gene expression patterns in the resulting embryo [80]. An oocyte-specific DNA methyltransferase, DNMT1o, has been identified and is now believed to play a critical role in maintenance of these methyl marks. *Dnmt1o*-null females are almost entirely infertile, with most conceptuses dying between embryonic day (E)14 and E21. Offspring of *Dnmt1o*-deficient females exhibit apparently normal global methylation, but display a suppression of methylation at ~50% of allele specific imprints [81]. Based on the observation that DNMT1o is targeted to the nucleus of 8-cell-stage embryos, this methyltransferase is thought to maintain methylation at imprints at that 8-cell stage. Interestingly, Hirasawa *et al.* generated conditional knockouts for both *Dnmt1o* and *Dnmt1s* genes and found that the resulting embryos showed a complete loss of methylation at imprinted loci, indicating that, in addition to DNMT1o, DNMT1s also appears to play an important role in maintenance of imprints during preimplantation development [82].

STELLA

Stella (*Dppa3*) is expressed in primordial germ cells, oocytes, cleavage stage embryos, and pluripotent cells. Analysis of *Stella*-null female mice found that while oogenesis, ovulation, and fertilization appeared normal, these animals were markedly subfertile, due to a developmental arrest in preimplantation stage embryos [83, 84]. *Stella* encodes a protein with a DNA-binding SAP motif and a splicing factor domain, thus suggesting this factor plays a role in embryonic gene transcription and/or mRNA processing. Functional studies indicated that, in collaboration with RanBP5, Stella also appears to protect several loci (including imprinted genes) from demethylation, thus implicating *Stella* in the maintenance of DNA methylation patterns following fertilization [85]. *Stella* has also been implicated in germline specification; however, defects of this nature were not observed in mutant *Stella* mice [83].

Subcortical maternal complex

In addition to PADI6 and MATER's role in lattice formation and maturation-induced organelle redistribution in oocytes, analysis of mutant mice finds these two maternal factors are also essential for progression of development beyond the 2-cell stage [44, 86]. Likewise, FLOPED (which is required for lattice formation) is also essential for early development [50]. Interestingly, MATER and FLOPED were previously identified as members of a high-molecular-weight complex, named the subcortical maternal complex (SCMC). This complex was also found to contain two other maternal genes encoding the proteins FILIA and TLE6 and was also predicted to contain PADI6 [50]. The precise relationship between the lattices and the SCMC is currently being investigated as is the role of the lattices and the SCMC in pre- and post-fertilization events. Interestingly, in morula stage embryos, members of the SCMC have been found to localize to the non-opposed cytocortex of outer blastomeres while apparently being excluded from the inner cells. This restricted localization pattern has led to the hypothesis that the SCMC may provide a molecular marker of embryonic cell lineages and possibly play a role in cell fate decisions during early development [48, 50].

Conclusions and future directions

This chapter has focused on reviewing recent advances in oocyte maturation and fertilization and has also discussed the role that stored maternal factors play in mediating the oocyte-to-embryo transition. Over the last decade, the use of mouse genetic models and "omic" technologies such as transcriptomics and proteomics have greatly increased our understanding of how the oocyte sets the stage for early development. Perhaps one of the biggest black boxes that remains to be elucidated in this area is how these events are ied together and regulated. In particular, while the signaling pathways driving meiotic resumption and completion are fairly well fleshed out, the signaling mechanisms that mediate cytoplasmic maturation (structural and molecular) are almost completely unknown. A better understanding of these pathways will help us understand how the egg prepares for fertilization and activation of development. Likewise, while the mechanisms of sperm–oolemmal binding and fusion and oocyte activation are now being elucidated, it seems likely that a multitude of additional signaling pathways are activated following gamete fusion; thus further investigations into these events would likely be productive. For example, while CD9 is clearly a critical "player" in sperm–oolemmal binding and fusion, the observation that the tetraspanin web is often associated with actin filaments suggests that CD9 may have additional, yet to be defined, roles in signaling to the oocyte cytoskeleton. Lastly, the recent use of mouse genetic models to investigate the function of a number of oocyte-restricted/abundant gene products has led to the finding that many of these molecules are essential for female fertility via their role in post-fertilization events. Given that many, if not all, of these genes are conserved in humans, a better understanding of these factors and the complexes and structures that they form will undoubtedly aid in our understanding of the oocyte-to-embryo transition and also potentially shed light on the mechanisms underlying human fertility and infertility.

References

1. Eppig JJ. Coordination of nuclear and cytoplasmic oocyte maturation in eutherian mammals. *Reprod Fertil Dev* 1996; **8**(4): 485–9.
2. Van Blerkom J, Runner MN. Mitochondrial reorganization during resumption of arrested meiosis in the mouse oocyte. *Am J Anat* 1984; **171**(3): 335–55.
3. Kline D, Mehlmann L, Fox C, Terasaki M. The cortical endoplasmic reticulum (ER) of the mouse egg: localization of ER clusters in relation to the generation of repetitive calcium waves. *Dev Biol* 1999; **215**(2): 431–42.
4. Schultz RM. Regulation of zygotic gene activation in the mouse. *Bioessays* 1993; **15**(8): 531–8.
5. Van Blerkom J. Microtubule mediation of cytoplasmic and nuclear maturation during the early stages of resumed meiosis in cultured mouse oocytes. *Proc Natl Acad Sci USA* 1991; **88**(11): 5031–5.
6. Wassarman PM, Jovine L, Litscher ES. A profile of fertilization in mammals. *Nat Cell Biol* 2001; **3**(2): E59–64.
7. Li L, Zheng P, Dean J. Maternal control of early mouse development. *Development* 2010; **137**(6): 859–70.
8. Downs SM. The influence of glucose, cumulus cells, and metabolic coupling on ATP levels and meiotic control in the isolated mouse oocyte. *Dev Biol* 1995; **167**(2): 502–12.
9. Dumollard R, Duchen M, Sardet C. Calcium signals and mitochondria at fertilisation. *Semin Cell Dev Biol* 2006; **17**(2): 314–23.
10. Calarco PG. Polarization of mitochondria in the unfertilized mouse oocyte. *Dev Genet* 1995; **16**(1): 36–43.
11. Nagai S, Mabuchi T, Hirata S, *et al.* Correlation of abnormal mitochondrial distribution in mouse oocytes with reduced developmental competence. *Tohoku J Exp Med* 2006; **210**(2): 137–44.
12. Stojkovic M, Machado SA, Stojkovic P, *et al.* Mitochondrial distribution and adenosine triphosphate content of bovine oocytes before and after in vitro maturation: correlation with morphological criteria and developmental capacity after in vitro fertilization and culture. *Biol Reprod* 2001; **64**(3): 904–9.
13. Torner H, Brussow KP, Alm H, *et al.* Mitochondrial aggregation patterns and activity in porcine oocytes and apoptosis in surrounding cumulus cells depends on the stage of pre-ovulatory maturation. *Theriogenology* 2004; **61**(9): 1675–89.
14. Wilding M, Dale B, Marino M, *et al.* Mitochondrial aggregation patterns and activity in human oocytes and preimplantation embryos. *Hum Reprod* 2001; **16**(5): 909–17.
15. Brevini TA, Vassena R, Francisci C, Gandolfi F. Role of adenosine triphosphate, active mitochondria, and microtubules in the acquisition of developmental competence of parthenogenetically activated pig oocytes. *Biol Reprod* 2005; **72**(5): 1218–23.
16. Van Blerkom J, Davis P. Mitochondrial signaling and fertilization. *Mol Hum Reprod* 2007; **13**(11): 759–70.
17. Kan R, Yurttas P, Kim B, *et al.* Regulation of mouse oocyte microtubule and organelle dynamics by PADI6 and the cytoplasmic lattices. *Dev Biol* 2011; **350**(2): 311–22.
18. Hirokawa N, Noda Y, Okada Y. Kinesin and dynein superfamily proteins in organelle transport and cell division. *Curr Opin Cell Biol* 1998; **10**(1): 60–73.
19. Boldogh IR, Pon LA. Mitochondria on the move. *Trends Cell Biol* 2007; **17**(10): 502–10.

20. Yu Y, Dumollard R, Rossbach A, Lai FA, Swann K. Redistribution of mitochondria leads to bursts of ATP production during spontaneous mouse oocyte maturation. *J Cell Physiol* 2010; **224**(3): 672–80.

21. Lee B, Yoon SY, Fissore RA. Regulation of fertilization-initiated $[Ca^{2+}]i$ oscillations in mammalian eggs: a multi-pronged approach. *Semin Cell Dev Biol* 2006; **17**(2): 274–84.

22. Mehlmann LM, Kline D. Regulation of intracellular calcium in the mouse egg: calcium release in response to sperm or inositol trisphosphate is enhanced after meiotic maturation. *Biol Reprod* 1994; **51**(6): 1088–98.

23. Ajduk A, Malagocki A, Maleszewski M. Cytoplasmic maturation of mammalian oocytes: development of a mechanism responsible for sperm-induced Ca^{2+} oscillations. *Reprod Biol* 2008; **8**(1): 3–22.

24. Kline D. Attributes and dynamics of the endoplasmic reticulum in mammalian eggs. *Curr Top Dev Biol* 2000; **50**: 125–54.

25. FitzHarris G, Marangos P, Carroll J. Cell cycle-dependent regulation of structure of endoplasmic reticulum and inositol 1,4,5-trisphosphate-induced Ca^{2+} release in mouse oocytes and embryos. *Mol Biol Cell* 2003; **14**(1): 288–301.

26. Dumollard R, Carroll J, Dupont G, Sardet C. Calcium wave pacemakers in eggs. *J Cell Sci* 2002; **115**(Pt 18): 3557–64.

27. FitzHarris G, Marangos P, Carroll J. Changes in endoplasmic reticulum structure during mouse oocyte maturation are controlled by the cytoskeleton and cytoplasmic dynein. *Dev Biol* 2007; **305**(1): 133–44.

28. Duchen MR. Mitochondria and calcium: from cell signalling to cell death. *J Physiol* 2000; **529** Pt 1: 57–68.

29. Dumollard R, Marangos P, Fitzharris G, *et al.* Sperm-triggered $[Ca^{2+}]$ oscillations and Ca^{2+} homeostasis in the mouse egg have an absolute requirement for mitochondrial ATP production. *Development* 2004; **131**(13): 3057–67.

30. Campbell K, Swann K. Ca^{2+} oscillations stimulate an ATP increase during fertilization of mouse eggs. *Dev Biol* 2006; **298**(1): 225–33.

31. Liu L, Hammar K, Smith PJ, Inoue S, Keefe DL. Mitochondrial modulation of calcium signaling at the initiation of development. *Cell Calcium* 2001; **30**(6): 423–33.

32. Bachvarova R. Gene expression during oogenesis and oocyte development in mammals. *Dev Biol (NY 1985)* 1985; **1**: 453–524.

33. Paynton BV, Rempel R, Bachvarova R. Changes in state of adenylation and time course of degradation of maternal mRNAs during oocyte maturation and early embryonic development in the mouse. *Dev Biol* 1988; **129**(2): 304–14.

34. Vitale AM, Calvert ME, Mallavarapu M, *et al.* Proteomic profiling of murine oocyte maturation. *Mol Reprod Dev* 2007; **74**(5): 608–16.

35. Eichenlaub-Ritter U, Peschke M. Expression in in-vivo and in-vitro growing and maturing oocytes: focus on regulation of expression at the translational level. *Hum Reprod Update* 2002; **8**(1): 21–41.

36. Racki WJ, Richter JD. CPEB controls oocyte growth and follicle development in the mouse. *Development* 2006; **133**(22): 4527–37.

37. Suh N, Baehner L, Moltzahn F, *et al.* MicroRNA function is globally suppressed in mouse oocytes and early embryos. *Curr Biol* 2010; **20**(3): 271–7.

38. Zamboni L. Ultrastructure of mammalian oocytes and ova. *Biol Reprod Suppl* 1970; **2**: 44–63.

39. Capco DG, Gallicano GI, McGaughey RW, Downing KH, Larabell CA. Cytoskeletal sheets of mammalian eggs and embryos: a lattice-like network of intermediate filaments. *Cell Motil Cytoskeleton* 1993; **24**(2): 85–99.

40. Bachvarova R, De Leon V, Spiegelman I. Mouse egg ribosomes: evidence for storage in lattices. *J Embryol Exp Morphol* 1981; **62**: 153–64.

41. Weakley BS. Initial stages in the formation of cytoplasmic lamellae in the hamster oocyte and the identification of associated electron-dense particles. *Z Zellforsch Mikrosk Anat* 1969; **97**(3): 438–48.

42. Yurttas P, Vitale AM, Fitzhenry RJ, *et al.* Role for PADI6 and the cytoplasmic lattices in ribosomal storage in oocytes and translational control in the early mouse embryo. *Development* 2008; **135**(15): 2627–36.

43. Wright PW, Bolling LC, Calvert ME, *et al.* ePAD, an oocyte and early embryo-abundant peptidylarginine deiminase-like protein that localizes to egg cytoplasmic sheets. *Dev Biol* 2003; **256**(1): 73–88.

44. Esposito G, Vitale AM, Leijten FP, *et al.* Peptidylarginine deiminase (PAD) 6 is essential for oocyte cytoskeletal sheet formation and female fertility. *Mol Cell Endocrinol* 2007; **273**(1–2): 25–31.

45. Kim B, Kan R, Anguish L, Nelson LM, Coonrod SA. Potential role for MATER in cytoplasmic lattice formation in murine oocytes. *PLoS One* 2010; **5**(9): e12587.

46. Tashiro F, Kanai-Azuma M, Miyazaki S, *et al.* Maternal-effect gene Ces5/Ooep/Moep19/Floped is essential for oocyte cytoplasmic lattice formation and

embryonic development at the maternal-zygotic stage transition. *Genes Cells* 2010; **15**(8): 813–28.

47. Tong ZB, Nelson LM, Dean J. Mater encodes a maternal protein in mice with a leucine-rich repeat domain homologous to porcine ribonuclease inhibitor. *Mamm Genome* 2000; **11**(4): 281–7.

48. Herr JC, Chertihin O, Digilio L, *et al.* Distribution of RNA binding protein MOEP19 in the oocyte cortex and early embryo indicates pre-patterning related to blastomere polarity and trophectoderm specification. *Dev Biol* 2008; **314**(2): 300–16.

49. Tong ZB, Gold L, De Pol A, *et al.* Developmental expression and subcellular localization of mouse MATER, an oocyte-specific protein essential for early development. *Endocrinology* 2004; **145**(3): 1427–34.

50. Li L, Baibakov B, Dean J. A subcortical maternal complex essential for preimplantation mouse embryogenesis. *Dev Cell* 2008; **15**(3): 416–25.

51. Fernandes R, Tsuda C, Perumalsamy AL, *et al.* NLRP5 mediates mitochondrial function in mouse oocytes and embryos. *Biol Reprod* 2012; 86(5): 138, 1–10.

52. Ikawa M, Inoue N, Benham AM, Okabe M. Fertilization: a sperm's journey to and interaction with the oocyte. *J Clin Invest* 2010; **120**(4): 984–94.

53. Wassarman PM. Mammalian fertilization: molecular aspects of gamete adhesion, exocytosis, and fusion. *Cell* 1999; **96**(2): 175–83.

54. Bleil JD, Greve JM, Wassarman PM. Identification of a secondary sperm receptor in the mouse egg zona pellucida: role in maintenance of binding of acrosome-reacted sperm to eggs. *Dev Biol* 1988; **128**(2): 376–85.

55. Gahlay G, Gauthier L, Baibakov B, Epifano O, Dean J. Gamete recognition in mice depends on the cleavage status of an egg's zona pellucida protein. *Science* 2010; **329**(5988): 216–19.

56. Burkart AD, Xiong B, Baibakov B, Jimenez-Movilla M, Dean J. Ovastacin, a cortical granule protease, cleaves ZP2 in the zona pellucida to prevent polyspermy. *J Cell Biol* 2012; **197**(1): 37–44.

57. Inoue N, Ikawa M, Okabe M. The mechanism of sperm-egg interaction and the involvement of IZUMO1 in fusion. *Asian J Androl* 2011; **13**(1): 81–7.

58. Herrero MB, Mandal A, Digilio LC, *et al.* Mouse SLLP1, a sperm lysozyme-like protein involved in sperm-egg binding and fertilization. *Dev Biol* 2005; **284**(1): 126–42.

59. Sachdev M, Mandal A, Mulders S, *et al.* Oocyte specific oolemmal SAS1B involved in sperm binding through intra-acrosomal SLLP1 during fertilization. *Dev Biol* 2012; **363**(1): 40–51.

60. Boucheix C, Rubinstein E. Tetraspanins. *Cell Mol Life Sci* 2001; **58**(9): 1189–205.

61. Chen MS, Tung KS, Coonrod SA, *et al.* Role of the integrin-associated protein CD9 in binding between sperm ADAM 2 and the egg integrin alpha6beta1: implications for murine fertilization. *Proc Natl Acad Sci USA* 1999; **96**(21): 11830–5.

62. Kaji K, Oda S, Shikano T, *et al.* The gamete fusion process is defective in eggs of Cd9-deficient mice. *Nat Genet* 2000; **24**(3): 279–82.

63. Miyado K, Yamada G, Yamada S, *et al.* Requirement of CD9 on the egg plasma membrane for fertilization. *Science* 2000; **287**(5451): 321–4.

64. Le Naour F, Rubinstein E, Jasmin C, Prenant M, Boucheix C. Severely reduced female fertility in CD9-deficient mice. *Science* 2000; **287**(5451): 319–21.

65. Jegou A, Ziyyat A, Barraud-Lange V, *et al.* CD9 tetraspanin generates fusion competent sites on the egg membrane for mammalian fertilization. *Proc Natl Acad Sci USA* 2011; **108**(27): 10946–51.

66. Rubinstein E, Ziyyat A, Prenant M, *et al.* Reduced fertility of female mice lacking CD81. *Dev Biol* 2006; **290**(2): 351–8.

67. Zhu GZ, Miller BJ, Boucheix C, *et al.* Residues SFQ (173–175) in the large extracellular loop of CD9 are required for gamete fusion. *Development* 2002; **129**(8): 1995–2002.

68. Runge KE, Evans JE, He ZY, *et al.* Oocyte CD9 is enriched on the microvillar membrane and required for normal microvillar shape and distribution. *Dev Biol* 2007; **304**(1): 317–25.

69. Miyado K, Yoshida K, Yamagata K, *et al.* The fusing ability of sperm is bestowed by CD9-containing vesicles released from eggs in mice. *Proc Natl Acad Sci USA* 2008; **105**(35): 12921–6.

70. Coonrod SA, Naaby-Hansen S, Shetty J, *et al.* Treatment of mouse oocytes with PI-PLC releases 70-kDa (pI 5) and 35- to 45-kDa (pI 5.5) protein clusters from the egg surface and inhibits sperm-oolemma binding and fusion. *Dev Biol* 1999; **207**(2): 334–49.

71. Alfieri JA, Martin AD, Takeda J, *et al.* Infertility in female mice with an oocyte-specific knockout of GPI-anchored proteins. *J Cell Sci* 2003; **116**(Pt 11): 2149–55.

72. Perreault SD, Barbee RR, Elstein KH, Zucker RM, Keefer CL. Interspecies differences in the stability of mammalian sperm nuclei assessed in vivo by sperm

microinjection and in vitro by flow cytometry. *Biol Reprod* 1988; **39**(1): 157–67.

73. Shintomi K, Iwabuchi M, Saeki H, *et al.* Nucleosome assembly protein-1 is a linker histone chaperone in *Xenopus* eggs. *Proc Natl Acad Sci USA* 2005; **102**(23): 8210–15.

74. Philpott A, Leno GH, Laskey RA. Sperm decondensation in *Xenopus* egg cytoplasm is mediated by nucleoplasmin. *Cell* 1991; **65**(4): 569–78.

75. Inoue A, Ogushi S, Saitou M, Suzuki MG, Aoki F. Involvement of mouse nucleoplasmin 2 in the decondensation of sperm chromatin after fertilization. *Biol Reprod* 2011; **85**(1): 70–7.

76. Burns KH, Viveiros MM, Ren Y, *et al.* Roles of NPM2 in chromatin and nucleolar organization in oocytes and embryos. *Science* 2003; **300**(5619): 633–6.

77. Wu X, Viveiros MM, Eppig JJ, *et al.* Zygote arrest 1 (Zar1) is a novel maternal-effect gene critical for the oocyte-to-embryo transition. *Nat Genet* 2003; **33**(2): 187–91.

78. Wu X, Wang P, Brown CA, Zilinski CA, Matzuk MM. Zygote arrest 1 (Zar1) is an evolutionarily conserved gene expressed in vertebrate ovaries. *Biol Reprod* 2003; **69**(3): 861–7.

79. Hu J, Wang F, Zhu X, *et al.* Mouse ZAR1-like (XM_359149) colocalizes with mRNA processing components and its dominant-negative mutant caused two-cell-stage embryonic arrest. *Dev Dyn* 2010; **239**(2): 407–24.

80. Reik W, Dean W, Walter J. Epigenetic reprogramming in mammalian development. *Science* 2001; **293**(5532): 1089–93.

81. Howell CY, Bestor TH, Ding F, *et al.* Genomic imprinting disrupted by a maternal effect mutation in the Dnmt1 gene. *Cell* 2001; **104**(6): 829–38.

82. Hirasawa R, Chiba H, Kaneda M, *et al.* Maternal and zygotic Dnmt1 are necessary and sufficient for the maintenance of DNA methylation imprints during preimplantation development. *Genes Dev* 2008; **22**(12): 1607–16.

83. Payer B, Saitou M, Barton SC, *et al.* Stella is a maternal effect gene required for normal early development in mice. *Curr Biol* 2003; **13**(23): 2110–17.

84. Bortvin A, Goodheart M, Liao M, Page DC. Dppa3 / Pgc7 / stella is a maternal factor and is not required for germ cell specification in mice. *BMC Dev Biol* 2004; **4**: 2.

85. Nakamura T, Arai Y, Umehara H, *et al.* PGC7/Stella protects against DNA demethylation in early embryogenesis. *Nat Cell Biol* 2007; **9**(1): 64–71.

86. Tong ZB, Gold L, Pfeifer KE, *et al.* Mater, a maternal effect gene required for early embryonic development in mice. *Nat Genet* 2000; **26**(3): 267–8.

Chapter 15

Egg activation: initiation and decoding of Ca^{2+} signaling

John Carroll and Karl Swann

ntroduction

:gg activation refers to the early events that occur in he egg (or oocyte) that start embryo development. The most significant of these events in mammals is the esumption of meiosis, which is evident as the emission of a second polar body and then the formation of two polar bodies. However, egg activation in mammals also includes the exocytosis of cortical granules which leads to modifications of the zona pellucida, and changes in the pattern of protein and RNA synthesis. In mammals the sperm initiates the events of egg ctivation. Egg activation can also be initiated by various chemical and physical stimuli, and by modulating the activity of some key cell-cycle proteins. These rtificial agents lead to egg activation in the absence of a sperm, which is termed parthenogenetic activaion. We review the sequence and mechanism of egg ctivation in mammals, concentrating upon data in the nouse.

Sperm-induced Ca^{2+} oscillations

The key change in the egg that initiates the events of egg activation is an increase in the cytosolic free Ca^{2+} oncentration. It was shown more than 25 years ago hat fertilization of mouse and hamster eggs is associated with a series of cytosolic Ca^{2+} oscillations [1, 2]. An example of such oscillations at fertilization in a mouse egg is shown in Figure 15.1. It can be seen hat each Ca^{2+} increase lasts about a minute but that here are repeated Ca^{2+} transients that last for several hours. In mouse eggs these oscillations persist up until the time of the formation of pronuclei [3]. Similar Ca^{2+} oscillations have now been reported in fertilizing eggs of a number of other different mammalian species uch as pigs, cows, horse, rats, and humans. There are slight differences in the exact form of the Ca^{2+} increase and in their frequency. In all cases the Ca^{2+} spikes, or transient oscillations, are separated by at least 10 minutes, and the series as a whole lasts for several hours. In mouse eggs, the oscillations have been shown to be essential for the key events of activation since the introduction of Ca^{2+} chelators into the cytosol blocks meiotic resumption and exocytosis [4]. Furthermore, we know these Ca^{2+} increases are sufficient for egg activation because causing an artificial increase in intracellular Ca^{2+} by applying a Ca^{2+} ionophore, or by microinjecting Ca^{2+} directly into the eggs, triggers development up to the blastocyst stage [1].

The first Ca^{2+} increase starts about a minute after sperm–egg fusion in the mouse. This initial Ca^{2+} increase is often seen in the form of a wave that crosses the egg from the point of sperm entry [5]. This wave can be initiated in the absence of extracellular Ca^{2+} and is due to Ca^{2+} release from intracellular stores. The waves at fertilization start off taking about 6 seconds to cross the egg, but as oscillations develop they speed up and after a few transients they cross the egg in less than 1 second [2, 5]. The direction of each wave is variable and does not appear to be of any significance with respect to egg polarity. It is, however, significant that the whole egg cytoplasm undergoes Ca^{2+} increases repetitively.

Some of the events of egg activation are episodic and reflect the periodic increase in cytosolic Ca^{2+}. In some cases these episodic events may be used as an indicator of the underlying Ca^{2+} increases. Cortical granule exocytosis occurs in a series of pulses that are directly timed and triggered by the first few Ca^{2+} increases [6]. Most of the granules seem to undergo release with the first Ca^{2+} increase. In some fertilizing eggs, such as those of hamster and rabbit, there

Biology and Pathology of the Oocyte, 2nd edn., ed. Alan Trounson, Roger Gosden, and Ursula Eichenlaub-Ritter.

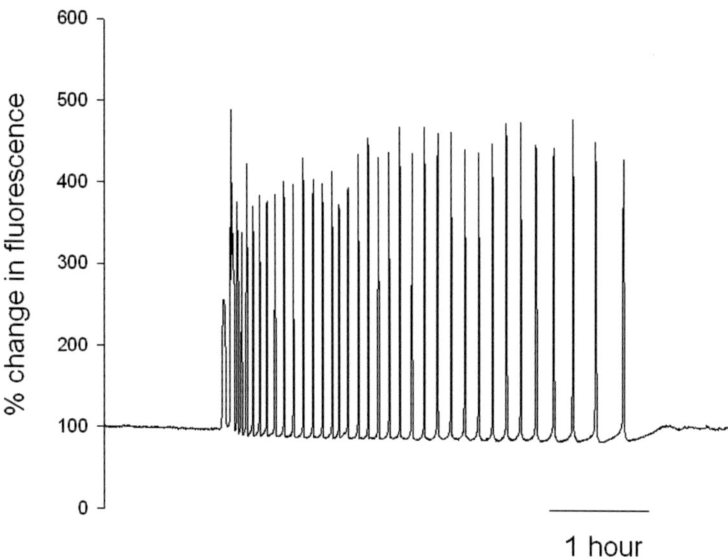

Figure 15.1 Ca^{2+} oscillations in mouse eggs at fertilization. A recording from a single mouse egg during in vitro fertilization. The egg was injected with a Ca^{2+}-sensitive fluorescent dye (Rhod-dextran). The increases in fluorescence represent increases in intracellular free Ca^{2+}, and it is plotted as the fluorescence divided by the "resting" fluorescence before fertilization (hence F/F_0). Repetitive Ca^{2+} transients or oscillations occur for several hours after sperm–egg interaction. The amplitudes and intervals show some slight variation.

are also membrane potential hyperpolarizations that are driven by Ca^{2+}-activated potassium channels [2]. The membrane potential hyperpolarizations in hamster eggs track the timing and amplitude of Ca^{2+} transients so closely that they were used as a simple way of monitoring Ca^{2+} oscillations. Ca^{2+} increases in the egg cytosol also lead to increases in mitochondrial Ca^{2+} and this stimulates increased reduction of flavin adenine dinucleotide (FAD) to FADH which is readily detected as increases in egg auto-fluorescence [7]. Consequently the series of Ca^{2+} oscillations leads to a series of auto-fluorescence oscillations. In mouse and human eggs, it has also been shown that each Ca^{2+} transient is associated with small movements of the egg cytoplasm [5, 8]. The series of cytoplasmic movements can be detected with particle tracking software and provides another way of monitoring the presence of Ca^{2+} oscillations without using invasive fluorescent dyes [8].

PLCζ and Ca^{2+} oscillations in mammalian eggs

The Ca^{2+} oscillations in mammalian eggs involve repeated release from intracellular stores. In mouse and bovine eggs there is clear evidence that Ca^{2+} release is mediated entirely via the inositol trisphosphate (IP_3) receptor, which forms a Ca^{2+} channel in the endoplasmic reticulum membrane [2, 9]. It has also been shown that there is distinct down-regulation of IP_3 receptors at fertilization, and since this can only occur in response to IP_3 levels, it is clear that the sperm generates IP_3. Several lines of evidence suggest that the sperm causes IP_3 production in the egg by introducing a protein factor after sperm–egg membrane fusion. Injecting sperm extracts into eggs of a variety of mammalian species can trigger Ca^{2+} oscillations very similar to those seen during fertilization [10, 11]. During the clinical procedure of ICSI (intracytoplasmic sperm injection), Ca^{2+} oscillations are also observed [12]. The active factor in extracts, and after ICSI has been shown to be protein based. After extensive research the protein factor in sperm extracts, and after ICSI, that causes Ca^{2+} oscillations was shown to be a novel phospholipase C (PLC) named PLCζ (zeta) [13, 14].

PLCζ is a sperm-specific form of PLC that hydrolyzes phosphatidylinositol 4,5-bisphosphate (PIP_2) to generate IP_3. It has been shown to be the sperm factor in sperm extracts that causes Ca^{2+} release in eggs [11, 13]. Significantly, the microinjection of PLCζ cRNA, or the recombinant protein into eggs causes a series of Ca^{2+} oscillations similar to those seen at fertilization. PLCζ has been shown to be effective in causing such Ca^{2+} oscillations in mouse, rat, cow, pig, and human eggs and to trigger development up to at least the blastocyst stage [9, 11]. The amount of PLCζ in sperm from mice and bulls has been shown to be sufficient to explain the generation of the Ca^{2+} oscillations at fertilization ᴾLCζ is found in the head of mouse sperm around he post-acrosomal region, which is where the sperm irst fuses with the egg. The localization in the sperm ead is consistent with the ability of mouse sperm eads, but not tails, to activate eggs after ICSI [14]. nterestingly in horse sperm, PLCζ is located in both he sperm head and tail regions and, unlike the mouse, oth sperm head and tail can cause activation when njected into eggs [15].

As yet there is no definitive proof that PLCζ is he only factor used by the sperm to activate the nammalian egg. A PLCζ knockout mouse has been eported, but PLCζ $^{-/-}$ male mice do not make mature perm so they cannot be used to determine the role of PLCζ in fertilization [16]. We do know that PLCζ nust play some role in fertilization since the knock-lown of PLCζ levels in sperm, using transgenic mice xpressing RNA interference (RNAi) against PLCζ, eads to a reduction in Ca^{2+} oscillations at fertilization 17]. We also know that the sperm signal for activa-ion is entirely via the IP_3 and Ca^{2+} signaling system, o any other candidate molecules involved in egg acti-ation would have to cause or modulate Ca^{2+} oscil-ations in eggs. There are no data to show that any other sperm-specific proteins cause Ca^{2+} oscillations n mammalian eggs, and PLCζ alone is sufficient to ccount for activation at fertilization.

The generation of Ca^{2+} oscillations by PLCζ clearly nvolves IP_3 production since, just like the sperm, the njection of PLCζ causes marked down-regulation of P_3 receptors [18]. The way in which PLCζ generates P_3 appears to involve a positive feedback from Ca^{2+}. ᴾLCζ is about 50% active at resting Ca^{2+} levels and small increase in Ca^{2+} leads to further increase in ᴾLCζ activity [11, 19]. Hence, during Ca^{2+} oscillations t is expected that there will also be IP_3 oscillations, and uch IP_3 oscillations have been shown to be an essen-ial part of the cycle of Ca^{2+} release [19].

It is not clear what other factors regulate the activity of PLCζ. It appears that PLCζ is autonomously active t resting Ca^{2+} levels since its introduction into eggs s a recombinant protein causes Ca^{2+} release within econds [20]. However, PLCζ can be expressed at high evels in cultured cells without any obvious effect upon Ca^{2+} levels [21]. Furthermore, the ectopic expression of PLCζ in a transgenic mouse was found to have no clear effect in somatic tissues. The only obvious ffect in these mice was in oocytes within ovaries, vhich became activated and led to teratoma forma-ion [22]. These data suggest that PLCζ is not active in most cells. Interestingly, the injection of cells, or cell extracts expressing PLCζ, back into mouse eggs leads to the immediate induction of Ca^{2+} oscillations [21]. So PLCζ may be inactive in cell lines because it is missing some factor or factors present in eggs. This cell context-dependent activity is an important property of PLCζ as it allows sufficient concentrations of the enzyme to be stored in the head of the sperm without stimulating unregulated Ca^{2+} release.

The site of action of PLCζ may be distinct from other PLCs. Somatic PLCs of the β, γ, or δ class hydrolyze PIP_2 in the plasma membrane, but fluorescently tagged PLCζ does not show any localization in the plasma membrane [23]. However, immunostaining of PLCζ has now shown that it is localized to intracellular vesicles that are dispersed throughout the cytoplasm [23]. It also appears that mouse eggs contain a considerable amount of PIP_2 in such intracellular vesicles. This intracellular PIP_2 appears to be important since depleting the vesicular PIP_2 inhibits Ca^{2+} oscillations triggered by sperm or PLCζ [23]. In contrast, depleting plasma membrane PIP_2 does not affect the Ca^{2+} oscillations caused by sperm or PLCζ, and yet this can block Ca^{2+} oscillations triggered by PLCδ1 [23]. These data suggest that PLCζ diffuses into the egg after gamete fusion, bypassing any signaling in the plasma membrane, and that PLCζ then binds to intracellular vesicles containing PIP_2. The Ca^{2+}-dependent hydrolysis of this PIP_2 then generates the IP_3 that causes Ca^{2+} release (see Figure 15.2).

PLCζ is also distinct in that it is the smallest of the mammalian PLCs. Its primary structure reveals that it consists of an X–Y catalytic domain, which is common to all PLCs, and then four Ca^{2+}-binding EF hand domains, and a C2 domain that is important for membrane targeting when Ca^{2+} is elevated [13]. The catalytic domain is critical to activity and mutation of an amino acid residue that is conserved in PLCs and shown to be essential for catalytic activity in PLCδ1, for example, leads to a loss of PLCζ function [11]. Interestingly, there are now mutations reported in the catalytic domain of human PLCζ in men whose sperm were unable to activate eggs after ICSI [24]. This supports the essential role of PLCζ in egg activation and suggests that mutations in PLCζ are a novel cause of infertility [24]. The EF hand domains of PLCζ appear to be significant in binding Ca^{2+} and conferring the extraordinary Ca^{2+} sensitivity. One of the unusual features of PLCζ is its lack of pleckstrin homology (PH) domain. Such domains are found in all

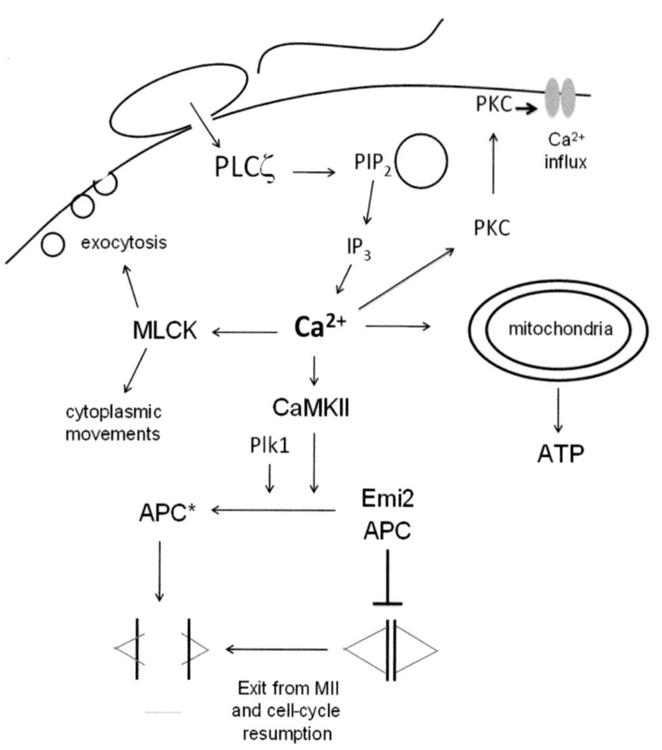

Figure 15.2 Ca^{2+} release mechanisms and downstream signaling in eggs. A schematic diagram of some of the key signaling pathways involved in egg activation. The sperm introduces PLCζ into the egg after sperm–egg membrane fusion. The hydrolysis of PIP_2 generates IP_3, which releases Ca^{2+} from the (ER) endoplasmic reticulum. The Ca^{2+} increases activate downstream signaling events. The central pathway is via calmodulin-dependent protein kinase II (CamKII), which phosphorylates early mitotic inhibitor 2 (Emi2), making it a substrate for polo-like kinase 1 (Plk1). Emi2 is then destroyed, releasing the anaphase-promoting complex (APC) to destroy cyclin B and securin, thereby promoting exit from arrest at metaphase II and progression into interphase. Ca^{2+} transients also stimulate conventional protein kinase C (cPKC) to be recruited to the plasma membrane where it may contribute to Ca^{2+} influx. Exocytosis of cortical granules and cytoplasmic movements are triggered via Ca^{2+}-mediated activation of myosin light chain kinase (MLCK). Finally Ca^{2+} increases are transduced to mitochondria, where ATP production is stimulated, providing energy for the events of egg activation.

other mammalian phosphatidylinositol-specific PLCs. The PH domain of PLCs generally mediates interaction with the plasma membrane, either via specific binding proteins, or via interaction with PIP_2. The lack of a PH domain in PLCζ therefore implies that other domains play a role of membrane binding.

Within the primary structure of PLCζ there is a region between the X and Y catalytic domains that appears to be significant, in that it binds with high affinity to PIP_2 [11]. This so-called X–Y linker region is considered to be unstructured and is essential in conferring high enzymatic activity on PLCζ. This is again in contrast to other mammalian somatic PLCs where the X–Y linker region appears to play a role in auto-inhibition of PLC activity [11]. The X–Y linker region is also of interest since it contains a nuclear localization sequence [25]. In the mouse, this has been shown to be responsible for the sequestration of PLCζ in the pronuclei as soon as they form [25]. The localization of PLCζ in the pronuclei, and its removal from the cytoplasm, then provides an explanation of why the Ca^{2+} oscillations stop just as pronuclear formation occurs in mouse zygotes. In the mouse zygote, there are also Ca^{2+} oscillations during the first mitosis [3]. PLCζ may also be responsible for these mitotic Ca^{2+} oscillations since it will be released back into the cytoplasm after nuclear envelope breakdown, which is when the mitotic oscillations are re-initiated [25]. The nuclear localization of PLCζ has been clearly demonstrated in mouse eggs, but it does not seem to occur in other mammalian species, so it is possible that other mechanisms are responsible for the termination of oscillations [26].

Ca^{2+}: a messenger that coordinates events of egg activation

The events of egg activation take place across timescales from seconds to hours. Initiation of exocytosis of cortical granules is within seconds of the first Ca^{2+} increase while the resumption of meiosis takes minutes to hours and longer-term effects on development occur over hours and days. The ability of the fertilization Ca^{2+} signal to coordinate these events is an inherent property of the initiation and duration of the Ca^{2+} signal (discussed above) as well as the properties of the signaling events downstream of Ca^{2+}. In the next sections we focus on the Ca^{2+}-induced activation of protein kinase C (PKC) and calmodulin-dependent protein kinase II (CaMKII) s well as Ca^{2+}-mediated activation of mitochondrial netabolism. These three examples provide a framevork that illustrates the ability of Ca^{2+} signaling to ct as a master coordinator of fast and slow events in gg activation.

a^{2+} and its partners, PKC and CaMKII

a^{2+} oscillations in cells are often discussed in the ontext of high frequency Ca^{2+} signals that lead to cumulative increase in enzyme activity (frequency nodulation). However, at fertilization, the relatively ow frequency of most of the Ca^{2+} oscillations supports mode of downstream activation where the enzyme ctivity returns to basal levels prior to the initiation f the subsequent Ca^{2+} transient. Nevertheless, as disussed above, the initial Ca^{2+} increase at fertilizaion in mammals has a distinct profile that favors a requency-modulated activation of downstream targets. It comprises an initial increase in Ca^{2+} from asal levels to around 800 nM and then a series of scillations superimposed on the initial increase [27, 8]. These oscillations occur at a relatively high freuency of one spike every 20–30 seconds and have an mplitude in the region of 3–4 μM [27, 28]. This high requency, high amplitude Ca^{2+}signal provides the cope for integrating the activation of Ca^{2+}-sensitive nzymes. PKC is one such enzyme that has the abilty to show frequency-dependent modulation [29]. In he presence of Ca^{2+}, conventional PKC (cPKC) is ecruited to the membrane by the C2 domain where he C1 domain engages diacylglycerol (DAG), retainng it at the membrane where it is activated [29]. Some vidence that the high frequency, high amplitude oscilations seen on the initial Ca^{2+} signal can lead to requency-dependent activation of PKC comes from tudies in which Ca^{2+} and cPKC-GFP translocation to he membrane (a proxy for PKC activation) are monioed dynamically in fertilizing eggs [28]. These studies evealed that each high frequency spike of Ca^{2+} leads o recruitment of cPKC to the plasma membrane. The igh frequency of these oscillations leads to an addiive – frequency-modulated – recruitment of cPKC to he plasma membrane that would be expected to result n strong and sustained enzyme activation. The subequent slow-frequency Ca^{2+}oscillations cause small ransient recruitment of cPKC to the membrane but he retention at the membrane does not significantly utlast the duration of the Ca^{2+} transient [28].

Direct measurement of PKC activation at fertilization has been performed using single time point assays to measure the phosphorylation of PKC substrates [30–32]. These studies show that PKCs are activated at fertilization, and in addition, that a novel PKC, PKCδ, appears to be active during oocyte maturation [33, 34]. Recently the use of a Forster resonance energy transfer (FRET)-based probe, in which a PKC substrate epitope is straddled by cyan fluorescent protein (CFP) and yellow fluorescent protein (YFP) has allowed dynamic measurement of PKC activity during fertilization [35]. The results point to some novel aspects of Ca^{2+} and PKC signaling at fertilization. Firstly, in contrast to the membrane recruitment of PKC–GFP, phosphorylation of cPKC substrates appears to persist for 2–3 minutes beyond the duration of each individual Ca^{2+} transient. This prolonged activation does not persist until the subsequent Ca^{2+} transient so the pattern of PKC activation is episodic, rising and falling after each Ca^{2+} spike [35]. Secondly, the cytoplasmic change was consistently larger than that at the plasma membrane where cPKC is activated [35]. Although there are a number of possible explanations, one possibility is that the cytoplasmic signal is arising from activation of nuclear PKCs (nPKCs) such as PKCδ via PLCζ-mediated production of DAG on intracellular vesicles [23] as we have discussed above. This idea is further supported by the detection of oscillations in PKCδ activity at fertilization [35]. The details on the mode of PKC activation may not be fully elucidated but it is now clear that physiological Ca^{2+} signals at fertilization are sufficient to activate PKC. The functions of PKC at fertilization remain somewhat confounded by the nature of the tools and agents available to manipulate PKC activity ([36–38] for reviews). On balance it would appear that cPKCs may not be necessary for egg activation but may be important for regulation of Ca^{2+} influx during fertilization [28, 38].

CaMKII and its role in egg activation is much better defined than for PKC. It was first shown in *Xenopus* eggs to mediate all Ca^{2+}-dependent events that caused exit from metaphase arrest [39]. The original experiments in *Xenopus* showed that CaMKII is activated at fertilization and that it was both necessary and sufficient to break the metaphase II arrest [39]. This landmark study was elegantly summarized in an accompanying news and views entitled "Sharper than a needle," a title that at the same time praises the work and points to the fact that recombinant CaMKII is a smarter and more effective approach to inducing egg activation than the traditional needle-mediated prick activation technique [40]. Further experiments would prove it was similarly effective in mammalian eggs.

Xenopus eggs undergo activation in response to a single long-lasting Ca^{2+} transient so it was important to understand the dynamics of CaMKII activation during the repetitive Ca^{2+} oscillations at fertilization in mammalian eggs. CaMKII activity has been shown to increase in response to Ca^{2+}-induced egg activation [41–44] and one study performed the impressive feat of measuring CaMKII activity in single oocytes picked at specific stages of the Ca^{2+} oscillation cycle. These experiments revealed that each Ca^{2+} transient triggered an accompanying increase in CaMKII activity and that the level of activity correlated with the size of the increase in Ca^{2+} [44]. Further, pharmacological inhibition of CaMKII inhibited egg activation [42, 44], providing strong evidence that CaMKII could be considered as a universal intermediary of Ca^{2+}-induced egg activation. Finally, proof that CaMKII is sufficient to transduce the downstream events of Ca^{2+} in mammalian eggs is provided by the findings that injection of constitutively active CaMKII causes exit from metaphase arrest, pronucleus formation, mRNA recruitment and development to the blastocyst stage [45, 46]. Interestingly, cortical granule exocytosis did not take place normally [46], suggesting roles for other Ca^{2+}-modulated proteins such as myosin light chain kinase [47] or synaptotagmin [48]. It was also unclear as to whether CaMKII-mediated activation is compatible with longer-term development [46] and further studies are needed to evaluate the full developmental capacity of CaMKII-activated eggs. Certainly, the pattern of CaMKII-mediated activation after injection of the active enzyme will not be physiological and it would be interesting to know whether oscillations in activity are required for longer-term development. The discovery that there is a single CaMKII isoform (CaMKIIγ3) responsible for mediating egg activation [49, 50] will provide an excellent tool for studying the impact of CaMKII dynamics on egg activation.

The mechanism of action of CaMKII in egg activation was finally revealed when the cell cycle and cell signaling fields intersected with the discovery of early mitotic inhibitor 2 (Emi2) and its regulation by CaMKII. In order to achieve exit from metaphase II (MII) arrest, Ca^{2+} is required to trigger the anaphase-promoting complex (APC) to initiate the degradation of cyclin B1 [51, 52]. The arrest at MII is mediated by an inhibition of the APC by a biochemical activity known as cytostatic factor (CSF), a component of which is the mos/MAPK (mitogen-activated protein kinase) pathway ([6, 53] for reviews). However, the fact that meiosis I is not sensitive to MAPK activity and that it remains active right through until pronucleus formation provided a suggestion that other factors may be involved. The key discovery was that Emi2 (Erp1 in *Xenopus*), a potent inhibitor of the APC, is destroyed in a Ca^{2+}-dependent manner and that this destruction is necessary for exit from MII arrest [54]. In mammalian eggs, Emi2 protein first appears close to the time of MII arrest and its destruction is also initiated after triggering of Ca^{2+} oscillations [55]. Furthermore, ablation of Emi2 during oocyte maturation causes a failure of MII arrest [56]. All these data point to Ca^{2+}-mediated Emi2 degradation as being the main requirement for release from MII arrest. To understand the role of CaMKII in Emi2 degradation we need to return to the *Xenopus* system. CaMKII was found to phosphorylate Emi2, which enabled its interaction with polo-like kinase I (Plk1). Phosphorylation of Emi2 by Plk1 induces its ubiquitination and destruction by the proteasome [54, 57–59]. Emi2 degradation therefore releases the brake on the APC, unleashing its ability to promote the destruction of cyclin B1 (and other mitotic substrates such as securin), leading to exit from metaphase and entry into the first mitotic cell cycle.

Thus, there is now a clear path from a sperm-induced Ca^{2+} increase to exit from arrest at MII, although it may be that some details differ in the mammalian oocyte [60]. The functional implications of perturbations in this pathway have not yet been fully explored or modeled [61] but are likely to be important in understanding the detailed mechanisms of egg activation and why it goes wrong in a number of clinical scenarios.

Ca^{2+}: coupling energy supply and demand at fertilization

Egg activation involves a rapid and dramatic increase in cellular activity, including Ca^{2+} homeostasis, exocytosis, cell-cycle resumption, organelle redistribution, and recruitment of mRNA and protein synthesis, all of which have an increased demand for ATP. One of the major developments in the Ca^{2+} signaling field over he past 10 years is the appreciation that close cou-ling of the ER and mitochondria allows mitochon-lrial Ca^{2+} uptake when there is an increase in cytoso-ic Ca^{2+} [62]. In many cell types, Ca^{2+} uptake has een found to activate mitochondrial metabolism via timulating enzymes (including pyruvate dehydroge-ase) in the tricarboxylic acid (TCA) cycle, ultimately eading to an increase in mitochondrial ATP produc-ion ([62] for review). At fertilization, such a mech-nism provides a means of increasing ATP supply, hereby matching the increased demand at the onset f development. There is now strong evidence that his functional coupling is active at fertilization. Ca^{2+}-lependent changes in the levels of FAD^{2+} and NADH t fertilization provide an increased supply of reduced ubstrates for the electron transport chain [63]. The hanges in FAD^{2+} and NADH accompany each Ca^{2+} ise and persist for much of the inter-spike interval 63]. The increase in mitochondrial activity is accom-anied by an increase in mitochondrial and cytosolic ATP that continues to increase over the first 1–2 hours f fertilization before falling to baseline levels when Ca^{2+} oscillations stop [63, 64].

Although mitochondrial ATP production is essen-ial for maintaining basal Ca^{2+} levels and for main-aining Ca^{2+} oscillations at fertilization [63, 65], the ole of the Ca^{2+}-induced increase in ATP production as not been formally tested. Inhibition of mitochon-lrial Ca^{2+} uptake has proved difficult due to the tox-city of available inhibitors. The recent identification f the mitochondrial Ca^{2+} uniporter [66] may pro-ide a genetic means of inhibiting mitochondrial Ca^{2+} ptake and effects on subsequent development. The Ca^{2+}-mediated matching of ATP supply and demand rovides a regulatory system that allows mitochondria o function at the required basal rate of activity rather han at a level necessary to meet the peak demand. This may also have the advantage of minimizing pro-luction of potentially harmful reactive oxygen species vhile the egg is arrested at MII. This physiological reg-lation of energy supply is consistent with the cen-ral idea in the "quiet embryo hypothesis" where it as been proposed that embryos that maintain a low evel of metabolism during the preimplantation period ave the best developmental potential [67]. At fertil-zation, the regulated supply of energy to meet spe-ific needs provides the framework for maintaining netabolism at the lowest rate for a given physiological ontext.

The mark of egg activation upon later development

A conventional view of egg activation is that it provides a stimulus that takes development from meiotic arrest up to the pronuclear stage, and that thereafter the role of the Ca^{2+} signal is over. However, it has become apparent that the pattern of Ca^{2+}oscillations has a longer-term influence upon later development. Different patterns of Ca^{2+} transients have been artificially imposed in mouse eggs using repeated electrical permeabilization [68]. There are clear differences in the size and morphology of post-implantation embryos when fertilizing eggs are exposed to a long train of Ca^{2+} pulses versus a single Ca^{2+} transient [68]. These effects are correlated with changes in gene expression [68, 69]. Other studies have shown that effects of different patterns of Ca^{2+} transients during activation influence post-implantation parthenogenetic development in rabbit embryos [70]. Unlike the events of meiotic resumption that we have described above, the mechanism that links Ca^{2+} signals in the first few hours of development with much later events in embryogenesis is unclear. However, it is possible that egg activation is not an all or nothing event and that different degrees of egg activation have an effect upon embryo development days or weeks later. Clearly, the role of Ca^{2+} in coordinating the signaling pathways discussed in this chapter, as well as pathways yet to be fully elucidated is of major importance not only in the initiation of development but in longer-term development and physiological functions.

References

1. Swann K, Ozil JP. Dynamics of the calcium signal that triggers mammalian egg activation. *Int Rev Cytol* 1994; **152**: 183–222.
2. Miyazaki S, Shirakawa H, Nakada K, Honda Y. Essential role of the inositol 1,4,5-trisphosphate/Ca^{2+} release channel in Ca^{2+} waves and Ca^{2+} oscillations at fertilization of mammalian eggs. *Dev Biol* 1993; **58**: 62–78.
3. Marangos P, FitzHarris G, Carroll J. Ca^{2+} oscillations at fertilization in mammals are regulated by the formation of pronuclei. *Development* 2003; **130**: 1461–72.
4. Kline D, Kline T. Repetitive calcium transients and the role of calcium in exocytosis and cell cycle activation in the mouse egg. *Dev Biol* 1992; **149**: 80–9.

5. Deguchi R, Shirakawa H, Oda S, Mohri T, Miyazaki S. Spatiotemporal analysis of Ca^{2+} waves in relation to the sperm entry site and animal-vegetal axis during Ca^{2+} oscillations in fertilized mouse eggs. *Dev Biol* 2000; **218**: 299–313.
6. Ducibella T, Fissore R. The roles of Ca^{2+}, downstream protein kinases, and oscillatory signalling in regulating fertilization and the activation of development. *Dev Biol* 2007; **315**: 257–79.
7. Dumollard R, Marangos P, Fitzharris G, *et al.* Sperm triggered Ca^{2+} oscillations and Ca^{2+} homeostasis in the mouse egg have an absolute requirement for mitochondrial ATP production. *Development* 2004; **131**: 3057–67.
8. Ajduk A, Ilozue T, Windsor S, *et al.* Rhythmic actomyosin-driven contractions induced by sperm entry predict mammalian embryo viability *Nat Commun* 2011; **2**: 417.
9. Lee S, Yoon Y, Fissore RA, Regulation of fertilization-initiated $[Ca^{2+}]$i oscillations in mammalian eggs: a multi-pronged approach. *Semin Cell Dev Biol* 2006; **17**: 274–84.
10. Swann K. A cytosolic sperm factor stimulates repetitive calcium increases and mimics fertilization in hamster oocytes. *Development* 1990; **110**: 1295–302.
11. Nomikos M, Swann K, Lai FA. Starting a new life: sperm PLC-zeta mobilizes the Ca^{2+} signal that induces egg activation and embryo development: an essential phospholipase C with implications for male infertility. *Bioessays* 2012; **34**: 126–34.
12. Nakano Y, Shirakawa H, Mitsuhashi N, Kuwubara Y, Miyazaki S. Spatiotemporal dynamics of intracellular calcium in the mouse egg injected with a spermatozoon. *Mol Hum Reprod* 1997; **3**: 1087–93.
13. Saunders CM, Larman MG, Parrington J, *et al.* PLCζ: a sperm-specific trigger of Ca^{2+} oscillations in eggs and embryo development. *Development* 2002; **129**: 3533–44.
14. Fujimoto S, Yoshida N, Fukui T, *et al.* Mammalian phospholipase Cz induces oocyte activation from the sperm perinuclear matrix. *Dev Biol* 2004; **274**: 370–83.
15. Bedford-Guaus SJ, McPartlin LA, Xie J, *et al.* Molecular cloning and characterization of phospholipase C zeta in equine sperm and testis reveals species-specific differences in expression of catalytically active protein. *Biol Reprod* 2011; **85**: 78–88.
16. Ito M, Ngaoka K, Kuroda K, *et al.* Arrest of spermatogenesis at round spermatids in PLCz1 deficient mice. Abstract at the 11th *International Symposium on Spermatology*. Okinawa, Japan, 2010.
17. Knott JG, Kurokawa M, Fissore RA, Schultz RM, Williams CJ. Transgenic RNAi reveals role for mouse sperm phospholipase Cz in triggering Ca^{2+} oscillations during fertilization. *Biol Reprod* 2005; **72**: 992–6.
18. Lee BS, Yoon Y, Malcuit C, Parys JB, Fissore RA, Inositol 1,4,5-trisphosphate receptor 1 degradation in mouse eggs and impact on $[Ca^{2+}]$i oscillations. *J Cell Physiol* 2010; **222**: 238–47.
19. Swann K, Yu Y. The dynamics of Ca^{2+} oscillations that activate mammalian eggs. *Int J Dev Biol* 2008; **52**: 585–94.
20. Nomikos M, Yu Y, Elgmati K, *et al.* Phospholipase Cζ rescues failed oocyte activation in a protptype of male factor infertility. *Fert Steril* 2013; **99**: 76–85.
21. Phillips SV, Yu Y, Rossbach A, *et al.* Divergent effect o mammalian PLCζ in generating Ca^{2+} oscillations in somatic cells compared with eggs. *Biochem J* 2011; **438** 545–53.
22. Yoshida N, Amani M, Kajikawa E, *et al.* Broad, extopic expression of the sperm protein PLCZ1 induces parthenogenesis and ovarian tumours in mice. *Development* 2007; **134**: 3941–52.
23. Yu Y, Nomikos M, Theodoridou M, *et al.* PLCζ causes Ca^{2+} oscillations in mouse eggs by targeting intracellular and not plasma membrane PI(4,5)P(2). *Mol Biol Cell* 2012; **23**: 371–80.
24. Kashir J, Heindryckx B, Jones C, *et al.* Oocyte activation, phospholipase C zeta and human infertility *Hum Reprod Update* 2010; **16**: 690–703.
25. Larman MG, Saunders CM, Carroll J, Lai FA, Swann K. Cell cycle-dependent Ca^{2+} oscillations in mouse embryos are regulated by nuclear targeting of PLCzeta *J Cell Sci* 2004; **117**: 2513–21.
26. Ito M, Shikano T, Oda S, *et al.* Difference in Ca^{2+} oscillation-inducing activity and nuclear translocation ability of PLCZ1, an egg-activating sperm factor candidate, between mouse, rat, human, and medaka fish. *Biol Reprod* 2008; **78**: 1081–90.
27. Cuthbertson KS, Whittingham DG, Cobbold PH. Free Ca^{2+} increases in exponential phases during mouse oocyte activation. *Nature* 1981; **294**: 754–7.
28. Halet G, Tunwell R, Parkinson SJ, Carroll J. Conventional PKCs regulate the temporal pattern of Ca^{2+} oscillations at fertilisation in mouse eggs. *J Cell Biol* 2004; **164**: 1033–44.
29. Oancea E, Meyer T. Protein kinase C as a molecular machine for decoding calcium and diacylglycerol signals. *Cell* 1998; **95**: 307–18.
30. Gallicano GI, McGaughey RW, Capco DG. Activation of protein kinase C after fertilization is required for remodelling in the mouse egg into the *zygote. Mol Reprod Dev* 1997; **46**: 587–601.

31. Tatone C, DelleMonarche S, Francione A, *et al.* Ca^{2+}-independent protein kinase C signalling in mouse eggs during the early phases of fertilization. *Int J Dev Biol* 2003; **47**: 327–33.

32. Kalive M, Faust JJ, Koeneman BA, Capco DG. Involvement of the PKC family in regulation of early development. *Mol Reprod Dev* 2010 **77**: 95–104.

33. Viveiros MM, Hirao Y, Eppig JJ. Evidence that protein kinase C (PKC) participates in the meiosis I to meiosis II transition in mouse oocytes. *Dev Biol* 2001; **235**: 330–42.

34. Viveiros MM, O'Brien M, Wigglesworth K, Eppig JJ. Characterization of protein kinase C-δ in mouse oocytes throughout meiotic maturation and following egg activation. *Biol Reprod* 2003; **69**: 1494–9.

35. Gonzalez-Garcia JR, Machaty Z, Lai FA, Swann K. The dynamics of PKC-induced phosphorylation triggered by Ca^{2+} oscillations in mouse eggs. *J Cell Physiol* 2013; **228**: 110–19.

36. Halet G. PKC signaling at fertilization in mammalian eggs. *Biochem Biophys Acta* 2004; **1742**: 185–9.

37. Jones KT. Protein kinase C action at fertilization: overstated or undervalued? *Rev Reprod* 1998; **3**: 7–12.

38. Yu Y, Halet.G, Lai FA, Swann K. Regulation of diacylglycerol production and protein kinase C stimulation during sperm- and PLCzeta-mediated mouse egg activation. *Biol Cell* 2008; **100**: 633–43.

39. Lorca T, Cruzalegui FH, Fesquet D, *et al.* Calmodulin-dependent protein kinase II mediates inactivation of MPF and CSF upon fertilization of *Xenopus* eggs. *Nature* 1993; **366**: 270–3.

40. Whitaker M. Sharper than a needle. *Nature* 1993; **366**: 211–12.

41. Winston NJ, Maro B. Calmodulin-dependent protein kinase II is activated transiently in ethanol-stimulated mouse oocytes. *Dev Biol* 1995; **170**: 350–2.

42. Johnson J, Bierle BM, Gallicano GI, Capco DG. Calcium/calmodulin-dependent protein kinase II and calmodulin: regulators of the meiotic spindle in mouse eggs. *Dev Biol* 1998; **204**: 464–77.

43. Markoulaki S, Matson S, Abbott AL, Ducibella T. Oscillatory CaMKII activity in mouse egg activation. *Dev Biol* 2003; **258**: 464–74.

44. Markoulaki S, Matson S, Ducibella T. Fertilization stimulates long-lasting oscillations of CaMKII activity in mouse eggs. *Dev Biol* 2004; **272**: 15–25.

45. Madgwick S, Levasseur M, Jones KT. Calmondulin-dependent protein kinase II, and not protein kinase C, is sufficient for triggering cell-cycle resumption in mammalian eggs. *J Cell Sci* 2005; **118**: 3849–59.

46. Knott JG, Gardner AJ, Madgwick S, *et al.* Calmodulin-dependent protein kinase II triggers mouse egg activation and embryo development in the absence of Ca^{2+} oscillations. *Dev Biol* 2006; **296**: 388–95.

47. Matson S, Markoulaki S, Ducibella T, Antagonists of myosin light chain kinase and of myosin II inhibit specific events of egg activation in fertilized mouse eggs. *Biol Reprod* 2006; **74**: 169–76.

48. Leguia M, Conner S, Berg L, Wessel GM. Synaptotagmin 1 is involved in the regulation of cortical granule exocytosis in the sea urchin. *Mol Reprod Dev* 2006; **73**: 895–905.

49. Backs J, Stein P, Backs T, *et al.* The gamma isoform of CaM kinase II controls mouse egg activation by regulating cell cycle resumption. *Proc Natl Acad Sci USA* 2010; **107**: 81–6.

50. Chang HY, Minahan K, Merriman JA, Jones KT. Calmodulin-dependent protein kinase gamma 3 (CamKIIgamma3) mediates the cell cycle resumption of metaphase II eggs in mouse. *Development* 2009; **136**: 4077–81.

51. Nixon VL, Levasseur M, McDougall A, Jones KT. Ca^{2+} oscillations promote APC/C-dependent cyclin B1 degradation during metaphase arrest and completion of meiosis in fertilizing mouse eggs. *Curr Biol* 2002; **12**: 746–50.

52. Marangos P, Carroll J. Fertilization and InsP3-induced Ca^{2+} release stimulate a persistent increase in the rate of degradation of cyclin B1 specifically in mature mouse oocytes. *Dev Biol* 2004; **272**: 26–38.

53. Tunquist BJ, Maller JL. Under arrest: cytostatic factor (CSF)-mediated metaphase arrest in vertebrate eggs. *Genes Dev* 2003; **17**: 683–710.

54. Rauh NR, Schmidt A, Bormann J, Nigg EA, Mayer TU. Calcium triggers exit from meiosis II by targeting the APC/C inhibitor XErp1 for degradation. *Nature* 2005; **437**: 1048–52.

55. Madgwick S, Hansen DV, Levasseur M, Jackson PK, Jones KT. Mouse Emi2 is required to enter meiosis II by reestablishing cyclin B1 during interkinesis. *J Cell Biol* 2006; **174**: 791–801.

56. Shoji S, Yoshida N, Amanai M, *et al.* Mammalian Emi2 mediates cytostatic arrest and transduces the signal for meiotic exit via Cdc20. *EMBO J* 2006; **25**: 834–45.

57. Liu J, Maller JL. Calcium elevation at fertilization coordinates phosphorylation of XErp1/Emi2 by Plx1 and CaMK II to release metaphase arrest by cytostatic factor. *Curr Biol* 2005; **15**: 1458–68.

58. Tung JJ, Hansen DV, Ban KH, *et al.* A role for the anaphase-promoting complex inhibitor Emi2/XErp1, a homolog of early mitotic inhibitor 1, in cytostatic factor arrest of *Xenopus* eggs. *Proc Natl Acad Sci USA* 2005; **102**: 4318–23.

59. Hansen DV, Tung JJ, Jackson PK. CaMKII and polo-like kinase 1 sequentially phosphorylate the cytostatic factor Emi2/XErp1 to trigger its destruction and meiotic exit. *Proc Natl Acad Sci USA* 2006; **103**: 608–13.

60. Suzuki T, Suzuki E, Yoshida N, *et al.* Mouse Emi2 as a distinctive regulatory hub in second meiotic metaphase. *Development* 2010; **137**: 3281–91.

61. Dupont G, Heytens E, Leybaert L. Oscillatory Ca^{2+} dynamics and cell cycle resumption at fertilization in mammals: a modelling approach. *Int J Dev Biol* 2010; **54**; 655–65.

62. Rizzuto R, De Stefani D, Raffaello A, Mammucari C. Mitochondria as sensors and regulators of calcium signalling. *Nat Rev Mol Cell Biol* 2012; **13**: 566–78.

63. Dumollard R, Marangos P, Fitzharris G, *et al.* Sperm-triggered $[Ca^{2+}]$ oscillations and Ca^{2+} homeostasis in the mouse egg have an absolute requirement for mitochondrial ATP production. *Development* 2004; **131**: 3057–67.

64. Campbell K, Swann K. Ca^{2+} oscillations stimulate an ATP increase during fertilization of mouse eggs. *Dev Biol* 2006; **298**: 225–33.

65. Liu L, Hammar K, Smith PJ, Inoue S, Keefe DL. Mitochondrial modulation of calcium signaling at the initiation of development. *Cell Calcium* 2001; **30**: 423–33.

66. De Stefani D, Raffaello A, Teardo E, Szabò I, Rizzuto R. A forty-kilodalton protein of the inner membrane i the mitochondrial calcium uniporter. *Nature* 2011; **476**: 336–40.

67. Leese HJ. Metabolism of the preimplantation embryo: 40 years on. *Reproduction* 2012; **143**: 417–27.

68. Ozil JP, Banrezes B, Tóth S, Pan H, Schultz RM. Ca^{2+} oscillatory pattern in fertilized mouse eggs affects gen expression and development to term. *Dev Biol* 2006; **300**: 534–44.

69. Rogers NT, Halet G, Piao Y, *et al.* The absence of a Ca^{2+} signal during mouse egg activation can affect parthenogenetic preimplantation development, gene expression patterns, and blastocyst quality. *Reproduction* 2006; **132**: 45–57.

70. Ozil JP, Huneau D. Activation of rabbit oocytes: the impact of the Ca^{2+} signal regime on development. *Development* 2001; **128**: 917–28.

Section 3 Developmental biology

Chapter 16

In vitro growth and differentiation of oocytes

Hang Yin and Roger Gosden

Introduction

Recent advances in oocyte culture technology from the primordial follicle stage give hope of generating more human oocytes for infertility treatment and fertility preservation for cancer patients. Several methods have already been valuable for studying the biology of oogenesis and folliculogenesis. Healthy mouse pups have been produced by growing oocytes entirely in vitro, and the challenge now is to translate this technology for human oocytes, which faces many problems: availability of research material, small follicle harvest, multistage culture systems. Nevertheless, growth from the secondary to early tertiary follicle stage has already succeeded, and there can be little doubt that complete success will be achieved eventually. The research focus will then turn to the question of whether the oocytes were appropriately programmed during development to be safely used for reproduction. There is a maximum number of oocytes that can be potentially generated in vitro determined by the primordial follicle store, which declines with age. Recent research indicates that this cap might be overcome using stem cell technology, which could, in theory, take away from oocytes the distinction of being the rarest cells in the body and a major limitation for fertility.

Prospects for growing oocytes in vitro

Oocyte culture is a natural companion technology for in vitro fertilization, like cryopreservation and preimplantation genetic testing, but it presents a high bar to the ultimate goal of encompassing the entire process of oogenesis. However, animal models are showing the way, in vitro maturation (IVM) is already in clinical practice, progress is being made at early stages of human follicle development, and eventually germline stem cells (GSCs) may open new territory. An emerging platform of technologies will undoubtedly have major impacts, addressing chronic shortages of this rare cell type and enabling many applications (Table 16.1).

Table 16.1. Potential applications of oocyte culture technologies

1. Treatment of infertility, including (a) ART without gonadotropin stimulation of the ovaries, (b) oocyte donation, (c) preimplantation genetic diagnosis/screening, (d) spindle/pronuclear transfer to avoid transmitting mitochondrial disease
2. Rescue of residual, small follicles in ovaries with premature ovarian insufficiency
3. Fertility preservation for cancer patients, including oocyte and ovarian tissue cryopreservation
4. Conservation of endangered species and rare animal breeds
5. Farm and domestic animal production
6. Cloning technologies involving somatic cell nuclear transfer to oocytes
7. Research on oocyte biology, pathology, contraceptive targeting, and reproductive toxicology

ART, assisted reproductive technology.

At the end of the continuum of follicle development, oocytes at the germinal vesicle stage are fully grown, possess a molecular program of mRNAs and proteins stored in the cytoplasm, and are prepared to resume meiosis to metaphase II [1]. When the cumulus mass is transferred to culture conditions, the process of nuclear maturation is initiated spontaneously, proceeding to completion in a physiological time frame of 30–40 hours. Edwards originally considered IVM as a strategy for generating mature human oocytes for in vitro fertilization (IVF) treatment, and although his vision was superceded by ovarian stimulation with gonadotropins it may be realized again when in vitro growth of oocytes (IVG) followed by IVM is proven

Biology and Pathology of the Oocyte, 2nd edn., ed. Alan Trounson, Roger Gosden, and Ursula Eichenlaub-Ritter.
Published by Cambridge University Press.

safe and efficient [2]. Practical and economic advantages will emerge from more-efficient use of the limited follicle store and avoiding the risks of ovarian hyperstimulation. On the other hand, optimism should be guarded until the safety of IVG–IVM technology is fully proven. A surgical procedure is needed to recover material for culture, but even a small biopsy from a young ovary will likely contain enough oocytes for multiple IVF treatment cycles, cryopreservation, and perhaps even oocyte donation [3].

Most follicles are wasted by atresia, which starts with apoptosis in granulosa cells and progresses to the oocyte [4]. The fate of a given follicle, whether recruitment for growth or atresia, is determined by a balance of growth and survival factors, serum follicle-stimulating hormone (FSH) being notably important for antral (tertiary) follicle stages (see Chapter 5). If atresia is, as widely presumed, a mechanism primarily serving to regulate the cohort of advancing follicles in normal ovaries, we can be more confident that the technology will not rescue unhealthy germ cells whose fate would otherwise be elimination.

Setting aside whole organ perfusion and incubation, which are time-limited by necrosis, IVG requires follicle excision from tissues for extended culture. The first three centers reporting progress with IVG adopted different strategies, and methods continue to evolve [5–7]. The field now witnesses an explosion of research activity around the globe, and although rodent ovaries originally served as founder models, advances are now being made with farm and companion animals, and even sub-human primate and human tissues.

Biological and technical challenges

Full development of human oocytes in culture from the primordial follicle stage presents a greater challenge than IVF and embryo culture. This is not to underrate the huge obstacles faced by pioneering embryologists in the 1960s and 1970s when culture methods and materials were so much more rudimentary. But follicles are structurally more complex than embryos, consisting of three basic cell types, and develop over a longer time course during which growth and differentiation have stage-specific requirements. Except at early stages, follicles are much larger than embryos, supported in a cortical stroma with the theca continuously perfused by the ovarian circulation. As a rule of thumb in physiology, solid tissues cannot satisfy their requirements for oxidative metabolism by gaseous diffusion above ~1 mm in diameter. Cells inside small tissue fragments can survive culture for a few days, especially follicles close to the periphery, but not long enough for a full growth span. Since the maximum diameter of preantral (secondary) follicles never exceeds 0.3–0.4 mm, diffusion should always satisfy their requirements after isolation in vitro. But since antral stages in most species are >1 mm, approaching 20 mm at maturity in humans, their needs cannot be met, especially near the center where the oocyte resides. Culture methods have sustained farm animal and primate follicles up to 1–2 mm, that is, close to the theoretical limit [8–10], but this size range may fall short of the threshold when oocytes are competent to resume meiosis. The intrafollicular pO_2 gradient could be increased in a hyperbaric chamber, but this carries the risk of oxygen toxicity.

Oocytes develop in a niche created by an envelope of granulosa cells forming a developmental unit. Thus, naked oocytes have limited growth potential, never becoming competent for meiosis in vitro [11]. Nutrients and regulatory molecules are supplied by diffusion across the basal lamina and granulosa layers to the perivitelline space, and transzonal projections (TZPs) extending to junctional complexes on the oolemma are critical for metabolic cooperation and regulation (see Chapter 8). In conclusion, culture conditions must satisfy the metabolic and trophic needs of both cell types as well as preserving TZPs with patent gap junctions.

The full span of follicle growth in vivo ranges from 3 weeks to 6 months or more, according to species. Such lengthy periods are not unusual when culturing homogeneous cell lines and stem cells, but are challenging for solid tissues and follicles. The problem is not only management, supplying nutrition, and preventing infection, but potentially oxidative stress and a culture environment which at best is always non-physiological. Chief concerns are to safeguard the fidelity of future meiotic divisions and epigenetic programming.

Culture methods are most likely to be successful if they support normal tissue architecture and mimic physiological requirements, which change over time. Hence, protocols for growth across the entire follicle spectrum have adopted multiple stages [12, 13]. In some cases, three stages have been used to match the major developmental transitions (primordial, primary, secondary, and tertiary follicles). Advances in hysiology will continue to instruct an evolving technology and address outstanding questions. How to ptimize follicle harvests from human ovaries? Are pecies-specific culture systems required for culture? Iow many stages are needed? Should culture media e formulated primarily to address the needs of granulosa cells or of oocytes? Should culture conditions e guided more by empirical results (i.e., trial and rror) than knowledge of follicular physiology and netabolism? Can this technology become safe enough or clinical applications?

ulture strategies

Iarvesting and isolating follicles nd oocytes

Vhereas fully grown oocytes from Graafian follies are aspirated for IVM, isolation of small follies for IVG requires either microdissection to retain heca–stroma cells or disaggregation using proteolytic nzymes to yield granulosa–oocyte complexes (GOCs) fter removing those cells. Enzymatic methods prouce larger harvests from delicate organs, but fibrous varies need a combination of methods, sometimes by training tissue through a stainless steel mesh.

Whole organs or cortical slices are chopped into mall fragments with sterile blades before vigorously haking or pipetting in an enzyme solution at 37 °C uffered with HEPES, PBS, or Leibovitz L-15 media. ince trypsin–EDTA and pronase are rather harsh, the nore specific digestion provided by collagenase type I s preferable, with DNase I added to avoid cells sticking together with DNA released from damaged cells 7, 14–16]. Large numbers of preantral follicles can be ecovered within 30 minutes from immature rodent varies, but far fewer from adult ages (Figure 16.1A). The process is more protracted with adult primate nd farm animal ovaries, which may require microdisection after semi-digestion to avoid excessive expoure to enzymes. Preantral follicles are widely scatered throughout the fibrous cortex of these ovaries, nly the primordial stage being abundant. According o live/dead cell staining and electron microscopy, 71% nd 91%, respectively, of granulosa cells and oocytes rom human follicles were viable, with similar harvests rom cryopreserved tissues [17]. Despite such encourging data, more follicles are now known to sustain njury which only becomes fully apparent in culture [18]. Damage to the basal lamina and the integrity of granulosa layers and TZPs compromise oocyte viability; sometimes they become completely denuded. To minimize the problem, crude collagenase preparations are being replaced by Liberase, purified to GMP quality [19, 20].

As soon as follicles or GOCs are freed, they must be quickly washed to remove cellular debris and enzymes. Small samples can be sorted according to size using calibrated pipettes [21]. For larger harvests, centrifugal elutriation enabled recovery of up to 30 × 10^3 viable primordial follicles from newborn piglet ovaries [16], but comparable harvests have never been reported for adult animals of any large species. Since density gradient columns and antibody-labeling methods are too slow and unreliable for efficient separation, microdissection with fine needles after semi-digestion is necessary for extraction from fibrous ovaries.

Culture from the primordial follicle stage is the ultimate goal, since this is the most abundant stage at all postnatal ages. Whereas the diminutive follicle in rodents (<20 μm) is too small, dissection is feasible with primordial follicles in cat and rabbit ovaries (45–50 μm), and avoids damaging enzyme treatment [12]. This stage in human ovaries can also be dissected, although slow-yielding, and for reasons discussed below cultures are normally initiated in cortical explants.

Culture systems and substrata

Among the methods available, culturing GOCs on membranes was one of the first and still among the best, in part because it reduces barriers for diffusion to the oocyte. The first wave of follicle growth produces a cohort of small, preantral follicles with midsized oocytes in 10- to 12-day-old mouse ovaries. After disaggregation, GOCs can be pipetted into wells containing a collagen-impregnated membrane immersed in medium, sometimes covered with mineral oil to prevent evaporative losses [5, 15]. The granulosa cells, largely denuded of basal lamina by enzyme digestion, anchor to the substratum without spreading, and over a 10-day period oocytes grow out on stalks corresponding to the cumulus oophorus in follicular fluid (Figure 16.1B). The merits of this system lie in simplicity and the relatively large numbers of oocytes that can be managed, but applications to human and farm animal ovaries have been limited because GOCs are not

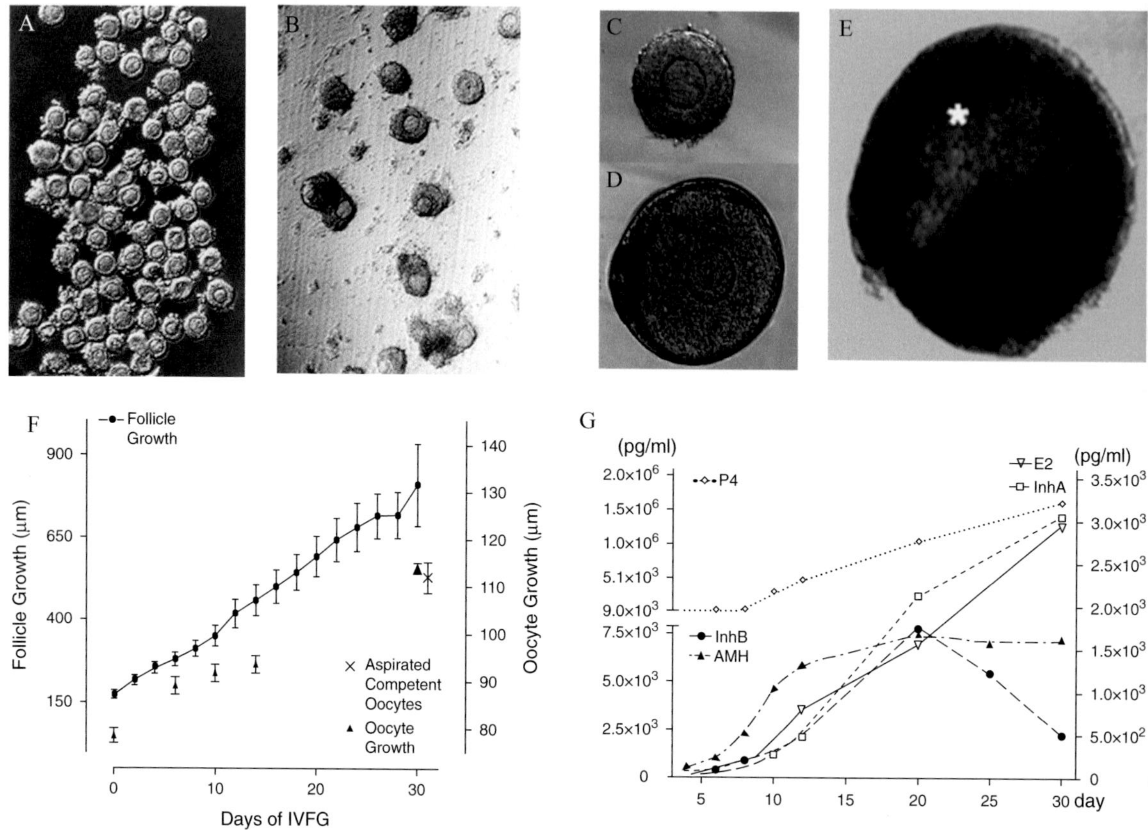

Figure 16.1 (A) Large harvests of granulosa–oocyte complexes (GOCs) can be obtained after disaggregating immature mouse ovaries with collagenase. (B) GOCs growing on a collagen-impregnated membrane. (C–E) Mouse follicles encapsulated in alginate at small preantral stage grow to antral sizes after 8 days with competent oocytes and a differentiated theca layer [52]. (F) Human follicles with 2–3 layers cultured in an alginate scaffold developed fully grown oocytes in 30 days (means ± SEM). (G) In the same scaffold, follicles secreted a physiological profile of estrogen (E2), progesterone (P4), anti-Müllerian hormone (AMH), inhibin A and B (InhA & InhB) [57]. Reprinted with kind permission from *Tissue Engineering* and *Human Reproduction*.

easily harvested in bulk and lose viability during organ disaggregation.

In other early studies, groups of GOCs or intact follicles from rodent ovaries were grown in agar or collagen gel to provide three-dimensional support [6, 7, 22]. The media enabled observation, and measurement and diffusion of metabolites, but neither substrate provided an ideal physical scaffold, and agar, a plant-based polymer, and collagen, purified from rat tail tendons or other sources, require adjustment of the pH to gelate, and protease activity caused collagen gels to contract during culture. Nevertheless, GOCs developed new layers during a 1- to 2-week period, though never progressing to the antral stage, and stroma sometimes overgrew, competing for space and nutrients [7]. These limitations let an attractive principle down until alginate hydrogels were introduced.

Alginate offers similar advantages but greater robustness and flexibility in which GOCs or intact follicles from rodents and even primates can grow for 30 days or longer, with better outcomes than other gel-based methods (Figure 16.1C–E). Physiologically important matrix proteins can be incorporated into gels, whose properties were optimal with 0.25–0.50% sodium alginate with or without fibrin [23]. Recently promising results have also been obtained using tyramine-based hyaluronan hydrogels [24]. Oocyte diameter can be continuously monitored through the transparent gel until the oocyte is obscured during antrum formation, and metabolites assayed from spent medium (Figures 16.1F and 16.1G). Finally, unless oocytes have already resumed meiosis within their follicles, they can be recovered by follicle puncture for IVM and IVF.

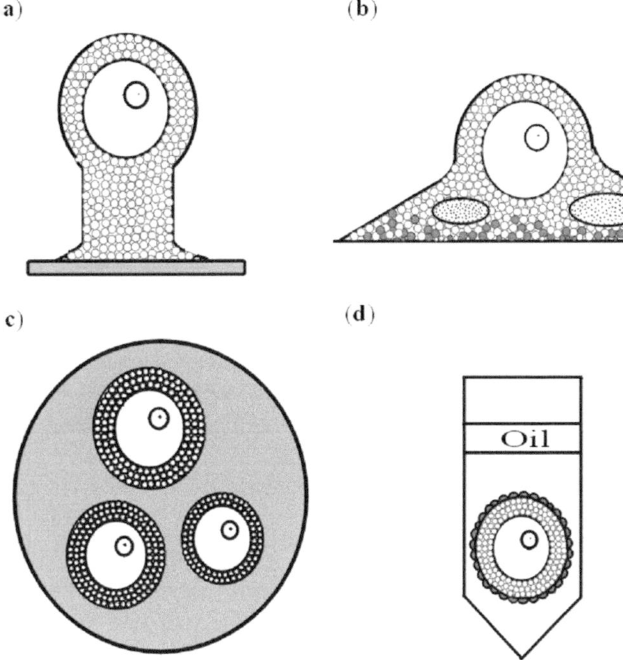

Figure 16.2 Diagrammatic representation of four culture methods: (a) granulosa–oocyte complexes on a membrane, (b) small follicles attaching to a plastic dish, (c) intact follicles in a hydrogel scaffold (agar or collagen gel or, generally nowadays, alginate) maintain a 3-D architecture, (d) intact follicles in microwells under a layer of mineral oil. Reprinted from [12] with kind permission from *Human Reproduction Update*.

Competent mouse oocytes from intact follicle cultures have also been generated in "free-floating" and conventional culture dishes. Preantral mouse follicles ranging from 140 to 170 μm were grown in the upper chambers of wells divided by a porous hydrophobic membrane to prevent sticking and spreading [25]. By draining the upper chamber to leave only a thin film covering the follicles, gas exchange was optimized. Boland *et al.* used 96-well, plastic microtiter plates to culture follicles in microdroplets of medium under a layer of oil (Figure 16.2) [26]. Minute volumes (10–20 μl) enabled cells to condition their own medium, although they required daily replenishment by transferring to successive rows of fresh medium. Transfer also avoided follicles sticking to the wells, which persisted even with untreated plastic surfaces lacking a charge. This method could only fully succeed with individual follicles because only one developed when a pair was cultured in close contact, the other remaining arrested in a non-atretic state [27]. While time-consuming, this method has found recent application with human follicles [9].

Cortvrindt *et al.* developed another method for intact mouse follicles using plastic culture dishes that are somewhat easier to manage and revealed that normal three-dimensional architecture is not mandatory for oocyte health [28]. In the presence of serum and FSH, follicles spread across the surface (Figure 16.2), the oocytes becoming competent for meiosis within 2 weeks [29, 30].

Other methods to avoid follicle adhesion, such as hanging drops and roller tubes, have gained less attention. In theory, microfluidics offers great potential for capillary tube cultures in parallel because of the expanded opportunities for monitoring development under more closely controlled conditions, perhaps rendering antibiotics unnecessary and applying physiological gradients to avoid step-changes required by multistage culture.

But none of these methods has yet satisfied the primordial follicle stage. After enzyme treatment, they tend to release their oocytes, although reaggregation with lectins and alginate may restore development [31, 32]. More commonly, primordial follicle cultures are started in organ fragments or slices from which most of the stroma has been stripped and the larger follicles removed. After initiating growth, they reach a sufficient size after 8–10 days for extraction using enzyme or mechanical methods [33]. Rather than culturing in a dish, which creates a dead space underneath, it is preferable to rest solid tissues on porous hydrophobic membranes covered with a film of medium. Since only a small fraction of the total number spontaneously start to grow in vivo on a given day, it is fortunate that the transition to the primary follicle stage is up-regulated in culture, for reasons that are still not entirely clear although local factors evidently operate [9, 34, 35]. A balance exists between inhibitory factors, notably phosphatase and tensin homolog (PTEN) and anti-Müllerian hormone (AMH), as opposed to stimulatory factors, such as mTOR [36]. In future, this growth wave might be reinforced pharmacologically [37].

Culture media

In the absence of detailed knowledge of follicle metabolism, culture media were first chosen for a broad spectrum of constituents to ensure that all cellular needs were met. But this strategy was likely to expose cells to compounds or concentrations they are not normally exposed to, which is more likely in media originally developed for non-mammalian species (e.g., Medium 199 with Earle's salts formulated for chick embryonic fibroblasts). Nowadays, chemically simpler media, such as Minimal Essential Medium (MEM) Eagle, are preferred although versions enriched with non-essential amino acids, vitamins, and nucleosides are often used to satisfy growth requirements (e.g., α-MEM). Nevertheless, all media provide the same basic requirements, namely, a physiologically balanced salt solution with glucose for energy and bicarbonate-CO_2 as a buffer system. They generally contain serum (either fetal or donor calf in origin), which is heat-inactivated to destroy complement activity and renders the need for supplements of micronutrients, trace minerals and perhaps even growth factors somewhat less important.

Transitioning to chemically defined conditions offers many benefits, including more rigorous interpretation of experimental data and greater safety for clinical applications. Use of serum-free media with recombinant proteins to replace natural sources eliminates potential risks of xenobiotic contamination from unknown compounds, viruses, and prions. Recombinant gonadotropins are the prime examples, but not all proteins of potential value are available in this form. Fetuin, a multifunctional, calcium-binding protein used to inhibit zona hardening in serum-free cultures, is still derived from serum sources. With exceptions, follicle cultures succeed better with serum, homologous sources being preferred, but the goal is universal serum-free conditions.

Intact follicles require more complex media than cleaving embryos, which carry the nutrient and informational molecules for the first 3–5 days of development when little or no net growth occurs. GOCs are expected to have less stringent requirements in culture than whole follicles, and grow successfully in serum-free conditions without FSH [8, 33]. Common replacements for serum in these cultures are human or bovine albumin plus a mixture of insulin, selenium, and transferrin, marketed in a fixed composition known as "ITS." Whether transferrin is necessary in the presence of expression by granulosa cells is unclear, and concentrations of insulin and selenite must negotiate a narrow range between sufficiency and overstimulation. Pyruvate, a requirement for oocyte metabolism and possibly other functions, is often present in the basic formula but is also secreted by cumulus cells [38]. While neither the rate of follicle growth nor estradiol production was affected by ascorbate, it protected the basal lamina of intact follicles and may serve as a beneficial antioxidant when serum is absent [39]. Oocytes in GOC cultures often undergo spontaneous germinal vesicle breakdown, which can be inhibited by hypoxanthine to maintain elevated cAMP levels in the cells until they are cytoplasmically mature [15].

FSH deserves special mention because physiological requirements for intact follicles are well understood [8, 25, 40]. FSH is an obligatory survival factor from the late secondary follicle stage (though not for GOCs) promoting antrum formation and enabling luteinizing hormone (LH)-induced ovulation [26]. Superphysiological FSH concentrations have often been used in culture, possibly because the threshold for biological actions was increased by diffusion across cell layers. High levels may, however, present a risk of premature differentiation, which is revealed by LH receptor expression, and the loss of cellular synchrony could impair oocyte quality [41]. Intact follicles reaching maturity can ovulate in vitro in response to LH although LH receptors are absent at earlier stages when this gonadotropin is not required [29, 42]. Epidermal growth factor (EGF) is required neither for ovulation nor for nuclear maturation, but is frequently added to improve cumulus expansion for IVF [43]. Whether FF-MAS, a follicular fluid sterol, provides any benefit is uncertain (see Chapter 10). Addition of estradiol, androstenedione, and progesterone has little impact, at least on mouse follicles, although high levels of estradiol impaired fertilization and affected global methylation [44]. In conclusion, endogenous production of steroids may be sufficient for auto- and paracrine functions, and supplementation might be detrimental.

Maintenance of pH close to neutrality, so critical for all mammalian cells, is determined by the CO_2–HCO_3^- balance except during culture preparation, when buffers should be compatible with ambient air. Monitoring pH changes with phenol red is more difficult in microdroplet cultures, for which alternative colorimetric methods or pH microelectrodes are sought. While follicles depend on glycolysis for their energy budget, oxygen is still essential for viability. Incubator concentrations vary from 5% to 20% oxygen depending on the type of culture, with intact follicles probably having a higher requirement [45–48]. Lastly, temperatures inside Graafian follicles have been recorded in some species to be lower than the body core, which was attributed to unknown endothermic processes [49]. Since IVM has produced optimal outcomes by incubating oocytes at 37 °C, it seems prudent to continue the same for all follicle stages.

Goals and outcomes

The first studies had comparatively modest aims. Growth of the oocyte, increased numbers of granulosa cells (or total DNA), and hormone secretion were all encouraging signs that development was proceeding normally, especially when matched by a physiological time frame. If oocytes failed to reach the same size as in vivo culture conditions were presumed to be suboptimal, even if they were becoming competent for resumption of meiosis, which is acquired stepwise. Germinal vesicle breakdown is a less reliable indicator than attaining metaphase II, which in turn is a weaker criterion than post-fertilization development. The gold standard is production of full-term, healthy offspring after IVG and IVM. This seemed a distant goal 20 years ago, at least for human primordial follicles, but live pups have been generated from small follicles of laboratory rodents from the early days, and technology is extending to other species, including humans.

Membrane, gel, and tube cultures have all produced apparently healthy pups from small- to mid-sized preantral follicles. It is difficult – perhaps pointless – to compare methods too strictly because the 'best' depends on the experimental goal, the species, and degrees of manipulative skill. If large numbers of competent oocytes are needed, they can be derived from GOCs from immature mouse ovaries [5]. Fetuin to inhibit zona hardening under serum-free conditions was necessary because mouse oocytes are extremely sensitive to conventional microinjection, requiring piezo-electric methods [50]. There would be wider application of this method if follicle harvesting was more productive in other species and at adult ages; nevertheless, GOCs have found roles in some studies of human and farm animal oocytes [8, 9].

Sometimes the chief goal is to create a physiological model for investigating follicle biology. Intact follicles, although in smaller numbers, serve very well, and the individual attention they demand suits the need for culturing more precious human and macaque oocytes. Preantral mouse follicles normally reach Graafian size after a week or two in culture (Figure 16.1E), when they become responsive to LH/hCG (human chorionic gonadotropin), producing metaphase II oocytes inside expanded cumulus cells, sometimes after ovulating into the medium [26]. Whether cultured in microwells or on culture plates, 50–80% of follicles grow under these conditions, with up to two-thirds reaching metaphase II after IVM for IVF, and 25% to close to 50% of 2-cell embryos becoming blastocysts [27, 28, 51]. It is clear, however, from GOCs that the oocyte does not have to develop inside an intact follicle to become fertile.

Nevertheless, alginate gels have become one of the preferred methods because of their versatility and support of normal follicular architecture. In 8–12 days, >80% of mouse follicles developed an antrum and secreted steroid hormones and 70% of oocytes reached metaphase II, with a similar percentage becoming 2-cell embryos from which a few pups were born [52]. Importantly, alginate encapsulation seems to succeed much better with primate follicles than agar or collagen gel [6, 7, 22].

Eppig and O'Brien were the first to produce a pup from an oocyte grown entirely in vitro from the primordial follicle stage [33]. Using a multiphase system, they initiated culture with ovarian fragments, transitioning to GOCs before IVM. The pup, eponymously called Eggbert, died as a young adult with obesity, diabetes, lymphosarcoma, and neurological problems, which raised concern about the general safety of IVG–IVM. But an optimized medium containing FSH, glucose, and ascorbate, with EGF at the final stage, so improved the outcome that a considerable number of healthy pups have now been produced [41, 53]. Initiating primordial follicle growth in tissue explants has become standard practice not only in rodents but for primates because it avoids damage at a tender stage [9, 54, 55]. But the problem of oocyte emission from damage to primordial follicles during their isolation might eventually be turned to an advantage if they can be recombined in a culture system that is easier to manage and avoids multiple stages.

Rodent follicles, so valuable for pioneering work, cannot serve as full and adequate models for every species. For one thing, their growth span is a mere fraction of that in primates and, for another, scheduling of oocyte growth, and probably imprinting too, is different. The most rapid phase of growth in mice occurs at the primordial-to-primary follicle transition when transcriptional activity is maximal [56], whereas oocyte growth in humans and farm animals is more gradual, continuing at antral stages, with meiotic competence acquired later. There is also a question of whether data from mice are even representative of the same species, since most studies were carried out with exceptionally vigorous F_1 hybrids. Nevertheless, this model has produced impressive results that paved the way for intermediate model species.

The ovaries of adult farm animals are valuable research models because they have bulky, fibrous stroma as in primates, but unlike primates they are freely available from abattoirs. Preantral sheep follicles (190–240 μm) isolated as GOCs for serum-free culture in multi-well plates grew in 30 days to ~1 mm with large oocytes, but were still too immature to resume meiosis [8]. Hirao *et al.* aspirated GOCs from small antral cow follicles for 14 days in plate cultures containing serum and polyvinylpyrrolidone (PVP) [40], which produced enlarged oocytes from which embryos and a live calf were generated. This result provided much encouragement, as have data from McLaughlin and Telfer working from the opposite end of the follicle spectrum. They used a two-stage system, transitioning from bovine cortical slices to isolated secondary follicles to obtain substantial oocyte growth in 2–3 weeks, depending on the balance of FSH and activin [10].

These advances provided leverage for progress with human and sub-human primate oocytes at the currently leading centers in Edinburgh and Northwestern Universities. Healthy young adult tissue consented for research is rare, but a few centers receive a trickle from patients undergoing ovarian tissue cryopreservation for fertility preservation, transgender operations, or even from ovarian biopsies during Caesarian section.

The Northwestern group used alginate encapsu lation to culture intact human follicles in the pres ence of FSH. Follicles grew from ~150 μm to antra stages, reaching 1 mm after 30 days but progress ing no further. Fully grown oocytes (130 μm) wer embedded in and connected to cumulus cells via TZP (Figure 16.1F) [57], and some were competent t resume meiosis to metaphase II. Typical profiles o steroid and protein hormone secretion were observe by assaying spent culture medium (Figure 16.1G) Follicle culture for 5 weeks or longer was also success ful for rhesus macaques in their collaborators' labo ratory in Oregon [58], taking technology beyond ear lier achievements made elsewhere with marmoset [59]. Since a few simian oocytes grown in vitro hav already reached the 8-cell stage, it will probably no be long before live-born monkeys are produced. For tunately for applications to fertility preservation, thes culture methods have succeeded almost as well wit cryopreserved tissue as fresh tissue, especially afte vitrification [60].

The Edinburgh group has made dramatic progres with human follicles grown by a different strategy [9 18, 36]. Primordial follicles initiated growth sponta neously in explants of cortical tissue: after a wee (longer periods caused excess necrosis) small follicle appeared at the surface which could be dissected fo transfer to V-wells for a further 10 days in cultur before extraction as GOCs (Figure 16.3). This proto col generated antral follicles secreting steroids wit a growing, morphologically normal oocyte, but at a faster rate than has been estimated in vivo. Accelerate development could be an advantage, but oocyte qual ity requires close examination. Since follicles grow a different rates in vivo, perhaps because of their loca tion in the ovarian parenchyma, accelerated growt may be more apparent than real by representing th extreme end of the distribution where inhibitory con straints are minimal.

The genuine optimism that now instills this fiel should be guarded. Demonstration of fertility in ani mal models is only a first step, and oocytes that hav reached advanced post-fertilization stages are still a tiny minority of the numbers started in culture. Sinc material is so scarce, high efficiency and quality ar everything for a human oocyte technology. Even i short-term cultures for IVM, only 40–80% of huma oocytes are competent, and clinical pregnancy rate vary between centers [61]. Moreover, the overlap o IVG with a critical period for imprinting is worryin

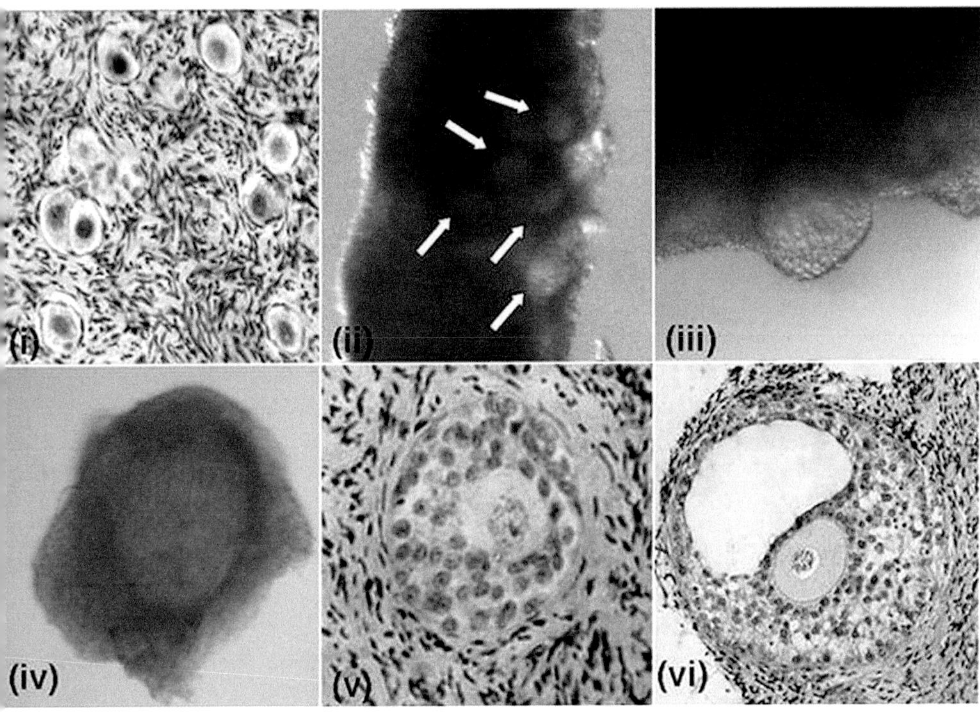

igure 16.3 (i) A cluster of quiescent follicles in freshly fixed human ovary. (ii) After 6 days in culture, growing follicles *(arrows)* appeared on ne surface of a cultured fragment of human ovarian cortex. (iii) A growing follicle protrudes from the edge of a fragment of cultured human ortex. (iv) Secondary follicle with a presumptive theca layer revealed by dissection after culture. (v) Histology of a secondary follicle growing 1 a cortical fragment after 6 days in culture. (vi) Histology of a small antral follicle after a total of 10 days in tube culture [18]. Reprinted with ind permission from *Seminars in Reproductive Medicine*.

see Chapter 37), and safety has been questioned for ome methods [62]. While limited evidence to date for VG and IVM is mostly reassuring [63], sub-human rimate models will be very important for assessing he physical health and behavior of offspring generted by these techniques. Screening the epigenome and nonitoring cardiovascular and metabolic factors will e priorities too, while the briefer lives of rodents proide early opportunities to test fertility and determine ongevity and causes of death. But in view of other ssisted reproductive technologies (ARTs) revealing he "forgiving nature" of the reproductive system, we an hope that safe protocols for IVG–IVM will evenually be found.

Germline stem cells (GSCs)

Vhen a mature technology is available for growing ocytes routinely from the primordial follicle stage o competent gametes, the next goal will be to generate them from earlier stages in the germ line. The potential gain is huge because GSCs can proliferate, which could at last make more eggs available for applications. Recent progress gives hope that a technology can be realized, although the sources of precursor cells are still debated.

When mouse embryonic stem cells (ESCs) were first isolated three decades ago they were shown to contribute to the germ line of chimeras, but only in the past decade has the existence of GSCs in differentiating cultures been noted [64, 65]. The first observations were hard to reproduce and the cells never progressed further than early meiosis, perhaps because factors needed for germ cell differentiation were absent, for example bone morphogenetic protein 4 (BMP4). But under more physiological conditions the original findings have confirmed beyond reasonable doubt that primordial germ cells are present in embryoid bodies from ESCs, where they intermingle among early somatic lineages. When putative GSCs were flow-sorted to separate them from pluripotent stem cells, then transplanted with somatic cells from neonatal ovaries to immunodeficient mice, structures resembling unilaminar follicles were formed, although development was stalled [66].

In the past year, however, the full potency of ESC-derived germ cells has been proven in both sexes by Hayashi *et al.* [67]. *Blimp1* and *Stella* reporter genes were used in epiblast cell cultures, representing the niche from which germ cells originate in vivo [68]. By aggregating candidate GSCs with day 13 fetal ovarian cells after flow-sorting, followed by a further period in culture with transplantation to a host mouse, germinal vesicle stage oocytes were obtained. Although the size and ploidy of the oocytes were sometimes abnormal, embryos generated after IVM and IVF became healthy offspring after transfer to host uteri.

Any strategy for utilizing ESCs will need to overcome some major obstacles, both technical and ethical, before patient-specific oocytes can be created for clinical treatment. The generation of ESCs for patients will require somatic cell nuclear transfer (SCNT), which was recently demonstrated using donor oocytes after a long quest [69]. It seems perverse to use precious donor oocytes for this purpose when they are desperately needed for the highly successful and standard practice of egg donation.

A remarkable solution to this dilemma was presented in the same paper reporting live offspring from ESC-derived germ cells [67]. By creating induced pluripotent stem cells (iPSCs) from embryonic fibroblasts expressing a *Pou5fl* reporter gene to identify candidate GSCs by flow-sorting, followed by culture and transplantation, fertile oocytes were generated. Their genetic provenance was confirmed after IVF by genotyping the pups, which were proven fertile and had normal imprints. It is too early to predict the future course and prospect of this technology until this breakthrough is confirmed, but the practical advantages of iPSCs are obvious, not least the abundance of potential precursor cells and avoidance of donor oocytes for SCNT.

Before closing, it is important to note recent claims that GSCs persist in postnatal ovaries, which conflict with a large body of experimental and clinical evidence since Zuckerman's seminal paper showing that oogenesis is restricted to pre- or perinatal life [70]. New data from adult mice [71, 72] and more limited observations from adult human ovaries [73] suggest that GSC candidate cells isolated using antibodies to the germ cell-specific protein, DDX4, form colonies in culture that can generate oocytes after transplantation. In one study the oocytes generated full-term offspring [72]. Like the studies of ESCs and iPSCs, these data await confirmation from independent laboratories before we can be sure of the best path to a new technology for oogenesis. At least they give greater confidence than the surprising finding of oocyte-like cells emerging spontaneously and rapidly in vitro from supposedly sterile organs, which we presume to be culture artifacts [74, 75]. Eventually, the strategies that require transplantation to realize fertility will no longer be needed to bridge stages that are difficult to culture. Then we can hope to witness the emergence of a complete technology for oogenesis, unfolding another revolution in reproductive technology.

Acknowledgments

Many scientists are engaged in developing these technologies, but Roger Gosden would like to acknowledge with gratitude those who have worked with him on this endeavor: Ronit Abir, Nicola Boland, J.-P. de Bruin, John Carroll, Helen Picton, Alison Murray, Helen Newton, Norah Spears, Evelyn Telfer, and Colin Torrance.

References

1. Gosden R, Lee B. Portrait of an oocyte: our obscure origin. *J Clin Invest* 2010; **120**: 973–83.
2. Edwards RG. Maturation in vitro of mouse, sheep, cow, pig, rhesus monkey and human ovarian oocytes. *Nature* 1965; **208**: 349–51.
3. Lambalk CB, de Koning CH, Flett A, *et al.* Assessment of ovarian reserve. Ovarian biopsy is not a valid method for the prediction of ovarian reserve. *Hum Reprod* 2004; **19**: 1055–9.
4. Manabe N, Goto Y, Matsuda-Minehata F, *et al.* Regulation mechanism of selective atresia in porcine follicles: regulation of granulosa cell apoptosis during atresia. *J Reprod Dev* 2004; **50**: 493–514.
5. Eppig JJ, Schroeder AC. Capacity of mouse oocytes from preantral follicles to undergo embryogenesis and development to live young after growth, maturation, and fertilization in vitro. *Biol Reprod* 1989; **41**: 268–76.
6. Roy SK, Greenwald GS. Hormonal requirements for the growth and differentiation of hamster preantral follicles in long-term culture. *J Reprod Fertil* 1989; **87**: 103–14.

7. Torrance C, Telfer E, Gosden RG. Quantitative study of the development of isolated mouse pre-antral follicles in collagen gel culture. *J Reprod Fertil* 1989; **87**: 367–74.

8. Newton H, Picton H, Gosden RG. In vitro growth of oocyte-granulosa cell complexes isolated from cryopreserved ovine tissue. *J Reprod Fertil* 1999; **115**: 141–50.

9. Telfer EE, McLaughlin M, Ding C, *et al.* A two-step serum-free culture system supports development of human oocytes from primordial follicles in the presence of activin. *Hum Reprod* 2008; **23**: 1151–8.

0. McLaughlin M, Telfer EE. Oocyte development in bovine primordial follicles is promoted by activin and FSH within a two-step serum-free culture system. *Reproduction* 2010; **139**: 971–8.

1. Honda A, Hirose M, Inoue K, *et al.* Large-scale production of growing oocytes in vitro from neonatal mouse ovaries. *Int J Dev Biol* 2009; **53**: 605–13.

2. Gosden RG, Mullan J, Picton HM, *et al.* Current perspective on primordial follicle cryopreservation and culture for reproductive medicine. *Hum Reprod Update* 2002; **8**:105–10.

3. Picton HM, Danfour MA, Harris SE, *et al.* Growth and maturation of oocytes in vitro. *Reprod Suppl* 2003; **61**: 445–62.

4. Roy SK, Greenwald GS. An enzymatic method for dissociation of intact follicles from the hamster ovary: histological and quantitative aspects. *Biol Reprod* 1985; **32**: 203–15.

5. Eppig JJ, Downs SM. The effect of hypoxanthine on mouse oocyte growth and development in vitro: maintenance of meiotic arrest and gonadotropin-induced oocyte maturation. *Dev Biol* 1987; **119**: 313–21.

6. Lazzari G, Galli C, Moor RM. Centrifugal elutriation of porcine oocytes isolated from the ovaries of newborn piglets. *Anal Biochem* 1992; **200**: 31–5.

7. Oktay K, Nugent D, Newton H, *et al.* Isolation and characterization of primordial follicles from fresh and cryopreserved human ovarian tissue. *Fertil Steril* 1997; **67**: 481–6.

8. Telfer EE, McLaughlin M. In vitro development of ovarian follicles. *Semin Reprod Med* 2011; **29**: 15–23.

9. Dolmans MM, Michaux N, Camboni A, *et al.* Evaluation of Liberase, a purified enzyme blend, for the isolation of human primordial and primary ovarian follicles. *Hum Reprod* 2006; **21**: 413–20.

0. Kristensen SG, Rasmussen A, Byskov AG, *et al.* Isolation of pre-antral follicles from human ovarian medulla tissue. *Hum Reprod* 2011; **26**: 157–66.

21. Roy SK, Greenwald GS. Methods of separation and in-vitro culture of pre-antral follicles from mammalian ovaries. *Hum Reprod Update* 1996; **2**: 236–45.

22. Roy SK, Treacy BJ. Isolation and long-term culture of human preantral follicles. *Fertil Steril* 1993; **59**: 783–90.

23. Shikanov A, Xu M, Woodruff TK, *et al.* A method for ovarian follicle encapsulation and culture in a proteolytically degradable 3 dimensional system. *J Vis Exp* 2011; (49): doi:pii: 2695. 10.3791/2695.

24. Desai N, Abdelhafez F, Calabro A, *et al.* Three dimensional culture of fresh and vitrified mouse pre-antral follicles in a hyaluronan-based hydrogel: a preliminary investigation of a novel biomaterial for in vitro follicle maturation. *Reprod Biol Endocrinol* 2012; **10**: 29.

25. Nayudu PL, Osborn SM. Factors influencing the rate of preantral and antral growth of mouse ovarian follicles in vitro. *J Reprod Fertil* 1992; **95**: 349–62.

26. Boland NI, Humpherson PG, Leese HJ, *et al.* Pattern of lactate production and steroidogenesis during growth and maturation of mouse ovarian follicles in vitro. *Biol Reprod* 1993; **48**: 798–806.

27. Spears N, Boland NI, Murray AA, *et al.* Mouse oocytes derived from in vitro grown primary ovarian follicles are fertile. *Hum Reprod* 1994; **9**: 527–32.

28. Cortvrindt R, Smitz J, Van Steirteghem AC. In-vitro maturation, fertilization and embryo development of immature oocytes from early preantral follicles from prepubertal mice in a simplified culture system. *Hum Reprod* 1996; **11**: 2656–66.

29. Cortvrindt R, Hu Y, Smitz J. Recombinant luteinizing hormone as a survival and differentiation factor increases oocyte maturation in recombinant follicle stimulating hormone-supplemented mouse preantral follicle culture. *Hum Reprod* 1998; **13**: 1292–302.

30. Hu Y, Cortvrindt R, Smitz J. Effects of aromatase inhibition on in vitro follicle and oocyte development analyzed by early preantral mouse follicle culture. *Mol Reprod Dev* 2002; **61**: 549–59.

31. Muruvi W, Picton HM, Rodway RG, *et al.* In vitro growth of oocytes from primordial follicles isolated from frozen-thawed lamb ovaries. *Theriogenology* 2005; **64**: 1357–70.

32. Hornick JE, Duncan FE, Shea LD, *et al.* Isolated primate primordial follicles require a rigid physical environment to survive and grow in vitro. *Hum Reprod* 2012; **27**: 1801–10.

33. Eppig JJ, O'Brien MJ. Development in vitro of mouse oocytes from primordial follicles. *Biol Reprod* 1996; **54**: 197–207.

34. Nilsson EE, Skinner MK. Kit ligand and basic fibroblast growth factor interactions in the induction of ovarian primordial to primary follicle transition. *Mol Cell Endocrinol* 2004; **214**: 19–25.

35. Carlsson IB, Laitinen MP, Scott JE, *et al.* Kit ligand and c-Kit are expressed during early human ovarian follicular development and their interaction is required for the survival of follicles in long-term culture. *Reproduction* 2006; **131**: 641–9.

36. Telfer EE, McLaughlin M. Strategies to support human oocyte development in vitro. *Int J Dev Biol* 2013; **56**: 901–7.

37. Li J, Kawamura K, Cheng Y, *et al.* Activation of dormant ovarian follicles to generate mature eggs. *Proc Natl Acad Sci USA* 2010; **107**: 10280–4.

38. Harris SE, Leese HJ, Gosden RG, *et al.* Pyruvate and oxygen consumption throughout the growth and development of murine oocytes. *Mol Reprod Dev* 2009; **76**: 231–8.

39. Murray AA, Molinek MD, Baker SJ, *et al.* Role of ascorbic acid in promoting follicle integrity and survival in intact mouse ovarian follicles in vitro. *Reproduction* 2001; **121**: 89–96.

40. Hirao Y, Itoh T, Shimizu M, *et al.* In vitro growth and development of bovine oocyte-granulosa cell complexes on the flat substratum: effects of high polyvinylpyrrolidone concentration in culture medium. *Biol Reprod* 2004; **70**: 83–91.

41. Eppig JJ, O'Brien MJ, Pendola FL, *et al.* Factors affecting the developmental competence of mouse oocytes grown in vitro: follicle-stimulating hormone and insulin. *Biol Reprod* 1998; **59**: 1445–53.

42. Spears N, Murray AA, Allison V, *et al.* Role of gonadotrophins and ovarian steroids in the development of mouse follicles in vitro. *J Reprod Fertil* 1998; **113**: 19–26.

43. Boland NI, Gosden RG. Effects of epidermal growth factor on the growth and differentiation of cultured mouse ovarian follicles. *J Reprod Fertil* 1994; **101**: 369–74.

44. Murray AA, Swales AK, Smith RE, *et al.* Follicular growth and oocyte competence in the in vitro cultured mouse follicle: effects of gonadotrophins and steroids. *Mol Hum Reprod* 2008; **14**: 75–83.

45. Smitz J, Cortvrindt R, Van Steirteghem AC. Normal oxygen atmosphere is essential for the solitary long-term culture of early preantral mouse follicles. *Mol Reprod Dev* 1996; **45**: 466–75.

46. Cecconi S, Barboni B, Coccia M, *et al.* In vitro development of sheep preantral follicles. *Biol Reprod* 1999; **60**: 594–601.

47. Gigli I, Byrd DD, Fortune JE. Effects of oxygen tension and supplements to the culture medium on activation and development of bovine follicles in vitro. *Theriogenology* 2006; **66**: 344–53.

48. Hirao Y, Shimizu M, Iga K, *et al.* Optimization of oxygen concentration for growing bovine oocytes in vitro: constant low and high oxygen concentrations compromise the yield of fully grown oocytes. *J Reprod Dev* 2012; **58**: 204–11.

49. Hunter RH, Grøndahl C, Greve T, *et al.* Graafian follicles are cooler than neighbouring ovarian tissues and deep rectal temperatures. *Hum Reprod* 1997; **12**: 95–100.

50. Liu J, Rybouchkin A, Van der Elst J, *et al.* Fertilization of mouse oocytes from in vitro-matured preantral follicles using classical in vitro fertilization or intracytoplasmic sperm injection. *Biol Reprod* 2002; **67**: 575–9.

51. Adriaens I, Cortvrindt R, Smitz J. Differential FSH exposure in preantral follicle culture has marked effects on folliculogenesis and oocyte developmental competence. *Hum Reprod* 2004; **19**: 398–408.

52. Xu M, Kreeger PK, Shea LD, *et al.* Tissue-engineered follicles produce live, fertile offspring. *Tissue Eng* 2006 **12**: 2739–46.

53. O'Brien MJ, Pendola JK, Eppig JJ. A revised protocol for in vitro development of mouse oocytes from primordial follicles dramatically improves their developmental competence. *Biol Reprod* 2003; **68**: 1682–6.

54. Wandji SA, Srsen V, Nathanielsz PW, *et al.* Initiation of growth of baboon primordial follicles in vitro. *Hum Reprod* 1997; **12**: 1993–2001.

55. Picton HM, Gosden RG. In vitro growth of human primordial follicles from frozen-banked ovarian tissue *Mol Cell Endocrinol* 2000; **166**: 27–35.

56. Pan H, O'Brien MJ, Wigglesworth K, *et al.* Transcript profiling during mouse oocyte development and the effect of gonadotropin priming and development in vitro. *Dev Biol* 2005; **286**: 493–506.

57. Xu M, Barrett SL, West-Farrell E, *et al.* In vitro grown human ovarian follicles from cancer patients support oocyte growth. *Hum Reprod* 2009; **24**: 2531–40.

58. Xu J, Xu M, Bernuci MP, *et al.* Primate follicular development in vitro. In: Kim S, ed. *Oocyte Biology in Fertility Preservation*. New York, NY: Springer Science Business Media, 2013 (in press).

59. Nayudu PL, Wu J, Michelmann HW. In vitro development of marmoset monkey oocytes by pre-antral follicle culture. *Reprod Domest Anim* 2003; **38**: 90–6.

0. Ting AY, Yeoman RR, Lawson MS, *et al.* In vitro development of secondary follicles from cryopreserved rhesus macaque ovarian tissue after slow-rate freeze or vitrification. *Hum Reprod* 2011; **26**: 2461–72.

1. Nogueira D, Sadeu JC, Montagut J. In vitro oocyte maturation: current status. *Semin Reprod Med* 2012; **30**: 199–213.

2. Mainigi MA, Ord T, Schultz RM. Meiotic and developmental competence in mice are compromised following follicle development in vitro using an alginate-based culture system. *Biol Reprod* 2011; **85**: 269–76.

3. Anckaert E, De Rycke M, Smitz J. Culture of oocytes and risk of imprinting defects. *Hum Reprod Update* 2013; **19**: 52–66.

4. Hübner K, Fuhrmann G, Christenson LK, *et al.* Derivation of oocytes from mouse embryonic stem cells. *Science* 2003; **300**: 1251–6.

5. Geijsen N, Horoschak M, Kim K, *et al.* Derivation of embryonic germ cells and male gametes from embryonic stem cells. *Nature* 2004; **427**: 148–54.

6. Nicholas CR, Haston KM, Grewall AK, *et al.* Transplantation directs oocyte maturation from embryonic stem cells and provides a therapeutic strategy for female infertility. *Hum Mol Genet* 2009; **18**: 4376–89.

7. Hayashi K, Ogushi S, Kurimoto K, *et al.* Offspring from oocytes derived from in vitro primordial germ cell-like cells in mice. *Science* 2012; **338**: 971–5.

68. Huang Y, Osorno R, Tsakiridis A, *et al.* In vivo differentiation potential of epiblast stem cells revealed by chimeric embryo formation. *Cell Rep* 2012; **2**: 1571–8.

69. Tachibana M, Amato P, Sparman M, *et al.* Human embryonic stem cells derived by somatic cell nuclear transfer. *Cell* 2013; **153**: 1228–38.

70. Zuckerman S. The number of oocytes in the mature ovary. *Recent Prog Horm Res* 1951; **6**: 63–109.

71. Johnson J, Canning J, Kaneko T, *et al.* Germline stem cells and follicular renewal in the postnatal mammalian ovary. *Nature* 2004; **428**: 145–50.

72. Zou K, Yuan Z, Yang Z, *et al.* Production of offspring from a germline stem cell line derived from neonatal ovaries. *Nat Cell Biol* 2009; **11**: 631–6.

73. White YA, Woods DC, Takai Y, *et al.* Oocyte formation by mitotically active germ cells purified from ovaries of reproductive-age women. *Nat Med* 2012; **18**: 413–21.

74. Dyce PW, Wen L, Li J. In vitro germline potential of stem cells derived from fetal porcine skin. *Nat Cell Biol* 2006; **8**: 384–90.

75. Virant-Klun I, Zech N, Rožman P, *et al.* Putative stem cells with an embryonic character isolated from the ovarian surface epithelium of women with no naturally present follicles and oocytes. *Differentiation* 2008; **76**: 843–56.

Chapter 17

Metabolism of the follicle and oocyte in vivo and in vitro

Helen M. Picton and Karen E. Hemmings

Introduction

Oocyte metabolism reflects other aspects of the unique biology of this important cell type. The protracted process of mammalian oogenesis exacts a huge metabolic toll on the presumptive gamete. To ensure that the nutritional needs of oocytes are met oogenesis occurs in concert with folliculogenesis. Folliculogenesis is a lengthy process beginning with a primordial oocyte surrounded by a small number of flattened pregranulosa cells and ending with the ovulation of a fully grown, metaphase II oocyte, some weeks or months later. Throughout their development, oocytes and follicle cells are physically and metabolically linked via a complex network of homologous and heterologous gap junctions [1]. Metabolic coupling of oocytes and somatic cells facilitates the transfer of molecules of <1 kDa, including ions, amino acids, pyruvate and glucose, molecules such as adenosine triphosphate (ATP) [2], and other signaling molecules and meiosis-arresting signals from the somatic compartment of the follicle to the oocyte and *vice versa* to provide the physiological basis for oocyte and follicle development [3]. While the metabolic cooperativity between oocytes and their companion granulosa cells is dynamic, discrete differences exist between the nutritional needs of oocytes and somatic granulosa cells and throughout their development oocytes are exposed to a changing nutritional environment as the follicular cells undergo proliferation, antral cavity formation, differentiation, and ovulation. In turn, oocytes have been shown to regulate apoptosis and cholesterol biosynthesis and metabolism by the follicular cells and so impact on follicular development [4].

Efforts to understand the metabolic and nutritional requirements of follicles and oocytes have tended to focus on the carbohydrate metabolism of fully grown oocytes during the final stages of meiotic maturation in vitro. While follicular metabolism is the sum of the net metabolism of the oocyte and its surrounding complement of somatic cells, such measurements mask the metabolic contribution and requirements of the oocyte. As a result the majority of the metabolic studies of oocytes across the different stages of follicle development have been conducted on denuded gametes, which may subject the cell to stresses and unphysiological deprivations of nutrients and signaling molecules. Nevertheless, studies of denuded oocytes are valuable and have revealed that oocyte metabolism plays a critical role in supporting oocyte nuclear and cytoplasmic maturation and subsequent developmental competence via multiple mechanisms. During the final stages of maturation, cumulus–oocyte complexes (COCs) require a range of substrates, including fatty acids, amino acids, electrolytes, purines and pyrimidines, and other metabolites [5–9]. In marked contrast, knowledge of the patterns of metabolic activity in immature oocytes and early stage follicles is far more limited and has largely been pieced together from a small number of studies of glucose and pyruvate metabolism during the in vitro growth of murine follicles or the culture of the individual cellular compartments which make up the follicle. Collectively the analysis of metabolism during follicle and oocyte development indicates that the metabolic needs and energy sources for these different cell types change during growth and differentiation and are influenced by both systemic hormones and local regulatory peptides (Figure 17.1). This chapter will therefore focus on the metabolic pathways present in oocytes and their supporting follicular granulosa cells and will explore how metabolism changes during follicle and oocyte growth and maturation in vivo and in vitro.

Biology and Pathology of the Oocyte, 2nd edn., ed. Alan Trounson, Roger Gosden, and Ursula Eichenlaub-Ritter.
Published by Cambridge University Press.

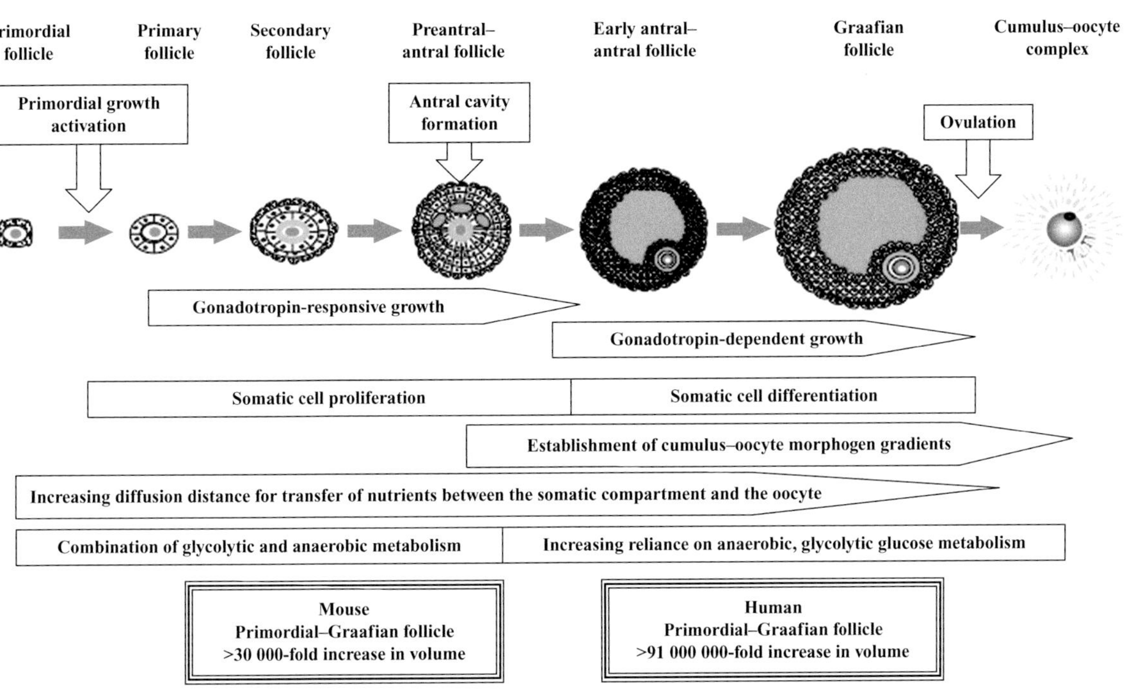

'igure 17.1 Overview of energy metabolism during key developmental events in mammalian folliculogenesis.

Metabolic pathways utilized by oocytes and ovarian follicles

:nergy metabolism

The metabolic needs of both the oocyte and its companion follicular cells must be met to support the production of a fertile gamete. Both pyruvate and glucose are important energy sources for these cell types. Glucose is metabolized via either glycolysis or the tricarboxylic acid (TCA) cycle. Glycolysis involves the stepwise breakdown of glucose into two molecules of the α-keto acid pyruvate. When oxygen is plentiful, aerobic glucose metabolism is possible and the net yield of pyruvate produced by glycolysis is metabolized through the TCA cycle to produce energy in the form of ATP. Alternatively, under anaerobic conditions pyruvate is less efficiently converted to lactate by the cytosolic enzyme lactate dehydrogenase. The glycolytic pathway therefore accounts for a large proportion of glucose metabolism by COCs and the production of ATP and metabolites such as pyruvate and lactate that can be readily utilized by the oocyte [10–12]. Additionally, a limited amount of glucose can be metabolized by the pentose phosphate pathway (PPP) to produce NADPH which is utilized for cytoplasmic integrity and redox state through the reduction of glutathione and ribose-5-phosphate which can either re-enter the glycolytic pathway or be used for nucleotide biosynthesis and the control of nuclear maturation. Glucose can also be utilized for nucleic acid and purine synthesis [13] and, via the hexosamine biosynthesis pathway (HBP), it can be used for *O*-linked glycosylation of proteins and the synthesis of extracellular matrix [14]. Finally, under hyperglycemic conditions the polyol pathway in granulosa cells can oxidize glucose to sorbitol and fructose so providing oocytes with a potential alternative energy source [14].

Glucose enters cells by sodium-coupled glucose transporters (SGLTs) or through sodium-independent, facilitative glucose transporters (GLUTs) [15]. Although SGLTs have been detected in oocytes most evidence suggests that their role is minimal in this cell type [16]. In contrast, multiple members of the GLUT gene family are expressed in reproductive cells and a few play key roles in the production of a fertile gamete [16]. For example, the glucose transporter genes *Slc2a1–2, Slc2a4–10* are expressed in murine oocytes, whereas *SLC2A1, SLC2A3* and *SLC2A8* are expressed by ovine, bovine, primate, and human oocytes [17–19]. Cumulus cells express an additional transporter gene – *SLC2A4* [20]. Glucose uptake by granulosa cells is known to be regulated by the pituitary gonadotropins luteinizing hormone (LH) and follicle-stimulating hormone (FSH) and by moderate oxygen tension [12, 21, 22]. Furthermore, glucose transporters SLC2A4 and SLC2A8 are sensitive to regulation by insulin and a collection of insulin signaling genes consistent with the presence of the phosphatidylinositol 3-kinase (PI3K)/AKT-dependent signaling pathways that have been reported in primate and murine oocytes [3, 19, 23].

Pyruvate is widely acknowledged to be the preferred energy substrate for mammalian oocytes. Indeed, the requirement of oocytes for pyruvate may originate in the primordial germ cells [24]. Oxidation of pyruvate through the TCA cycle and oxidative phosphorylation results in much greater ATP production than glycolysis; it is essential for the completion of oogenesis and serves as a vital source of energy for the nuclear and cytoplasmic maturation of oocytes [25]. Oocyte ATP concentration increases during maturation [26] and in some, but not all species, ATP concentrations are associated with oocyte developmental competence [27]. In mature human oocytes, for example, gametes with >2 pmol ATP/oocyte have a greater potential for development and implantation [28]. Although pyruvate is their preferred substrate, the machinery for glycolytic metabolism is present in oocytes and both pyruvate and glucose carrier-mediated uptake have been demonstrated [12, 29, 30]. Oocyte glucose consumption may be important for species such as pigs and rhesus monkeys and the presence of hexose kinase [31], glucose-6-phosphate dehydrogenase [32], and the PPP all suggest a possible involvement of glucose metabolism in some oocyte functions. However, oocytes from the majority of mammalian species, including humans, have been shown to have very limited capacity for glucose uptake and metabolism [10, 12, 30, 33–35]. Manipulation of the PPP has been shown to affect oocyte meiotic progression, and developmental competence [10]; however, this pathway only accounts for <3% of the small amount of glucose metabolized by murine oocytes [34]. Additionally, oocytes demonstrate low levels of phosphofructokinase activity, which is a rate-limiting enzyme in the glycolytic pathway [36], with the consequence that oocytes have a low glycolytic capacity [11]. When glucose uptake occurs naturally in COCs, the nutrient is first taken up by the cumulus cell's GLUT system before being transferred to the oocyte via gap junctions, where it is metabolized to pyruvate or lactate before it can be utilized by the oocyte [3, 14].

Oocyte metabolism is influenced by a number of different factors, including the mixture of exogenous nutrients either in the follicular environment in vivo or the culture medium in vitro, as well as oxygen levels; the rate of conversion of nutrients in the cytoplasm to substrates that can feed the TCA cycle; and the number, distribution, and activity of key organelles such as mitochondria [37, 38]. While oocytes are reliant upon mitochondrial ATP production to ensure their growth and development, at the same time excessive mitochondrial energy production in oocytes can lead to the generation of reactive oxygen species (ROS), which if left unchecked can lead to oxidative damage, impaired mitochondrial function, and free radical formation, all of which can adversely affect oocyte health [39]. Interestingly, some energy substrates such as pyruvate can act as free radical scavengers and so may help protect the cells from the damaging effects of ROS [40].

Other endogenous energy stores such as glycogen and lipids may be used as building blocks for oocyte growth and development in some species. Although relatively little is known about lipid metabolism as an energy source during oocyte development, the close proximity between lipid droplets and mitochondria during oocyte maturation suggests that fatty acid oxidation may be a source of ATP during gamete production [7, 8]. In cow and pig oocytes lipid droplets accumulate during oogenesis and fatty acid oxidation generates high numbers of ATP molecules, making lipids a potentially valuable energy source for oocyte growth and maturation. Furthermore, in support of this idea, the triglyceride content of porcine and bovine oocytes decreased and lipase activity increased during oocyte in vitro maturation (IVM) [7, 36]. However, it must be noted that oocyte lipid content varies greatly between species. Nevertheless the up-regulation of the β-oxidation pathway is required for meiotic resumption during the IVM of murine oocytes [41–43]. Finally, oocyte lipid metabolism has been shown to be hormonally regulated in vivo [42, 44].

Amino acid metabolism

Amino acids serve many roles in cells. Some amino acids, such as glutamine and glycine, act as energy substrates in the TCA cycle [35] while others such as glycine, alanine, and glutamate function as chelators of heavy metal ions or osmolytes, or they facilitate intracellular pH regulation and the elimination of ammonia [45]. Little is known about amino acid metabolism across oogenesis and folliculogenesis. Radioactive tracer studies have identified approximately 18 amino acid transport systems in murine oocytes and embryos, indicating the capacity of these cells for amino acid uptake [46, 47]. Metabolic cooperativity exists between cumulus cells and oocytes with regard to the uptake of some, but not all, amino acids. Indeed, cumulus-enclosed mouse oocytes take up more radiolabeled glycine, alanine, proline, serine, tyrosine, glutamate, and lysine than their denuded counterparts [48]. In contrast, cooperativity does not appear to exist for the uptake of valine, leucine, and phenylalanine. An increased activity of some of the enzymes involved in amino acid metabolism, such as aspartate- and alanine-aminotransferase and malate dehydrogenase, has been observed in cumulus cells [49]. These enzymes mediate the production of substrates for the TCA cycle such as pyruvate, oxaloacetate, and malate, forming the malate–aspartate shuttle, which is important for the transfer of NADH between the mitochondria and the cellular cytosol. During folliculogenesis the uptake of key amino acids also varies between preantral, antral, and preovulatory stages of follicle development [50] and appears to be dependent on oocyte maturational status [49, 46].

Details of the amino acid transporter systems present in mammalian oocytes and follicular cells are limited. Amino acid transporters generally transport groups of multiple related amino acids as defined by the transporter's substrate binding site structure. A transporter of the L system is thought to be responsible for the amino acid uptake observed in denuded oocytes [48]. Further work has demonstrated that the oolemma of growing murine oocytes possesses both system L and system ASC transporter activity, with system L being the more prevalent [46, 51]. While the uptake of amino acids by the cumulus cells is an energy-requiring process, growing oocytes retain the capacity to fine tune the balance between the external environment and free amino acid intracellular pools with minimal energy expenditure [51]. System A and N transporters couple the transport of amino acids with that of Na^+ ions. Transcripts encoding the β subunit are present in the oocyte and early embryo; however, the α subunit required for expression is not expressed until the blastocyst stage [52]. The lack of a functional Na^+/K^+ATPase pump in oocytes means that uptake of glutamine must occur via another system. Although the activity of the system A and N transporters has not yet been confirmed in mammalian oocytes [46], *Slc38a3* has been found to be strongly expressed in the cumulus cells of murine oocytes and expression is strong in fully grown germinal vesicle (GV) stage oocytes, but not growing oocytes [53]. The presence of mRNA encoding *Slc7a1* and *Slc7a2* has been identified in murine oocytes [47, 54] whereas *SLC7A9* appears to be highly expressed in human metaphase II (MII) oocytes [55]. These cationic amino acid transporters transport arginine, lysine, and ornithine however they have differing affinities for each amino acid [56]. Recent research on germinal vesicle (GV) and bovine MII oocytes and cumulus and mural granulosa cells has confirmed the presence of mRNA encoding *SLC7A1–3, SLC7A5–7, SLC3A2,* and *SLC7A9* in mature oocytes and has detected the expression of *SLC7A1, SLC7A2, SLC7A5, SLC38A2,* and *SLC38A5* in cumulus cells, and *SLC7A1, SLC7A2, SLC7A5,* and *SLC38A2* in granulosa cells (Figure 17.2). In order for *SLC7A5–8* to be active the transporters must be expressed in conjunction with their corresponding heavy chain *SLC3A2* [57]. Expression of *SLC7A6* and *SLC7AY,* also referred to as system *y*+L, mediates the transfer of arginine and lysine. The data in Figure 17.2 also support the idea that the granulosa cells play a key role in transporting nutrients to the oocyte during maturation.

Metabolism during follicle and oocyte development and maturation

Primordial follicles and oocytes

Primordial follicles are the most abundant stage of follicle development present in the mammalian ovary. Primordial follicles form the building blocks of the ovarian reserve and are characterized by the presence of a central oocyte arrested at prophase I of meiosis, surrounded by flattened pregranulosa cells [58]. It has long been considered that primordial follicles are metabolically quiescent. However, for their size, these follicles exhibit relatively high levels of metabolism in order to remain viable for extended periods and to facilitate the conduct of essential subcellular "housekeeping" activities such as transcription and

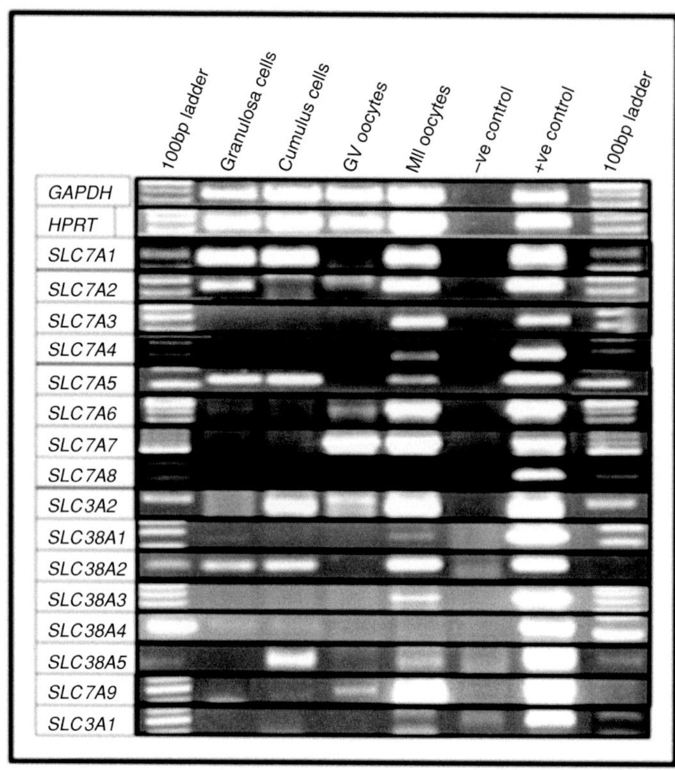

Figure 17.2 Patterns of amino acid transporter transcript RNA expression in bovine oocytes, granulosa cells, and cumulus cells as determined by RT-PCR.

translation, protein synthesis, and sodium pumping. Furthermore, using mouse cells as a model for mammalian oogenesis, measurement of carbohydrate metabolism by intact primordial follicles has revealed that these cells consume glucose and pyruvate in relatively large amounts and produce lactate [59]. As the primordial oocyte occupies a large proportion of the volume of each primordial follicle, it is tempting to speculate that it is the oocyte that drives pyruvate consumption by primordial follicles and that the fate of this pyruvate is oxidation. Indeed, the potential ATP produced by oxidation of pyruvate would more than cover the energy demands of protein synthesis at this stage of development. However, when oocyte volume is taken into account, primordial oocyte pyruvate consumption is higher than during the later stages of oocyte development and maturation (Figures 17.3A and 17.3B). Importantly, denuded primordial oocytes do not take up glucose [60] due to insufficient glucose transporters, hexose kinase, or phosphofructokinase [61, 62]. This evidence suggests that glucose consumption by primordial follicles is due to the presence of the pregranulosa cells rather than to the oocyte.

Although primordial follicles maintain the capacity for both glycolytic and aerobic metabolism, anaerobic glycolysis appears to be the major fate of any glucose taken up at this stage of follicle development [59]. Indeed, the amount of pyruvate consumption by primordial follicles in vitro is two times greater than the amount of glucose consumed, demonstrating that in addition to glycolysis, energy production in primordial follicles also occurs via pathways such as the TCA cycle. Furthermore, as lactate production by cultured primordial follicles exceeds that which can be generated from glucose alone, additional energy substrates such as glycogen may also be metabolized by primordial follicles. It is also possible that some of the pyruvate consumed by primordial follicles is converted to lactate which is subsequently exported to help regulate intracellular pH [63]. Alternatively lactate may be mobilized from intracellular glycogen stores as required.

Growing follicles and oocytes

Once primordial follicle growth has been initiated, the granulosa cells proliferate, forming multilaminar, preantral follicles which subsequently form a

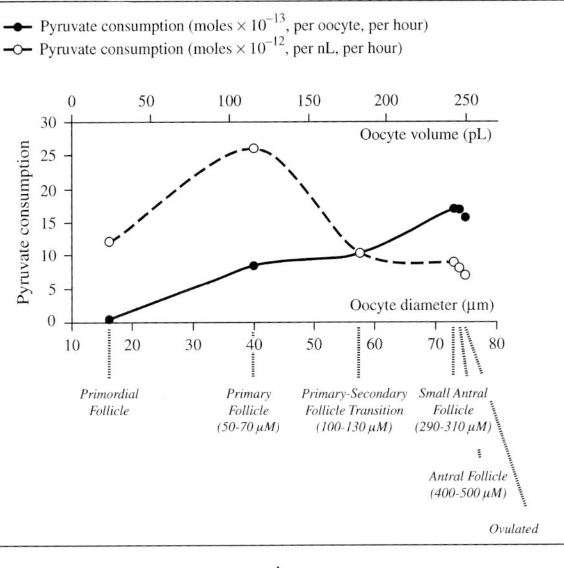

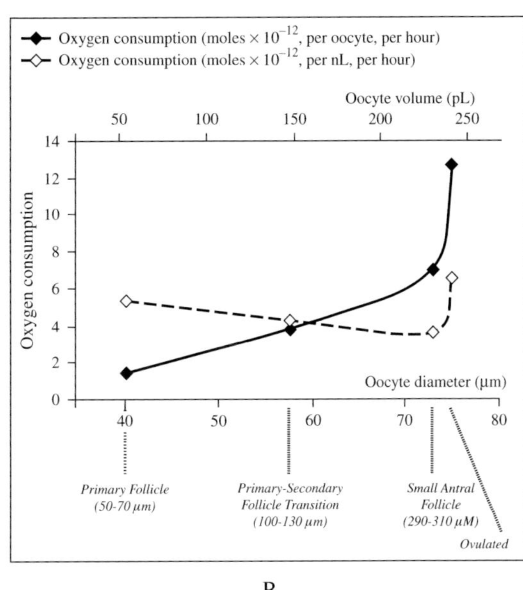

igure 17.3 Rates of pyruvate (A) and oxygen (B) consumption by non-growing, growing and mature mouse oocytes. Reproduced from larris and Picton [59] with permission.

luid-filled antral cavity and a vascularized theca layer. ollicular growth is a lengthy process and in long-lived pecies such as humans, sheep, and cattle it may take 6– months to complete with the majority of this time (3 nonths) being spent in the preantral stages of development [64]. Preantral follicle development is accompanied by oocyte growth during which time the oocytes teadily accumulate RNA and proteins required to support meiotic maturation and fertilization of the preumptive gamete as well as early embryogenesis prior o embryonic genome activation. Oocyte growth is lso accompanied by the replication and redistribution f key cytoplasmic organelles such as the mitochonria, endoplasmic reticulum and cortical granules all f which are vital to the acquisition of oocyte develpmental competence (see Chapter 18 of this volume or further details). A continuous supply of nutrients nd energy is required to support both the growth proesses themselves and the evolution of differentiated unction in the different cellular compartments of the ollicle.

Oocytes are obligate aerobes. Consequently, growng oocytes consume large amounts of pyruvate and xygen, whereas glucose consumption is frequently oo low to be detectable [30, 59]. Indeed, developing nouse oocytes show a steady increase in pyruvate and xygen consumption which parallels the increases in ocyte size as growth progresses (Figure 17.3) [12]. Consumption peaks during the resumption of meiosis in the mature gamete. Interestingly, when gamete substrate consumption/production is corrected for oocyte volume, primary oocytes are found to consume four times more pyruvate than ovulatory oocytes (Figure 17.3) [59]. The high levels of pyruvate and oxygen consumed by growing oocytes suggest that the TCA cycle coupled with highly efficient oxidative phosphorylation are the major ATP-contributing pathways during growth rather than glycolysis or the PPP [34, 65]. Indeed, accelerated metabolism is immediately needed to sustain the increases in protein and RNA synthesis which follow the activation of primordial growth as well as the longer-term synthesis and accumulation of the molecules required for gamete developmental competence [66]. Pyruvate may also act as a free radical scavenger during follicle and oocyte growth [40]. In addition to pyruvate, growing oocytes take up many other substrates to supplement energy production, including the amino acids alanine, lysine, choline, glycine, and histidine [48, 53].

With regard to the regulation of metabolism during follicular development, following the activation of primordial growth, glucose consumption and lactate production appear to increase as follicle development progresses beyond preantral and antral stages and into the periovulatory period [11]. By quantifying the amount of glucose consumed that accounts for lactate production it is possible to access the relative contribution of glycolysis to glucose metabolism during follicle growth. Accordingly, measurement of metabolism in murine preantral/early antral follicles in vitro suggests that in preantral follicles with two to four layers of granulosa cells where oxygen is not limiting, glycolytic glucose metabolism is not a major contributor to follicular energy production [11]. However, as the number of granulosa cell layers increases so the distance between the oocyte and its follicular blood supply extends and antral cavity formation occurs. Nutrient and oxygen diffusion gradients are established across the granulosa cell compartment [67]. To accommodate the energy demands of the oocyte as folliculogenesis progresses beyond antrum formation follicles switch their metabolic strategy and become increasingly reliant upon glycolytic glucose breakdown [11]. By the late stages of antral follicle development in mice, anaerobic glycolysis accounts for 76–100% of glucose metabolism [11, 12]. This strategy has the advantage that it conserves oxygen for use by the oocyte, whose ATP production is predominantly confined to the catabolism of pyruvate. Recent evidence suggests that the oocyte plays a key role in pushing this follicular metabolic switch [68, 69]. The establishment of gradients of oocyte-derived growth factors helps to define the steroidogenic and metabolic phenotype of the somatic cells in the immediate vicinity of the oocyte [69]. In support of this idea cumulus cells' cholesterol metabolism and glycolysis appear to be modulated by differential gradients of oocyte-secreted factors such as growth differentiation factor 9 [68, 69]. Several additional lines of evidence support the idea of metabolic cooperativity between the cellular compartments during growth and the switch to glycolytic glucose metabolism as development progresses beyond antrum formation. Measurement of the nutrient composition of follicular fluid indicates that the pyruvate content can be several-fold higher than that found in blood [70, 71], whereas the glucose concentration of follicular fluid is substantially lower than that of plasma and is inversely related to lactate content [72]. During growth, oocytes promote the uptake of amino acids, including glutamate, histidine, and alanine, by cumulus cells which are then transferred to the oocyte via heterologous gap junctions [53]. Finally, the follicular endocrine environment regulates somatic glucose consumption. For example, FSH has been shown to promote metabolism in cultured rat granulosa cells [73] as well as murine and bovine COCs [14, 74]. Gonadotropin-stimulated follicular glucose metabolism is influenced by insulin [75] and ovarian growth factors [76, 77] and these endocrine effects appear to be mediated by alteration of the expression and translocation of glucose transporters to the cell membrane [78] as well as the increased activity of glucose metabolic pathways [74, 79].

The periovulatory period

The final stages of preovulatory follicle development are characterized by cellular processes which require increased ATP production. During the terminal stages of murine and bovine COC development oxygen consumption decreases just as glycolytic activity increases [10] and ovarian glucose uptake peaks [11]. Indeed during ovulation induction in mouse follicles in vitro glucose consumption and lactate production are enhanced by up to twofold. Both FSH and LH stimulate glucose consumption by murine and bovine COCs [10, 14]. Just as occurs during growth these actions are mediated by the up-regulation of glucose transporters [80] and glycolytic enzymes [79]. Indeed, translocation of GLUT4 to the cell membrane [78] and hexose kinase activity increase in response to FSH, which provides intermediates for glycolysis, the TCA cycle, and the PPP [74]. The principal metabolic consequence of FSH in vitro is to alter the glycolytic rate of the cumulus cells of mature COCs, while oocyte-derived regulatory factors such as bone morphogenetic protein 15 act via the cumulus cells to regulate oxidative phosphorylation in the oocyte [81]. The preovulatory peak in follicular lactate production serves to increase the lactate concentration in follicular fluid so pushing down the pH of the fluid bathing the oocyte. It has been shown that the meiotic maturation of the murine COCs is suppressed in more acidic conditions [82].

The availability and utilization of glucose and pyruvate are vital during the terminal stages of oocyte development as the concentrations and combinations of these nutrients affect cumulus expansion, oocyte meiotic progression, and ultimately oocyte developmental competence. Indeed the nuclear status of the oocyte determines both the pyruvate consumption and turnover of key amino acids [9, 11, 35]. Overall an increased consumption of oxidizable substrates is required during oocyte maturation to facilitate spindle formation, chromosome condensation and segregation, protein synthesis, and extrusion of the first polar body. To support these increased energy demands cumulus cells have been shown to produce increased pyruvate from glucose in response to stimulation by FSH, which creates a localized increase in pyruvate in the immediate vicinity of the oocyte [74]. The increased supply of pyruvate may also serve to reduce oxidative stress in the gamete during the periovulatory period. During oocyte maturation cumulus glucose and glutamine support the synthesis of purines. Similarly, within the oocyte the increased activity of the PPP generates a precursor of phospho-ribosyl-pyrophosphate which is an essential metabolite for *de novo* purine synthesis [83, 84]. The timing and duration of these synthetic activities determines whether oocyte meiotic resumption will be suppressed or promoted [85]. Finally, the up-regulation of β-oxidation of fatty acids during oocyte maturation may increase the availability of glucose for non-ATP-producing pathways such as redox regulation, nucleic acid production and hyaluronic acid synthesis, and cumulus expansion [44]. Once meiotic maturation has been completed the metabolic needs and hence pyruvate consumption by the COCs drop [86, 87] while glycolytic activity increases substantially, suggesting that the mature cumulus–oocyte complex becomes more reliant upon glycolytic, rather than oxidative, glucose metabolism [10].

Future prospects and clinical implications

An improved understanding of the metabolic processes associated with follicle and oocyte growth and maturation has many clinical applications. Indeed, oocyte metabolic competence and the accumulation of oxidative damage are key factors in defining oocyte quality. In pathologies affecting metabolism, such as diabetes or polycystic ovary syndrome (PCOS), follicle and oocyte metabolism may be perturbed. Indeed, glucose uptake has recently been shown to be aberrant in oocytes collected from infertile women with PCOS [30]. In COCs from diabetic mice FSH-stimulated PPP activity is compromised as during hyperglycemia, hexose kinase becomes saturated, which forces glucose along the alternative polyol metabolic pathway which generates molecules which suppress meiotic maturation [88, 89]. Defects of oocyte meiotic regulation in these animals can also be attributed to reduced communication between the somatic and germ cell compartments, decreased *de novo* purine and cAMP production, as well as structural, spatial, and metabolic dysfunction of oocyte mitochondria that leads to spindle defects and chromosome misalignment [90]. Cultures of bovine follicles deprived of insulin have impaired maturation rates compared to their insulin-treated counterparts [91].

A detailed knowledge of oocyte and granulosa metabolism during oocyte growth and meiotic maturation is highly relevant to human assisted reproductive technology and will support the development of new generation culture media to improve the efficiency of the IVM and fertilization of oocytes. In recent years the non-invasive measurement of energy and protein metabolism has attracted significant interest as a potential strategy for assessment of the developmental competence of oocytes and embryos in humans and other mammalian species [92]. Recently, the turnover of key amino acids during the IVM of bovine oocytes has been found to be predictive of oocyte fertile potential and developmental competence prior to activation of the embryonic genome [9]. Furthermore, while the potential for the in vitro growth and maturation of mammalian follicles and oocytes for fertility preservation strategies is well recognized [93], this goal is only likely to be achieved if these technologies are underpinned by a detailed understanding of the nutritional and metabolic needs of oocytes and follicles across all stages of development [11]. Indeed, the concentration of glucose and the rapidity of nutrient uptake and depletion from the culture environment itself may regulate oocyte metabolic activity and so have a profound impact on the subsequent oocyte nuclear and cytoplasmic maturation and developmental competence. Furthermore, the ratio of nutrients such as lactate and pyruvate and the oxygen tension during culture must be balanced so as to avoid altering the redox state of the presumptive gamete. More extensive studies of the nutrient requirements of large animal and human oocytes and follicles across oogenesis and folliculogenesis are therefore needed if the therapeutic potential of in vitro growth and maturation of oocytes is ever to be realized.

References

1. Kidder GM, Vanderhyden BC. Bidirectional communication between oocytes and follicle cells: ensuring oocyte developmental competence. *Can J Physiol Pharmacol* 2010; **88**: 399–413.

2. Heller DT, Schultz RM. Ribonucleoside metabolism by mouse oocytes: metabolic cooperativity between the fully grown oocyte and cumulus cells. *J Exp Zool* 1980; **214**: 355–64.

3. Wang Q, Chi MM, Schedl T, *et al.* An intracellular pathway for glucose transport into mouse oocytes. *Am J Physiol Endocrinol Metab* 2012; **302**: E1511–18.

4. Su YQ, Suguira K, Eppig JJ. Mouse oocytes control granulosa cell development and function: paracrine regulation of cumulus cell metabolism. *Semin Reprod Med* 2009; **27**: 32–42.

5. Homa ST Racowsky C, McGaughley RW. Lipid analysis of immature pig oocytes. *J Reprod Fertil* 1986; **77**: 425–34.

6. McEvoy TG, Coull GD, Broadbent PJ, *et al.* Fatty acid composition of lipids in immature cattle, pig and sheep oocytes with intact zona pellucida. *J Reprod Fertil* 2000; **118**: 163–70.

7. Ferguson EM, Leese HJ. A potential role for triglyceride as an energy source during bovine oocyte maturation and early embryo development. *Mol Reprod Dev* 2006; **73**: 1195–201.

8. Sturmey RG, Reis A, Leese HJ, *et al.* Role of fatty acids in energy provision during oocyte maturation and early embryo development. *Reprod Domest Anim* 2009; **44** Suppl 3: 50–8.

9. Hemmings KE, Leese HJ, Picton HM. Amino acid turnover by bovine oocytes provides an index of oocyte developmental competence in vitro. *Biol Reprod* 2012; **86**: 165, 1–12.

10. Downs SM, Utecht AM. Metabolism of radio labelled glucose by mouse oocytes and oocyte cumulus cell complexes. *Biol Reprod* 1999; **60**: 1446–52.

11. Harris SE, Adriens I, Leese HJ, *et al.* Carbohydrate metabolism by murine ovarian follicles and oocytes grown *in vitro*. *Reproduction* 2007; **134**: 415–24.

12. Harris SE, Leese HJ, Gosden RG, *et al.* Pyruvate and oxygen consumption throughout the growth and development of murine oocytes. *Mol Reprod Dev* 2009; **76**: 231–8.

13. Sutton ML, Gilchrist RB, Thompson JG. Effects of in vivo and in vitro environments on the metabolism of the cumulus-oocyte complex and its influence on oocyte developmental capacity. *Hum Reprod Update* 2003; **9**: 35–48.

14. Sutton-McDowall ML, Gilchrist RB, Thompson JG. The pivotal role of glucose metabolism in determining oocyte developmental competence. *Reproduction* 2010; **139**: 685–95.

15. Wood IS, Trayhurn P. Glucose transporters (GLUT and SGLT): expanded families of sugar transport proteins. *Br J Nutr* 2003; **89**: 3–9.

16. Purcell SH, Moley KH. Glucose transporters in gametes and preimplantation embryos. *Trends Endocrinol Metab* 2009; **20**: 483–9.

17. Dan-Goor M, Sasson S, Davarashvili A. Expression of glucose transporter and glucose uptake in human oocytes and preimplantation embryos. *Hum Reprod* 1997; **12**: 2508–10.

18. Augustin R, Pocar P, Navarrete-Santos A, *et al.* Glucose transporter expression is developmentally regulated in in vitro derived bovine preimplantation embryos. *Mol Reprod Dev* 2001; **60**: 370–6.

19. Zheng P, Vasenna R, Latham KE. Effects of *in vitro* oocyte maturation and embryo culture on the expression of glucose transporters, glucose metabolism and insulin signalling in rhesus monkey oocytes and preimplantation embryos. *Mol Hum Reprod* 2007; **13**: 361–71.

20. Nishimoto H, Matsutani R, Yamamoto S, *et al.* Gene expression of glucose transporter (GLUT) 1, 3 and 4 in bovine follicle and corpus luteum. *J Endocrinol* 2006; **188**: 111–19.

21. Seamark RF, Amoto F, Hendrickson S, *et al.* Oxygen uptake, glucose utilization, lactate release and adenine nucleotide content of sheep ovarian follicles in culture effect of human chorionic goadotrophin. *Aust J Biol Sc* 1976; **29**: 557–63.

22. Boland NJ, Humpherson PG, Leese HJ, *et al.* The effec of glucose metabolism on murine follicle development and steroidogenesis *in vitro*. *Hum Reprod* 1994; **9**: 617–23.

23. Benomar Y, Naour N, Aubourg A, *et al.* Insulin and leptin induce Glut4 plasma membrane translocation and glucose uptake in a human neuronal cell line by a phosphatidylinositol 3-kinase-dependent mechanism. *Endocrinology* 2006; **147**: 2550–6.

24. Brinster RL, Harstad H. Energy metabolism in primordial germ cells of the mouse. *Exp Cell Res* 1997; **109**: 111–17.

25. Johnson NT, Freeman EA, Gardner DK, *et al.* Oxidative metabolism of pyruvate is required for meiotic maturation of murine oocytes *in vivo*. *Biol Reprod* 2007; **77**: 2–8.

26. Duran HE, Simsek-Duran F, Oehninger SC, *et al.* The association of reproductive senescence with mitochondrial quantity, function, and DNA integrity in human oocytes at different stages of maturation. *Fertil Steril* 2011; **96**: 384–8.

7. Krisher RL, Brad AM, Herrick JR, *et al.* A comparative analysis of metabolism and viability in porcine oocytes during in vitro maturation. *Anim Reprod Sci* 2007; **98**: 72–96.

8. Van Blerkom J, Davis PW, Lee J. ATP content of human oocytes and developmental potential and outcome after in vitro fertilization and embryo transfer. *Hum Reprod* 1995; **10**: 415–24.

9. Hardy K, Hooper MA, Handyside AH, *et al.* Non-invasive measurement of glucose and pyruvate uptake by individual human oocytes and preimplantation embryos. *Hum Reprod* 1989; **4**: 188–91.

0. Harris SE, Maruthini D, Tang T, *et al.* Metabolism and karyotype analysis of oocytes from patients with PCOS. *Hum Reprod* 2010; **25**: 2305–15.

1. Tsutsumi O, Yano T, Satoh K, *et al.* Studies of hexose kinase activities in human and mouse oocytes. *Am J Obstet Gynecol* 1990; **162**: 1301–4.

2. Mangia F, Epstein CJ. Biochemical studies of growing mouse oocytes: preparation of oocytes and analysis of glucose-6-phosphate dehydrogenase and lactate dehydrogenase activities. *Dev Biol* 1975; **45**: 211–20.

3. Biggers JD, Whittingham DG, Donahue RP. The pattern of energy metabolism in the mouse oocyte and zygote. *Zoology* 1967; **58**: 560–7.

4. Urner F, Sakkas D. A possible role for the pentose phosphate pathway of spermatogenesis in gamete fusion in the mouse. *Biol Reprod* 1999; **60**: 733–9.

5. Reiger D, Luskutoff N. Changes in the metabolism of glucose, pyruvate, glutamine and glycine during maturation of cattle oocytes in vitro. *J Reprod Fertil* 1994; **100**: 257–62.

6. Cetica P, Pintos L, Dalvit G, Beconi M. Activity of key enzymes involved in glucose and triglyceride metabolism during bovine oocyte maturation in vitro. *Reproduction* 2002; **124**: 675–81.

7. Wilding M, Dale B, Marino M, *et al.* Mitochondrial aggregation patterns and activity in human oocytes and preimplantation embryos. *Hum Reprod* 2001; **16**: 909–17.

8. Almeida Santos T, El Shourbagy S, St John JC. Mitochondrial content reflects oocytes variability and fertilisation outcome. *Fertil Steril* 2005; **85**: 584–91.

9. Van Blerkom J. Mitochondria in human oogenesis and preimplantation embryogenesis: engines of metabolism, ionic regulation and developmental competence. *Reproduction* 2004; **128**: 269–80.

0. O'Donnel-Tormey J, Nathan CF, Lanks K, *et al.* Secretion of pyruvate. An antioxidant defence of mammalian cells. *J Exp Med* 1987; **165**: 500–14.

41. Downs SM, Mosey JL, Klinger J. Fatty acid oxidation and meiotic resumption in mouse oocytes. *Mol Reprod Dev* 2009; **76**: 844–53.

42. Dunning JR, Cashman K, Russell DL, *et al.* Beta-oxidation is essential for mouse oocyte developmental competence and early embryo development. *Biol Reprod* 2010; **83**: 909–18.

43. Somfai T, Kaneda M, Akagi S, *et al.* Enhancement of lipid metabolism with L-carnitine during in vitro maturation improves nuclear maturation and cleavage ability of follicular porcine oocytes. *Reprod Fertil Dev* 2011: **23**: 912–20.

44. Sutton-McDowell ML, Feil D, Robker RL, *et al.* Utilisation of endogenous fatty acid stores for energy production in bovine preimplantation embryos. *Theriogenology* 2012; **77**: 1632–41.

45. Leese HJ. Metabolism of the preimplantation mammalian embryo. *Oxf Rev Reprod Biol* 1991; **13**: 35–72.

46. Pelland AMD, Corbett HE, Baltz JM. Amino acid transport mechanisms in mouse oocytes during growth and meiotic maturation. *Biol Reprod* 2009; **81**: 1041–54.

47. Van Winkle LJ. Amino acid transport regulation and early embryo development. *Biol Reprod* 2001; **64**: 1–12.

48. Colonna R, Mangia F. Mechanisms of amino acid uptake in cumulus enclosed mouse oocytes. *Biol Reprod* 1983; **28**: 797–803.

49. Cetica P, Pintos L, Dalvit G, Beconi M. Involvement of enzymes of amino acid metabolism and tricarboxylic acid cycle in bovine oocyte maturation in vitro. *Reproduction* 2003; **126**: 753–63.

50. Chand AR, Legge M. Amino acid transport system L activity in developing mouse ovarian follicles. *Hum Reprod* 2011; **26**: 3102–8.

51. Colonna R, Cecconi S, Buccione R, Mangia F. Amino acid transport systems in growing mouse oocytes. *Cell Biol Int Rep* 1983; **7**: 1007–15.

52. Watson AJ, Pape C, Emanuel JR, Levenson R, Kidder GM. Expression of Na, K-ATPase alpha subunit and beta subunit genes during preimplantation development of the mouse. *Dev Genet* 1990; **11**: 41–8.

53. Eppig JJ, Pendola FL, Wigglesworth K, Pendola JK. Mouse oocytes regulate metabolic cooperativity between granulosa cells and oocytes: amino acid transport. *Biol Reprod* 2005; **73**: 351–7.

54. Choi HW, Shin MR, Lee HS, *et al.* Differential expression of amino acids transporter genes in mouse blastocysts and embryonic stem cells. *Fertil Steril* 2005; **84**: S393–4.

55. Bermudez M, Wells D, Malter H, *et al.* Expression profiles of individual human oocytes using microarray technology. *Reprod Biomed Online* 2004; **8**: 325–37.

56. Closs EI, Simon A, Vekony N, Rotmann A. Plasma membrane transporters for arginine. *J Nutr* 2004; **134**: 2752S–9S.

57. Verrey F, Meier C, Rossier G, Kuhn LC. Glycoprotein-associated amino acid exchangers: broadening the range of transport specificity. *Pflugers Arch* 2000; **440**: 503–12.

58. Picton HM. Activation of follicle development: the primordial follicle, its activation and possible use as source of female genetic material. *Theriogenology* 2001; **55**: 1193–210.

59. Harris SE, Picton HM. Metabolism of follicles and oocytes during growth and maturation. In: Tan SL, Chian RC, Buckett W, eds. *In-Vitro Maturation of Human Oocytes: Basic Science to Clinical Application.* Oxon: Informa Health. 2007; 15–36.

60. Eppig J. Analysis of mouse oogenesis *in vitro*. Oocyte isolation and the utilization of exogenous energy sources by growing oocytes. *J Exp Zool* 1976; **198**: 375–82.

61. Barbehenn EK, Wales RG, Lowry OH. The explanation for the blockade of glycolysis in early mouse embryos. *Proc Natl Acad Sci USA* 1974; **71**: 1056–60.

62. Barbehenn EK, Wales RG, Lowry OH. Measurement of metabolites in single preimplantation embryos; a new means to study metabolic control in early embryos. *J Embryol Exp Morphol* 1978; **43**: 29–46.

63. Butcher L, Coates A, Martin KL, *et al.* Metabolism of pyruvate by the early human embryo. *Biol Reprod* 1998; **58**: 1054–6.

64. Gougeon A. Regulation of ovarian follicular development in primates – facts and hypotheses. *Endocr Rev* 1996; **17**: 121–55.

65. Dumollard R, Duchen M, Carroll J. The role of mitochondrial function in the oocyte and embryo. *Curr Top Dev Biol* 2007; **77**: 21–49.

66. Conti M, Hsieh M, Zamah AM, *et al.* Novel signaling mechanisms in the ovary during oocyte maturation and ovulation. *Mol Cell Endocrinol* 2012; **356**: 65–73.

67. Gosden RG, Byatt-Smith JG. Oxygen concentration gradient across the ovarian follicular epithelium: model, predictions and implications. *Hum Reprod* 1986; **1**: 65–8.

68. Sugiura K, Pendola FL, Eppig JJ. Oocyte control of metabolic cooperativity between oocytes and companion granulosa cells: energy metabolism. *Dev Biol* 2005; **279**: 20–30.

69. Gilchrist RB, Lane M, Thompson JG. Oocyte secreted factors: regulators of cumulus function and oocyte quality. *Hum Reprod Update* 2008; **14**: 159–77.

70. Harris SE, Gopichandran N, Picton HM, *et al.* Nutrient concentrations in murine follicle, oviduct and uterine fluids. *Theriogenology* 2005; **64**: 992–1006.

71. Orsi NM, Gopichandran N, Leese HJ, *et al.* Fluctuations in bovine ovarian follicular fluid composition throughout the oestrous cycle: a comparison with plasma and a TCM-199-based maturation medium. *Reproduction* 2005; **192**: 219–28.

72. Leese HJ, Lenton EA. Glucose and lactate in human follicular fluid: concentration and inter relationships. *Hum Reprod* 1990; **5**: 915–19.

73. Hillier SG, Purohit A, Reichert LE, Jr. Control of granulosa cell lactate production by follicle-stimulating hormone and androgen. *Endocrinology* 1985; **116**:1163–7.

74. Downs SM, Humpherson PG, Martin KL, *et al.* Glucose utilization during gonadotropin-induced meiotic maturation in cumulus cell-enclosed mouse oocytes. *Mol Reprod Dev* 1996; **44**: 121–31.

75. Lin Y, Fridstrom M, Hillensjo T. Insulin stimulation of lactate accumulation in isolated human granulosa-luteal cells: a comparison between normal and polycystic ovaries. *Hum Reprod* 1997; **12**: 2469–72.

76. Nilsson L. Acute effects of gonadotrophins and prostaglandins on the metabolism of isolated ovarian follicles from PMSG-treated immature rats. *Acta Endocrinol (Copenh)* 1974; **77**: 540–58.

77. Hillensjo T. Oocyte maturation and glycolysis in isolated pre-ovulatory follicles of PMS-injected immature rats. *Acta Endocrinol (Copenh)* 1976; **82**: 809–30.

78. Roberts R, Stark J, Iatropoulou A, *et al.* Energy substrate metabolism of mouse cumulus-oocyte complexes: response to follicle-stimulating hormone is mediated by the phosphatidylinositol 3-kinase pathway and is associated with oocyte maturation. *Biol Reprod* 2004; **71**: 199–209.

79. Roy SK, Terada DM. Activities of glucose metabolic enzymes in human preantral follicles: *in vitro* modulation by follicle-stimulating hormone, luteinizing hormone, epidermal growth factor, insulin-like growth factor I, and transforming growth factor beta1. *Biol Reprod* 1999; **60**: 763–8.

80. Brogan RS, MacGibeny M, Mix S, *et al.* Dynamics of intra-follicular glucose during luteinization of macaque ovarian follicles. *Mol Cell Endocrinol* 2011; **332**: 189–95.

81. Sutton-McDowall ML, Mottershead DG, Gardner DK, *et al.* Metabolic differences in bovine cumulus oocyte complexes matured in vitro in the presence or absence of follicle stimulating hormone and bone morphogenetic protein 15. *Biol Reprod.* 2012; **87**: 1–8.

82. Downs SM, Mastropolo AM. Culture conditions affect meiotic regulation in cumulus cell-enclosed mouse oocytes. *Mol Reprod Dev* 1997; **46**: 551–66.

83. Shim C, Lee DK, Lee CC, *et al.* Inhibitory effect of purines in meiotic resumption of denuded mouse oocytes. *Mol Reprod Dev* 1992; **314**: 280–6.

84. Downs SM. Adenosine blocks hormone-induced meiotic maturation by suppressing purine *de novo* synthesis. *Mol Reprod Dev* 2000; **56**: 172–9.

85. Downs SM, Verhoeven A. Glutamine and the maintenance of meiotic arrest in mouse oocytes: influences of culture medium, glucose and cumulus cells. *Mol Reprod Dev* 2003; **66**: 90–7.

86. Billig H, Magnusson C. Gonadotropin-induced inhibition of oxygen consumption in rat oocyte-cumulus complexes: relief by adenosine. *Biol Reprod* 1985; **33**: 890–8.

87. Downs SM, Houghton FD, Humpherson PG, *et al.* Substrate utilization and maturation of cumulus cell-enclosed mouse oocytes: evidence that pyruvate oxidation does not mediate meiotic induction. *J Reprod Fertil* 1997; **110**: 1–10.

88. Colton SA, Humpherson PG, Leese HJ, *et al.* Physiological changes in oocyte-cumulus cell complexes from diabetic mice that potentially influence meiotic regulation. *Biol Reprod* 2003; **69**: 761–70.

89. Colton SA, Downs SM. Potential role for the sorbitol pathway in the meiotic dysfunction exhibited by oocytes from diabetic mice. *J Exp Zool A Comp Exp Biol* 2004; **301**: 439–48.

90. Wang Q, Ratchford AM, Chi MM, *et al.* Maternal diabetes causes mitochondrial dysfunction and meiotic defects in murine oocytes. *Mol Endocrinol* 2009; **23**: 1603–12.

91. Landau S, Braw-Tal R, Kaim M, *et al.* Preovulatory follicular status and diet affect the insulin and glucose content of follicles in high-yielding dairy cows. *Anim Reprod Sci* 2000; **64**: 181–97.

92. Leese HJ. Metabolism of the preimplantation embryo: 40 years on. *Reproduction* 2012; **143**: 417–27.

93. Picton HM, Harris SE, Muruvi W, Chambers EL. The *in vitro* growth and maturation of follicles. *Reproduction* 2008; **136**: 703–15.

Section 3 Developmental biology

Chapter 18

Improving oocyte maturation in vitro

Jeremy G. Thompson and Robert B. Gilchrist

Introduction

Successful infertility treatment, especially in vitro fertilization (IVF) and accompanying clinical and laboratory technologies, has to be one of the great medical success stories of the late twentieth and early twenty-first centuries. In the space of 35 years of development, assisted reproduction through IVF now contributes up to 4% of all births in developed nations, with these figures set to increase further due to the influence of increasing maternal age to first conception, lifestyle choices, and the exposure to environmental toxins. The success of current technology utilized in an IVF cycle is dependent on gonadotropic hormone hyperstimulation of the ovary to generate large numbers of mature oocytes (Figure 18.1). Nevertheless, hormonal stimulation of the ovary by follicle stimulating hormone (FSH), or an analog, is associated with various risks and financial costs. These include: a health risk to women caused by severe ovarian hyperstimulation syndrome (OHSS), which affects 0.5–5% of gonadotropin-treated women [1]; a risk to oocyte and resulting embryo health (e.g., embryo aneuploidy [2] and perturbed genomic imprinting [3]); and a significant financial burden placed on couples and/or healthcare providers due to the cost of the gonadotropin treatment. Furthermore, FSH has dose-dependent adverse effects on subsequent embryo quality, endometrial protein expression, and pregnancy rates in adult, cycling female mice [4, 5]. Therefore, safe, reliable alternatives to the current clinical IVF practices that remove the need for hyperstimulatory FSH treatment, accompanied with increased treatment options for women, is highly attractive. This would be particularly so for women who suffer from the very prevalent condition of polycystic ovaries (estimated to be around 20% of women of reproductive age), who are particularly susceptible to OHSS and as a result, at times have limited IVF treatment options.

In vitro maturation of oocytes

Although the in vitro meiotic maturation of a mammalian oocyte was first described in the 1930s [6] it was not until 1984 that in vitro maturation (IVM) was shown to be able to support the birth of live (mouse) offspring [7]. It was a further 7 years before the first report of a successful human pregnancy to term was published in which the oocyte had been matured in vitro from unstimulated ovaries [8]. Today IVM is a highly successful procedure for advanced cattle artificial breeding, where an estimated half a million embryos are produced per annum [9]. However in humans, IVM is far less developed and less efficient, with rates of oocyte maturation, on-time embryo development, implantation, and live birth rates all notably lower than from oocytes matured in vivo. This poor performance of IVM relative to IVF has been the most significant factor preventing the widespread adoption of IVM into clinical practice. Much of this poor performance of IVM cycles relative to hyperstimulated IVF cycles has been attributed to the poor competence of the IVM-derived mature oocyte, even though initial fertilization and early development of meiotically matured IVM oocytes largely does not differ from hyperstimulated mature oocytes.

Why do IVM-derived oocytes have this reduced developmental capacity? Oocyte developmental competence (also described as "oocyte quality") refers to the biochemical and molecular state required of a mature oocyte to support development to firstly a differentiating embryo and ultimately a healthy infant at term [10]. Over many years of fundamental research this has been characterized as the synthesis of mRNA

Biology and Pathology of the Oocyte, 2nd edn., ed. Alan Trounson, Roger Gosden, and Ursula Eichenlaub-Ritter. Published by Cambridge University Press.

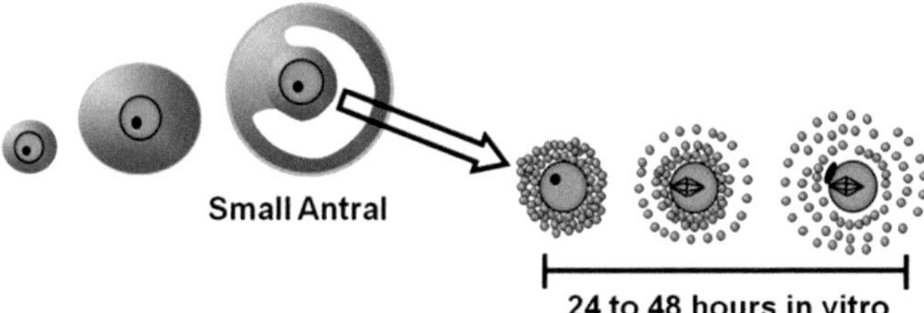

Figure 18.1 In vitro maturation (IVM) generates mature oocytes without patient hormone stimulation but oocytes are less developed at collection. In traditional IVF systems, which rely on ovarian hyperstimulation using follicle-stimulating hormone (FSH), oocytes are recovered after the ovulatory surge has been triggered in periovulatory (large) antral follicles. In contrast, IVM is conducted utilizing oocytes collected from (mostly) non-stimulated small antral follicles.

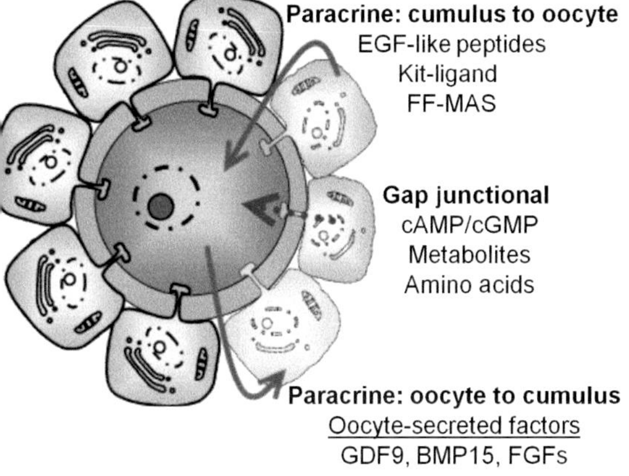

igure 18.2 Modes of cell–cell communication between the oocyte and surrounding cumulus cells in the cumulus–oocyte omplex (COC). Examples of factors which interact between these wo cell types are listed, but this is by no means a complete escription. Reprinted (with modifications from [22]) with ermission from Oxford University Press. BMP15, bone norphogenetic protein 15; EGF, epidermal growth factor; GDF9, rowth differentiation factor 9; FF-MAS, follicular fluid neiosis-activating sterol; FGFs, fibroblast growth factors.

nd proteins within the growing oocyte, whilst the oocyte itself is in an arrested stage of prophase 1 of neiosis, commonly known as the germinal vesicle GV) stage. Within the ovarian follicle, the oocyte is urrounded by specialized somatic cells, the cumulus ells, forming the cumulus–oocyte complex (COC). Bidirectional communication between the oocyte and surrounding cumulus cells, via physical contact (gap junctions) and two-way paracrine signaling, is essential for oocyte development (Figure 18.2) (for recent reviews see [11, 12]). Through gap junctions, cumulus cells provide the oocyte with both energy metabolites (e.g., [13]) and small signaling molecules for the control of maturation (e.g., cyclic adenosine 3′, 5′-monophosphate [cAMP] [14]). We and others have proposed that the impact of IVM under conditions where these signaling systems are not preserved is to rapidly silence them. This effect may be even more acute within oocytes collected from smaller follicles. Therefore, both the paracrine signaling between cumulus and the oocyte, as well as the physical connection allowing small-molecule exchange have, to us at least, been logical targets to focus on when considering mediators of oocyte developmental competence that may be manipulated to improve oocyte developmental competence during IVM.

Ovaries of women contain ~400 000 oocytes at puberty that have varying potential to mature, ovulate, fertilize, and develop into viable offspring. The great majority of oocytes fail to gain the opportunity to ovulate as only 0.1% are selected for this process. Ovarian hyperstimulation during IVF treatment exploits this by "rescuing" growing follicles from atresia during a wave of follicular development. It is well established across mammalian species, including humans, that

Table 18.1. Oocyte developmental competence is determined by follicle size, donor hormonal stimulation, and mode of oocyte maturation in all species studied

	In vitro maturation (IVM)		Conventional IVF
	Less developed COC[a]	**Developed COC[b]**	**Developed COC**
Hormonal stimulation of donor	None	Partial	Full
Follicle size at COC collection[c]	Small–medium antral	Medium antral	Large antral
Active oocyte transcription	Yes	Minimal	No
Oocyte dev. competence: blastocyst	Low	Moderate	High
Oocyte dev. competence: term	Low	Low	High

[a] COC is still not fully competent in vivo at collection – typical clinical IVM scenario.
[b] COC is fully competent in vivo at collection. Examples of this may include mild stimulation of patients or, in mouse oocyte biology, include the classic model of collecting COCs 46 hours after hyperstimulation of prepubertal mice with 5 IU eCG (equine chorionic gonadotropin).
[c] In patients: small–medium antral (4–10 mm), medium antral (10–14 mm), large antral (14–18 mm).

ovarian follicle size is associated with oocyte developmental competence, with the periovulatory follicle containing a fully grown and competent oocyte (Table 18.1). By contrast, there is minimal or no hormonal stimulation of the patient in clinical IVM, so most oocytes are collected from small antral follicles (5–12 mm in humans) [15]. These oocytes are generally fully grown but are nonetheless not fully developed or fully competent from a molecular perspective and as such have a poorer capacity to support embryo and fetal development compared to oocytes from periovulatory follicles (Table 18.1) [16, 17]. Therefore, a critical need in clinical IVM is to understand the molecular deficiencies in less developed COCs from small antral follicles and to facilitate capacitation of these oocytes in vitro.

Current clinical and laboratory practices in IVM

Although improved from early attempts, current implantation rates from clinical IVM remain low, at around 10–15% following embryo transfer on day 3, especially compared to best practice IVF rates (approximately 30–40% implantation rate). Furthermore, subsequent miscarriage rates remain higher than for IVF. Current typical practices for IVM in patients differ significantly from those conducted within other mammalian species. In particular, administering patients a large bolus of human chorionic gonadotropin (hCG), usually 10 000 IU, pioneered by Chian and Tan [18], has become a very common IVM practice over the past decade, but notably is unique to IVM in humans. Administration of hCG is conducted in acyclic polycystic ovary syndrome (PCOS) patients or in cycling patients where the lead (dominant) follicle is tracked, and reaches 10–12 mm in diameter, with oocyte retrieval conducted 36 hours later. This usually provides two types of oocytes: usually one or two that have expanding cumulus masses and have completed meiosis in vivo (correlating to those derived from the dominant and any other large follicle[s]), and a larger cohort of unexpanded cumulus-enclosed immature (GV or early GV breakdown [GVBD]) oocytes. The protocol requires two time points for cumulus cell removal and insemination (via intracytoplasmic sperm injection [ICSI]). For oocytes collected with an expanded cumulus mass, cumulus removal occurs at approximately 4 hours post-retrieval (to assess polar body extrusion, indicating meiosis completion to MII) and for oocytes with an unexpanded cumulus mass at collection; they are examined for MII at approximately 24–30 hours following retrieval [19]. In both cases, insemination only occurs if a polar body has been extruded and this may require further tracking of the oocyte up to 44 hours post-retrieval, with the latter stages of maturation for these oocytes conducted in the absence of cumulus cells. In all other species, and most notably in cattle, the bolus of hCG is not administered and oocytes can be collected at any stage of the cycle, although in cattle it is well known that oocyte collection in the presence of a large dominant follicle reduces developmental competence of oocytes from the smaller subordinate follicles [20]. The effect of the hCG bolus is controversial and largely unknown, as even 10–12 mm ovarian follicles should be refractory to hCG treatment, although clearly this is not the case as the hCG advances oocyte meiotic esumption without affecting cumulus expansion [19], ndicating some luteinizing hormone (LH) recepor activity. Another possibility is that hCG priming and the subsequent ovarian response also assists n endometrial priming, improving the likelihood of mplantation. Again uniquely, human IVM has been onducted with the aim of returning at least one mbryo to the patient in the same cycle as oocyte etrieval. This is not the case in animal breeding, where embryos produced from the donor are invaribly transferred to a recipient animal or frozen for torage, allowing multiple collections from a donor to ccur, even on a weekly basis in the case of cattle.

In respect to media and incubation systems utized for clinical IVM, this has been mostly translated rom the animal breeding sector, especially cattle IVM. Both Tissue Culture Medium 199 (TCM-199) and -Minimal Essential Medium (with Earle's salts; MEM) have been widely used and are now commerially provided by several companies that manufacure and market IVM/IVF media systems. Their IVM nedia are generally supplemented with homologous erum and cumulus expansion in vitro is maintained r initiated (depending on the extent of cumulus xpansion at the time of collection) with supplemenal FSH and often supplemental hCG. Although some esearch has been conducted on optimizing physical onditions, such as O_2 concentration [21], most laboatories utilize a common incubation environment of % CO_2 in air at 37 °C.

There is no doubt that relative to IVF, IVM cretes additional demands within the clinical laboraory. Firstly, the preferred method of insemination is ia ICSI as there are fears that the IVM procedure nay induce zona hardening and render the oocyte less apable of sperm penetration. Secondly, if the hCGriming clinical protocol is used, multiple inseminaion times are required to prevent oocyte aging prior o insemination.

New insights into oocyte biology and regulation of oocyte maturation in vivo

Cellular regulation of oocyte developmental competence

At the cellular level, oocyte developmental compeence is achieved via exchange of molecules between oocytes and their companion somatic cells in the follicle (Figure 18.2) [22], with cumulus cells acting to relay directly maternal endocrine signals to support oocyte development. Communication between the oocyte and cumulus cells is mediated by gap junctions and by bidirectional paracrine signaling (Figure 18.2). Over the past decade, fundamental discoveries have been made in understanding the regulation of meiosis and acquisition of oocyte developmental competence prior to, and following, the LH surge and the importance to this process of these small regulatory molecules. These molecules are transferred from granulosa cells to cumulus cells and then to the oocyte via gap junctions (Figure 18.2) [14, 23, 24]. As the COC gradually develops in the growing ovarian follicle, the vast array of maternal nutrients that enable the oocyte to grow and develop sufficiently to support the next generation are passed to the oocyte via cumulus cells. In addition, the oocyte is transcriptionally active at this stage and generates maternal mRNA that is stored in the fully developed oocyte, to eventually support early embryo and fetal development (Table 18.1) [25].

Oocyte-secreted factors

The concept that oocytes actively regulate granulosa and cumulus cell functions is now an established paradigm in reproductive biology (reviews: [12, 26]). Oocytes regulate a broad range of cell functions associated with growth and differentiation, through the secretion of soluble growth factors, oocyte-secreted factors (OSFs), which in antral follicles act directly on cumulus cells to promote cellular growth, prevent cell death, modulate steroidogenesis and metabolism, and regulate cumulus cell expansion (see Figure 18.2) (reviews: [12, 22]). Over the past decade, we and others have focused efforts into dissecting apart this paracrine communication axis to identify the key rate-limiting growth factors, and have established that novel members of the transforming growth factor-β (TGFβ) superfamily are the primary mediators of oocyte paracrine signaling. Two key oocyte-secreted growth factors are growth differentiation factor 9 (GDF9) and bone morphogenetic protein 15 (BMP15), which are closely related, are coexpressed in the oocyte only, and exhibit remarkable combined synergistic interactions [27] (please refer to Chapter 10). While other factors are involved, in particular fibroblast growth factor 8 (FGF8, [28]) and perhaps BMP6 [29], GDF9 and BMP15 are clearly critical. Earlier genetic deficiency studies, either spontaneous mutations (sheep) or targeted gene knockouts (mice), revealed that there are striking species differences between the relative importance for follicle growth and development of GDF9 and BMP15. Only GDF9 is required for fertility in mice, whereas both GDF9 and BMP15 are required in sheep, and furthermore there are notable gene dosage effects in sheep but not mice [30–33]. More recently, it has been discovered that the expression ratios of GDF9 and BMP15 by the oocyte are species specific, are tightly regulated within a species, but differ substantially between species [34]. Furthermore, human GDF9 is produced in a latent form whereas mouse GDF9 is not [35]. These species-specific differences in the expression and bioactivity of growth factors are highly unusual for TGFβ superfamily proteins, and are probably very important as they may underpin the fundamental mechanism regulating mammalian ovulation rate and fecundity.

The role of lipid metabolism during oocyte maturation

The oocytes of most mammalian species have high lipid content. Nevertheless, until recently, for both oocyte maturation and embryo development, the contribution and importance of lipid metabolism has been an enigma [36]. Even though the potential ATP production from intra-oocyte and embryo lipid stores has long been recognized, direct proof of the importance of fatty acid oxidation to oocyte maturation and developmental competence has only just been established [37, 38]. This has partly been through the recognition that most media lack L-carnitine, a key cofactor required for fatty acid transport across the mitochondrial membrane. Addition of carnitine to IVM medium significantly improves mouse oocyte developmental competence [38].

cAMP and cGMP are the master regulators of oocyte maturation

A critically important regulatory molecule in the COC is cAMP, which is synthesized in the oocyte by constitutively active G protein-coupled receptors [39] and is also supplied to the oocyte by cumulus cells through gap junctions (Figure 18.2) [14]. The granulosa and cumulus cells also supply cyclic guanidine monophosphate (cGMP) to the oocyte [24, 40] which inhibit the oocyte's phosphodiesterase (PDE), the enzyme that degrades cAMP. As the oocyte acquires developmental competence prior to ovulation, moderate levels of oocyte cAMP keep the oocyte meiotically arrested via activation of protein kinase A (PKA) and subsequent inhibition of maturation-promoting factor. Artificial removal of an immature COC from the follicle, as occurs during IVM, causes loss of granulosa-supplied cGMP, leading to activation of the oocyte PDE, hydrolysis of cAMP, and inactivation of PKA, culminating in the resumption of meiosis [24, 41]. This is referred to as spontaneous oocyte maturation (cf. induced maturation) as it occurs without ligand stimulation and independently of cumulus cells. Although spontaneous oocyte IVM was first described in 1935 [6], the mechanism underlying this process has just recently been revealed [24, 41].

How the LH surge mediates the ovulatory cascade in vivo

The preovulatory surge of LH induces oocyte maturation in the follicle, leading to ovulation; however fully developed COCs do not express LH receptors and are incapable of responding directly to the LH surge. A series of significant papers has provided important new insights into the regulation of mouse oocyte maturation in vivo. The ovulatory gonadotropin surge causes: [1] a decrease in granulosa/cumulus cell C-type natriuretic peptide (CNP) levels [42, 43], leading to a fall in cumulus and oocyte cGMP; [2] the removal of the cGMP-mediated inhibition of the oocyte PDE, which allows PDE activity to resume and to degrade cAMP, leading to the resumption of oocyte maturation [24, 41]; and [3] an induction of a secondary cascade of epidermal growth factor (EGF)-like peptides across the follicle [44]. In response to the LH surge, mural granulosa cells rapidly up-regulate expression of the three major EGF-like peptides; amphiregulin, epiregulin, and betacellulin. These peptides activate the principal EGF receptor-1 on granulosa and cumulus cells which activates p38 and Erk1/2 MAPKs (mitogen-activated protein kinases) and prostaglandin cascades that in turn lead to cumulus autocrine production of the EGF-like peptides [44–47]. LH-mediated activation of this extensive EGF network in vivo coordinates cumulus expansion, oocyte maturation, and ovulation [48].

New insights and opportunities in IVM laboratory practice

With the benefit of these major recent insights into mouse oocyte maturation in vivo, it is now clear that IVM, as it has been conducted for the past 40 years, occurs in the absence of the full molecular cascade that normally regulates oocyte maturation in vivo. As the maternal contribution from the granulosa/cumulus compartment (e.g., the EGF cascade) is required to coordinate major oocyte meiotic and cytoplasmic events, it is perhaps not surprising that current clinical IVM procedures compromise oocyte quality and subsequent embryo and fetal development [11, 49]. The challenge now for scientists and clinicians practicing IVM is to capitalize on these new discoveries, to modernise clinical IVM, in order to improve its efficiency and clinical application.

Application of GDF9 and BMP15 to IVM

As GDF9 and BMP15 are the fundamental determinants of cumulus cell differentiation, they are likely to be important to oocyte developmental competence and in IVM [11]. Several lines of evidence suggested to us that IVM causes a loss of paracrine cumulus cell–oocyte communication, which most likely is reflected in a decrease in OSFs. Firstly, OSF activity on cumulus cells is strongest for cells adjacent to the oocyte and decreases in a gradient fashion [29]. Secondly, several microarray studies (including our own [50]), comparing cumulus cell gene expression between in vivo and in vitro matured COCs, revealed that many OSF-regulated genes, such as *Has2, Ptx3*, etc., are down-regulated in IVM-derived cumulus cells, compared with cumulus cells from in vivo matured oocytes. Thirdly, in other candidate gene or microarray studies, these same genes have been reported as markers of oocyte competence, especially in human cumulus cells [51, 52]. Based on the hypothesis that OSF activity is impaired by IVM, we exposed COCs to additional OSFs during oocyte IVM. In bovine IVM cultures we: [1] exposed COCs to an uncharacterized mix of native OSFs by co-culturing COC with denuded oocytes, or [2] we treated COC with in-house produced recombinant GDF9 or BMP15. Both modes of supplementing oocyte factors increased rates of blastocyst development and quality as adjudged by cell number and allocation (inner cell mass/trophectoderm) [53, 54]. This approach has since been validated by others using native OSFs in goats, pigs, and cattle [55–57]. Furthermore, following IVM with GDF9, the number of surviving mouse fetuses after blastocyst transfer to foster mothers was significantly increased, without adverse effects on fetal or placental morphology [54]. It has yet to be determined if levels of protein for these growth factors, or their conformational structure, differ between in vivo and in vitro maturing oocytes, due to a lack of appropriate antibodies to either GDF9 or BMP15. Nevertheless, tantalizing but incomplete evidence that OSF bioactivity and GDF9 and BMP15 protein levels alter during the time course of spontaneous IVM in cattle oocytes [58], coupled with the evidence described above, suggests that there is a deficiency in OSF signaling during IVM, which can be overcome by exogenous application of recombinant oocyte-specific factors. This has immediate relevance for improving clinical IVM outcomes. However, given the striking differences between species in the role and activities of GDF9 and BMP15 [34, 35], caution may be required in the application of the correct type and form of OSF(s) in IVM.

Manipulation of cAMP during IVM affects oocyte–cumulus functions and developmental competence

Essentially all clinics (human and veterinary) practicing IVM allow oocytes to undergo spontaneous maturation in vitro. By simply removing the COC from the follicle, this causes an immediate drop in intra-oocyte cAMP, leading to activation of the oocyte cell cycle, which culminates in meiotic maturation. Hence, under standard clinical IVM procedures, IVM occurs at basal oocyte cAMP levels (Figure 18.3), in contrast to the pulse of high cAMP that occurs during in vivo oocyte maturation. Several laboratories, including our own, have focused on preventing spontaneous oocyte maturation during IVM, by using cAMP modulators, including PDE inhibitors, to increase oocyte cAMP and maintain oocyte–cumulus gap junctional communication. This approach has shown that modulating cAMP during IVM improves oocyte developmental competence across a broad range of species including mouse, pig, cattle, and human [49]. In contrast, other methods of arresting meiosis during a lengthened meiotic arrest with cell-cycle inhibitors,

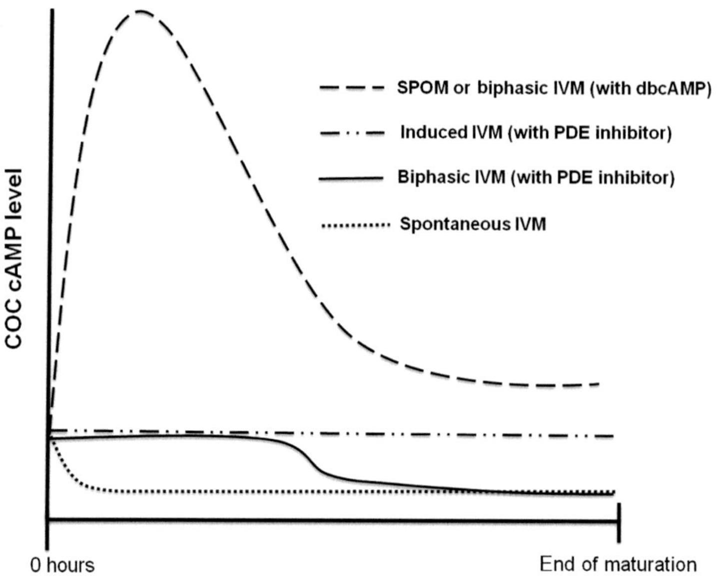

Figure 18.3 Different approaches to managing COC cAMP levels (theoretical) in different IVM systems to improve oocyte developmental competence. Spontaneous IVM (the standard clinical IVM system) allows cAMP levels to fall and not recover, thereby allowing oocyte maturation to occur. Biphasic IVM systems use an agent either to preserve cAMP levels (e.g., PDE inhibitors) or to increase cAMP levels (e.g., dbcAMP) to prevent oocyte maturation, but then in a second IVM phase the agent is washed out, which allows maturation to then proceed. Induced IVM systems use an agent to preserve (e.g., PDE inhibitor) or even increase cAMP levels which would normally inhibit meiotic maturation but in combination with a ligand such as FSH or EGF, meiosis is stimulated or induced. Simulated physiological oocyte maturation (SPOM [62]) has a short prematuration phase that significantly increases COC cAMP levels, followed by ligand-induced maturation in the presence of a cAMP preserving agent, such as a PDE inhibitor.

such as tyrosine kinase inhibitors, have generally produced oocytes with poor developmental competence [10].

Although the principle of manipulating cAMP is a common basis which has been found to improve oocyte competence during IVM, there are several different approaches, which are schematically described in Figure 18.3. These can be broadly divided into two categories: [1] those that protect cAMP degradation using PDE inhibitors such that COC cAMP levels are low to moderate, but nonetheless higher than during spontaneous IVM (e.g., [59–61]), and [2] those that stimulate high COC cAMP levels at the start or throughout IVM (e.g., [62–65]). Based on principles established by our own laboratory and those of others, in 2010 we published a new approach to IVM (SPOM: simulated physiological oocyte maturation; [62]). We propose that a fundamental principle required to maintain or enhance developmental competence of oocytes during IVM is that they are exposed to an initial pulse of cAMP, as occurs during in vivo maturation, which bestows a cumulus cell signaling cascade that appropriately coordinates major oocyte–cumulus cell maturation events. This is then followed by an "induced meiotic maturation," widely used within mouse oocyte IVM but uncommon in other species. In this phase, cAMP-mediated inhibition of meiosis is overcome by a ligand-induced stimulus, such as FSH or EGF. This differs from spontaneous IVM, where oocyte maturation occurs without ligand stimulation and under basal oocyte cAMP levels.

The first hour following COC recovery

In addition to work conducted on OSFs and manipulation of cAMP levels during IVM, most work conducted in optimizing IVM media composition has focused on addition of gonadotropins and growth factors. In addition, methods for increasing COC reduced glutathione concentrations to facilitate protection from reactive oxygen species, and protamine removal following fertilization have made an important impact on improving oocyte competence (for review, see [66]). However, we have observed that in many published reports seemingly standard IVM conditions yield poor embryo development. Some of this loss in competence may be attributed to how COCs are recovered and handled for the first hour after recovery. There are several lines of evidence that suggest COCs are particularly sensitive to the environment that they encounter immediately following removal from the follicle. In particular, if COC cAMP levels are not managed during COC collection, especially in the absence of adenylate cyclase activators, the rapid reduction in cAMP levels has a profound impact on the COC, including immediate loss of oocyte–cumulus cell gap junctional communication, cessation of oocyte transcription, and spontaneous meiotic resumption [67]. Our own observations have extended to the presence or absence of key metabolic compounds during the first hour, such as glucose. We have observed that an absence of glucose in the collection medium for the first hour after liberation of the COC from the follicle can have significantly detrimental effects on subsequent embryo development, even if maturation is conducted in the presence of glucose and normal cumulus expansion is observed (L. Frank, R. B. Gilchrist, and J. G. Thompson, unpublished observations, 2012). These insights have particular relevance for clinics that recover COCs in saline or phosphate-buffered saline, usually in the domestic animal IVM/IVF, but this is also known to occur in human IVM programs, where saline is often used to flush and prime catheters and needles.

Which temperature to use?

There are now several reports that the temperature within a large preovulatory follicle is approximately 1–2 °C lower than core body temperature in several species. It remains unclear what mechanism causes this, but the relevance to IVM cannot be ignored [68]. Indeed, Leese *et al.* [69] have proposed this may facilitate the "quiet embryo" hypothesis, by providing a less metabolically active environment in vivo, due to a reduction in temperature, which should be examined in vitro.

Which concentration of oxygen to use?

It is now well accepted that early embryo development to the blastocyst stage should be conducted in vitro under reduced O_2 atmospheres from 5% to 7%, unless a co-culture environment is used. However, the same accepted paradigm cannot be applied to IVM and there is debate as to which concentration is suitable. Early work [70] found that low concentrations (5% O_2 vs. 20% O_2) for cattle IVM was highly detrimental. In contrast, Hashimoto *et al.* [71] found that 5% O_2 could be beneficial if glucose concentrations were raised significantly. In the mouse there are also conflicting data. Preis *et al.* [72] compared IVM under 5% and 20% (air) concentrations of O_2 and examined post-fertilization consequences, demonstrating that 5% produced better quality blastocysts by virtue of increased cell numbers. However, in a paper examining four concentrations of O_2 during mouse COC IVM (2, 5, 10, and 20% O_2), Banwell *et al.* [21] found that although early development morphological parameters appeared to be improved under 5% O_2, this was not true of post-transfer survival measures, which revealed that 5% O_2 produced the smallest fetuses. Mathematical modeling by us has revealed that little O_2 is utilized by cumulus cells in comparison with the oocyte, whereas the opposite is the case for glucose [73]. This has led us to develop a "nutrient partitioning" hypothesis, where cumulus cells use little O_2 to allow the oocyte to have a metabolic preference for oxidative phosphorylation, yet glycolytically active cumulus cells have a high capacity for glucose consumption, protecting the oocyte from glucose and enabling an adequate supply of carboxylic acids to the oocyte for metabolism.

New insights into clinical practice

Clinical practices in human IVM are unique compared to other species, both in patient treatment prior to oocyte retrieval and then subsequent embryo transfer strategies. In particular, the administration of hCG prior to an IVM pick-up [18] is not performed in any other species. In addition, the practice of transferring an embryo(s) within the same cycle as oocytes are retrieved is not generally practiced in other species. Two recent reports from De Vos and colleagues in Belgium have seriously questioned this clinical approach. In both studies, they performed IVM without hCG priming, and compared embryo transfer in the pick-up cycle with transfer in a new cycle following vitrification of all good quality day 3 embryos produced from the oocyte retrieval [15, 74]. The results are remarkable in that implantation rates were raised from 1% to 15% in fresh embryo transfer cycles to over 30% in the vitrify-all transfer in the next cycle approach. The results are more remarkable in that: all patients were PCOS, an hCG bolus was not administered; ICSI was performed at just one time point [40 hours maturation), and in the latter publication, embryos were generated from oocytes recovered from 6 mm or smaller follicles. This provides two significant insights: firstly, IVM using oocytes from small antral follicles can lead to highly competent embryos; and secondly, the most significant rate-limiting factor in human IVM is appropriate endometrial preparation.

As vitrification of mature oocytes is increasingly adopted due to the improved success rates [75], coupled with improvements to cryopreservation and regrafting of ovarian tissue, the capacity to successfully preserve fertility in girls and women suffering cancer has advanced significantly [76]. As it is still difficult to successfully cryopreserve immature COCs, IVM has the potential to play a key role in fertility preservation, either as a means to generate mature oocytes from antral follicles following ovarian tissue collection or after in vitro follicle culture.

Conclusions

Knowledge of how to mature oocytes in vitro from unstimulated ovaries has existed for more than 40 years. Whilst IVM is a routine and highly successful assisted reproductive technology (ART) in cattle, IVM has not been widely adopted in human ART despite the clear medical and financial advantages over typical current ART practices. Hence, is there any future for IVM in the treatment of human infertility? The lower efficiency of IVM appears to be the only clear impediment to clinical application. Major advances in mammalian oocyte biology have been made in the past 10 years, which have settled long-standing controversies in the world of mouse oocyte biology. During this time, clinical and laboratory IVM practices have improved little, so it is now incumbent on both clinicians and scientists to modernize IVM methodologies and procedures to capitalize on this opportunity.

References

1. Delvigne A, Rozenberg S. Epidemiology and prevention of ovarian hyperstimulation syndrome (OHSS): a review. *Hum Reprod Update* 2002; **8**(6): 559–77.
2. Baart EB, Martini E, Eijkemans MJ, *et al.* Milder ovarian stimulation for in-vitro fertilization reduces aneuploidy in the human preimplantation embryo: a randomized controlled trial. *Hum Reprod* 2007; **22**(4): 980–8.
3. Market-Velker BA, Zhang L, Magri LS, Bonvissuto AC, Mann MR. Dual effects of superovulation: loss of maternal and paternal imprinted methylation in a dose-dependent manner. *Hum Mol Genet* 2010; **19**(1): 36–51.
4. Edwards LJ, Kind KL, Armstrong DT, Thompson JG. Effects of recombinant human follicle-stimulating hormone on embryo development in mice. *Am J Physiol Endocrinol Metab* 2005; **288**(5): E845–51.
5. Kelley RL, Kind KL, Lane M, *et al.* Recombinant human follicle-stimulating hormone alters maternal ovarian hormone concentrations and the uterus and perturbs fetal development in mice. *Am J Physiol Endocrinol Metab* 2006; **291**(4): E761–70.
6. Pincus G, Enzmann EV. The comparative behavior of mammalian eggs in vivo and in vitro : I. The activation of ovarian eggs. *J Exp Med* 1935; **62**(5): 665–75.
7. Schroeder AC, Eppig JJ. The developmental capacity o mouse oocytes that matured spontaneously in vitro is normal. *Dev Biol* 1984; **102**(2): 493–7.
8. Cha KY, Koo JJ, Ko JJ, *et al.* Pregnancy after in vitro fertilization of human follicular oocytes collected from nonstimulated cycles, their culture in vitro and their transfer in a donor oocyte program. *Fertil Steril* 1991; **55**(1): 109–13.
9. Stroud B. The year 2010 worldwide statistics of embryo transfer in domestic farm animals. *International Embryo Transfer Newsletter* 2011; **29**(4): 14–23.
10. Gilchrist RB, Thompson JG. Oocyte maturation: emerging concepts and technologies to improve developmental potential in vitro. *Theriogenology* 2007; **67**(1): 6–15.
11. Gilchrist RB. Recent insights into oocyte-follicle cell interactions provide opportunities for the development of new approaches to in vitro maturation. *Reprod Fertil Dev* 2011; **23**(1): 23–31.
12. Gilchrist RB, Lane M, Thompson JG. Oocyte-secreted factors: regulators of cumulus cell function and oocyte quality. *Hum Reprod Update* 2008; **14**(2): 159–77.
13. Sutton ML, Gilchrist RB, Thompson JG. Effects of in-vivo and in-vitro environments on the metabolism of the cumulus-oocyte complex and its influence on oocyte developmental capacity. *Hum Reprod Update* 2003; **9**(1): 35–48.
14. Anderson E, Albertini DF. Gap junctions between the oocyte and companion follicle cells in the mammalian ovary. *J Cell Biol* 1976; **71**(2): 680–6.
15. Guzman L, Ortega-Hrepich C, Albuz FK, *et al.* Developmental capacity of in vitro-matured human oocytes retrieved from polycystic ovary syndrome ovaries containing no follicles larger than 6 mm. *Fertil Steril* 2012; **98**(2): 503-7.e1–2.
16. Fair T, Hyttel P, Greve T. Bovine oocyte diameter in relation to maturational competence and transcriptional activity. *Mol Reprod Dev* 1995; **42**(4): 437–42.
17. Hyttel P, Fair T, Callesen H, Greve T. Oocyte growth, capacitation and final maturation in cattle. *Theriogenology* 1997; **47**: 23–32.
18. Chian RC, Gulekli B, Buckett WM, Tan SL. Priming with human chorionic gonadotropin before retrieval of immature oocytes in women with infertility due to the polycystic ovary syndrome [letter] [published erratum appears in *N Engl J Med* 2000; **342**(3): 224]. *N Engl J Med* 1999; 341(21): 1624, 1626.

9. Chian RC, Buckett WM, Tulandi T, Tan SL. Prospective randomized study of human chorionic gonadotrophin priming before immature oocyte retrieval from unstimulated women with polycystic ovarian syndrome. *Hum Reprod* 2000; **15**(1): 165–70.

0. Hagemann LJ. Influence of the dominant follicle on oocytes from subordinate follicles. *Theriogenology* 1999; **51**(2): 449–59.

1. Banwell KM, Lane M, Russell DL, Kind KL, Thompson JG. Oxygen concentration during mouse oocyte in vitro maturation affects embryo and fetal development. *Hum Reprod* 2007; **22**(10): 2768–75.

2. Gilchrist RB, Ritter LJ, Armstrong DT. Oocyte-somatic cell interactions during follicle development in mammals. *Anim Reprod Sci* 2004; **82**–83: 431–46.

3. Thomas RE, Armstrong DT, Gilchrist RB. Bovine cumulus cell-oocyte gap junctional communication during in vitro maturation in response to manipulation of cell-specific cyclic adenosine 3′,5′-monophosophate levels. *Biol Reprod* 2004; **70**(3): 548–56.

4. Norris RP, Ratzan WJ, Freudzon M, *et al.* Cyclic GMP from the surrounding somatic cells regulates cyclic AMP and meiosis in the mouse oocyte. *Development* 2009; **136**(11): 1869–78.

5. Fair T, Hulshof SC, Hyttel P, Greve T, Boland M. Nucleus ultrastructure and transcriptional activity of bovine oocytes in preantral and early antral follicles. *Mol Reprod Dev* 1997; **46**(2): 208–15.

6. McNatty KP, Moore LG, Hudson NL, *et al.* The oocyte and its role in regulating ovulation rate: a new paradigm in reproductive biology. *Reproduction* 2004; **128**(4): 379–86.

7. Mottershead DG, Ritter LJ, Gilchrist RB. Signalling pathways mediating specific synergistic interactions between GDF9 and BMP15. *Mol Hum Reprod* 2012; **18**(3): 121–8.

8. Sugiura K, Su YQ, Diaz FJ, *et al.* Oocyte-derived BMP15 and FGFs cooperate to promote glycolysis in cumulus cells. *Development* 2007; **134**(14): 2593–603.

9. Hussein TS, Froiland DA, Amato F, Thompson JG, Gilchrist RB. Oocytes prevent cumulus cell apoptosis by maintaining a morphogenic paracrine gradient of bone morphogenetic proteins. *J Cell Sci* 2005; **118**(Pt 22): 5257–68.

0. Dong J, Albertini DF, Nishimori K, *et al.* Growth differentiation factor-9 is required during early ovarian folliculogenesis. *Nature* 1996; **383**(6600): 531–5.

1. Yan C, Wang P, DeMayo J, *et al.* Synergistic roles of bone morphogenetic protein 15 and growth differentiation factor 9 in ovarian function. *Mol Endocrinol* 2001; **15**(6): 854–66.

32. Galloway SM, McNatty KP, Cambridge LM, *et al.* Mutations in an oocyte-derived growth factor gene (BMP15) cause increased ovulation rate and infertility in a dosage-sensitive manner. *Nat Genet* 2000; **25**(3): 279–83.

33. Hanrahan JP, Gregan SM, Mulsant P, *et al.* Mutations in the genes for oocyte-derived growth factors GDF9 and BMP15 are associated with both increased ovulation rate and sterility in Cambridge and Belclare sheep (*Ovis aries*). *Biol Reprod* 2004; **70**: 900–9.

34. Crawford JL, McNatty KP. The ratio of growth differentiation factor 9: bone morphogenetic protein 15 mRNA expression is tightly co-regulated and differs between species over a wide range of ovulation rates. *Mol Cell Endocrinol* 2012; **348**(1): 339–43.

35. Simpson CM, Stanton PG, Walton KL, *et al.* Activation of latent human GDF9 by a single residue change (Gly391Arg) in the mature domain. *Endocrinology* 2012; **153**(3): 1301–10.

36. Sturmey RG, Reis A, Leese HJ, McEvoy TG. Role of fatty acids in energy provision during oocyte maturation and early embryo development. *Reprod Domest Anim* 2009; **44** Suppl 3: 50–8.

37. Downs SM, Mosey JL, Klinger J. Fatty acid oxidation and meiotic resumption in mouse oocytes. *Mol Reprod Dev* 2009; **76**(9): 844–53.

38. Dunning KR, Cashman K, Russell DL, *et al.* Beta-oxidation is essential for mouse oocyte developmental competence and early embryo development. *Biol Reprod* 2010; **83**(6): 909–18.

39. Mehlmann LM, Jones TL, Jaffe LA. Meiotic arrest in the mouse follicle maintained by a Gs protein in the oocyte. *Science* 2002; **297**(5585): 1343–5.

40. Tornell J, Billig H, Hillensjo T. Regulation of oocyte maturation by changes in ovarian levels of cyclic nucleotides. *Hum Reprod* 1991; **6**(3): 411–22.

41. Vaccari S, Weeks JL, 2nd, Hsieh M, Menniti FS, Conti M. Cyclic GMP signaling is involved in the luteinizing hormone-dependent meiotic maturation of mouse oocytes. *Biol Reprod* 2009; **81**(3): 595–604.

42. Zhang M, Su YQ, Sugiura K, Xia G, Eppig JJ. Granulosa cell ligand NPPC and its receptor NPR2 maintain meiotic arrest in mouse oocytes. *Science* 2010; **330**(6002): 366–9.

43. Kawamura K, Cheng Y, Kawamura N, *et al.* Pre-ovulatory LH/hCG surge decreases C-type natriuretic peptide secretion by ovarian granulosa cells to promote meiotic resumption of pre-ovulatory oocytes. *Hum Reprod* 2011; **26**(11): 3094–101.

44. Park JY, Su YQ, Ariga M, *et al.* EGF-like growth factors as mediators of LH action in the ovulatory follicle. *Science* 2004; **303**(5658): 682–4.

45. Shimada M, Hernandez-Gonzalez I, Gonzalez-Robayna I, Richards JS. Paracrine and autocrine regulation of epidermal growth factor-like factors in cumulus oocyte complexes and granulosa cells: key roles for prostaglandin synthase 2 and progesterone receptor. *Mol Endocrinol* 2006; **20**(6): 1352–65.

46. Fan HY, Liu Z, Shimada M, *et al.* MAPK3/1 (ERK1/2) in ovarian granulosa cells are essential for female fertility. *Science* 2009; **324**(5929): 938–41.

47. Downs SM, Chen J. EGF-like peptides mediate FSH-induced maturation of cumulus cell-enclosed mouse oocytes. *Mol Reprod Dev* 2008; **75**(1): 105–14.

48. Conti M, Hsieh M, Musa Zamah A, Oh JS. Novel signaling mechanisms in the ovary during oocyte maturation and ovulation. *Mol Cell Endocrinol* 2011; **356**(1–2): 65–73.

49. Smitz JE, Thompson JG, Gilchrist RB. The promise of in vitro maturation in assisted reproduction and fertility preservation. *Semin Reprod Med* 2011; **29**(1): 24–37.

50. Kind KL, Banwell KM, Gebhardt KM, *et al.* Microarray analysis of mRNA from cumulus cells following in vivo or in vitro maturation of mouse cumulus-oocyte complexes. *Reprod Fertil Dev* 2013; **25**(2): 426–58.

51. Wathlet S, Adriaenssens T, Segers I, *et al.* Cumulus cell gene expression predicts better cleavage-stage embryo or blastocyst development and pregnancy for ICSI patients. *Hum Reprod* 2011; **26**(5): 1035–51.

52. Gebhardt KM, Feil DK, Dunning KR, Lane M, Russell DL. Human cumulus cell gene expression as a biomarker of pregnancy outcome after single embryo transfer. *Fertil Steril* 2011; **96**(1): 47–52 e2.

53. Hussein TS, Thompson JG, Gilchrist RB. Oocyte-secreted factors enhance oocyte developmental competence. *Dev Biol* 2006; **296**(2): 514–21.

54. Yeo CX, Gilchrist RB, Thompson JG, Lane M. Exogenous growth differentiation factor 9 in oocyte maturation media enhances subsequent embryo development and fetal viability in mice. *Hum Reprod* 2008; **23**(1): 67–73.

55. Romaguera R, Morato R, Jimenez-Macedo AR, *et al.* Oocyte secreted factors improve embryo developmental competence of COCs from small follicles in prepubertal goats. *Theriogenology* 2010; **74**(6): 1050–9.

56. Gomez MN, Kang JT, Koo OJ, *et al.* Effect of oocyte-secreted factors on porcine in vitro maturation, cumulus expansion and developmental competence of parthenotes. *Zygote* 2012; **20**(2): 135–45.

57. Dey SR, Deb GK, Ha AN, *et al.* Coculturing denuded oocytes during the in vitro maturation of bovine cumulus oocyte complexes exerts a synergistic effect on embryo development. *Theriogenology* 2012; **77**(6): 1064–77.

58. Hussein TS, Sutton-McDowall ML, Gilchrist RB, Thompson JG. Temporal effects of exogenous oocyte-secreted factors on bovine oocyte developmental competence during IVM. *Reprod Fertil Dev* 2011; **23**(4): 576–84.

59. Nogueira D, Cortvrindt R, De Matos DG, Vanhoutte L, Smitz J. Effect of phosphodiesterase type 3 inhibitor on developmental competence of immature mouse oocytes in vitro. *Biol Reprod* 2003; **69**: 2045–52.

60. Thomas RE, Thompson JG, Armstrong DT, Gilchrist RB. Effect of specific phosphodiesterase isoenzyme inhibitors during in vitro maturation of bovine oocyte on meiotic and developmental capacity. *Biol Reprod.* 2004; **71**(4): 1142–9.

61. Nogueira D, Albano C, Adriaenssens T, *et al.* Human oocytes reversibly arrested in prophase I by phosphodiesterase type 3 inhibitor in vitro. *Biol Reprod* 2003; **69**(3): 1042–52.

62. Albuz FK, Sasseville M, Lane M, *et al.* Simulated physiological oocyte maturation (SPOM): a novel in vitro maturation system that substantially improves embryo yield and pregnancy outcomes. *Hum Reprod* 2010; **25**(12): 2999–3011.

63. Funahashi H, Cantley TC, Day BN. Synchronization of meiosis in porcine oocytes by exposure to dibutyryl cyclic adenosine monophosphate improves developmental competence following in vitro fertilization. *Biol Reprod* 1997; **57**(1): 49–53.

64. Guixue Z, Luciano AM, Coenen K, Gandolfi F, Sirard MA. The influence of cAMP before or during bovine oocyte maturation on embryonic developmental competence. *Theriogenology* 2001; **55**(8): 1733–43.

65. Luciano AM, Pocar P, Milanesi E, *et al.* Effect of different levels of intracellular cAMP on the in vitro maturation of cattle oocytes and their subsequent development following in vitro fertilization. *Mol Reprod Dev* 1999; **54**(1): 86–91.

66. Banwell KM, Thompson JG. In vitro maturation of mammalian oocytes: outcomes and consequences. *Semin Reprod Med* 2008; **26**(2): 162–74.

67. Luciano AM, Franciosi F, Modina SC, Lodde V. Gap junction-mediated communications regulate chromatin remodeling during bovine oocyte growth and differentiation through cAMP-dependent mechanism(s). *Biol Reprod* 2011; **85**(6): 1252–9.

68. Hunter RH. Temperature gradients in female reproductive tissues. *Reprod Biomed Online* 2012; **24**(4): 377–80.

69. Leese HJ, Baumann CG, Brison DR, McEvoy TG, Sturmey RG. Metabolism of the viable mammalian embryo: quietness revisited. *Mol Hum Reprod* 2008; **14**(12): 667–72.

70. Pinyopummintr T, Bavister BD. Optimum gas atmosphere for in vitro maturation and in vitro fertilization of bovine oocytes. *Theriogenology* 1995; **44**(4): 471–7.

71. Hashimoto S, Minami N, Takakura R, *et al.* Low oxygen tension during in vitro maturation is beneficial for supporting the subsequent development of bovine cumulus-oocyte complexes. *Mol Reprod Dev* 2000; **57**(4): 353–60.

72. Preis KA, Seidel GE, Jr., Gardner DK. Reduced oxygen concentration improves the developmental competence of mouse oocytes following in vitro maturation. *Mol Reprod Dev* 2007; **74**(7): 893–903.

73. Clark AR, Stokes YM, Lane M, Thompson JG. Mathematical modelling of oxygen concentration in bovine and murine cumulus-oocyte complexes. *Reproduction* 2006; **131**(6): 999–1006.

74. De Vos A, Van de Velde H, Joris H, Van Steirteghem A. In-vitro matured metaphase-I oocytes have a lower fertilization rate but similar embryo quality as mature metaphase-II oocytes after intracytoplasmic sperm injection. *Hum Reprod* 1999; **14**(7):1859–63.

75. Edgar DH, Gook DA. A critical appraisal of cryopreservation (slow cooling versus vitrification) of human oocytes and embryos. *Hum Reprod Update* 2012; **18**(5): 536–54.

76. Smitz J, Dolmans MM, Donnez J, *et al.* Current achievements and future research directions in ovarian tissue culture, in vitro follicle development and transplantation: implications for fertility preservation. *Hum Reprod Update* 2010; **16**(4): 395–414.

Chapter 19

Human genes modulating primordial germ cell and gamete formation

Valerie L. Baker, Ruth Lathi, and Renee A. Reijo Pera

Introduction

Although 10–15% of couples are infertile [1], relatively few studies to date have probed the developmental genetics of human germ cell formation and differentiation in spite of the fact that poor germ cell production (poor quality and/or insufficient quantity) is a leading cause of infertility. Historically, the inaccessibility of germ cell development to studies in vivo and the lack of tools to study the pathways in vitro have limited progress in understanding human germ cell development. In recent years, however, with advances in human genetics, derivation of human embryonic stem cells (hESCs), reprogramming of somatic cells to induced pluripotent stem cells, and advances in clinical progress in in vitro fertilization, studies of human germ cell formation and differentiation are feasible and promise to enhance understanding of the unique pathways of germ cell development and their contribution to preimplantation, fetal, and postnatal development.

Rationale for studies of human germ cell formation and development per se

The examination of human germ cell development remains an important objective in spite of elegant studies in model systems that provide a foundation for understanding the divergence of the somatic and germ cell lineages early in human embryo development. Indeed, there are several unique aspects to human germ cell development that merit investment in these tools: firstly, genes and gene dosages required for human germ cell development differ from those of mice, including both autosomal and sex chromosomal genes and dosages [2–10]. Secondly and most importantly to human health, humans are rare among species in that infertility is remarkably common relative to other species, with nearly half of all infertility cases linked to faulty germ cell development [11]. Moreover, pathologies associated with meiotic errors are numerous in human development relative to other species. Indeed, meiotic chromosome segregation errors occur in as many as 5–20% of human germ cells depending on sex and age [12, 13]. This is in contrast to frequencies of approximately 1/10 000 cells in yeast, 1/1000 cells in flies, and 1/100 cells in mice. Finally, advances in pluripotent stem cell biology provide a unique opportunity to incorporate new strategies into our analysis of human germ cell development. This review addresses fundamental questions regarding human germline origins, function, and pathology and provides a foundation for considering rational therapeutics and diagnostics that inform clinical decisions.

Lessons from germ cell development in vivo in model systems

In animals, there are two apparently divergent methods of germ cell specification and maintenance [14–17]. Firstly, in non-mammalian species, germ cell fate is determined by the inheritance of germ plasm, microscopically distinct oocyte cytoplasm that is particularly rich in RNAs and RNA-binding proteins and segregates with cells destined to become germ cells [14–17]. Secondly, in mammalian species and a subset of other animals, both male and female germ cells are specified independently of germ plasm via inductive signaling [18–23]. In the mouse, germ cells are definitively recognized at c. 7.2 days postcoitum (dpc)

Biology and Pathology of the Oocyte, 2nd edn., ed. Alan Trounson, Roger Gosden, and Ursula Eichenlaub-Ritter.
Published by Cambridge University Press.

as an extraembryonic cluster of cells that express tissue non-specific alkaline phosphatase, *Oct4,* and *Stella*, at the base of the allantois [24–28]. Subsequently, the nascent primordial germ cells (PGCs) migrate out of the embryo proper and reside in extraembryonic tissues. Following extensive somatic differentiation in the embryo, the cells re-enter the embryo, and migrate to and invade the genital ridges. There they colonize, proliferate mitotically, and begin the process of resetting genomic imprints by erasure (embryonic day [E]9.5–11.5) [29, 30]. Subsequently, the differentiation of the genital ridges to testes or ovaries signals the germ cells to develop as either male or female germ cells and re-establishment of diagnostic sex-specific imprinting patterns begins [14].

The elaborate reprogramming that occurs in the germ cell lineage distinguishes cells of the germ line from somatic cells [26, 31]. Recent studies have documented that one of the first signs of reprogramming consists of the loss of histone H3 lysine 9 dimethylation (H3K9me2) from E7.75 concomitant with a global increase of H3 lysine 27 trimethylation (H3K27me3) by E9.5 [26, 31]. These early histone changes are accompanied by changes in methylation status, with evidence for site-specific erasure of methylation at 5-methylcytosine residues (5MeC) as well as modification of 5MeC to 5-hydroxylmethylcytosine throughout the genome during germline formation and during the oocyte-to-embryo transition [26, 31]. Subsequently, the site-specific epigenomic reorganization appears to serve as a prequel to the genome-wide erasure of DNA methylation and extensive chromatin remodeling that is observed in PGCs as they enter the gonads at approximately E10.5 in mice.

Development of pluripotent stem cell systems to directly modulate gene function in human germ cell development

Classically, hESCs are derived from the inner cell mass (ICM), are capable of contributing to all three germ layers, as well as the germ line, and are characterized by specific cell markers, epigenetic and genetic status, and growth requirements [32–34]. Recent studies indicate that mouse epiblast stem cells (mEpiSCs) are more similar to hESCs in terms of cell signaling and culture conditions, molecular signature, and morphological characteristics, than mouse ESCs (mESCs) derived from the ICM [35, 36]. Other studies have similarly suggested that hESCs bear resemblance to early progeny of the epiblast, the PGCs [37–39]. More recently, cells with extensive similarities to mESCs and hESCs have been derived via reprogramming of fetal and adult fibroblasts [40–45]. In general, by introducing a cocktail of three to six factors, somatic cells can be reprogrammed to an ESC-like fate distinguished by classic criteria of hESC identity.

Differentiation of germ cells from embryonic stem cells in vitro

Several studies have shown that mESCs (derived from the ICM of the blastocyst prior to epiblast formation) are capable of differentiating into female and male germ cells in [38, 46–50]. Oocyte differentiation from mESCs was obtained via spontaneous differentiation of adherent cultures, as indicated by analysis of germ cell-specific markers such as *Vasa*, *Gdf9,* and *Scp3*, and as corroborated by analysis of morphology and follicular steroidogenic enzyme production [46, 47]. Similarly, male germ cell differentiation was demonstrated via differentiation of mESCs into embryoid bodies (EBs) and analysis of germ cell-specific markers [48–50]. In one study, putative PGCs were then transplanted to testes where they formed sperm [48]. In a second study, the authors demonstrated that the imprinting status of genes such as *Igfr2* was diagnostic of PGCs and that haploid male gametes derived from ESCs in vitro were capable of fertilizing oocytes and activating development to blastocysts [49]. In addition, another group suggested that mESC-derived male gametes can generate offspring in mice, thus potentially bringing the work full circle to the ultimate proof of functional gametogenesis in vitro [50]. Nonetheless, skepticism remained about the legitimacy of germ cell development in vitro and success in transplantation of germ cells was limited in both the mouse and human systems.

Subsequently, Saitou and colleagues reported the generation of what they termed PGCLCs (primordial germ cell-like cells) [25]. These cells were generated from mESCs via generation of epiblast-like cells (EpiLCs), which are thought to bear more resemblance to hESCs than mESCs [35, 36]. The authors found that these cells were highly efficient in generating PGCs that possessed the global transcription profiles, epigenetic status, and cellular dynamics that distinguish PGCs from other cell types of the body. The cells could be prospectively isolated via use of the cell surface markers SSEA1 and integrin-β3. Isolated cells were characterized by reduced tumorigenic potential with increased capacity for spermatogenesis, post-transplantation to the testis. Efforts to extend studies to hESCs and human iPSCs are underway in several laboratories.

Concurrent with the mouse studies described above, others sought evidence that multiple, independently derived hESC lines could contribute to germ cell formation in vitro [38, 47, 51–53]. In these studies, hESCs were differentiated either via formation of EBs or in adherent cultures and differentiated cells were assessed for morphology, expression of germ cell markers, meiotic progression and ploidy. Markers included those from studies of mouse germ cell differentiation to allow comparisons between mice and humans [46, 48, 49]. In addition, several studies have documented that human germ cell formation in vitro is responsive to factors that are implicated in murine germ cell formation, such as members of the bone morphogenetic protein (BMP) and fibroblast growth factor (FGF) gene families [47, 52–54].

Studies on differentiation of human germ cells in vitro have also been used to examine the genetic function of genes linked to male infertility, especially those that lack homologs in mouse models, such as the Y-chromosome genes linked to male infertility and production of gametes beyond the PGC stage (meiotic and post-meiotic). In these studies, Kee *et al.* used a germ cell reporter to quantitate and isolate PGCs derived from both male and female hESCs [55]. Then, these authors silenced and overexpressed genes of the *DAZ (Deleted in AZoospermia)* gene family that encode germ cell-specific cytoplasmic RNA-binding proteins (not transcription factors). Via manipulation of members of the *DAZ* gene family, human germ cell formation and developmental progress could be modulated, as assessed by a panel of assays that distinguish germ cells from somatic cells and diagnose developmental stages of germ cell development (Figure 19.1). The authors were able to demonstrate that the human *DAZL (Deleted in AZoospermia-Like)* gene functions in PGC formation, whereas closely related genes, Y-chromosome *DAZ* and autosomal *BOULE,* promote later stages of meiosis and development of haploid gametes.

Differentiation of germ cells from human induced pluripotent stem cells in vitro

As described above, in 2006 and 2007, Yamanaka and colleagues reported the reprogramming of murine and adult somatic cells to pluripotent stem cells [41, 42, 56]. An obvious question regarding the potential of iPSCs was whether they could contribute to the differentiation of the germ cell lineage. This question was answered via germline transmission in mice, with several reports following the announcements of reprogramming with evidence of germline transmission [40, 43]. However, in humans, assessment of ability to form germ cells must be accomplished in vitro for obvious reasons. The first study to report germ cell differentiation from iPSCs was reported by Park *et al.* using reprogrammed fetal cells and fetal gonadal feeders, which provided a significant improvement in PGC differentiation relative to previous methods [57]. Subsequent reports used similar methods with reprogrammed adult cells and extended observations to the production of haploid cells; moreover, methods in these later studies paralleled those reported by Kee *et al.* [55] with use of overexpression of translational regulators to promote meiotic entry and progression [58, 59].

Recent studies have examined whether overexpression of intrinsic germ cell translational, rather than transcriptional, factors might be limited to the use of DAZ and DAZL to drive germline formation and/or differentiation from human pluripotent stem cells in vitro. In these studies, Medrano *et al.* observed that overexpression of VASA (DDX4) protein, an evolutionarily distant RNA-binding protein, mimicked the action of DAZ and DAZL in promoting both hESC and iPSC differentiation to PGCs and maturation and progression through meiosis [59]. Still other studies, however, reported complete meiosis in in vitro-derived germ cells based on purification of spontaneous differentiated germ cells and subsequent further culture with a cocktail of growth factors, in the absence of genetic manipulation [60]. However, the efficiency of formation of haploid cells in all these reports is very low and further research is needed.

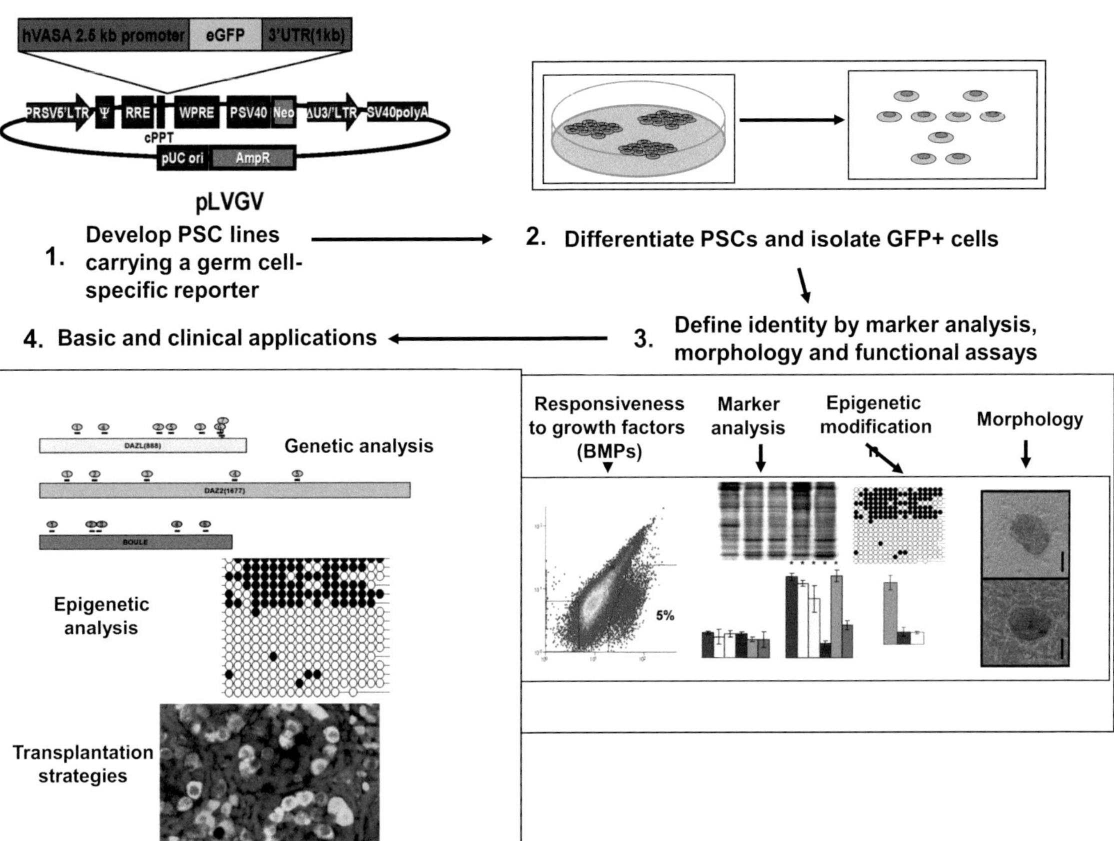

Figure 19.1 Experimental overview of the system used to probe landmark events and genetic requirements for human germ cell formation and differentiation in both the human embryonic stem cell (hESC) and induced pluripotent stem cell (iPSC) systems. Methods are as reported by Kee *et al.* [55], Panula *et al.* [58], and Medrano *et al.* [59]. Essentially, (1) a germ cell reporter (VASA:GFP) was created and stably integrated into hESCs. (2) Adherent or embryoid body differentiation is used to achieve efficient recovery of early germ cells for fluorescence activated cell sorting (FACS) isolation and characterization. (3) Multiple molecular and functional assays are conducted to characterize GFP+ cells after FACS isolation, including quantitative analysis of GFP+ by FACS under various culture conditions to examine the responsiveness of hESCs to BMPs, expression analysis, methylation of genomic DNA by three independent analyses, and ability to propagate embryonic germline (EG) cells. (4) Results are of value for both potential clinical and basic applications.

Special challenges with differentiation of female germ cells

As noted briefly above, Hubner *et al.* differentiated mESCs to the germ cell lineage and reported the production of oocytes; their approach to germ cell differentiation involved the use of mESCs that were genetically modified with a germ cell-specific *Oct4* promoter driving GFP reporter construct [46]. *Oct4*-GFP was obviously expected to be expressed in undifferentiated ESCs but the concept was that the expression would disappear in somatic cells and persist in the germ cell lineage. The authors report that approximately 25% of cells maintained expression of *Oct4*-GFP after 4 days of differentiation, with an increase to 40% after 7 days. The cells that differentiated were analyzed for expression of cKit and *Oct4*-GFP expression by FACS (fluorescence activated cell sorting) to identify those cells that co-express both markers and were most likely to be cells of the germ cell lineage. The authors report that as adherent differentiation was continued, they observed the formation of GFP+ and Vasa+ colonies by day 12 [46]. As reported in both the mouse and human, Vasa remains one of the most reliable markers of germ cell differentiation in pluripotent stem cell colonies [46]. Small aggregates of cells that expressed Vasa, and lacked *Oct4*-GFP expression, then detached from the adherent culture and were found in the supernatant. These floating aggregates developed into morphologically visible follicular structures that were termed putative oocytes. By day 16, other signs of oocyte differentiation were also noted including the presence of nuclear Scp-3. Follicular structures were reported to express growth differentiation factor 9 (GDF9), steroidogenic enzymes, and produce estrogen. These studies also reported that follicles released oocytes of 50–70 μm in diameter that expressed Zp-2/3 and Figla. Upon extended culture, preimplantation stage embryos were observed and were likely the result of abnormal parthenogenic oocyte activation.

Notably, however, both XX and XY mESC lines produced oocytes. Moreover, the functionality of these oocytes remained unclear as tests regarding their ability to be integrated into ovarian tissue and/or produce offspring were not reported.

Subsequently, other authors followed up on this work, including Novak *et al.*; these authors reproduced the Hubner protocol and also found follicular-like aggregates and estrogen production [61]. Notably, however, this group reported that Scp-3 nuclear localization was variable and that in most cases incomplete alignment of Scp-3 along the chromosomes was observed, indicative of abnormal meiotic prophase. Thus, along with other evidence provided, these authors suggested that the ESC-derived oocyte-like cells produced by the Hubner protocol appeared defective and not capable of proper progression through meiotic prophase I. Another study by Qing *et al.* reported an alternative method to differentiate oocyte-like cells from mESCs in two separate steps [62]. These authors reported the use of retinoic acid (RA) to promote differentiation, and co-culture of EBs with ovarian granulosa cells and conditioned media to promote oocyte maturation. The authors used FACS to isolate Ssea1 and cKit double-positive cells and found that they represented 25% of the cells in the EBs and were re-plated on feeders in the presence of 2 μM RA for 7 days to differentiate persisting ESCs and enrich for ESC-derived germ cells. After RA treatment, alkaline phosphatase-positive germ cell colonies were observed in double-positive cell cultures but rarely detected in double-negative cell populations. Still other reports describe differentiation protocols with a germ cell-specific Stella promoter driving GFP reporter construct or a Gdf9 promoter [63, 64]. Although these methods enriched for germ cell production, follicle-like structures were difficult to detect and any oocyte like cells that were generated appeared to quickly degenerate.

Transplantation as a means to promote oocyte maturation from pluripotent stem cell-derived germ cells

The field of germ cell differentiation has struggled to document fundamental properties of differentiation, making it difficult to determine the physiological relevance of differentiated germ cells. The most complete descriptions of oocyte differentiation from pluripotent stem cells remain a pair of reports from Nicholas *et al.* [65, 66]. These authors used transplantation of mESC-derived germ cells in efforts to overcome deficiencies in meiotic progression and in order to direct functional integration, recruitment of endogenous granulosa cells, and maturation of ESC-derived oocytes in physiological ovarian follicles to the primary stage. They demonstrated bona fide oocyte differentiation from ESCs using functional parameters that were complementary to each other and probed multiple milestones of endogenous oocyte development that are distinguishable from undifferentiated ESCs. Functional properties included ESC-derived germ cell responsiveness to media supplementation with defined germ cell maturation factors, requirement of an active *Dazl* gene along an endogenous developmental timeline, entry and partial progression through meiosis, and recruitment of endogenous somatic granulosa cells to support follicle formation and development following transplantation into a synchronized ovarian niche [65, 66]. Notably, primordial germ cells were distinquished from undifferentiated ESCs by the lower level of intensity of Oct4-GFP and down-regulatation of the expression of SSEA1 by day 14 of in vitro differentiation. In addition, the authors were able to confirm germ cell identity via analysis of single cells and found that germ cells were characterized by the expression of multiple germ cell markers within the same cell. The production of these cells was induced by the use of supplemented media and validated by the observation that a null mutation in the *Dazl* gene, required for germ cell differentiation in vivo, resulted in severe reductions of germ cell development in vitro [65, 67]. Finally, these authors also noted aberrant synaptonemal complex formation in vitro and sought to direct successful mESC-derived oocyte maturation in ovarian follicles by transplantation into a physiological and synchronized ovarian niche [65, 66]. They found that following transplantation, ESC-derived oocytes integrated into the ovarian niche, recruited somatic granulosa cells from the mouse ovary, and directed follicle formation and development; thereby confirming endogenous oocyte-comparable identity, function, and potential, and providing a solid foundation for extension to the hESC system for studies of human oocyte development and clinical translation.

Transplantation is a rigorous test of cell identity and function in diverse stem cell systems. However, considerable research remains to be done before it is likely that pluripotent stem cell-derived oocytes will be optimized for basic, translational, and clinical applications. Formation of teratomas in grafts remains common, the efficiency of differentiation of germ cells remains very low, and in clinical applications, a demonstration that ESC-derived oocytes can support the development of healthy offspring is needed once the efficiency of oocyte maturation is improved. Nonetheless it is clear that pluripotent stem cells from mouse and human, both ESCs and iPSCs, can differentiate to the germ cell lineage and that maturation via transplantation to an endogenous niche provides critical support for physiologically relevant, endogenous sperm and egg development and future clinical utility. The clinical need is great.

Future applications and prospects

One of the hopes for studies of human germ cell development in vitro is to elucidate the developmental genetics of human germ cell formation, maintenance, differentiation, and function. The role of genetics in infertility, and the relationship of genetics to poor sperm and oocyte quality, came to the forefront beginning in the 1970s with studies of azoospermia in men and premature ovarian failure in women with Turner syndrome. In the mid 1970s, Tiepolo and Zuffardi proposed that some cases of male infertility might be linked to the deletion of a gene or genes on the human Y chromosome [68]. Historically infertility was not considered to be genetically based; yet, when Tiepolo and Zuffardi karyotyped 1170 azoospermic and oligospermic men (with no sperm or less than 20 million sperm per ml, respectively), they observed that six azoospermic men had microscopic deletions of the long arm of the Y chromosome and when tested, their fathers did not [68]. Numerous studies confirmed these findings over the next two decades; however, it was equally likely that large microscopic deletions might be polymorphic in men, linked to disruption of meiotic chromosome pairing and/or might disrupt essential "fertility genes." It was not until the mid 1990s that the term "genetic infertility" was coined [3]. The discovery of interstitial deletions was made possible by the complete mapping of the Y chromosome with PCR-based markers that were useful for comprehensive deletion analysis [69, 70]. The frequency immediately indicated that Y chromosome deletions were an unexpectedly common cause of infertility in men [2, 71, 72]. Subsequent studies by many laboratories confirmed our results and identified two additional, less-frequent deletions [4]. Still later, sequencing of the human Y chromosome demonstrated that it has 156 transcription units that encode 27 proteins [5]. Genotype:phenotype correlations indicate that deletions of the *AZFc* region (a large region on the distal long arm of the Y chromosome) is associated with phenotypes that vary from the production of no sperm (Sertoli cell only [SCO] syndrome) to the production of a few hundred thousand sperm, in general. Phenotypes are entirely restricted to infertility associated with few or no germ cells, with no somatic abnormalities observed.

The need for a full complement of the sex chromosomes, XX or XY, is also further illustrated by the phenotypes associated with Turner syndrome (45, XO) in women [8, 73, 74]. The presence of just a single X chromosome (without the second X or Y chromosome) is one of the most common chromosomal abnormalities compatible with live birth (though >99% of XO infants are miscarried); postnatal phenotypes, often associated with mosaic XO cell composition, include abnormalities of cardiac development and aortic function, amenorrhea, and ovarian failure [75, 76]. Natural birth by those with pure, non-mosaic XO karyotype is rare, with less than a handful of cases reported. Logically, genes thought to be important for germ cell formation and differentiation are those that escape X-inactivation and potentially have a Y chromosome homolog given that both XX and XY individuals form germ cells in approximately similar quantity and developmental time frames [8, 73, 74].

In the last two decades, numerous genes and pathways have been implicated in human infertility and germ cell development [77, 78]. Genes span the entire developmental pathways of both sexes, including somatic sex determination; germ cell sex determination; primordial germ cell formation; migration of the primordial germ cells to the gonad; proliferation of initial populations of gonocytes; entry, progression, and completion of meiosis; and morphogenesis, culminating in sperm formation and folliculogenesis. Mutations and polymorphisms implicated in germline development include those in non-coding RNAs, translational and transcriptional factors as well as hormonal and paracrine regulators [77, 78].

Infertility and primary ovarian insufficiency

As noted above, infertility is very common [1]. The most common cause of infertility in the male is a quantitative and/or qualitative defect in sperm production. In most cases, an underlying etiology for spermatogeneic failure is not known but as described above in a subset of cases, genetic causes can be determined, including Y-chromosome deletions. In women, causes for infertility are diverse and can be linked to somatic and germline (oocyte) etiologies often associated with ovarian aging. In addition, a subset of women may experience primary ovarian insufficiency (POI). POI is the preferred term for the condition that was previously referred to as premature menopause or premature ovarian failure (POF). While specific diagnostic criteria have not been established, POI in its most severe form is typically considered to be present when a woman who is less than 40 years of age has experienced amenorrhea or irregular menses for 4 months or more and has had two serum follicle-stimulating hormone (FSH) levels (taken at least 1 month apart) in the menopausal range [79, 80]. This condition differs from naturally occurring menopause because POI is occurring prematurely and does not necessarily indicate the complete or permanent cessation of menstruation. Instead, POI involves varying and unpredictable ovarian function, most often accompanied by decreased ovarian reserve (oocyte number) [81–83].

Currently, there are large gaps in knowledge regarding molecular and genetic causes of POI and potential treatments. One cause of POI, first identified in the late 1990s, is premutations in the *fragile X mental retardation-1 (FMR1)* gene; premutations are associated with variable degrees of ovarian dysfunction with some women displaying overt POI and others demonstrating normal ovarian and reproductive function [84]. Strategies to assist women with POI are relatively few; however, two strategies may come to light in the years to come: (1) Recruitment of oocytes from the dormant rather than the cycling pool as described by Li and colleagues [85]. (2) Fertility preservation and/or restoration measures based on generation of immature oocytes for maturation post-transplantation or maturation in vitro [86]. Although the latter efforts are experimental and lack current ability to generate mature oocytes, efforts are moving forward with recruitment of oocytes from the dormant pool and seem likely to succeed if risks of miscarriage and chromosomal abnormalities can be minimized.

Essentially, Hsueh and colleagues (see Chapter 6) devised a novel method to activate dormant follicles via treatment of ovarian cortex (containing immature primordial follicles) with phosphatase and tensin homolog (PTEN) inhibitors and phosphatidylinositol 3-kinase (PI3K) activators in vitro [85]. These studies recognize that the majority of ovarian follicles stay dormant in mammals, including women; indeed the follicles remain dormant up to several decades in women and it is the depletion of the dormant pool that is linked to menopause. Typically in women, mechanisms that are still poorly understood result in the activation of approximately 1000 primordial follicles per month and the rest remain quiescent. As noted by Hsueh and colleagues, once recruited, primordial follicles continue growth to the early antral stage with minimal loss and readily respond to hormonal stimulation, leading to maturation for fertilization [85]. Studies in mice have shown that the PTEN gene, which encodes a phosphatase enzyme that negatively regulates the PI3K and Akt signaling pathway, is required for growth of all primordial follicles [87, 88]. Thus in key studies, Hsueh and colleagues exposed mouse ovaries transiently to PTEN inhibitors and a PI3K-activating peptide in vitro; subsequently they transplanted treated and control ovaries under the kidney capsule of FSH-treated adult recipients. They observed that they could obtain mature murine oocytes that were capable of contributing to IVF, blastocyst formation, and subsequent live births [85]. In addition, these authors demonstrated the efficacy of the PTEN inhibitor in activating dormant human primordial follicles in cortical strips donated by a cancer patient to yield mature oocytes. Translation of these studies to women may involve an in vitro follicle activation approach, followed by auto-transplantation, to enable retrieval of functional mature oocytes for infertile women with diminishing ovarian reserve and for cancer patients requiring fertility preservation. Future development, however, would focus on development of primordial follicles to the antral stage, followed by the generation of mature oocytes, in vitro, if possible. In addition, there will be a need to assess the frequency of aneuploidy in oocytes that are obtained via novel methods.

Need to assess aneuploidy

Indeed, aneuploidy is a major factor contributing to reproductive failure and adverse pregnancy outcomes in natural and IVF conceptions. Fetal aneuploidy is the most common cause of first trimester miscarriage and is present in 50–60% of miscarriages [89–91]. Although embryonic aneuploidy could be the result of missing chromosomes from either the ooctye or the sperm, the majority of numeric chromosomal abnormalities, miscarriages, and live births are maternal in origin [12, 13, 91–93]. Although classic studies examining the types of aneuploidy in live births and miscarriages have shown the preponderance to be due to maternal meiosis errors affecting a single chromosome, examinations of human embryos have shown a higher rate of complex aneuploidies and mosaicism [94, 95]. Maternal age and parental translocations are the only undisputed risk factors for chromosomal abnormalities in embryos. However, studies that examined preimplantation embryos have shown that women with recurrent pregnancy loss and those with diminished ovarian reserve have higher rates of aneuploidy in the embryos created by assisted reproductive technology (ART) than age-matched controls [96].

There are two well-described mechanisms for abnormal chromosome segregation in oocyte maturation, meiotic non-disjunction and premature separation of sister chromatids. In meiotic non-disjunction, homologous whole chromosomes fail to separate, leading to a polar body with either all four sets of sister chromatids from the affected chromosome (two from each homologous chromosome) or no copies of the affected chromosome because both copies of the homologous chromosomes are left in the oocyte. If meiosis II occurs normally, then this will lead to whole chromosome loss or gain in the oocyte. The second mechanism of abnormal chromosome separation in oocytes has been termed premature separation of sister chromatids (PSSC). In PSSC, homologous chromosomes align but the sister chromatids prematurely separate in M1, and the polar body and oocyte receive three or one chromatid from the affected chromosome [96, 97]. In this case, it is possible that the abnormality could correct in M2 or could persist and form an unbalanced gamete and aneuploid embryo. Although several studies in the recent literature have shown a high incidence of abnormalities in both PB1 and PB2, the rate and mechanism of correction after an abnormal first meiotic division is unknown [94]. Abundant efforts are aimed at identifying errors in chromosome segregation prior to transfer in order to increase the probability of a full-term, successful pregnancy. Recently, in light of the limitations of day 3 biopsies, the benefits of polar body biopsy and trophectoderm biopsy have been explored in much more detail [98, 99]. In parallel, time-lapse image analysis of early embryonic behavior has also been shown to have the potential to increase the probability of selecting a viable embryo [100]. Robust methods are needed to diagnose normal and abnormal developmental patterns if the full value of alternative strategies to generate human germline cells is to be realized for both basic and clinical applications. The studies of Hayashi and colleagues elegantly bring the differentiation of murine germ cells to completion with the production of pups derived not only from sperm but also oocytes *in vitro* [101]. Clearly, we are entering a new era for basic science and potentially clinical applications.

References

1. Hull MGR, Glazener CMA, Kelly NJ, *et al.* Population study of causes, treatment, and outcome of infertility. *Brit Med J* 1985; **291**: 1693–7.
2. Reijo R, Alagappan RK, Patrizio P, Page DC. Severe oligospermia resulting from deletions of the *Azoospermia Factor* gene on the Y chromosome. *Lancet* 1996; **347**: 1290–3.
3. Reijo R, Lee TY, Salo P, *et al.* Diverse spermatogenic defects in humans caused by Y chromosome deletions encompassing a novel RNA-binding protein gene. *Nat Genet* 1995; **10**(4): 383–93.
4. Vogt PH, Edelmann A, Kirsch S, *et al.* Human Y chromosome azoospermia factors (AZF) mapped to different subregions in Yq11. *Hum Mol Gene* 1996; **5**(7): 933–43.
5. Skaletsky H, Kuroda-Kawaguchi T, Minx PJ, *et al.* The male-specific region of the human Y chromosome is a mosaic of discrete sequence classes. *Nature* 2003; **423**: 825–37.
6. Repping S, van Daalen S, Brown L, *et al.* High mutation rates have driven extensive structural polymorphism among human Y chromosomes. *Nat Genet* 2006; **38**: 463–7.

7. Repping S, Skaletsky H, Lange J, *et al.* Recombination between palindromes P5 and P1 on the human Y chromosome causes massive deletions and spermatogenic failure. *Am J Hum Genet* 2002; **71**: 906–22.

8. Zinn AR, Page DC, Fisher EMC. Turner syndrome: the case of the missing sex chromosome. *Trends Genet* 1993; **9**: 90–3.

9. Hendry AP, Wenburg JK, Bentzen P, Volk EC, Quinn TP. Rapid evolution of reproductive isolation in the wild: evidence from introduced salmon. *Science* 2000; **290**: 516–18.

10. Swanson WJ, Vacquier VD. The rapid evolution of reproductive proteins. *Nat Rev Genet* 2002; **3**: 137–44.

11. Menken J, Larsen U. Estimating the incidence and prevalence and analyzing the correlates of infertility and sterility. *Ann NY Acad Sci* 1994; **709**(249): 249–65.

12. Hassold T, Hunt P. To err (meiotically) is human: the genesis of human aneuploidy. *Nat Rev Genet* 2001; **2**: 280–91.

13. Hunt PA, Hassold TJ. Sex matters in meiosis. *Science* 2002; **296**: 2181–3.

14. Saffman EE, Lasko P. Germline development in vertebrates and invertebrates. *Cell Mol Life Sci* 1999; **55**: 1141–63.

15. Houston DW, King ML. A critical role for *Xdazl,* a germ plasm-localized RNA, in the differentiation of primordial germ cells in *Xenopus. Development* 2000; **127**: 447–56.

16. Houston DW, King ML. Germ plasm and molecular determinants of germ cell fate. *Curr Top Dev Biol* 2000; **50**: 155–81.

17. Wylie C. Germ cells. *Curr Opin Genet Dev* 2000; **10**: 410–13.

18. McLaren A. Primordial germ cells in the mouse. *Dev Biol* 2003; **262**: 1–15.

19. McLaren A. Signalling for germ cells. *Genes Dev* 1999; **13**: 373–6.

20. Ying Y Liu, XM, Marble A Lawson KA, Zhao GQ. Requirement of Bmp8b for the generation of primordial germ cells in the mouse. *Mol Endocrinol* 2000; **14**: 1053–63.

21. Lawson KA, Dunn NR, Roelen BA, *et al. Bmp4* is required for the generation of primordial germ cells in the mouse embryo. *Genes Dev* 1999; **13**: 424–36.

22. Yoshimizu T Obinata M, Matsui Y. Stage-specific tissue and cell interactions play key roles in mouse germ cell specification. *Development* 2001; **128**: 481–90.

23. Tam P, Zhou S. The allocation of epiblast cells to ectodermal and germ-line lineages is influenced by position of the cells in the gastrulating mouse embryo. *Dev Biol* 1996; **178** 124–32.

24. Chiquoine A. The identification, origin and migration of the primordial germ cells in the mouse embryo. *Anat Rec* 1954; **118**: 135–46.

25. Hayashi K, Ohta H, Kurimoto K, Aramaki S, Saitou M. Reconstitution of the mouse germ cell specification pathway in culture by pluripotent stem cells. *Cell* 2011; **146**: 519–32.

26. Seki Y, Yamaji M, Yabuta Y, *et al.* Cellular dynamics associated with the genome-wide epigenetic reprogramming in migrating primordial germ cells in mice. *Development* 2007; **134**: 2627–38.

27. Ohinata Y, Payer B, O'Carroll D, *et al.* Blimp1 is a critical determinant of the germ cell lineage in mice. *Nature* 2005; **436**: 207–13.

28. Payer B, Saitou M, Barton S, *et al.* Stella is a maternal effect gene required for normal early development in mice. *Curr Biol* 2003; **13**: 2110–17.

29. Gomperts M, Garcia-Castro M, Wylie C, Heasman J. Interactions between primordial germ cells play a role in their migration in mouse embryos. *Development* 1994; **120**: 135–41.

30. Hajkova P, Erhardt S, Lane N, *et al.* Epigenetic reprogramming in mouse primordial germ cells. *Mech Dev* 2002; **117**: 15–23.

31. Hackett J, Zylicz J, Surani M. Parallel mechanisms of epigenetic reprogramming in the germline. *Trends Genet* 2012; **28**: 164–74.

32. Thomson J, Itskovitz-Eldor J, Shapiro S, *et al.* Embryonic stem cell lines derived from human blastocysts. *Science* 1998; **282**: 1145–7.

33. Chavez S, Meneses J, Nguyen H, Kim S, Reijo Pera RA. Characterization of six new human embryonic stem cell lines (HSF-7, -8, -9, -10, -12 and -13) derived in minimal animal-component conditions. *Stem Cells Dev* 2008; **17**: 535–46.

34. Adewumi O, Aflatoonian B, Ahrlund-Richter L, *et al.* Characterization of human embryonic stem cell lines by the International Stem Cell Initiative. *Nat Biotechnol* 2007; **25**(7): 803–16.

35. Brons I, Smithers L, Trotter M, *et al.* Derivation of pluripotent epiblast stem cells from mammalian embryos. *Nature* 2007; **448**: 191–5.

36. Tesar P, Chenoweth J, Brook F, *et al.* New cell lines from mouse epiblast share defining features with human embryonic stem cells. *Nature* 2007; **448**: 196–9.

37. Abeyta M, Clark AT, Rodriguez R, *et al.* Unique gene expression signatures of independently-derived human embryonic stem cell lines. *Hum Mol Genet* 2004; **13**: 601–8.

38. Clark AT, Bodnar MS, Fox MS, *et al.* Spontaneous differentiation of germ cells from human embryonic stem cells in vitro. *Hum Mol Genet* 2004; **13**: 727–39.

39. Zwaka T, Thomson J. A germ cell origin of embryonic stem cells? *Development* 2005; **132**: 227–33.

40. Okita K, Ichisaka T, Yamanaka S. Generation of germline-competent induced pluripotent stem cells. *Nature* 2007; **448**: 313–18.

41. Takahashi K, Tanabe K, Ohnuki M, *et al.* Induction of pluripotent stem cells from adult human fibroblasts by defined factors. *Cell* 2007; **131**: 861–72.

42. Takahashi K, Yamanaka S. Induction of pluripotent stem cells from mouse embryonic and adult fibroblast cultures by defined factors. *Cell* 2006; **126**: 663–76.

43. Wernig M, Meissner A, Foreman R, *et al.* In vitro reprogramming of fibroblasts into a pluripotent ES-cell-like state. *Nature* 2007; **448**: 318–25.

44. Yu J, Vodyanik M, Smuga-Otto K, *et al.* Induced pluripotent stem cell lines derived from human somatic cells. *Science* 2007; **318**: 1917–20.

45. Park I, Zhao R, West J, *et al.* Reprogramming of human somatic cells to pluripotency with defined factors. *Nature* 2008; **451**: 141–6.

46. Hubner K, Fuhrmann G, Christenson L, *et al.* Derivation of oocytes from mouse embryonic stem cells. *Science* 2003; **300**: 1251–6.

47. Lacham-Kaplan O, Chy H, Trounson A. Testicular cell conditioned medium supports differentiation of embryonic stem (ES) cells into ovarian structures containing oocytes. *Stem Cells* 2005; **24**: 266–73.

48. Toyooka Y, Tsunekawa N, Akasu R, Noce T. Embryonic stem cells can form germ cells *in vitro. Proc Natl Acad Sci USA* 2003; **100**: 11457–62.

49. Geijsen N, Horoschak M, Kim K, *et al.* Derivation of embryonic germ cells and male gametes from embryonic stem cells. *Nature* 2004; **427**: 148–54.

50. Nayernia K, Nolte J, Michelmann H, *et al.* In vitro-differentiated embryonic stem cells give rise to male gametes that can generate offspring mice. *Dev Cell* 2006; **11**: 125–32.

51. Clark AT, Rodriguez R, Bodnar M, *et al.* Human STELLAR, NANOG, and GDF3 genes are expressed in pluripotent cells and map to chromosome 12p13, a hot-spot for teratocarcinoma. *Stem Cells* 2004; **22**: 169–79.

52. Bucay N, Yebra M, Cirulli V, *et al.* A novel approach for the derivation of putative primordial germ cells and sertoli cells from human embryonic stem cells. *Stem Cells* 2009; **27**: 68–77.

53. Tilgner K, Atkinson S, Golebiewska A, *et al.* Isolation of primordial germ cells from differentiating human embryonic stem cells. *Stem Cells* 2008; **26**: 3075–85.

54. Kee K, Gonsalves J, Clark A, Pera RR. Bone morphogenetic proteins induce germ cell differentiation from human embryonic stem cells. *Stem Cells Dev* 2006; **15**: 831–7.

55. Kee K, Angeles V, Flores M, Nguyen H, Reijo Pera RA. Human DAZL, DAZ and BOULE genes modulate primordial germ cell and haploid gamete formation. *Nature* 2009; **462**: 222–5.

56. Takahashi K, Okita K, Nakagawa M, Yamanaka S. Induction of pluripotent stem cells from fibroblast cultures. *Nat Protoc* 2007; **2**(12): 3081–9.

57. Park T, Galic Z, Conway A, *et al.* Derivation of primordial germ cells from human embryonic and induced pluripotent stem cells is significantly improved by coculture with human fetal gonadal cells. *Stem Cells* 2009; **27**: 783–95.

58. Panula S, Medrano J, Kee K, *et al.* Human germ cell differentiation from fetal- and adult-derived induced pluripotent stem cells. *Hum Mol Genet* 2010; **20**: 752–62.

59. Medrano J, Ramathal C, Nguyen H, Simon C, Reijo Pera RA. Divergent RNA-binding proteins, DAZL and VASA, induce meiotic progression in human germ cells derived in vitro. *Stem Cells* 2012; **30**: 441–51.

60. Eguizabal C, Montserrat N, Vassena R, *et al.* Complete meiosis from human induced pluripotent stem cells. *Stem Cells* 2011; **29**: 1186–95.

61. Novak I, Lightfoot D, Wang H, *et al.* Mouse embryonic stem cells form follicle-like ovarian structures but do not progress through meiosis. *Stem Cells* 2006; **24**: 1931–6.

62. Qing T, Shi Y, Qin H, *et al.* Induction of oocyte-like cells from mouse embryonic stem cells by co-culture with ovarian granulosa cells. *Differentiation* 2007; **75**: 902–11.

63. Payer B, Chuva-de-Sousa-Lopes S, Barton S, *et al.* Generation of stella-GFP transgenic mice: a novel tool to study germ cell development. *Genesis* 2006; **44**: 75–83.

64. Salvador L, Silva C, Kostetskii I, Radice G, Strauss J. The promoter of the oocyte-specific gene, *Gdf9*, is active in population of cultured mouse embryonic stem cells with an oocytelike phenotype. *Methods* 2008; **45**: 172–81.

65. Nicholas C, Haston K, Grewall A, Longacre T, Reijo Pera RA. Transplantation directs oocyte maturation from embryonic stem cells and provides a therapeutic strategy for female infertility. *Hum Mol Genet* 2009; **18**: 4376–89.

66. Nicholas C, Haston K, Reijo Pera RA. Intact fetal ovarian cord formation promotes mouse oocyte survival and development. *BMC Dev Biol* 2010; **10**: 2.

67. Haston K, Tung J, Reijo Pera RA. Dazl functions in maintenance of pluripotency and genetic and epigenetic programs of differentiation in mouse primordial germ cells in vivo and in vitro. *PLoS One* 2009; **4**: e5654.

68. Tiepolo L, Zuffardi O. Localization of factors controlling spermatogenesis in the nonfluorescent portion of the human Y chromosome long arm. *Hum Genet* 1976; **34**: 119–24.

69. Foote S, Vollrath D, Hilton A, Page DC. The human Y chromosome: overlapping DNA clones spanning the euchromatic region. *Science* 1992; **258**: 60–6.

70. Vollrath D, Foote S, Hilton A, *et al.* The human Y chromosome: A 43-interval map based on naturally occurring deletions. *Science* 1992 **258**: 52–9.

71. Mulhall JP, Reijo R, Alaggappan R, *et al.* Azoospermic men with deletion of the *DAZ* gene cluster are capable of completing spermatogenesis: fertilization, normal embryonic development and pregnancy occur when retrieved testicular spermatozoa are used for intracytoplasmic sperm injection. *Hum Reprod* 1997; **12**(3); 503–8.

72. Page DC, Silber S, Brown LG. Men with infertility caused by AZFc deletion can produce sons by intracytoplasmic sperm injection, but are likely to transmit the deletion and infertility. *Hum Reprod* 1999; **14**: 1722–6.

73. Rappold GA. The pseudoautosomal regions of the human sex chromosomes. *Hum Genet* 1993; **92**: 315–24.

74. Fisher EMC, Beer-Romero P, Brown LG, *et al.* Homologous ribosomal protein genes on the human X and Y chromosomes: Escape from X inactivation and possible implications for Turner syndrome. *Cell* 1990; **63**: 1205–18.

75. Turner A. Syndrome of infantilism, congenital webbed neck, and cubitus valgus. *Endocrinology* 1938; **23**: 566–74.

76. Saenger P. Turner's syndrome. *N Engl J Med* 1996; **335**: 1749–54.

77. Roy A, Matzuk M. Deconstructing mammalian reproduction: using knockouts to define fertility pathways. *Reproduction* 2006; **131**: 207–19.

78. Matzuk M, Lamb D. Genetic dissection of mammalian fertility pathways. *Nat Cell Biol* 2002; **4** Suppl: 41–9.

79. Rebar R. Premature ovarian failure. *Obstet Gynecol* 2009; **113**: 1355–63.

80. Nelson L. Primary ovarian insufficiency. *N Engl J Med* 2009; **360**: 606–14.

81. Schuh-Huerta S, Johnson N, Rosen M, *et al.* Genetic variants and environmental factors associated with hormonal markers of ovarian reserve in Caucasian and African American women. *Hum Reprod* 2012; **27**: 594–608.

82. Rosen M, Sternfeld B, Schuh-Huerta S, *et al.* Antral follicle count – absence of significant midlife decline. *Fertil Steril* 2010; **94**: 2182–5.

83. Schuh-Huerta S, Johnson N, Rosen M, *et al.* Genetic markers of ovarian follicle number and menopause in women of multiple ethnicities. *Hum Genet* 2012; **131**: 1709–24.

84. Murray A. Premature ovarian failure and the FMR1 gene. *Semin Reprod Med* 2000; **18**: 59–66.

85. Li J, Kawamura K, Cheng Y, *et al.* Activation of dormant ovarian follicles to generate mature eggs. *Proc Natl Acad Sci USA* 2010; **107**: 10280–4.

86. Nicholas C, Chavez S, Baker V, Reijo Pera RA. Instructing an embryonic stem cell-derived oocyte fate: lessons from endogenous oogenesis. *Endocr Rev* 2009; **30**: 264–83.

87. Reddy P, Liu L, Adhikari D, *et al.* Oocyte-specific deletion of Pten causes premature activation of the primordial follicle pool. *Science* 2008; **319**(5863): 611–13.

88. Reddy P, Shen L, Ren C, *et al.* Activation of Akt (PKB) and suppression of FKHRL1 in mouse and rat oocytes by stem cell factor during follicular activation and development. *Dev Biol* 2005; **281**(2): 160–70.

89. Stephenson M, Awartani K, Robinson W. Cytogenetic analysis of miscarriages from couples with recurrent miscarriage: a case-control study. *Hum Reprod* 2002; **17**: 446–51.

90. Lathi R, Westphal L, Milki A. Aneuploidy in the miscarriages of infertile women and the potential benefit of preimplanation genetic diagnosis. *Fertil Steril* 2008; **89**: 353–7.

91. Hassold T, Takaesu N. Analysis of non-disjunction in human trisomic spontaneous abortions. *Prog Clin Biol Res* 1989; **311**: 115–34.

92. Koehler KE, Hawley RS, Sherman S, Hassold T. Recombination and nondisjunction in humans and flies. *Hum Mol Genet* 1996; **5** Spec No: 1495–504.

93. Hassold T, Sherman S, Hunt P. Counting cross-overs: characterizing meiotic recombination in mammals. *Hum Mol Genet* 2000; **9**: 2409–19.

94. Kuliev A, Zlatopolsky Z, Kirillova I, Spivakova J, Janzen JC. Meiosis errors in over 20,000 oocytes studied in the practice of preimplantation aneuploidy testing. *Reprod Biomed Online* 2011; **22**: 2–8.

95. Mantzouratou A, Mania A, Fragouli E, *et al.* Variable aneuploidy mechanisms in embryos from couples with poor reproductive histories undergoing preimplantation genetic screening. *Hum Reprod* 2007; **22**: 1844–53.

96. Vialard F, Boitrelle F, Molina-Gomes D, Selva J. Predisposition to aneuploidy in the oocyte. *Cytogenet Genome Res* 2011; **133**: 127–35.

97. Gabriel A, Thornhill A, Ottolini C, *et al.* Array comparative genomic hybridisation on first polar bodies suggests that non-disjunction is not the predominant mechanism leading to aneuploidy in humans. *J Med Genet* 2011; **48**: 433–7.

98. McArthur S, Leigh D, Marshall J, *et al.* Blastocyst trophectoderm biopsy and preimplantation genetic diagnosis for familial monogenic disorders and chromosomal translocations. *Prenat Diagn* 2008; **28**: 434–42.

99. McArthur S, Leigh D, Marshall J, de Boer KA, Jansen R. Pregnancies and live births after trophectoderm biopsy and preimplantation genetic testing of human blastocysts. *Fertil Steril* 2005; **84**: 1628–36.

100. Wong C, Loewke K, Bossert N, *et al.* Non-invasive imaging of human embryos before embryonic genome activation predicts development to the blastocyst stage. *Nat Biotechnol* 2010; **28**: 1115–21.

101. Hayashi K, Ogushi S, Kurimoto K, *et al.* Offspring from oocytes derived from in vitro primordial germ-like cells in mice. *Science* 2012; **338**: 971–5.

Chapter 20

In vitro differentiation of germ cells from stem cells

Fumihiro Sugawa, Karin Hübner, and Hans R. Schöler

Introduction

Germ cells are the only cell type in the body that can carry genetic information on to the next generation, and the somatic cell lineages give rise to the soma, or body [1]. The development of germ cells from primordial germ cells (PGCs) into mature gametes involves a series of complex biological processes that occur over a given time period and that can be subdivided into several steps: specification, migration, epigenetic reprogramming, sex differentiation, and meiosis, the last of which includes oogenesis or spermatogenesis. A complex program of genetic regulatory networks rigorously directs the precise sequence of developmental events. Some genes are expressed specifically in germ cells, whereas others are expressed specifically in the somatic component of the germ cell environment. Yet still others are expressed in both germ cells and somatic cells. Despite recognizing the importance of germ cells, the scientific community has not yet elucidated the molecular mechanisms underlying the individual steps of germ cell development – these remain poorly understood, owing in part to the lack of sufficient tools and quantities of cells for conclusive studies.

Embryonic stem cells (ESCs) are cells derived from the inner cell mass (ICM) of preimplantation blastocysts [2–4]. These cells have the ability to self-renew indefinitely while maintaining the feature of pluripotency, defined as the potential to differentiate into cell types of all three germ layers (ectoderm, endoderm, and mesoderm) and germ cells. The establishment of mouse ESCs (mESCs) and human ESCs (hESCs) brought great excitement not only to the scientific community, but also to the clinical setting, raising high expectations on the potential use of these cells to broaden our understanding of the mechanisms involved in development and disease. However, the controversy surrounding the derivation of ESCs from "human embryos" has limited the number of cell lines that could be derived. A breakthrough in the mid 2000s forever changed the field of stem cell research and has the potential to overcome this limitation. Somatic cells were discovered to be capable of being reprogrammed into so-called induced pluripotent stem cells (iPSCs) [5, 6] by the ectopic co-expression of the four transcription factors Oct4, Sox2, Klf4, and c-Myc – four factors that are known to sustain pluripotency in ESCs. This new technique enables the derivation of patient-specific iPSCs for disease modeling, drug screening, and investigations into the causative mechanisms underlying disease.

Over the past few years, several studies have demonstrated the successful in vitro differentiation of pluripotent stem cells, including iPSCs, from a variety of organisms into PGCs. Amazingly, some reports have also demonstrated further maturation of these germ cells into presumptive gametes, suggesting that in vitro differentiation models are a powerful tool for the study of reproductive biology. In this review, prior to examining in vitro germ cell development and gametogenesis in culture, a brief review into mammalian germline development using the mouse as a key model will be provided. This will be followed by an overview of the advances in germ cell differentiation using mouse and human stem cells to date, with a focus on the generation of oocytes. The chapter will end with a presentation of the challenges encountered in the successful generation of mature gametes.

Germ cell development in vivo

Current understanding of the mechanisms underlying germ cell determination and differentiation is based largely on studies performed in the mouse. As the series of sequential differentiation events to produce

Biology and Pathology of the Oocyte, 2nd edn., ed. Alan Trounson, Roger Gosden, and Ursula Eichenlaub-Ritter. Published by Cambridge University Press.

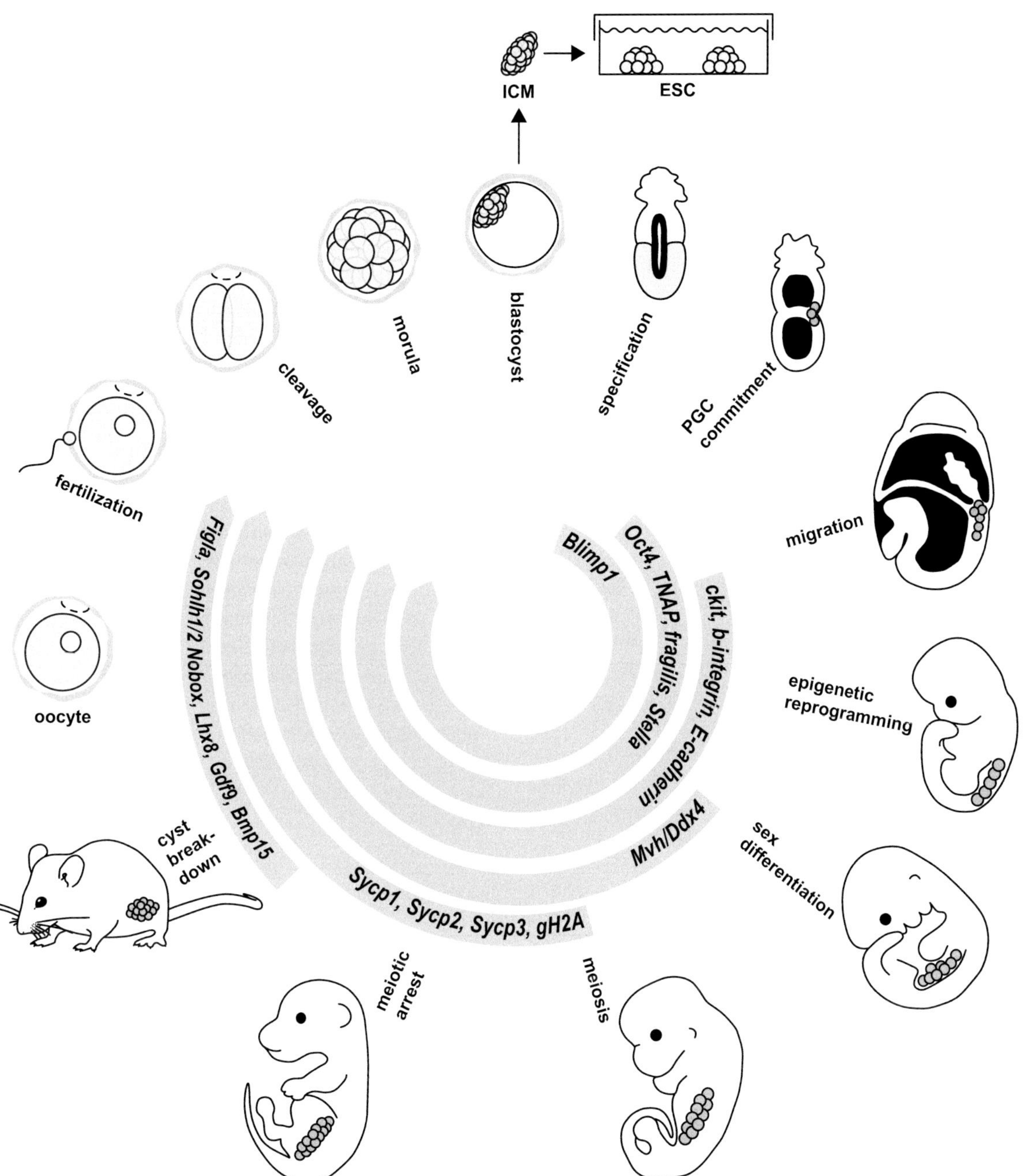

Figure 20.1 Schematic presentation of primordial germ cell development and oogenesis in the mouse.

germ cells is highly conserved among mammalian species, this section provides an overview of germ cell development in the mouse (Figure 20.1). A complex and as yet not fully understood network of transcriptional regulators directs the development of gametes and any disturbance of the fine-tuned gene expression program can lead to reproductive abnormalities and disease. Despite large numbers of essential sets of genes involved in gametogenesis, only a small subset of the genes known to play pivotal roles in germ cell development in vitro and in vivo will be outlined in this review.

Germ cell specification

The germ cell lineage is not allocated in the embryo proper of mammals before implantation – unlike the case of lower-order eukaryotes – as early epiblast cells injected into blastocysts have an equipotent ability to enter the mouse germ line [7, 8]. Cells within the proximal epiblast begin their commitment to become PGCs at the onset of gastrulation, between 5.5 and 6 days postcoitum (dpc) [9], with the entire epiblast retaining this germline plasticity as late as 7 dpc [10] in response to paracrine signaling from the extra-embryonic ectoderm (ExE) and visceral endoderm (VE) [11]. BMP2, BMP4, and BMP8, members of the bone morphogenetic protein family, induce Smad1, Smad5, and Smad8 signaling in the *Oct4*, *TNAP*, *fragilis* (also known as *Ifitm3*) triple-positive founding cell population of the proximal epiblast, which subsequently comprises approximately 45 committed PGCs by 7.25 dpc [12–15]. The expression of the transcriptional repressor *Blimp1* (also known as *Prdm1*) in PGC progenitor cells around 6.5 dpc marks the specification of the PGC lineage by repression of the homeobox genes (*Hox* genes), thus silencing the somatic program [16]. Committed PGCs reactivate regulators of pluripotency, such as *Oct4*, *Sox2*, *Nanog* [16–18], and activate the expression of germline-specific genes, such as *Blimp1*, *fragilis*, and *Stella* (also known as *Dppa3)* [17].

Germ cell migration

Subsequent to the commitment of PGCs at the proximal epiblast, as yet undefined mechanisms regulate the formation of functional gametes. Proliferating PGCs migrate through amoeboid-like movements toward the dorsal region of the fetus and reach the genital ridges at about 10.5 dpc. Genes that are expressed in the germ cells and in the soma ensure not only PGC survival, but also proper gonad formation. Signaling cascades from gonadal somatic cells and cell-to-cell interactions ensure PGC proliferation, survival, and colonization of the gonads. For example, expression of integrin-β1 and E-cadherin [19, 20] facilitates the interaction of PGCs with the extracellular matrix (ECM) and cell-to-cell adhesion via cellular processes. Receptor–ligand interactions, such as cKit signaling or chemokine responsiveness of PGCs to stromal cell-derived factor-1 (SDF1) signaling from the genital ridge, are crucial for germ cell development and subsequent maturation of PGCs into gametes [21, 22]. Concomitant with the arrival of PGCs at the genital ridges is the up-regulation of the mouse Vasa homolog (*Mvh*, *Vasa*, *Ddx4*) of the *Drosophila vasa* gene in PGCs – an exclusive marker for irreversibly committed cells of the germ line [23, 24].

Epigenetic reprogramming

The full commitment of cells toward the germ cell lineage is contingent upon the fine-tuned molecular mechanisms regulating the maintenance of genomic imprinting. DNA methylation, a key mechanism in this stage of development, regulates the imprinted allele-specific gene expression. Once established, the methylation status of the DNA is typically stable through generations. However, dynamic changes in the DNA methylation pattern of germ cells occur at specific time points in germ cell development – namely in fertilized embryos and in proliferating and migratory PGCs. Following fertilization, genome-wide demethylation may occur actively by enzymes and passively by non-methylation during replication of the paternal and maternal genome, followed by *de novo* DNA methylation. Similarly, DNA demethylation and erasure of imprinting occurs in PGCs at about 10.5 to 13.5 dpc [25]. Genomic methylation becomes subsequently reestablished in the sex-specific patterns (imprinting) in mature germ cells.

Sex differentiation

Upon colonization, the PGCs (now called gonia) are exposed to retinoic acid (RA), and interact with sex-specific somatic Sertoli or granulosa cells. The signals from these gonadal somatic cells precipitate the onset of sexual differentiation of the gonia at about 13.5 dpc. Consequently, in the male genital ridge, PGCs undergo mitotic arrest and become irreversibly committed to the spermatogenic cell fate by 14.5 dpc [26]. These spermatogonia resume cell proliferation at about 10 days post-partum (dpp) and continue spermatogenesis. In the female gonads, gonia reside in clusters, so-called germ cell cysts, enter meiosis at about 13.5 dpc, and transiently arrest at the diplotene stage of meiosis I as primary oocytes by 18.5 dpc.

Meiosis

Meiosis is a unique type of cell division that generates gametes with a haploid parental chromosome set. Specialized interactions between chromosomes and modifications of the cell-cycle machinery facilitate chromosome segregation – a precisely timed process involving complex pathways. Errors in meiosis are the leading cause of birth defects and infertility, and unraveling the mechanisms involved in the meiotic process represents one of the biggest challenges in developmental biology today. In the mouse, oocytes initiate meiosis in the fetal ovary between 13.5 and 16.5 dpc and arrest in the diplotene stage of meiotic prophase I by 18.5 dpc. At the onset of meiosis, germ cells express meiosis-specific proteins, such as synaptonemal complex protein 1, 2, and 3 (SYCP1, SYCP2, and SYCP3) or γH2AX, that play a role in axial core compaction, synapsis, and recombination. The down-regulation of *Sycp1* in oocytes coincides with the arrest of oocytes in the diplotene stage of prophase I and is thought to signal somatic cells to begin organizing the primordial follicles [27]. Oocytes resume meiosis I by entering into metaphase I during folliculogenesis a few weeks after birth to arrest again in the second meiotic division prior to ovulation.

The mechanisms underlying sex differentiation and initiation of meiosis of gonocytes remain poorly understood. One recent study identified RA as a meiosis-inducing signal expressed in the gonads. While RA triggers meiotic entry by inducing *Stra8* expression in germ cells of the fetal ovary, the protein is degraded by the cytochrome P450 enzyme CYP26B1 in the fetal testis, resulting in inhibition of germ cell entry into meiosis [28]. Another study identified fibroblast growth factor (FGF9) to be a negative regulator of meiosis in the fetal testis. RA and FGF9 act directly on germ cells to up-regulate *Stra8* expression and prevent *Stra8* up-regulation, respectively [29].

Folliculogenesis and oocyte maturation

Shortly after birth, germ cell cysts degenerate and about one-third of the oocytes become enclosed by granulosa cells and form primordial follicles, while the remaining oocytes undergo programmed cell death, or apoptosis [30]. Upon activation of the primordial follicle, the complex process of folliculogenesis ensues, where a bidirectional communication system between the oocyte and the companion granulosa cells directs follicle development [31, 32]. Primordial follicles transition to become primary follicles when the granulosa cells surrounding the oocyte turn into cuboidal granulosa cells. Steel factor (SCF), leukemia inhibitory factor (LIF), and basic fibroblast growth factor (bFGF) secreted by the somatic compartment and cKIT receptor, *Figla*, *Sohlh1*, *Sohlh2*, *Nobox*, and *Lhx8* expressed by the oocyte promote this transition and rapid growth of the oocyte. During the secondary follicle stage, proliferation of granulosa and theca cells is mediated by expression of *Gdf9* and *Bmp15* in the oocyte [33]. Subsequently, in response to follicle-stimulating hormone (FSH) and luteinizing hormone (LH), follicles form an antrum, initiating the process of steroidogenesis. Once the oocyte reaches maturity within the antral follicle, ovulation proceeds and meiosis resumes. Transcriptional regulators expressed in the soma of the ovary ensure ovarian determination. For example, the transcription factor *Foxl2* is expressed in granulosa cells throughout folliculogenesis, directing the differentiation of these cells and repressing testis-specific genes. Removal of *Foxl2* leads to somatic sex reprogramming of the ovary into testes [34].

In vitro differentiation of germ cells from mouse pluripotent stem cells

Over the past 10 years, a number of research groups have successfully generated germ cells in vitro (Table 20.1). The majority of publications report the generation of putative migratory or post-migratory PGCs from stem cells and subsequent attempts to further differentiate them into gametes (Figure 20.2). In 2003, Hübner *et al.* reported the generation of PGCs in vitro from mouse XY-ESCs that followed the oogenesis pathway upon extended culture conditions [35]. The authors differentiated ESCs as a feeder-free monolayer in the absence of LIF and observed *Oct4* and *Vasa* double-positive presumptive post-migratory germ cells after about 8 days of culture. Aggregates of VASA-positive and *Oct4*-negative cells were subsequently found to detach from the cell layer and produced large SYCP3-positive oocyte-like cells. After 30 days of culture, rare blastocyst-like structures were detected, indicative of parthenogenetic activation. However, the functionality of the presumptive oocytes was not shown. Shortly afterwards, Toyooka *et al.* published a study describing the differentiation of ESCs into male germ cells in vitro [36]. In that study, mESCs were co-aggregated with BMP4-producing cells to form embryoid bodies (EBs) and, interestingly, *Vasa*-positive presumptive post-migratory PGCs were detected within 1 day of co-aggregation. This observation indicates that a subpopulation of ESCs had already committed to the germ cell fate within the ESC culture, as the in vivo development of the ICM into post-migratory PGCs takes significantly longer. These *Vasa*-positive cells developed into sperm-like cells upon transplantation into

Table 20.1. Overview of germ cell differentiation procedures cited in this review

Reference (No.)	Origin	Approach/factors supplemented	Cell type observed/offspring
Hübner *et al.*, 2003 [35]	mESC	ML/-	PostPGC, oocyte, blastocyst
Toyooka *et al.*, 2003 [36]	mESC	EB/co-aggregate with TM4 secreting BMP4	PostPGC, sperm
Geijsen *et al.*, 2004 [37]	mESC	ML/-	Sperm, blastocyst (by ICSI)
Lacham-Kaplan *et al.*, 2006 [41]	mESC	EB/mouse testis-conditioned medium	Oocyte
Nayernia *et al.*, 2006 [40]	mESC	ML/retinoic acid (RA)	PostPGC, sperm, offspring[a] (abnormal)
Novak *et al.*, 2006 [38]	mESC	ML/-	Oocyte
Qing *et al.*, 2007 [42]	mESC	EB/co-culture with mouse granulosa cells	Oocyte
Nicholas *et al.*, 2009 [43]	mESC	EB/BMP4, CYP26 inhibitor, SDF1, SCF, bFGF, *N*-acetylcysteine, forskolin	PostPGC, oocyte
Hayashi *et al.*, 2011 [45]	mESC, miPSC	ML+EB/activin A, bFGF, BMP4, BMP8b, LIF, SCF, EGF	PrePGC, offspring[a]
Psathaki *et al.*, 2011 [39]	mESC	ML+EB/ITS, EGF, SCF, BMP4, LIF, FSH	Oocyte
Vincent *et al.*, 2011 [46]	mESC	EB/-	PrePGC
Clark *et al.*, 2004 [48]	hESC	EB	PostPGC
Kee *et al.*, 2006 [49]	hESC	EB/BMP4, BMP7, BMP8b	PostPGC
Tilgner *et al.*, 2008 [50]	hESC	ML/-	PostPGC
West *et al.*, 2008 [54]	hESC	ML/co-culture with MEF, bFGF	PostPGC
Bucay *et al.*, 2009 [57]	hESC	ML/co-culture with MEF, bFGF	PostPGC
Kee *et al.*, 2009 [51]	hESC	ML/BMP4, BMP7, BMP8b	PostPGC, sperm[b] (DAZ family)
Park *et al.*, 2009 [56]	hESC, hiPSC	ML/co-culture with hFGSCs	PostPGC
Eguizabal *et al.*, 2011 [58]	hESC, hiPSC	ML/co-culture with MEF, RA, bFGF, LIF, forskolin, R115866	Sperm
Medrano *et al.*, 2012 [53]	hESC, hiPSC	ML/-	PostPGC, sperm[b] (VASA)
Panula *et al.*, 2011 [52]	hESC, hiPSC	ML/BMP4, BMP7, BMP8b	PostPGC, sperm[b] (DAZ family)
West *et al.*, 2011 [55]	hESC	ML/co-culture with MEF, bFGF	PostPGC, sperm

[a] Upon transplantation into mouse.
[b] Upon overexpression of germ cell-related genes(s).
mESC, mouse embryonic stem cell; miPSC, mouse induced pluripotent stem cell; hESC, human embryonic stem cell; hiPSC, human induced pluripotent stem cell; ML, monolayer; EB, embryoid body; MEF, mouse embryonic fibroblast; hFGSC, human fetal gonad stromal cell; R115866, CYP26 inhibitor; postPGC, post-migratory PGC; prePGC, pre-migratory PGC; PGC, primordial germ cell.

mouse testis; however, fertilization was not reported to occur. Similarly, Geijsen *et al.* described the generation in vitro of male haploid cells from spontaneously differentiating EBs [37]. Upon intracytoplasmic injection of sperm into oocytes, the haploid cells developed into blastocysts, but offspring were not produced. Both studies demonstrated the generation of male germ cells, but as germ cells of both sexes share a common precursor, these cells might also be capable of developing into female germ cells under appropriate conditions. Taken together, these initial reports clearly demonstrated the differentiation capacity of mESCs into both male and female germ cells in culture, and spurred further efforts in the development of robust in vitro differentiation systems.

Those researchers have not yet been able to demonstrate proof of competence and functionality of the reported ESC-derived germ cells. In this context, Novak *et al.* reported that ESC-derived germ cells exhibit abnormal progression through meiosis [38]. Although the putative germ cells generated by those researchers exhibited SYCP3 protein expression, additional meiotic markers or homologous chromosome synapses specific for meiotic progression could not be detected. These data imply that the majority of in vitro-generated germ cells fail to undergo normal

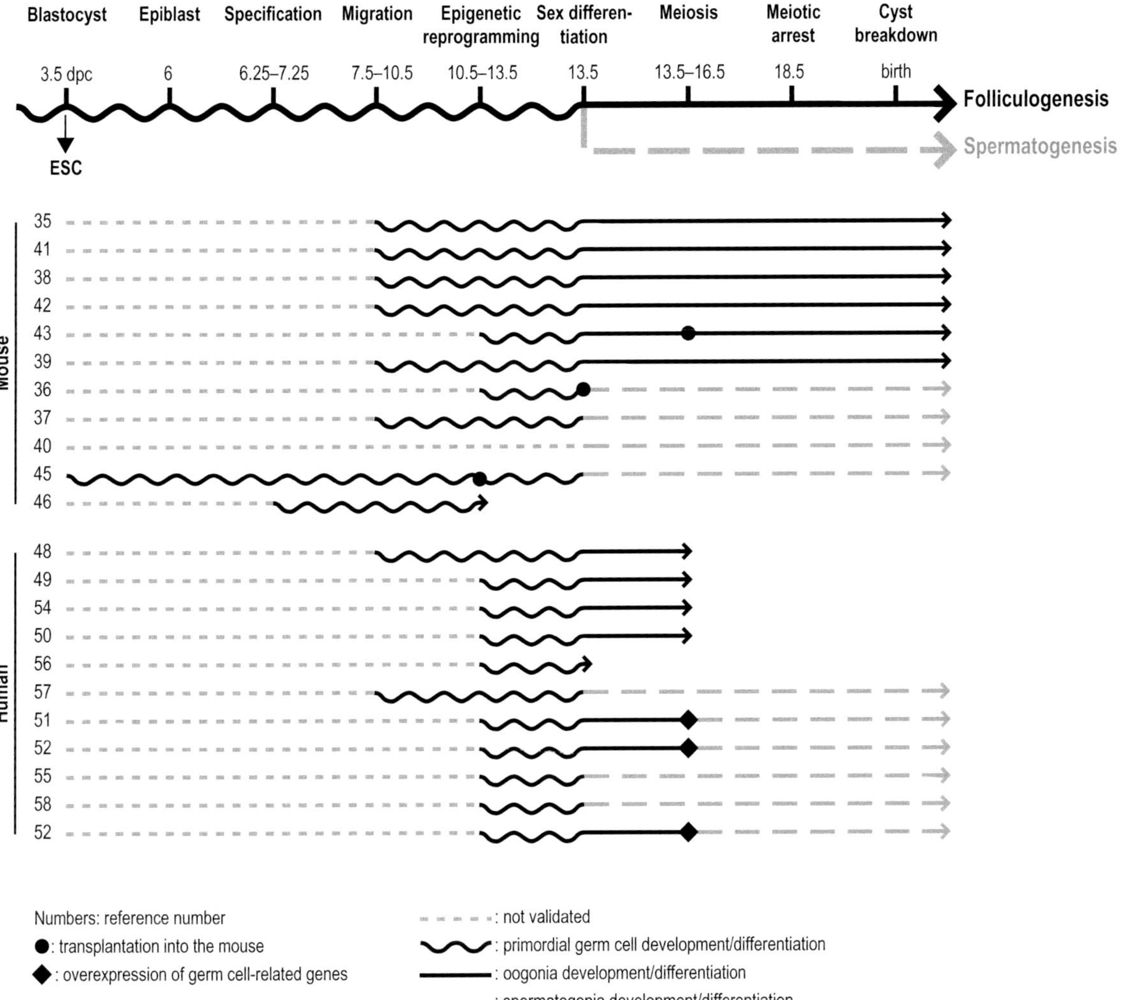

Figure 20.2 Chronology of mouse germ cell development and correlation of cited in vitro germ cell protocols.

meiosis, which may explain their failure to further differentiate into functional gametes. Nevertheless, a recent ultrastructural comparison between natural and ESC-derived oocytes and follicles by Psathaki *et al.* revealed that the oocytes exhibited remarkable similarities, as did, interestingly, the in vitro-produced granulosa-like cells. The aggregates analyzed in that study exhibited characteristics typical of natural follicles, that is, one or multiple oocyte-like cells, an ECM, and granulosa-like cells exhibiting transzonal projections (TZPs). These data suggest the presence of ongoing folliculogenesis with active interactions between germ cells and granulosa cells generated in vitro [39]. The competence and functionality of these oocytes, however, could not be investigated due to insufficient oocyte yields. To overcome this shortage, culture conditions that promote germ cell proliferation and meiosis more efficiently must be developed.

One report describes the in vitro differentiation of mature sperm, as ascertained by morphology and immunocytochemical staining for known sperm markers [40]. According to this report, stable germ cell-like cell lines were derived from mESCs carrying a *Stra8* reporter construct [40]. Upon differentiation on inactivated mouse embryonic fibroblasts (MEFs) and induction with RA, about 60% of the cells expressed *Stra8*, an RA-responsive gene involved in meiosis in the male mouse. The *Stra8*-positive cell population was further cultivated under non-inducing conditions, giving rise to stable cell lines with conserved *Stra8* and germ cell marker expression, including *Oct4*, *Stella*, and *Vasa*, indicative of spermatogonial stem cells (SSCs). After another course of RA treatment, acrosin-positive, haploid cells were detected in the medium, indicative of post-meiotic spermatids. However, analysis of these differentiated cells revealed incomplete epigenetic resetting. ESC-derived SSCs gave rise to sperm after implantation into testis and intracytoplasmic injection of this sperm into oocytes produced live offspring. However, the progeny had obvious growth abnormalities and died within 5 months. This report provides evidence for the potential derivation of male gametes in vitro, but the responsibility for generating live offspring with normal development remains with the scientific community.

Other approaches for the generation of germ cells from ESCs in vitro utilize co-cultures with gonadal somatic cells or cultures in conditioned medium. Lacham-Kaplan *et al.* reported the formation of ovary-like structures containing oocyte-like cells from differentiating EBs in testis-conditioned medium that were collected from testicular cell cultures of newborn mice [41]. After 2–5 days of differentiation, *Oct4*, *cKit*, and *Vasa* triple-positive presumptive PGCs were observed, which further developed into 15–30 μm large oocyte-like cells within follicle-like structures. Although expression of the oocyte markers *Figla* and *Zp3* was shown, neither meiotic progression nor functionality was confirmed. A similar report came from Qing *et al.*, demonstrating that co-culturing EBs with granulosa cells from newborn mice enhances female germ cell marker expression and oocyte-like cell formation [42]. Different from other publications is the reported expression of *Sycp1*, *Sycp2*, and *Sycp3* at the mRNA level in presumptive oocytes. However, SYCP3 was detected in the cytoplasm, while SYCP proteins colocalize with DNA during meiosis in natural germ cells. These presumptive oocytes reached a maximum size of approximately 25 μm in diameter. Taken together, these data suggested that factors secreted by the somatic component of the gonads and the direct interaction of gonadal somatic cells with in vitro-generated germ cells appear to have positive effects on in vitro germ cell differentiation. However, these effects could not give rise to mature and functional gametes. Nevertheless, the identification of factors that enhance germ cell differentiation in these culture systems would greatly enhance our understanding of germ cell development both in vivo and in vitro.

The lack of markers that can distinguish germ cells from ESCs likely constitutes the biggest limitation in the field of in vitro germ cell differentiation to date. PGCs and ESCs share most of the known markers of the germ cell lineage, hampering the ability to separate efficiently PGCs from ESCs or pluripotent cell populations. For example, stage-specific embryonic antigen 1 (SSEA1) is not only commonly used for the identification of undifferentiated mESCs, but also serves as a surface marker for the isolation of early PGCs from somatic cell populations. Nicholas *et al.* differentiated *Oct4*Δ PE-GFP-ESCs and reported that a combination of common markers can be used to distinguish early PGCs and late female germ cells from differentiating ESCs by the signal intensity during purification [43]. An isolated *Oct4* and SSEA1 double-positive (high signal) population was enriched within differentiation cultures with early germ cell markers, such as *Oct4*, *Stella*, *Nanos3*, and *Vasa*, while the corresponding *Oct4*-positive and SSEA1-negative (low signal) population expressed the meiotic marker *Stra8* and the oocyte-specific gene *Gdf9*, suggesting an oocyte identity. In addition, the expression of the meiotic markers was enhanced by the addition of BMP4, RA, and CYP26 inhibitor – factors known to stimulate meiosis. However, these in vitro ESC-derived oocyte-like cells showed blockage of meiotic progression, as indicated by only partial synaptonemal complex protein 3(SCP3) chromosomal alignment and absence of SCP1 elongation. To further assess the developmental capacity of the generated meiotic oocytes, co-aggregates with dissociated wild-type (wt) newborn ovarian tissues were transplanted into recipient female mice. The ESC-derived, green fluorescent protein (GFP)-positive oocytes were found to recruit somatic granulosa cells and develop up to the primary follicle stage. In addition, ESCs with knockout of the *Dazl* gene were found to give rise to fewer germ cells, compared with their wt counterparts, consistent with the function of Dazl in vivo in the maintenance of pluripotency, thus further confirming the germ cell identity of the cells. However, whether these follicles can progress further in development remains to be elucidated.

The difficulty of meiotic progression in vitro impedes the robust establishment of post-migratory germ cells, while the establishment of pre-migratory PGCs continues to advance. In 2009, Ohinata *et al.* established an *ex vivo* system for the generation of early PGCs from embryonic day (E)6.0 epiblast under serum- and feeder-free culture conditions in the presence of BMP4, BMP8B, LIF, and SCF. After 6 days of culture, a small cell population expressing exclusively early germ cell markers (including *Blimp1*, *Stella*, *Oct4*, and *Vasa*) had formed, indicative of migratory PGCs. Furthermore, upon injection of dissociated cultured epiblast cells into neonatal mouse testis, epiblast-derived PGCs were found to develop into sperm, which subsequently produced live offspring after intracytoplasmic injection into oocytes [44]. This study suggested that if epiblast-like cells can be obtained from other pluripotent cell types in vitro, the same protocol could be used to facilitate further differentiation into PGCs. Based on this report, Hayashi *et al.* introduced a two-step differentiation protocol for ESCs – an approach that closely recapitulates germ cell commitment in vivo. ESCs were first converted into epiblast-like cells (EpiLCs) by induction with activin A and bFGF, followed by differentiation into PGCs according to Ohinata *et al.* [44] Global gene expression profiling of EpiLCs and PGC-like cells revealed a high similarity to their in vivo counterparts. Interestingly, EpiLCs were similar to E5.75 epiblasts, but different from epiblast stem cells (EpiSCs). Consistent with this observation, EpiSCs did not give rise to PGCs under the same differentiation regime. In vitro-derived PGCs also exhibited epigenetic properties and cellular dynamics similar to those of in vivo PGCs. ESC-derived PGCs were injected into neonatal mouse testis to produce sperm, which subsequently produced live offspring after intracytoplasmic injection into oocytes [45]. To provide evidence for PGC specification, Vincent *et al.* performed in vitro loss-of-function experiments with *Blimp1*-knockout ESCs and demonstrated a reduced yield of PGCs in the EB differentiation system, as determined by cKit and SSEA1 expression. This study also showed that the in vitro system is sensitive enough to mimic in vivo development, as knockdown of *Blimp1* in vivo also resulted in loss of PGCs [46].

In vitro germ cell derivation from human pluripotent stem cells

A great deal of our knowledge on PGC specification and development has been borne out of studies in the mouse embryo and over the last decade in particular in mESC differentiation models. Due to the limited accessibility of pluripotent stem cell materials, difficulty in performing the experimental approaches, as well as ethical considerations associated with the derivation of hESCs, investigations into the development of early human germ cells have only recently gained headway with the increasing use of hESCs and iPSCs as experimental models. Human pluripotent stem cells differ significantly from mouse pluripotent stem cells, and the same is thought true for germ cells. Direct extrapolation of data obtained from animal models to the human system is obviously not possible and several studies have already identified a variety of fundamental differences. For example, a recent study found that SOX2 is not expressed in early germ cells in the human system [47]; however, Sox2 plays an important role in early germ cell development in the mouse.

One year after the first report of the differentiation of mESCs into germ cells in vitro, Clark *et al.* demonstrated that hESCs are also capable of differentiating into PGCs [48]. Firstly, those authors compared the gene expression of human homologs of known mouse germ cell markers in several hESC lines, the ICM of human blastocysts, and human testis, and observed that ESCs expressed early germ cell markers such as *STELLA* and *DAZL* but not the late germ cell markers such as *VASA, SYCP1, SYCP3, BOULE,* and *TEKT1*. After the spontaneous differentiation of EBs, the down-regulation of early germ cell markers and up-regulation of later germ cell markers confirmed the commitment of cells within the cultures to the germ cell lineage. In addition, a small number of VASA-positive cells, indicative of post-migratory germ cells, were detected at the border of the EBs. These encouraging findings spurred fervent interest in the discovery of more efficient differentiation protocols.

Although at that time – in 2004 – BMP proteins were known to be key regulators of mouse germ cell development, their role in the human system had not been elucidated. Kee *et al.* addressed this topic 2 years later and reported the inductive effect of BMP proteins on germ cell marker expression during the differentiation of hESCs into germ cells in vitro. [49]. BMP4 was found to induce *VASA* expression, whereas BMP7 and BMP8B did not show any individual effect, but rather enhanced the action of BMP4. Based on these data, the authors concluded that the combination of BMP4, BMP7, and BMP8B most strongly induces germ cell formation in vitro.

In contrast to the mouse system, a relatively small number of hESC reporter lines have been generated – even though these lines are deemed crucial for distinguishing germ cells from other cell types. Tilgner *et al.* reported the differentiation of germ cells from hESCs in monolayer cultures utilizing SSEA1 – which, in contrast to mESCs, is not expressed in hESCs – for the isolation of presumptive germ cells [50]. Although the isolated SSEA1-positive cell population was most probably not homogeneous, owing to known SSEA1 expression in some somatic cell types, up-regulation of germ cell markers such as *STELLA, VASA,* and *SYCP3* was still observed. The cell fraction analyzed exhibited post-migratory marker expression, but it did not show simultaneous features of histone modification, at least at significant levels. This may be attributed partly to the non-homogeneous cell population that was analyzed after fluorescence activated cell sorting (FACS) isolation.

Kee *et al.* reported the generation of human transgenic VASA-GFP ESC lines based on the observation that *VASA* is not expressed in ESCs [51]. Those authors differentiated transgenic ESCs in medium supplemented with BMP4, BMP7, and BMP8B based on their previous study [49]. After 2 weeks of culture, GFP-positive cells expressing *PRDM1, STELLA,* and *DAZL*, and showing initiation of imprinting erasure of the H19 locus were observed. However, the potential for meiotic progression and sexual bipotentiality of VASA-positive cells remained unclear, as most of the analyzed cells did not express SYCP3 or γH2AX proteins, which are required for meiotic recombination and binding to double-stranded DNA breaks. The authors then investigated the role of DAZ, DAZL, and BOULE in the differentiation of human PGCs by utilizing the same differentiation protocol but without BMPs. Knockdown of the genes by short hairpin RNA (shRNA) led to a decrease in the number of GFP-positive cells, whereas overexpression of the genes led to progression of meiosis, indicated by a punctuate or elongated SYCP3 signal at higher frequency than that observed in wt cells. These meiocytes differentiated further into ACROSIN-positive, male haploid cells. That same group subsequently reported that iPSCs could be differentiated into PGCs, similarly to hESCs, suggesting that iPSCs might depict a promising alternative to ESCs [52]. Interestingly, iPSC cultures contained more SYCP3-expressing cells than ESC lines under non-differentiating culture conditions, and one of the iPSC lines even contained a subpopulation of cells with elongated SYCP3 distribution. The authors suggested that iPSCs preferentially differentiate into the germ line, a phenomenon that might be associated with enhanced expression of pluripotency markers during the reprogramming process. Medrano *et al.* utilized the overexpression of *VASA* to enhance meiotic progression, and reported that even though VASA was not as effective as DAZL overexpression, VASA exhibited a synergistic effect with DAZL in ESCs and iPSCs [53].

Feeder-free human PGC differentiation protocols appear to be less effective than protocols employing co-cultures with feeder cells. West *et al.* reported the emergence of VASA-positive PGC-like cells when ESCs were differentiated on MEF cells in the presence of bFGF without being passaged for 10 days [54]. Amazingly, about 60% of the cells expressed OCT4 and VASA proteins by that time. However, VASA was localized to the nucleus – a phenomenon that needs to be explained and clarified, as it is typically expressed in the cytoplasm. The same group subsequently reported the establishment of a stable germ-like cell line (GLC) from those ESC-derived VASA-positive cells [55]. Extended culture of GLCs without passaging purportedly produced more than 70% of cells positive for the meiotic marker SYCP3 and the meiotic recombination protein MLH1. Upon further differentiation, cells showed increased expression of the male germ cell marker ACROSIN, with more than 6% of cells being haploid. Interestingly, this group and Nayernia *et al.*, who also generated haploid cells, reported similar data [40]. For instance, both groups established stable ESC-derived germ-like cell lines that expressed late germ cell markers (*VASA* and *Stra8*) and upon further differentiation produced SYCP3-expressing meiotic subpopulations. As the cell lines established by Nayernia *et al.* showed imprinting abnormality, it would be interesting to know the imprinting status of these GLCs.

Park *et al.* reported that co-culturing of ESCs and iPSCs with human fetal gonadal stromal cells (hFGSCs) enhances the generation of PGCs [56]. When differentiated on hFGSCs in the absence of bFGF, both ESCs and iPSCs produced cKIT, SSEA1, and VASA triple-positive cells that additionally co-expressed *PRDM1, STELLA,* and *DAZL* by day 7. PGCs generated from ESCs initiated imprinting erasure, whereas iPSC-derived PGCs did not, indicating that iPSC-derived PGCs may have compromised ability to undergo erasure of CpG methylation at imprinted genes. Of importance is that the induced differentiation of hFGSCs into PGCs is more efficient than that of placenta or liver stromal cells, suggesting that PGC induction is affected by not only the topology of the feeder cells, but also the specific cell type of the starting cell population.

Bucay *et al.* reported the co-differentiation of in vitro PGCs and Sertoli cells from ESCs [57]. ESCs were first differentiated into VASA and alkaline phosphatase (AP) double-positive PGC-like cells that revealed morphological characteristics of natural PGCs at the level of electron microscopy (EM). Upon further differentiation, these presumptive PGCs showed increased expression of the late male germ cell markers *VASA* and *ACROSIN* and the Sertoli cell markers *MIS*, *FSHR*, and *SOX9*. These Sertoli-like cells exhibited morphological features characteristic of their in vivo counterparts, as analyzed by EM. However, although 45% of cells within the differentiation cultures expressed VASA and 35% expressed follicle-stimulating hormone receptor (FSHR) at the protein level, haploid cells were not detected. Interestingly, this report mirrors the main findings of Psathaki *et al.*, who performed an ultrastructural analysis of co-differentiated presumptive oocytes and granulosa cells generated from mESCs [39].

Eguizabal *et al.* reported the spontaneous generation of haploid cells from iPSCs [58]. iPSCs were cultured on MEF feeder cells without bFGF for 3 weeks, followed by treatment with RA for 3 weeks. Early spermatogonia and spermatid marker-expressing cells were isolated and further cultivated in the presence of bFGF, LIF, forskolin, and CYP26 inhibitor for 3–4 weeks. By that time, VASA-expressing cells surrounded by somatic cells with marker expression typical of Sertoli and Leydig cells (VIMENTIN, NESTIN, and 3β-HSD) were observed. Upon differentiation for a period of 4 weeks in the presence of factors supporting meiosis, a subpopulation of cells showed expression of the meiotic markers SYCP3 and γH2AX and the post-meiotic marker ACROSIN, indicating formation of meiotic, that is, haploid, cells. Analysis of the methylation status revealed a male-specific hypermethylation pattern of the H19 locus. Of importance is that the differentiation protocol did not work the same way for ESCs – as ESCs produced only VASA and SYCP3 double-positive and γH2AX-negative cells, as in the report by Kee *et al.* [51]. These findings and the report by Panula *et al.* [52] suggest that certain iPSC lines differentiate preferentially toward the germ line.

Germ cell differentiation from adult somatic stem cells

Adult multipotent stem cells depict another possible source for the induction of germ cells and gametes in vitro and raise hopes for their utilization in unique clinical applications.

Dyce *et al.* reported the potential differentiation of somatic stem cells into oocyte-like cells [59]. Isolated multipotent stem cells from porcine fetal skin were cultured in ovarian fluid with gonadotropins and were observed to develop into oocyte-like cells and subsequently into blastocyst-like structures, suggesting that there was parthenogenetic activation. This study warranted more detailed evaluation of data but was nonetheless important, as it suggested readily accessible skin to be a source for germ cells and demonstrated that the in vitro derivation of germ cells is not confined to the mouse model.

For centuries it was believed that in the mammalian ovary, the number of primordial follicles formed shortly after birth in the mouse (or during midgestation in the human ovary) provides a pool of oocytes for the entire reproductive lifespan of the animal [60]. This belief was challenged in 2004 by an astonishing study, claiming postnatal *de novo* oogenesis from presumptive ovarian stem cells (OSCs) [61]. Johnson *et al.* observed 1% to 33% of immature degenerating follicles in mouse ovaries at any given time between postnatal days 8 and 42. The authors claimed that if there is no postnatal *de novo* oogenesis, the degeneration of follicles would completely exhaust the pool of follicles by young adulthood, considering that degenerated follicles are cleared from the ovaries within 3 days of apoptosis. The observation that mice generally possess immature follicles past 1 year of age led to the hypothesis that follicles must get replenished after birth. Supporting their hypothesis, the authors detected Vasa and 5′-bromodeoxyuridine (BrdU) double-positive cells, and concluded that these mitotic germ cells are indeed the source for the generation of postnatal *de novo* oocytes. One year later, the same research group provided evidence for putative germ cell precursors in the bone marrow by identifying a small population of Vasa-positive cells that are purportedly transported to the ovary by the peripheral blood [62]. When transplanted into recipient mice, these precursor cells developed into oocytes. These reports have since been heavily discussed, albeit with much skepticism, and considered controversial by both reproductive scientists and the general public alike. However, two other independent groups supported these data by cultivating presumptive OSCs in vitro and transplanting them into the ovaries of recipient mice to subsequently generate live offspring [63, 64]. Most recently, White *et al.* extended the hypothesis of Johnson *et al.* and claimed the establishment of OSC lines from mouse and human adult ovaries [65]. According to their data, human OSCs exhibited similar characteristics in terms of cell size, morphology, and gene expression profiles to their mouse counterparts. Injection of the human OSCs into adult human ovarian cortical tissue biopsies and subsequent xeno-transplantation into immunodeficient female mice led to OSC-derived oocyte development within follicles within 1–2 weeks. This rapid oocyte development is surprising, considering the time necessary for in vivo PGC development. In particular, the kinetics of in vitro oogenesis from cultured OSCs appears unusual, as the authors observed not only large oocytes-like cells within 24–48 hours of passage of mouse OSCs and 72 hours of human OSCs, but also haploid cells. Further analysis and additional data, for example epigenetic status, are required to provide unequivocal evidence for the identity of these presumptive oocytes. Overall, this study supports the idea that OSCs reside in the ovaries of mice and humans, which could have significant implications on clinical approaches to the autologous treatment of premature ovarian failure and age-related ovarian infertility. As exciting as this idea may be, scientists need to take a cautionary approach and first assess and confirm the existence of OSCs in the ovaries and then evaluate their potential as a new source for oocytes (also see Chapter 16).

Perspective

Many studies have been conducted over the past several years that have successfully advanced techniques for the derivation of germ cells from pluripotent stem cells in vitro. In the mouse model, differentiation of ESCs and iPSCs into male haploid germ cells has been successfully accomplished, while the generation of haploid oocytes still faces substantial hurdles. Although follicle-like structures have been observed, a comprehensive analysis of these structures is still missing. Post-meiotic oocytes from hESCs and iPSCs have not been reported to date, most likely reflecting our limited knowledge of the mechanisms involved in meiotic progression. Nevertheless, stem cell-based in vitro differentiation models for the generation of germ cells and subsequently gametes from human stem cell sources depict an extraordinarily powerful tool to unravel step by step the many unknown mechanisms in germ cell development. Optimized and robust differentiation systems that demonstrate full recapitulation of germ cell development in vivo will enable us eventually to perform detailed mechanistic analysis, drug screening, and disease modeling by utilizing patient-specific iPSCs from reproductively compromised patients. Future investigations in germ cell biology will reveal whether in vitro-derived gametes, irrespective of the source, ultimately prove suitable in the treatment for infertility in the clinical setting.

Acknowledgments

We apologize to all those whose studies could not be included due to space limitations. We thank Damir Illich and Guangming Wu for critically reading and Areti Malapetsas for editing the manuscript. Furthermore, we thank Jeanine Müller-Keuker for help with the artwork. This work was supported by the Max Planck Society and the DFG grant for Research Unit Germ Cell Potential (FOR 1041).

References

1. Weismann A. *The Germ-plasm; A Theory of Heredity.* New York, NY: Charles Scribner's Sons, 1893.
2. Evans MJ, Kaufman MH. Establishment in culture of pluripotential cells from mouse embryos. *Nature* 1981; **292**: 154–6.
3. Martin GR. Isolation of a pluripotent cell line from early mouse embryos cultured in medium conditioned by teratocarcinoma stem cells. *Proc Natl Acad Sci USA* 1981; **78**: 7634–8.
4. Thomson JA, Itskovitz-Eldor J, Shapiro SS, *et al.* Embryonic stem cell lines derived from human blastocysts. *Science* 1998; **282**: 1145–7.
5. Takahashi K, Yamanaka S. Induction of pluripotent stem cells from mouse embryonic and adult fibroblast cultures by defined factors. *Cell* 2006; **126**: 663–76.
6. Takahashi K, Tanabe K, Ohnuki M, *et al.* Induction of pluripotent stem cells from adult human fibroblasts by defined factors. *Cell* 2007; **131**: 861–72.
7. Rossant J, Gardner RL Alexandre HL. Investigation of the potency of cells from the postimplantation mouse embryo by blastocyst injection: a preliminary report. *J Embryol Exp Morphol* 1978; **48**: 239–47.

8. Gardner RL, Rossant J. Investigation of the fate of 4–5 day post-coitum mouse inner cell mass cells by blastocyst injection. *J Embryol Exp Morphol* 1979; **52**: 141–52.

9. Yoshimizu T, Obinata M, Matsui Y. Stage-specific tissue and cell interactions play key roles in mouse germ cell specification. *Development* 2001; **128**: 481–90.

10. Tam PP, Zhou SX. The allocation of epiblast cells to ectodermal and germ-line lineages is influenced by the position of the cells in the gastrulating mouse embryo. *Dev Biol* 1996; **178**: 124–32.

11. Ginsburg M, Snow MH, McLaren A. Primordial germ cells in the mouse embryo during gastrulation. *Development* 1990; **110**: 521–8.

12. Lawson KA, Dunn NR, Roelen BA, *et al.* Bmp4 is required for the generation of primordial germ cells in the mouse embryo. *Genes Dev* 1999; **13**: 424–36.

13. Fujiwara T, Dunn NR, Hogan BL. Bone morphogenetic protein 4 in the extraembryonic mesoderm is required for allantois development and the localization and survival of primordial germ cells in the mouse. *Proc Natl Acad Sci USA* 2001; **98**: 13739–44.

14. Ying Y, Liu XM, Marble A, *et al.* Requirement of Bmp8b for the generation of primordial germ cells in the mouse. *Mol Endocrinol* 2000; **14**: 1053–63.

15. Ying Y, Zhao GQ. Cooperation of endoderm-derived BMP2 and extraembryonic ectoderm-derived BMP4 in primordial germ cell generation in the mouse. *Dev Biol* 2001; **232**: 484–92.

16. Ohinata Y, Payer B, O'Carroll D, *et al.* Blimp1 is a critical determinant of the germ cell lineage in mice. *Nature* 2005; **436**: 207–13.

17. Yabuta Y, Kurimoto K, Ohinata Y, *et al.* Gene expression dynamics during germline specification in mice identified by quantitative single-cell gene expression profiling. *Biol Reprod* 2006; **75**: 705–16.

18. Yamaguchi S, Kimura H, Tada M, *et al.* Nanog expression in mouse germ cell development. *Gene Expr Patterns* 2005; **5**: 639–46.

19. Anderson R, Fassler R, Georges-Labouesse E, *et al.* Mouse primordial germ cells lacking beta1 integrins enter the germline but fail to migrate normally to the gonads. *Development* 1999; **126**: 1655–64.

20. Bendel-Stenzel MR, Gomperts M, Anderson R, *et al.* The role of cadherins during primordial germ cell migration and early gonad formation in the mouse. *Mech Dev* 2000; **91**: 143–52.

21. Molyneaux KA, Zinszner H, Kunwar PS, *et al.* The chemokine SDF1/CXCL12 and its receptor CXCR4 regulate mouse germ cell migration and survival. *Development* 2003; **130**: 4279–86.

22. Hutt KJ, McLaughlin EA, Holland MK. Kit ligand and c-Kit have diverse roles during mammalian oogenesis and folliculogenesis. *Mol Hum Reprod* 2006; **12**: 61–9.

23. Raz E. The function and regulation of vasa-like genes in germ-cell development. *Genome Biol* 2000; **1**: REVIEWS1017.

24. Noce T, Okamoto-Ito S, Tsunekawa N. Vasa homolog genes in mammalian germ cell development. *Cell Struct Funct* 2001; 26: 131–6.

25. Hajkova P, Erhardt S, Lane N, *et al.* Epigenetic reprogramming in mouse primordial germ cells. *Mech Dev* 2002; **117**: 15–23.

26. Ohta H, Wakayama T, Nishimune Y. Commitment of fetal male germ cells to spermatogonial stem cells during mouse embryonic development. *Biol Reprod* 2004; **70**: 1286–91.

27. Paredes A, Garcia-Rudaz C, Kerr B, *et al.* Loss of synaptonemal complex protein-1, a synaptonemal complex protein, contributes to the initiation of follicular assembly in the developing rat ovary. *Endocrinology* 2005; **146**: 5267–77.

28. Koubova J, Menke DB, Zhou Q, *et al.* Retinoic acid regulates sex-specific timing of meiotic initiation in mice. *Proc Natl Acad Sci USA* 2006; **103**: 2474–9.

29. Bowles J, Feng CW, Spiller C, *et al.* FGF9 suppresses meiosis and promotes male germ cell fate in mice. *Dev Cell* 2010; **19**: 440–9.

30. Pepling ME, Spradling AC. Mouse ovarian germ cell cysts undergo programmed breakdown to form primordial follicles. *Dev Biol* 2001; **234**: 339–51.

31. Eppig JJ. Oocyte control of ovarian follicular development and function in mammals. *Reproduction* 2001; **122**: 829–38.

32. Eppig JJ, Wigglesworth K, Pendola FL. The mammalian oocyte orchestrates the rate of ovarian follicular development. *Proc Natl Acad Sci USA* 2002; **99**: 2890–4.

33. Jagarlamudi K, Reddy P, Adhikari, *et al.* Genetically modified mouse models for premature ovarian failure (POF). *Mol Cell Endocrinol* 2010; **315**: 1–10.

34. Uhlenhaut NH, Jakob S, Anlag K, *et al.* Somatic sex reprogramming of adult ovaries to testes by FOXL2 ablation. *Cell* 2009; **139**: 1130–42.

35. Hübner K, Fuhrmann G, Christenson LK, *et al.* Derivation of oocytes from mouse embryonic stem cells. *Science* 2003; **300**: 1251–6.

36. Toyooka Y, Tsunekawa N, Akasu R, *et al.* Embryonic stem cells can form germ cells in vitro. *Proc Natl Acad Sci USA* 2003; **100**: 11457–62.

37. Geijsen N, Horoschak M, Kim K, *et al.* Derivation of embryonic germ cells and male gametes from embryonic stem cells. *Nature* 2004; **427**: 148–54.
38. Novak I, Lightfoot DA, Wang H, *et al.* Mouse embryonic stem cells form follicle-like ovarian structures but do not progress through meiosis. *Stem Cells* 2006; **24**: 1931–6.
39. Psathaki OE, Hubner K, Sabour D, *et al.* Ultrastructural characterization of mouse embryonic stem cell-derived oocytes and granulosa cells. *Stem Cells Dev* 2011; **20**: 2205–15.
40. Nayernia K, Nolte J, Michelmann HW, *et al.* In vitro-differentiated embryonic stem cells give rise to male gametes that can generate offspring mice. *Dev Cell* 2006; **11**: 125–32.
41. Lacham-Kaplan O, Chy H, Trounson A. Testicular cell conditioned medium supports differentiation of embryonic stem cells into ovarian structures containing oocytes. *Stem Cells* 2006; **24**: 266–73.
42. Qing T, Shi Y, Qin H, *et al.* Induction of oocyte-like cells from mouse embryonic stem cells by co-culture with ovarian granulosa cells. *Differentiation* 2007; **75**: 902–11.
43. Nicholas CR, Haston KM, Grewall AK, *et al.* Transplantation directs oocyte maturation from embryonic stem cells and provides a therapeutic strategy for female infertility. *Hum Mol Genet* 2009; **18**: 4376–89.
44. Ohinata Y, Ohta H, Shigeta M, *et al.* A signaling principle for the specification of the germ cell lineage in mice. *Cell* 2009; **137**: 571–84.
45. Hayashi K, Ohta H, Kurimoto K, *et al.* Reconstitution of the mouse germ cell specification pathway in culture by pluripotent stem cells. *Cell* 2011; **146**: 519–32.
46. Vincent JJ, Li Z, Lee SA, *et al.* Single cell analysis facilitates staging of blimp1-dependent primordial germ cells derived from mouse embryonic stem cells. *PLoS One* 2011; **6**: e28960.
47. Perrett RM, Turnpenny L, Eckert JJ, *et al.* The early human germ cell lineage does not express SOX2 during in vivo development or upon in vitro culture. *Biol Reprod* 2008; **78**: 852–8.
48. Clark AT, Bodnar MS, Fox M, *et al.* Spontaneous differentiation of germ cells from human embryonic stem cells in vitro. *Hum Mol Genet* 2004; **13**: 727–39.
49. Kee K, Gonsalves JM, Clark AT, *et al.* Bone morphogenetic proteins induce germ cell differentiation from human embryonic stem cells. *Stem Cells Dev* 2006; **15**: 831–7.
50. Tilgner K, Atkinson SP, Golebiewska A, *et al.* Isolation of primordial germ cells from differentiating human embryonic stem cells. *Stem Cells* 2008; **26**: 3075–85.
51. Kee K, Angeles VT, Flores M, *et al.* Human DAZL, DAZ and BOULE genes modulate primordial germ-cell and haploid gamete formation. *Nature* 2009; **462**: 222–5.
52. Panula S, Medrano JV, Kee K, *et al.* Human germ cell differentiation from fetal- and adult-derived induced pluripotent stem cells. *Hum Mol Genet* 2011; **20**: 752–62.
53. Medrano JV, Ramathal C, Nguyen HN, *et al.* Divergent RNA-binding proteins, DAZL and VASA, induce meiotic progression in human germ cells derived in vitro. *Stem Cells* 2012; 30: 441–51.
54. West FD, Machacek DW, Boyd NL, *et al.* Enrichment and differentiation of human germ-like cells mediated by feeder cells and basic fibroblast growth factor signaling. *Stem Cells* 2008; **26**: 2768–76.
55. West FD, Mumaw JL, Gallegos-Cardenas A, *et al.* Human haploid cells differentiated from meiotic competent clonal germ cell lines that originated from embryonic stem cells. *Stem Cells Dev* 2011; **20**: 1079–88.
56. Park TS, Galic Z, Conway AE, *et al.* Derivation of primordial germ cells from human embryonic and induced pluripotent stem cells is significantly improved by coculture with human fetal gonadal cells. *Stem Cells* 2009; **27**: 783–95.
57. Bucay N, Yebra M, Cirulli V, *et al.* A novel approach for the derivation of putative primordial germ cells and sertoli cells from human embryonic stem cells. *Stem Cells* 2009; **27**: 68–77.
58. Eguizabal C, Montserrat N, Vassena R, *et al.* Complete meiosis from human induced pluripotent stem cells. *Stem Cells* 2011; **29**: 1186–95.
59. Dyce PW, Wen L, Li J. In vitro germline potential of stem cells derived from fetal porcine skin. *Nat Cell Biol* 2006; **8**: 384–90.
60. Zuckerman S. The number of oocytes in the mature ovary. *Recent Prog Horm Res* 1951; **6**: 63–108.
61. Johnson J, Canning J, Kaneko T, *et al.* Germline stem cells and follicular renewal in the postnatal mammalian ovary. *Nature* 2004; **428**: 145–50.
62. Johnson J, Bagley J, Skaznik-Wikiel M, *et al.* Oocyte generation in adult mammalian ovaries by putative germ cells in bone marrow and peripheral blood. *Cell* 2005; **122**: 303–15.
63. Zou K, Yuan Z, Yang Z, *et al.* Production of offspring from a germline stem cell line derived from neonatal ovaries. *Nat Cell Biol* 2009; **11**: 631–6.

64. Pacchiarotti J, Maki C, Ramos T, *et al.* Differentiation potential of germ line stem cells derived from the postnatal mouse ovary. *Differentiation* 2010; **79**: 159–70.

65. White YA, Woods DC, Takai Y, *et al.* Oocyte formation by mitotically active germ cells purified from ovaries of reproductive-age women. *Nat Med* 2012; **18**: 413–21.

Chapter 21

Parthenogenesis and parthenogenetic stem cells

Tiziana A. L. Brevini and Fulvio Gandolfi

Parthenogenesis

Parthenogenesis is the process by which an egg can develop without being fertilized by the sperm and is a form of reproduction common to a variety of lower organisms such as ants, flies, lizards, snakes, fish, amphibia, and honeybees that may occasionally reproduce in this manner.

Although mammals are not spontaneously capable of this form of reproduction, mammalian ova can successfully undergo artificial parthenogenesis in vitro. Mimicking the calcium wave induced by the sperm at fertilization, with the use of a calcium ionophore or other stimuli, the mature oocyte is activated and begins to divide. Mammalian parthenotes can develop into different stages after oocyte activation, depending on the species, but never to term.

Parthenogenetic activation can be induced at different stages along oocyte meiosis, resulting in parthenotes with different chromosome complements.

When parthenogenetic activation is performed in oocytes at the second metaphase it results in the extrusion of the second polar body and leads to the formation of a haploid parthenote. This method is rarely used since, in this case, the developmental competence is reduced compared to normal embryos and to diploid parthenotes [1].

Diploid parthenotes can be obtained in two different ways. The most common consists in combining the activation of metaphase II oocytes with exposure to an actin polymerization inhibitor, usually cytochalasin B [2]. Alternatively, a diploid parthenote can be generated by preventing the extrusion of the first polar body. This protocol leads to the formation of tetraploid oocytes and the diploid status is then re-established at the end of oocyte maturation with the extrusion of the second polar body [3].

Using one or the other method has important consequences on the genetic makeup of the parthenotes. In fact, performing the oocyte activation before the inhibition of the second polar body extrusion determines the formation of highly homozygous parthenotes, since the diploid status of the parthenotes is obtained after the segregation of sister chromatids. On the contrary when the first polar body extrusion is inhibited parthenotes are genetically identical to each other and have the same heterozygosity as their mother [3].

Differences between parthenotes and embryos

Although a mammalian parthenote can be diploid and heterozygote, its genome is still substantially different from that of a biparental embryo.The difference lies in the fact that male and female genomes are not identical but complementary to each other thanks to the phenomenon known as imprinting [4]. This epigenetic modification modulates the expression of a number of genes so that either the maternal or the paternal alleles are transcribed. It follows that the presence of two female genomes, as in the case of a parthenote, determines the silencing of those genes that are physiologically expressed by the paternally derived alleles.

The parental-specific expression pattern of imprinted genes brings as a consequence the fact that mammalian parthenotes are unable to develop to term, as opposed to their lower vertebrate counterparts. In the mouse, the most advanced parthenotes survive to the early limb bud stage, have little extraembryonic tissue, and almost no trophoblast [5]. Parthenotes will not develop and will arrest development by day 10 in the mouse, day 11.5 in rabbit, day 21 in sheep,

Biology and Pathology of the Oocyte, 2nd edn., ed. Alan Trounson, Roger Gosden, and Ursula Eichenlaub-Ritter. Published by Cambridge University Press.

and day 29 in pigs (reviewed by [6]). However, the effect of genomic imprinting in parthenotes does not seem to be limited to a defective development of the trophoblast since even when supplied with trophoblast cells, parthenotes will stop and die [7]. Parthenote–embryo chimeras can go to term [8, 9] but their development is delayed and parthenote cells fail to contribute to tissues of mesodermal and endodermal origin such as skeletal muscle, liver, and pancreas [10].

Differences between embryos and parthenotes are not limited to the DNA but extend to a peculiar organelle, the centrosome, which consists of a pair of perpendicularly oriented cylindrical centrioles surrounded by a number of proteins that form an electron dense protein matrix known as pericentriolar material (PCM).

The centrosome acts as the microtubule-organizing center (MTOC) of the cell. During interphase it has a central role in several aspects of cell function including signal transduction and transport of organelles or macromolecules. During mitosis it forms the center of the mitotic poles and at the S-phase centrosomes duplicate in synchrony with DNA [11].

All somatic cells contain a typical centrosome, including spermatids and primary oocytes. However, during gametogenesis this organelle undergoes a profound modification, as happens to the gametes themselves, in order to meet the specific functions that these highly differentiated cells will perform at fertilization [12]. During male gametogenesis, spermatozoa retain the proximal centriole but lose most of the PMC as well as the distal centriole. In a complementary fashion, during early oogenesis centrioles are lost but the bulk of PCM is retained in the mature oocyte.

At the time of fertilization the proximal centriole forms the sperm aster and duplicates during the pronuclear stage. At syngamy a centriole is visible at both poles of the first mitotic spindle (except in zygotes of some rodents, such as in the mouse, see below) so that at the first cleavage a complete centrosome is restored in each blastomere. In this way the centrosomes of all somatic cells originate from the zygote centrosome [13]. From this description it emerges that the centrosome is contributed by both parents in a complementary way and, as a consequence, parthenogenesis prevents the physiological reconstitution of this organelle.

However, it is important to note that laboratory mice and rats represent a notable exception to the process of centrosome inheritance described above. In these species, in fact, spermatozoa centrioles degenerate completely. As a consequence, rodent zygotes rely on an exclusively maternal origin of the centrosome, a pattern substantially different from most other animal species including the human [14]. Therefore, cleavage divisions in mouse embryos take place in the absence of centrioles, which reappear at the blastocyst stage, initially limited to the polar trophoblast cells [15].

This is different from what happens in human and bovine embryos where centrioles are found throughout preimplantation development from the 1-cell stage to the hatching blastocyst [16, 17]. However, in rabbit embryos centrioles appear to degenerate rapidly immediately after fertilization and to become substituted by maternal cytoplasmic molecules [18]. A similar pattern is observed also in pigs, where paternal centrioles are lost immediately after fertilization and functional centrioles become visible again only at the blastocyst stage similarly to what has been described in rodent embryos [19].

The relationship between parthenogenesis and centrosome is not clear. Most of the information available has been collected in lower species and the possible consequences of the lack of paternal centriole in parthenotes is far from being understood (reviewed in [20]). In particular, detailed information on centriole appearance in mammalian parthenotes is very limited and contradictory. In the rabbit, parthenote centrioles become visible only at the blastocyst stage [21], similar to what has been described after fertilization. In bovine parthenotes the appearance of centrioles is delayed compared to fertilized embryos and functional centrosomes are organized only during the third cell cycle [22]. Although a detailed description of centriole biogenesis in mouse parthenotes is not available, some preliminary observations performed in our laboratory indicated that the appearance of centrioles follows the same timing observed in fertilized embryos. Therefore, rodent parthenotes may be less sensitive to the lack of the paternal centriole since this is physiologically missing anyway.

Whereas centrosome analysis during mammalian preimplantation development has been scarcely investigated more data are available on the incidence of chromosomal abnormalities during the initial steps of parthenogenetic development.

Extensive karyotype analyses of parthenogenetic bovine embryos showed that the majority display abnormal chromosomal complements [23–25]. Similarly, a recent study on sheep parthenotes described a minimum incidence of aneuploidy of 93.6% [26], and pig parthenotes showed a significant decrease of normal diploid blastocyst compared to in vitro fetilization (IVF) controls [27]. Evidence in the mouse is variable. Some reports describe a dramatic increase in the level of aneuploidy from 1% to 28% following ethanol activation [28]; other observations, in contrast with all other species, show that the level of aneuploidy in mouse parthenotes does not increase compared to the spontaneous rate observed in 1-cell fertilized embryos [29]. Data available for human parthenotes are extremely limited [30, 31] but indicate an incidence of aneuploidy (ranging from 72% to 100%) that exceeds the already high rate (over 50%) detected in preimplantation embryos, derived from assisted reproduction procedures [32].

Are the two components: lack of paternal contribution to the embryonic centrosome and high level of aneuploidy, somehow connected? Although a direct link at present has not been proved, several data clearly indicate that sperm centrosomal dysfunctions at the time of fertilization are a major cause of embryonic aneuploidy, polyploidy, and mosaicism [23, 26]. Therefore, it is reasonable to hypothesize that the complete lack of paternal centrosome components has a severe effect on the high incidence of chromosomal abnormalities observed in parthenotes. This appears to be an inevitable consequence of the fact that all microtubule formation throughout early embryonic development depends on sperm-derived centriolar integrity, the lack of paternal centriole–centrosome complex in the parthenote is likely to lead to abnormal chromosome separation (see Figure 21.1) with subsequent genomic instability, therefore compromising embryonic development [33].

A direct connection between abnormal parthenogenetic development and paternal centriole has only been achieved in amphibian eggs. If a *Xenopus* egg is activated by pricking with a fine needle it just begins to contract and no cleavage occurs, but normal cell division is restored if isolated centrioles are injected into the ooplasm [34]. A similar experiment has been performed in human oocytes that were injected with a sperm head together with a separated tail or with a sperm tail alone. Results indicated that all arising embryos were chromosome mosaics, suggesting that physical dissection damages the human sperm centriole or that a disruption in the pericentriolar material prevents a normal microtubule nucleation [35]. Unfortunately, at present, a similar experiment has not been performed in other mammalian species.

A much lower incidence of aneuploidy was observed in human benign ovarian teratomas (7 out of 95 cases) [36]. However, teratomas are thought to derive from germ cells, rather than mature oocytes, which retain a normal centriole [37], and this may mitigate the absence of the paternal component.

Despite these differences, diploid parthenotes can reach the blastocyst stage at rates substantially similar to those of embryos with no evident morphological and functional differences. Therefore parthenogenetic blastocysts have been used as a source of embryonic stem cells.

Mouse parthenogenetic stem cells

Parthenogenetic embryonic stem cell (PESC) lines have been derived from mouse embryos shortly after the establishment of the first traditional embryonic stem cells (ESCs) [38]. Interestingly, in these first attempts, haploid parthenotes were purposely selected but the resulting cell lines were invariably homogeneously diploid. It was soon clear that in standard ESC culture conditions haploid cells spontaneously diploidize. It was necessary to wait for 28 years before haploid mouse PESC lines were derived [39]. This was made possible by the use of a more recent and purposely developed culture medium (the so-called 2i medium) that enables the maintenance of the pluripotent state even in the presence of a haploid genome. Haploid PESCs largely maintain a normal mESC profile and can contribute substantially to both male and female chimeras. However, such contribution takes place only after the cells diploidize, confirming the fact that the haploid status is incompatible with the differentiation process. This is consistent with the fact that diploid parthenotes are more viable and explains why parthenogenetic cell lines are diploid in mouse and other species.

As discussed above, diploid parthenote development is limited by the lack of a symmetric genomic imprinting; therefore, the developmental potential of PESC lines has been investigated extensively from the early days, assessing cell differentiation potential both in vivo and in vitro. Using cultures at the early passages, Allen *et al.* [40] demonstrated that PESCs injected into fertilized blastocysts fail to contribute to some tissues, analogous to that observed when parthenote blastomeres were combined with fertilized embryos. However, growth retardation was not observed in injected embryos,

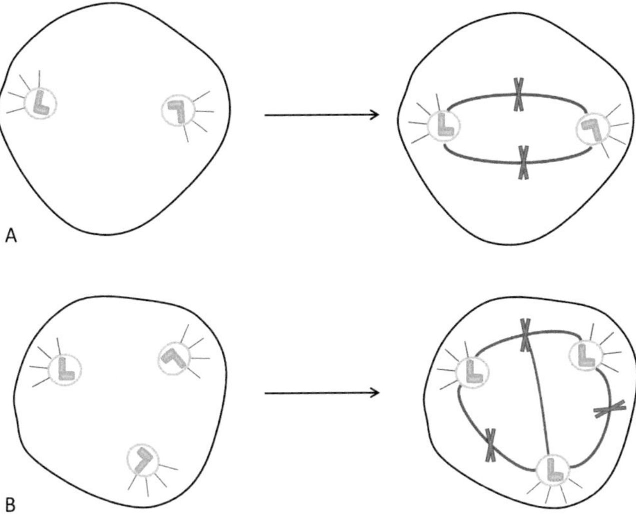

Figure 21.1 The correct number of centrioles in biparental cells ensures the establishment of bipolar mitotic spindles, with a correct chromosome segregation (A). The lack of paternal centriole–centrosome complex in parthenotes leads, by contrast, to the formation of supernumerary centrioles. This is likely to induce multipolar mitotic spindles causing abnormal chromosome separation, with subsequent genomic instability (B).

contrary to parthenote/embryo chimeras. Overall, abnormal genomic imprinting is gradually lost in culture, therefore attenuating the developmental defects linked to it [41, 42]. Consistent with the observation that prolonged culture spontaneously restores an epigenetic pattern progressively more similar to the biparental one, full-term pups have been generated by tetraploid embryo complementation [43]. However, even in this case restoration was incomplete since the parthenogenetic pups died within 1 day, rather than reaching adulthood as normally happens with tetraploid complementation embryos obtained by fertilized ESCs. An alternative, or additional, explanation for the rapid death of these pups may be linked to the loss of heterozygosity which typically amplifies any negative genetic component potentially present in the genotype.

A close relationship between uniparental origin of a cell line and tumorigenic potential has been described in mouse androgenetic and parthenogenetic fibroblasts. In this case the paternal-only cell lines formed tumors after a few passages in culture whereas parthenogenetic cells underwent a rapid process of senescence and died [44]. However, in the perspective of a clinical use of parthenogenetic stem cells, homozygosity can be a potential benefit because it reduces the immunogenicity of their derivatives. Furthermore, homozygosity has also been suggested to be an advantage that could be exploited in the perspective to provide a useful research tool for drug testing and development, selecting cell lines homozygous for drug response, disease, or cancer genes [45].

Parthenogenetic stem cells in non-rodent species

As described above there is a substantial divide between rodent and non-rodent species when fertilization and, consequently, parthenogenesis is concerned. This is mainly based on the mechanisms involved in the reconstitution of a functional centrosome after fertilization. The entirely maternal origin of the rodent centrosome eliminates an important difference between parthenotes and embryos. This results in a much lower incidence of aneuploidy in preimplantation parthenotes even if no direct connection between the two aspects has been established so far. Furthermore, differences in the epigenetic profile linked to imprinting are gradually lost in culture and diploidy is spontaneously restored upon transplantation in vivo. All this leads to a remarkable similarity of rodent PESCs with their biparental counterpart, as described in some detail in the previous paragraph.

Despite this negative background, PESCs have been derived in a number of non-rodent species including human, non-human primates, buffalo, cow, pig, and rabbit as summarized in a recent review [6].

In general PESCs show a morphology comparable to their biparental counterpart, express the most common pluripotency markers, and spontaneously differentiate in the derivatives of all three germ layers both in vitro and in vivo.

The reasons for deriving PESCs were the possibility of obtaining cell lines that would immunologically match with the oocyte donor and the less controversial nature of the activated oocyte as a source of stem cell compared with an embryo. The latter is largely debatable and we will not deal with this issue.

The first non-rodent PESCs were derived from *Macaca fascicularis* [46], followed a few years later by human cell lines as a result of improved protocols for the activation of human oocytes [47].

At present only a few laboratories have generated human parthenogenetic embryonic stem cells (hPESCs) and their functional characterization is just beginning [48–55].

Advantages and limitations of human parthenogenetic stem cells

The most common way to obtain hPESCs has been to induce oocyte activation followed by inhibition of the extrusion of the second polar body. This generates cell lines that are compatible with the oocyte donor but have a high degree of heterozygosity caused by meiotic recombination events taking place prior to cell line derivation. Typically in parthenogenetic cells the degree of heterozygosity is directly proportional to the distance from the centromeres [51, 52, 56]. Detailed analysis performed on rhesus monkey PESCs showed an average heterozygosity of 64% of the examined loci [57].

It was soon observed that adopting different activation strategies had a significant effect on the level of homozygosity. Similarly to what has been described in the mouse (see above), if haploid parthenotes are used as a source of cell lines, these spontaneously diploidize but, as opposed to the originally diploid parthenotes, the level of homozygosity is very high [50, 58]. This is certainly an advantage when human leukocyte antigens (HLA) patterns are considered since it considerably enhances the chances of a more extensive matching between cells and recipient. A specific combination of HLA genes is expressed on the somatic cell surface of each individual. The number of HLA proteins can vary between 12 and 14 and each one can have as many as several hundred alleles. The end result is a virtually endless amount of combinations (haplotypes). The success of either organ or cell transplantation is directly proportional to the degree of the matching between the donor and the recipient haplotypes. Having a cell line with all homozygous HLA greatly enhances the chances of finding suitable matches and, if this combination is included amongst the 200 most commonly found in the population, the cell line would be compatible with a large number of individuals. Whereas this is the good news, the bad news is that high homozygosity would dramatically increase the chance of amplifying the negative effect of any mutation that may occur in the genome. This would lead to loss of heterozygosity, which is a leading cause for malignant transformation and hardly a desirable feature for cells destined for regenerative medicine.

Another issue with PESCs is the role of genomic imprinting and how this epigenetic modification is maintained passing from the parthenote to the cell line. Indeed the maintenance of a maternal pattern of expression, with the expression of only the maternal alleles and the down-regulation of the paternal ones, as opposed to the physiological biparental pattern, has been used to demonstrate the parthenogenetic nature of the first hPESCs [50–52]. However, these data were limited to a small number of genes and only recently were confirmed by a wide-range study using human parthenogenetic induced puripotent stem cells (iPSCs) [59]. These cell lines were obtained by infecting with pseudoretroviruses expressing the four traditional reprogramming factors (*OCT4, SOX2, KLF4,* and *c-MYC*) fibroblasts derived from two diploid parthenogenetic teratomas. Genome-wide analysis indicated that, whether maternally imprinted genes were all expressed, 60% of paternally expressed genes were down-regulated and most of the remaining ones were not expressed at all. In addition this study revealed the existence of multiple imprinted miRNA, revealing a new dimension to the imprinting mechanism and its role in development. And, at the same time, it added a new abnormal aspect of parthenogenetic development and parthenogenetic cell lines.

But has all this an effect on the developmental potential of hPESCs?

We know that contributions from both maternal and paternal genomes are required for normal embryogenesis. Therefore, it was not surprising that studies performed on mouse parthenote–embryo chimeras and on mouse PESCs injected into fertilized blastocysts demonstrated that the developmental potential of parthenogenetic cells is limited (see above) and particularly affects tissues of mesodermal and endodermal origin (e.g., skeletal muscle, liver, pancreas). Consistent with this background, Stelzer *et al.* [59] confirmed that their human parthenogenetic

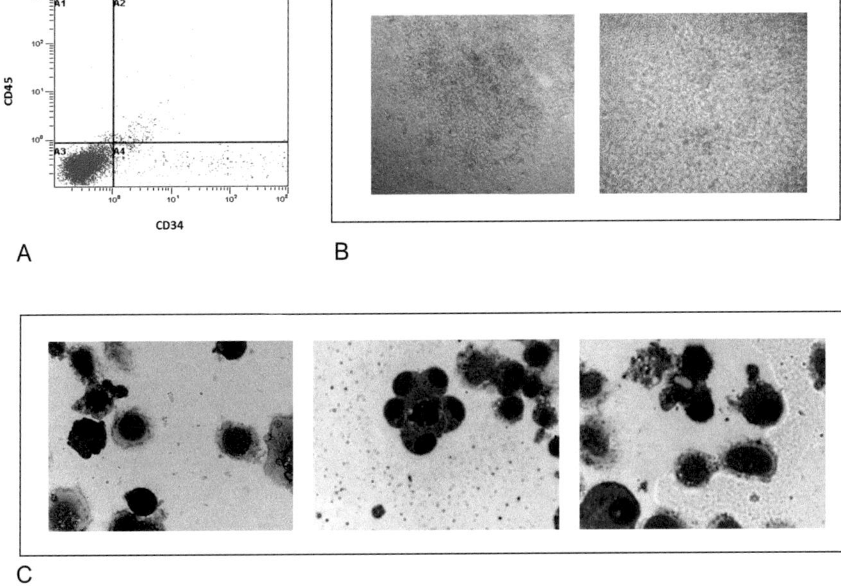

Figure 21.2 Exposure of hPESCs to a combination of thrombopoietin, stem cell factor, and interleukin and adequate culture conditions allowed for their commitment towards the hematopoietic lineage, with the generation of CD34/CD45-positive cells (A). These cells were able to form colonies in methylcellulose medium (B) and, upon further differentiation, they generated mature lymphoid, erythroid, and myeloid subpopulations (C).

iPSCs failed to give rise, both in vivo and in vitro, to endoderm derived tissues. In particular, liver was the most affected organ together with a consistent reduction of skeletal muscle and kidney development.

However, these were all spontaneous differentiation experiments and data on directed differentiation of human or other species PESCs are very limited.

The first demonstration of direct differentiation of hPESCs has been performed in our laboratory, towards the hematopoietic lineage [54]. We obtained a high rate of colony-forming cells by exposing hPESCs to a combination of thrombopoietin, stem cell factor, and interleukin. Upon further differentiation the cells generated mature lymphoid, erythroid, and myeloid subpopulations at a rate comparable to that obtainable from cord blood cells (see Figure 21.2).

More recently other attempts to direct differentiation have been described. The group led by Turovets described the direct differentiation of hPESCs into an enriched population of definitive endoderm. These results are somewhat surprising since they are in contrast to all other data; however, specific procedures were introduced to facilitate this process. In particular, cells were either exoposed to trichostatin A, a potent histone deacetylase inhibitor [60], or were cultured in a three-dimensional device in an attempt to mimic the transition through the primitive streak [61]. Although potentially interesting, these results need further confirmation, also considering that only very immature cell types were obtained.

The possibility of promoting the transition of hPESCs from the pluripotent state to a more limited multipotent level is also being currently explored. At present data have been presented describing the transformation of hPESCs into mesenchymal-like stem cells. Although most characteristics are similar to their biparental counterpart, parthenogenetic mesenchymal stem cells derived from hPESCs showed an altered differentiation potential which favors their osteogenic potential but reduces the adipogenic capacity [62]. This further indicates that the capacity of hPESCs to differentiate, even if transitioning through an intermediate stage, is abnormal and likely reflects the predominantly maternal gene expression pattern linked to their uniparental imprinting.

Multipotent neural stem cells have also been obtained from hPESCs showing a stable in vitro phenotype and some capacity to give rise to more differentiated neural cell types [63].

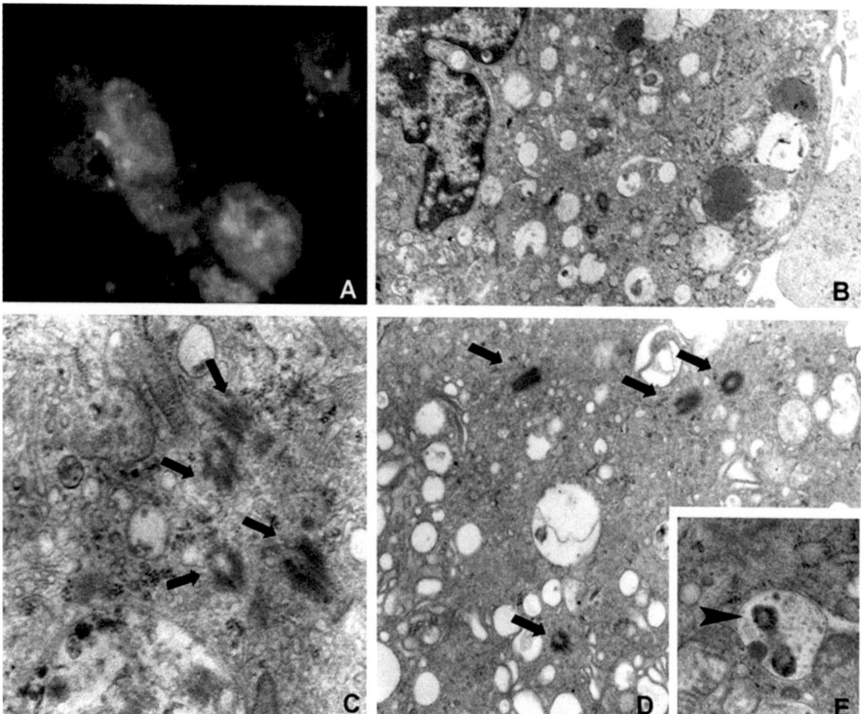

Figure 21.3 Immunohistochemical (A) and ultrastructural (B–E) analysis of hPESCs demonstrated the formation of supernumerary centrioles. These cells were characterized by massive autophagic processes (D) and cargoes that often contained centrioles (E). These observations suggest that autophagy is one of the resources used by these cells to eliminate supernumerary centrioles.

The parthenogenetic centrosome

One of the most striking differences between parthenotes and embryos, described in the initial part of this chapter, is the lack of paternal contribution to the newly formed centrosome. Given the fact that no paternal contribution is known to occur in laboratory rodents this aspect could not be investigated in these species even though PESCs have been derived for many decades.

However, recent research has highlighted the important role of the centrosome in stem cell division and differentiation [64]. Therefore, we considered it very interesting to investigate the centrosome biology in PESC lines of non-rodent species and in hPESCs in particular.

In our studies we observed the presence of centrosomal material loosely dispersed in the cytoplasm of the hPESC lines derived in our laboratory. Detailed ultrastructural analysis revealed the presence of supernumerary centrioles, generally associated with massive autophagic processes (see Figure 21.3). A similar pattern of abnormal centrosome re-aggregations, which is a common feature in parthenotes obtained in lower species, can also be seen in neoplastic cells and it is suggested as a possible cause of the abnormal mitosis and multipolar cells frequently observed in cancer [65]. Interestingly, however, the cargo of autophagic compartments observed in hPESCs often resembled partially damaged centrioles [54], suggesting that this process may be used as an active self-protective strategy in order to eliminate highly abnormal organelles, thus contributing to cell survival and ensuring the survival of a "normal" population [66].

The comparison of our hPESCs with biparental ESC lines revealed a much higher level of expression of *MAD1*, and of the related molecules *MAX* and *SIN3*, in parthenogenetic cells. These molecules are a central component of the spindle assembly checkpoint and recruitment of kinetochores [67–69] as well as active regulators of cell proliferation [70]. In contrast, low transcription for *TTK* and *CENP-E* was detected. These molecules are normally involved in kinetochore–microtubule binding, and in the correct chromosome congression and alignment as well as segregation, during mitosis. Their down-regulation suggests the possible onset of disturbances in the control of spindle formation and cell division. Taken together these observations indicate that as a consequence of the altered levels of such molecules anomalies in the control of proliferation and differentiation are likely to occur.

On the contrary, the main pathways controlling potency, self-renewal, and cell plasticity are active and functional in hPESCs and, in line with this, parthenogenetic cells are able to self-renew and maintain unaltered stable pluripotent cell colonies in vitro. Presumably this is due to the fact that when symmetric cell division is predominant, abnormal centrioles and chromosome malsegregations do not result in aberrant growth and/or dedifferentiation. The same seems to be true when hPESCs respond to differentiation media in vitro and give rise to populations representative of the three germ layers, switching between symmetric and asymmetric cell divisions in a timely and controlled manner. Our data suggest that autophagy is one of the resources that these cells utilize in order to eliminate supernumerary centrioles in these conditions. However, in some cases, this equilibrium is lost upon transplantation in severe compromised immunodeficient (SCID) mice, with the in vivo milieu that releases the cells from their normal patterns causing the unrestrained expansion of the stem cell compartment with the formation of malignant sarcomas [54].

Obviously this is not a general rule and we have no clear explanations for it but experiments on bovine parthenotes showed that the functional ability of maternal centrosomes differs from oocyte to oocyte, determining the developmental fate of each parthenote [71]. Similarly, Dighe *et al.* [57] observed that aberrant genomic imprinting and homozygosity levels are cell-line dependent. Therefore, further investigations are required to understand how individual variations can impact on the properties of each cell line and how undesirable anomalies can possibly be prevented.

Conclusions

PESCs have a number of desirable features that could be advantageously used for cell therapy as well as for studying some fundamental processes of embryonic development. The possibility to obtain monoparental, highly homozygous pluripotent cell lines is a very promising tool to investigate the epigenetic mechanisms of genomic imprinting and its role, not only in development but also in the onset of different diseases. Particularly innovative and rich of potential is the use of the parthenogenetic centrosome as a research tool, given the constantly growing interest in this organelle for its role in cell replication, genome instability, tumour formation, genetic diseases, and ciliopathies, a variety of complex diseases caused by absent or defective cilia [72].

At present, however, the balance between positive and negative features of PESCs is highly contradictory, with most experiments showing at least one or more potentially dangerous deviations from the norm. Therefore, we believe that remarks suggesting and supporting the use of these cells in regenerative medicine, currently accompanying many scientific papers, should be taken with a great degree of caution especially when dealing with human or other primate cell lines.

Acknowledgments

The work of the authors is supported by the Carraresi Foundation and Fondazione Istituto Nazionale Genetica Molecolare.

References

1. Henery CC, Kaufman MH. Cleavage rate of haploid and diploid parthenogenetic mouse embryos during the preimplantation period. *Mol Reprod Dev* 1992; **31**: 258–63.
2. Balakier H, Tarkowski AK. Diploid parthenogenetic mouse embryos produced by heat-shock and cytochalasin B. *J Embryol Exp Morphol* 1976; **35**: 25–39.
3. Kubiak J, Paldi A, Weber M, Maro B. Genetically identical parthenogenetic mouse embryos produced by inhibition of the first meiotic cleavage with cytochalasin D. *Development* 1991; **111**: 763–9.
4. Surani MA. Reprogramming of genome function through epigenetic inheritance. *Nature* 2001; **414**: 122–8.
5. Kaufman MH, Barton SC, Surani MA. Normal postimplantation development of mouse parthenogenetic embryos to the forelimb bud stage. *Nature* 1977; **265**: 53–5.
6. Brevini TA, Pennarossa G, Vanelli A, Maffei S, Gandolfi F. Parthenogenesis in non-rodent species: developmental competence and differentiation plasticity. *Theriogenology* 2012; **77**: 766–72.
7. Newman-Smith ED, Werb Z. Stem cell defects in parthenogenetic peri-implantation embryos. *Development* 1995; **121**: 2069–77.

8. Stevens LC, Varnum DS, Eicher EM. Viable chimaeras produced from normal and parthenogenetic mouse embryos. *Nature* 1977; **269**: 515–17.

9. Surani MA, Barton SC, Kaufman MH. Development to term of chimaeras between diploid parthenogenetic and fertilised embryos. *Nature* 1977; **270**: 601–3.

10. Fundele RH, Norris ML, Barton SC, *et al.* Temporal and spatial selection against parthenogenetic cells during development of fetal chimeras. *Development* 1990; **108**: 203–11.

11. Nigg EA, Stearns T. The centrosome cycle: centriole biogenesis, duplication and inherent asymmetries. *Nat Cell Biol* 2011; **13**: 1154–60.

12. Manandhar G, Schatten H, Sutovsky P. Centrosome reduction during gametogenesis and its significance. *Biol Reprod* 2005; **72**: 2–13.

13. Schatten H, Sun Q-Y. New insights into the role of centrosomes in mammalian fertilization and implications for ART. *Reproduction* 2011; **142**: 793–801.

14. Schatten G. The centrosome and its mode of inheritance: the reduction of the centrosome during gametogenesis and its restoration during fertilization. *Dev Biol* 1994; **165**: 299–335.

15. Calarco-Gillam PD, Siebert MC, Hubble R, Mitchison T, Kirschner M. Centrosome development in early mouse embryos as defined by an autoantibody against pericentriolar material. *Cell* 1983; **35**: 621–9.

16. Sathananthan AH, Ratnam SS, Ng SC, *et al.* The sperm centriole: its inheritance, replication and perpetuation in early human embryos. *Hum Reprod* 1996; **11**: 345–56.

17. Sathananthan AH, Lyons G, Dharmawardena V, *et al.* Centriolar dynamics in the bovine embryo: inheritance and perpetuation of the sperm centrosome during fertilization and development. *Protoplasma* 1999; **206**: 263–9.

18. Morita J, Terada Y, Hosoi Y, *et al.* Microtubule organization during rabbit fertilization by intracytoplasmic sperm injection with and without sperm centrosome. *Reprod Med Biol* 2005; **4**: 169–78.

19. Manandhar G, Feng D, Yi YJ, *et al.* Centrosomal protein centrin is not detectable during early pre-implantation development but reappears during late blastocyst stage in porcine embryos. *Reproduction* 2006; **132**: 423–34.

20. Schatten H, Sun QY. Centrosome dynamics during mammalian oocyte maturation with a focus on meiotic spindle formation. *Mol Reprod Dev* 2011; **78**: 757–68.

21. Szöllosi D, Ozil J-P. De novo formation of centrioles in parthenogenetically activated, diploidized rabbit embryos. *Biol Cell* 1991; **72**: 61–6.

22. Shin M-R, Kim N-H. Maternal gamma (γ)-tubulin is involved in microtubule reorganization during bovine fertilization and parthenogenesis. *Mol Reprod Dev* 2003; **64**: 438–45.

23. Winger QA, De La Fuente R, King WA, Armstrong DT, Watson AJ. Bovine parthenogenesis is characterized by abnormal chromosomal complements: implications for maternal and paternal co-dependence during early bovine development. *Dev Genet* 1997; **21**: 160–6.

24. Bhak J-S, Lee S-L, Ock S-A, *et al.* Developmental rate and ploidy of embryos produced by nuclear transfer with different activation treatments in cattle. *Anim Reprod Sci* 2006; **92**: 37–49.

25. Van De Velde A, Liu L, Bols PEJ, Ysebaert M-T, Yang X. Cell allocation and chromosomal complement of parthenogenetic and IVF bovine embryos. *Mol Reprod Dev* 1999; **54**: 57–62.

26. Alexander B, Coppola G, Di Berardino D, *et al.* The effect of 6-dimethylaminopurine (6-DMAP) and cycloheximide (CHX) on the development and chromosomal complement of sheep parthenogenetic and nuclear transfer embryos. *Mol Reprod Dev* 2006; **73**: 20–30.

27. Somfai T, Ozawa M, Noguchi J, *et al.* Diploid porcine parthenotes produced by inhibition of first polar body extrusion during in vitro maturation of follicular oocytes. *Reproduction* 2006; **132**: 559–70.

28. Kaufman MH. The chromosome complement of single-pronuclear haploid mouse embryos following activation by ethanol treatment. *J Embryol Exp Morphol* 1982; **71**: 139–54.

29. Henery CC, Kaufman MH. The incidence of aneuploidy after single pulse electroactivation of mouse oocytes. *Mol Reprod Dev* 1993; **34**: 299–307.

30. Santos F, Zakhartchenko V, Stojkovic M, *et al.* Epigenetic marking correlates with developmental potential in cloned bovine preimplantation embryos. *Curr Biol* 2003; **13**: 1116–21.

31. Combelles CM, Kearns WG, Fox JH, Racowsky C. Cellular and genetic analysis of oocytes and embryos in a human case of spontaneous oocyte activation. *Hum Reprod* 2011; **26**: 545–52.

32. Munne S, Chen S, Colls P, *et al.* Maternal age, morphology, development and chromosome abnormalities in over 6000 cleavage-stage embryos. *Reprod Biomed Online* 2007; **14**: 628–34.

33. Sathananthan AH. Human centriole: origin, & how it impacts fertilization, embryogenesis, infertility & cloning. *Indian J Med Res* 2009; **129**: 348–50.

34. Maller J, Poccia D, Nishioka D, *et al.* Spindle formation and cleavage in *Xenopus* eggs injected with

centriole-containing fractions from sperm. *Exp Cell Res* 1976; **99**: 285–94.

35. Palermo G, Colombero L, Rosenwaks Z. The human sperm centrosome is responsible for normal syngamy and early embryonic development. *Rev Reprod* 1997; **2**: 19–27.

36. Surti U, Hoffner L, Chakravarti A, Ferrell RE. Genetics and biology of human ovarian teratomas. I. Cytogenetic analysis and mechanism of origin. *Am J Hum Genet* 1990; **47**: 635–43.

37. Sathananthan AH, Selvaraj K, Girijashankar ML, *et al.* From oogonia to mature oocytes: inactivation of the maternal centrosome in humans. *Microsc Res Tech* 2006; **69**: 396–407.

38. Kaufman MH, Robertson EJ, Handyside AH, Evans MJ. Establishment of pluripotential cell lines from haploid mouse embryos. *J Embryol Exp Morphol* 1983; **73**: 249–61.

39. Leeb M, Wutz A. Derivation of haploid embryonic stem cells from mouse embryos. *Nature* 2011; **479**: 131–4.

40. Allen ND, Barton SC, Hilton K, Norris ML, Surani MA. A functional analysis of imprinting in parthenogenetic embryonic stem cells. *Development* 1994; **120**: 1473–82.

41. Horii T, Kimura M, Morita S, Nagao Y, Hatada I. Loss of genomic imprinting in mouse parthenogenetic embryonic stem cells. *Stem Cells* 2008; **26**: 79–88.

42. Li C, Chen Z, Liu Z, *et al.* Correlation of expression and methylation of imprinted genes with pluripotency of parthenogenetic embryonic stem cells. *Hum Mol Genet* 2009; **18**: 2177–87.

43. Chen Z, Liu Z, Huang J, *et al.* Birth of parthenote mice directly from parthenogenetic embryonic stem cells. *Stem Cells* 2009; **27**: 2136–45.

44. Hernandez L, Kozlov S, Piras G, Stewart CL. Paternal and maternal genomes confer opposite effects on proliferation, cell-cycle length, senescence, and tumor formation. *Proc Natl Acad Sci USA* 2003; **100**: 13344–9.

45. Lin H, Lei J, Wininger D, *et al.* Multilineage potential of homozygous stem cells derived from metaphase II oocytes. *Stem Cells* 2003; **21**: 152–61.

46. Cibelli JB, Grant KA, Chapman KB, *et al.* Parthenogenetic stem cells in nonhuman primates. *Science* 2002; **295**: 819.

47. Paffoni A, Brevini TA, Somigliana E, *et al.* In vitro development of human oocytes after parthenogenetic activation or intracytoplasmic sperm injection. *Fertil Steril* 2007; **87**: 77–82.

48. Brevini T, Cillo F, Tosetti V, *et al.* Human pluripotent stem cells derived by parthenogenesis. *Keystone Symposia on Stem Cells Whistler, BC* 2006; **54** (abstract).

49. Kim K, Lerou P, Yabuuchi A, *et al.* Histocompatible embryonic stem cells by parthenogenesis. *Science* 2007; **315**: 482–6.

50. Lin G, OuYang Q, Zhou X, *et al.* A highly homozygous and parthenogenetic human embryonic stem cell line derived from a one-pronuclear oocyte following in vitro fertilization procedure. *Cell Res* 2007; **17**: 999–1007.

51. Mai Q, Yu Y, Li T, *et al.* Derivation of human embryonic stem cell lines from parthenogenetic blastocysts. *Cell Res* 2007; **17**: 1008–19.

52. Revazova ES, Turovets NA, Kochetkova OD, *et al.* Patient-specific stem cell lines derived from human parthenogenetic blastocysts. *Cloning Stem Cells* 2007; **9**: 432–49.

53. Brevini TA, Gandolfi F. Parthenotes as a source of embryonic stem cells. *Cell Prolif* 2008; **41** Suppl 1: 20–30.

54. Brevini TA, Pennarossa G, Antonini S, *et al.* Cell lines derived from human parthenogenetic embryos can display aberrant centriole distribution and altered expression levels of mitotic spindle check-point transcripts. *Stem Cell Rev* 2009; **5**: 340–52.

55. Lu Z, Zhu W, Yu Y, *et al.* Derivation and long-term culture of human parthenogenetic embryonic stem cells using human foreskin feeders. *J Assist Reprod Genet* 2010; **27**: 285–91.

56. Kim K, Ng K, Rugg-Gunn PJ, *et al.* Recombination signatures distinguish embryonic stem cells derived by parthenogenesis and somatic cell nuclear transfer. *Cell Stem Cell* 2007; **1**: 346–52.

57. Dighe V, Clepper L, Pedersen D, *et al.* Heterozygous embryonic stem cell lines derived from nonhuman primate parthenotes. *Stem Cells* 2008; **26**: 756–66.

58. Revazova ES, Turovets NA, Kochetkova OD, *et al.* HLA homozygous stem cell lines derived from human parthenogenetic blastocysts. *Cloning Stem Cells* 2008; **10**: 1–14.

59. Stelzer Y, Yanuka O, Benvenisty N. Global analysis of parental imprinting in human parthenogenetic induced pluripotent stem cells. *Nat Struct Mol Biol* 2011; **18**: 735–41.

60. Turovets N, D'Amour KA, Agapov V, *et al.* Human parthenogenetic stem cells produce enriched populations of definitive endoderm cells after trichostatin A pretreatment. *Differentiation* 2011; **81**: 292–8.

61. Turovets N, Fair J, West R, *et al.* Derivation of high-purity definitive endoderm from human

parthenogenetic stem cells using an in vitro analog of the primitive streak. *Cell Transplant* 2012; **21**: 217–34.

62. Chen Y, Ai A, Tang ZY, *et al.* Mesenchymal-like stem cells derived from human parthenogenetic embryonic stem cells. *Stem Cells Dev* 2012; **21**: 143–51.
63. Isaev DA, Garitaonandia I, Abramihina TV, *et al.* In vitro differentiation of human parthenogenetic stem cells into neural lineages. *Regen Med* 2012; **7**: 37–45.
64. Schatten H, Sun Q-Y. The significant role of centrosomes in stem cell division and differentiation. *Microsc Microanal* 2011; **17**: 506–12.
65. Schatten H, Hueser CN, Chakrabarti A. From fertilization to cancer: the role of centrosomes in the union and separation of genomic material. *Microsc Res Tech* 2000; **49**: 420–7.
66. Mizushima N, Levine B, Cuervo AM, Klionsky DJ. Autophagy fights disease through cellular self-digestion. *Nature* 2008; **451**: 1069–75.
67. Chung E, Chen RH. Spindle checkpoint requires Mad1-bound and Mad1-free Mad2. *Mol Biol Cell* 2002; **13**: 1501–11.
68. Mayer C, Filopei J, Batac J, Alford L, Paluh JL. An extended anaphase signaling pathway for Mad2p includes microtubule organizing center proteins and multiple motor-dependent transitions. *Cell Cycle* 2006; **5**: 1456–63.
69. May KM, Hardwick KG. The spindle checkpoint. *J Cell Sci* 2006; **119**: 4139–42.
70. Grandori C, Cowley SM, James LP, Eisenman RN. The Myc/Max/Mad network and the transcriptional control of cell behavior. *Annu Rev Cell Dev Biol* 2000; **16**: 653–99.
71. Morito Y, Terada Y, Nakamura S, *et al.* Dynamics of microtubules and positioning of female pronucleus during bovine parthenogenesis. *Biol Reprod* 2005; **73**: 935–41.
72. Nigg EA, Raff JW. Centrioles, centrosomes, and cilia in health and disease. *Cell* 2009; **139**: 663–78.

Chapter 22

Epigenetic consequences of somatic cell nuclear transfer and induced pluripotent stem cell reprogramming

Jose Cibelli, Victoria L. Mascetti, and Roger A. Pedersen

Introduction and historical context

Work on amphibian embryos by Hans Spemann more than 80 years ago (see Chapter 1) raised the possibility that individual nuclei could maintain developmental integrity despite undergoing multiple cell divisions [1]. Subsequent work by Briggs and King amplified this concept through development and use of nuclear transfer to replace the nucleus of a frog oocyte with that of a later stage embryo [2]. While early blastula nuclei could support frog egg development, later nuclei did not, leading Briggs and King to conclude that nuclei lose their developmental potential as embryogenesis progresses [3]. Work by Gurdon, however, brought about a paradigm shift (see Chapter 1) from Briggs and King's view of decreasing nuclear potential to one of sustained nuclear potential, owing to his demonstration that fully differentiated tadpole intestinal nuclei could support *Xenopus laevis* development into a functional tadpole [4]. The possibility of sustained nuclear developmental potential was fully realized 35 years later when Wilmut and co-workers demonstrated that cultured cells derived from the adult sheep mammary gland could sustain development all the way to adulthood [5]. These insights into nuclear developmental potential were further amplified by the discovery of Yamanaka and co-workers that differentiated somatic cells could be reprogrammed into cells with developmental capacity equivalent to that of mouse embryonic stem cells (mESCs). This was achieved by administering to mouse fetal fibroblasts a limited set of transcription factors that were known to be expressed in mESCs [6]. The following year, Yamanaka and others extended their compelling observation to human somatic cells, demonstrating that these could be similarly reprogrammed to a pluripotent state [7–9]. The award of the 2012 Nobel Prize in Physiology or Medicine jointly to Gurdon and Yamanaka emphasized the importance of these discoveries.

We have used this chapter to summarize recent studies on the epigenetic characteristics of embryos generated by somatic cell nuclear transfer (SCNT) and pluripotent stem cells induced by reprogramming, as compared to their fertilization-derived counterparts. A recent review has addressed similar issues [10], and others have delineated the epigenetic features that would distinguish SCNT embryos and reprogrammed pluripotent stem cells from their counterparts derived by normal fertilization [11–15]. Accordingly, we forego reiterating the detailed methods for epigenetic analysis, focusing rather on the results from recent studies and their implication for potential applications of SCNT or reprogrammed cells in regenerative medicine.

SCNT unequivocally demonstrated that the metaphase II (MII) oocyte is capable of reprogramming somatic cells back to totipotent cells by generating embryos that when placed into the uterus of a recipient female can generate healthy offspring. After the first report in 1997 by Wilmut and collaborators, more than 20 different species have been cloned by other groups [5, 16]. Numerous reports have shown that cloned animals can be healthy and capable of reaching a normal lifespan. At the same time, it is quite clear that the efficiency of the technique remains low; depending on the species, it hovers around 1% and up to 10% when measured as the number of normal animals born over the number of reconstructed embryos transferred using fibroblast or fibroblast-like cells from an adult. It is evident that in those species in which assisted reproductive technologies have been implemented more successfully, that is, bovine, goat,

Biology and Pathology of the Oocyte, 2nd edn., ed. Alan Trounson, Roger Gosden, and Ursula Eichenlaub-Ritter. Published by Cambridge University Press.

and sheep, the efficiency of SCNT is the highest. And yet, it is still fourfold lower than other techniques such as in vitro fertilization (IVF). This does not apply in the mouse species in which regardless of the high efficiency of IVF, SCNT continues to be in the single digits. Several groups, including ours [17], were quick to point out that animals born by SCNT can be normal, at least for the physiological parameters measured. At the same time, the majority of the SCNT embryos that can reach blastocyst stage in vitro when transferred into the uterus fail to implant or when they do, frequently die in the uterus, or at, or around, birth.

All these deviations from the normal process of embryonic and fetal development are the result of the oocyte's inability to reprogram completely the nucleus of the somatic cell. At the molecular level such a process can be narrowed down to an array of epigenetic errors including deviant DNA methylation, histone acetylation, and histone methylation.

Pluripotent stem cells are capable of differentiating into all body tissues and are able to renew themselves through unlimited proliferation. Pluripotent stem cells were first derived in 1981 by growing the inner cell mass (ICM) of mouse embryos in tissue culture [18]. The functional capacity of mESCs and the tissues generated by their differentiation was assayed by formation of chimeras. This was achieved by introducing mESCs to an early mouse embryo and then transferring the embryo to the uterus of a foster female, for gestation and birth. Such studies definitively demonstrated the pluripotency of mESCs, as the stem cells contributed differentiated progeny to all organs and tissues, including the germ line. Importantly, this method of assessing pluripotent stem cell function has been limited mainly to animal stem cells (mostly mouse and rat), because such studies on human cells are practically and ethically challenging. The differentiative capacity of human pluripotent stem cells has been measured instead by transplanting them to ectopic sites (e.g., kidney capsule, leg muscle) of immunodeficient mice, where the stem cells undergo differentiation and extensive proliferation into tissues representing all major lineages (ectoderm, endoderm, and mesoderm). Despite the evidence from such studies for the pluripotency of human ESCs, it is now thought that these have a substantially different biological nature from pluripotent mESCs.

Human ESCs were first derived in 1998 by growing the ICM of human embryos in the same way mESCs had previously been derived. The similarity of the methods used in their derivation, together with the apparent pluripotency in teratoma assays led to the belief that hESCs were biologically equivalent to mESCs. Differences observed in the growth requirements for hESCs and mESCs were attributed to their species differences. Two studies [19, 20] established, however, that a novel type of pluripotent stem cell could be derived from the epiblast layer of mouse embryos after their implantation into the uterine wall (i.e., at post-implantation stages). Known as mouse epiblast stem cells (EpiSCs), these were shown to be pluripotent by the same assay used to demonstrate hESC pluripotency, but they did not incorporate efficiently into mouse embryos and were essentially unable to form chimeras. This and other key differences between mESCs and EpiSCs led to an understanding of the origin of the differences between mESCs and human pluripotent stem cells. Namely, EpiSCs and hESCs seemingly represent a pluripotent state equivalent to the epiblast layer of pre-gastrulation stage embryos, rather than the inner cell mass-like state of mESCs. Intriguingly, mouse induced pluripotent stem cells (iPSCs) recapitulate the pluripotent state of mESCs, whereas human iPSCs (hiPSCs) recapitulate that of hESCs and EpiSCs.

This distinction in pluripotent state between mESCs and EpiSCs influences the consequences of SCNT. ESCs derived from SCNT mouse embryos are indistinguishable from fertilized embryo-derived ESCs [21–23]. By contrast, EpiSCs derived from SCNT embryos show distinct abnormalities in transcription, with reduced expression of a number of imprinted genes mapped to mouse chromosome 11, including *Snrpn, Necdin, Impact, Mest,* and *Peg3*. Reduced expression of *Snrpn* correlated with increased DNA methylation of the SnrpN imprint control region, which likely explains the reduction in transcript levels for this gene [24]. Thus, there is a difference in how SCNT-derived epigenetic and transcriptional anomalies are either eliminated (mESCs) or persist (EpiSCs).

The transcriptional and developmental equivalence of mESCs derived from fertilized and SCNT blastocysts [21–23] suggests that epigenetic errors acquired during SCNT might be repaired during derivation of the pluripotent stem cells from the cultured ICM. The alternative possibility that epigenetic errors have been already been erased in the ICM itself cannot be reconciled with the existence of epigenetic abnormalities in SCNT-EpiSCs [24], because these are derived from the late epiblast, which comes from the ICM. Thus it appears that epigenetic errors generated by SCNT have different fates in pluripotent stem cells, depending on whether these are derived from the ICM (mESCs in which epigenetic errors are repaired) or from the late epiblast (EpiSCs in which epigenetic errors stably persist).

Epigenetic stability of mESCs and EpiSCs has been studied by comparing their expression of imprinted genes [25]. This confirmed previous studies showing imprinting instability in mESCs, causing them to lose repression of the imprinted (normally silent) allele and acquire biallelic gene expression [26, 27]. By contrast, mouse EpiSCs (mEpiSCs) generally maintained stable imprints, with resulting monoallelic expression of imprinted genes [25]. In this regard, mEpiSCs thus resembled hESCs, for which generally stable genomic imprinting has been demonstrated [28, 29]. When mouse iPSCs were compared using the same approach, they closely resembled mESCs, consistent with other studies in which there was striking similarity between iPSCs and mESCs. Nevertheless, the contrasting properties of mEpiSCs derived from fertilized and from SCNT embryos, together with the general stability of genomic imprinting in EpiSCs, suggest that epigenetic signatures of EpiSCs are handled differently than those of mESCs. This view is supported by the close similarity of mESCs derived from fertilized and from SCNT embryos and by the stability of imprinted gene signatures in both EpiSCs and hESCs. Moreover, the strong epigenetic resemblance of mouse iPSCs to mESCs leads to the prediction that hiPSCs would resemble hESCs in their epigenetic properties. Accordingly, the epigenetic consequences of reprogramming human somatic cells to a pluripotent state are likely to be different to those of reprogramming mouse somatic cells. Therefore, in seeking to understand the translational impact of such epigenetic consequences of reprogramming to pluripotency, it will be necessary to focus on human cells, as these are likely to be less "forgiving" of epigenetic errors than mouse iPSCs. The distinct state of hiPSCs may by analogy affect the outcomes of reprogramming, and accordingly this could have a significant impact on the future clinical utility of the differentiated progeny of hiPSCs in cell-based therapies.

Evidence for epigenetic alterations as a consequence of somatic cell nuclear transfer (SCNT)

Overview

A significant body of literature can be found describing the most common physiological defects affecting animals produced using SCNT techniques. More recently the source of such phenotypic manifestations has been discussed in reviews by others [30, 31]. In this chapter we focus on the most prevalent findings described in multiple species. These include perturbations in DNA methylation, histone acetylation, histone methylation, and X chromosome inactivation.

Perturbations of DNA methylation in SCNT embryos

The first indication of abnormal DNA methylation levels came from looking at the skin and placenta of cloned mice. These tissues showed abnormal methylation in somatic cell loci [32]. Further analysis has shown that mouse and bovine SCNT embryos display atypical dynamics during *de novo* methylation of DNA in the most critical stages of preimplantation development. While DNA demethylation at the 1-cell stage of cloned embryos resembled that observed in the male pronucleus of fertilized embryos, there is precocious *de novo* methylation one or two cell cycles sooner than normally expected (i.e., 4-cell instead of 8-cell stage and 8-cell instead of 16-cell stage for mouse and bovine embryos respectively) [26]. Of the DNA methyl transferases (DNMTs) present in bovine cloned embryos, the one that seems abnormally down-regulated when compared to IVF embryos at the same stage is DNMT1, which is normally associated with methylation maintenance in somatic cells. This finding seems to be counterintuitive considering that most studies point to hypermethylation of DNA in SCNT embryos. However, somatic cells used as donors for SCNT carry their own DNA methylation and therefore it may not be necessary to have active DNMT1 in cloned embryos. It is also relevant that functional studies have shown that down-regulation of DNMT1 does not affect the development of SCNT embryos to blastocyst stage [33].

Work published by Kang and collaborators demonstrated DNA hypermethylation in specific CpG-rich sequences of SCNT embryos reconstructed with fibroblasts that were actively growing or serum starved, as compared to the methylation in IVF or parthenogenetically activated blastocysts [34]. For the genomic regions analyzed, IVF blastocysts had a total dinucleotide methylation of 9% whereas in SCNT embryos it was 65%. The original somatic cells had 72% and parthenogenetic and in vivo isolated blastocysts had 3% and 5%, respectively, for the same regions. This group also reported that in some SCNT embryos methylation was as low as 25% but the majority were approaching the methylation levels of the donor somatic cell. This study clearly showed that demethylation of the somatic cell DNA does not follow that of fertilized embryos. Or if DNA demethylation does occur, as shown by Dean *et al.*, methylation is re-established at the level found in the original somatic cell. Only in rare events is a more "normal" demethylation observed, likely resulting in embryos that can develop into healthy adults [26].

More specific analysis of the DNA regions affected in cloned mice and pigs revealed that there are hotspots for aberrant methylation errors. In mice, Ohgane *et al* showed that the abnormal placenta of cloned fetuses presents, in almost 100% of the samples surveyed, hypermethylation in the Sall3 locus, previously associated with placental abnormalities in human [35].

Recent studies in pigs have shown that cloned animals may appear phenotypically normal with no significant differences in the transcriptome of certain tissues but still possess aberrant methylation in certain loci. This was demonstrated by looking at samples of liver and muscle isolated from 6-week-old cloned pigs as compared to age-matched control animals produced by fertilization. Transcriptional profiles of both tissues showed no significant differences between them; however, methylation-specific digital karyotyping (MMSDK) did show slightly elevated DNA methylation in cloned pigs [36].

Recent data comparing genome-wide methylation status of fertilized and SCNT mouse embryos clearly demonstrate that in turning the somatic cell DNA methylation pattern into that of a zygote, the oocyte accomplishes a remarkable albeit incomplete remodeling of the epigenetic landscape [37]. Reduced representation bisulfite sequencing was used to show that SCNT resulted in a lower scope of demethylation than fertilization, particularly for long interspersed nuclear elements (LINE) repetitive elements. Overall, these results suggest the intriguing conclusion that gametes enter development with specially conditioned DNA methylation in certain genomic regions that is destined for a different fate than the DNA methylation of these regions in donor somatic nuclei.

One of the fundamental questions about all the abnormalities observed in cloned animals is whether they are passed along to the progeny. This is particularly intriguing, as current evidence suggest that all the defects manifested in SCNT development are of epigenetic origin. The first evidence against such transmission emerged from studies in mice in which founder animals produced by SCNT had clear phenotypic defects associated with the procedure, such as obesity, hypertrophic placenta, and open eyelids at birth. None of these signs was observed in their offspring [38]. A bovine study also showed that embryos produced by natural fertilization from non-cloned founders had a pattern of methylation in the satellite I region of the genome – known to have a dozen conserved CpG sites – similar to that of embryos produced using oocytes and sperm from cloned founders [39].

While it is clear that 5-methylcytosine (5MeC) plays an important role during early embryonic development, the role of 5-hydroxymethylcytosine (5hMeC) has just surfaced, and is now starting to be elucidated in the context of preimplantation development [40]. With a few exceptions, all aforementioned studies have measured DNA methylation using bisulfite sequencing. This technique unfortunately cannot distinguish between DNA methylation and DNA hydroxymethylation at the same cytosine nucleotide. 5hMeC methylation is observed when a hydroxyl group is added to an already existent 5MeC, via an oxidative process mediated by TET proteins. It was previously thought that 5hMeC was an intermediate step of the demethylation process that takes place during active demethylation of the paternal pronuclei soon after fertilization. Strong evidence now indicates that 5hMeC may have a specific role on its own as an epigenetic modifier [41]. The enzymes responsible for the hydroxylation of 5MeC and TET 1, 2, and 3, show localized expression in different cell types. While TET3 is highly expressed in the oocyte and pronuclear stage embryos, TET1 is found in ESCs. Knockout mice for Tet1 are viable but show a mild phenotype, that is, a smaller body size. Tet1$^{-/-}$ ESCs have a tendency to differentiate more readily towards trophectoderm in vitro [42]. A recent study using tilling microarray and RNA sequencing has shown that 5hMeC is associated with the gene body of highly expressed genes and that the total level of 5hMeC is directly correlated with tissue type [43]. More concrete evidence that 5hMeC has an important role in early embryonic development came from studies using conditional knockout of Tet3 in mouse oocytes. Embryos resulting from the fertilization of these oocytes developed poorly and failed to implant. When SCNT was done using such Tet3-deficient oocytes, there was a lack of reactivation of endogenous Oct4 from the nucleus of the donor cell [44]. It is thus likely that 5hMeC and the enzymes responsible for this hydroxylation process play a key role in the outcome of the SCNT procedure with genetically normal oocytes.

Histone acetylation perturbations resulting from SCNT

Histone 3 acetylation at its lysine residue 9 (H3K9) is associated with active chromatin configurations. Studies in the bovine have demonstrated that when compared to fertilized embryos, the nuclei of SCNT embryos remain hyperacetylated throughout all the stages of preimplantation development. This phenomenon is not limited to the bovine since porcine and mouse SCNT embryos also have a similar phenotype. In seeming contrast to this observation, treatment of mouse SCNT embryos with trichostatin A (TSA), an inhibitor of histone deacetylases, can increase the efficiency of SCNT fivefold when measured as number of embryos reaching blastocyst stage as well as number of blastocysts from which ESCs can be derived [45]. However, this treatment (which is expected to increase acetylation) must be performed very early on in the SCNT process – at or during oocyte activation.

X inactivation and histone methylation

During normal preimplantation development, female embryos must inactivate one X chromosome to compensate levels of gene expression. This inactivation takes place during the earliest embryonic differentiation event, namely the formation of the blastocyst. It was clearly shown that in cloned bovine embryos, certain genes from both X chromosomes, rather than undergoing inactivation, remained activated, including certain imprinted genes. Of note, one of these was *Xist*, the gene responsible for initiation of X inactivation [46]. Inoue and collaborators observed that in cloned mouse embryos, the majority of genes significantly misregulated, as compared to fertilized embryos, mapped to the X chromosome, independently of the cell type origin used and sex. Notably, they found that *Xist* was overexpressed in SCNT embryos. They hypothesized that by down-regulating *Xist* expression the efficiency of cloning might be increased. Using a cell line in which one X chromosome had a *Xist* deletion, they performed SCNT and transferred the embryos into surrogate mothers. *Xist*-deficient embryos showed an increase in SCNT efficiency to 19%, almost tenfold over the expected level [47]. Similar results were obtained when siRNA for *Xist* was administered to preimplantation embryos. While some disregulation of *Xist* was also observed at later stages of development, preimplantation knockdown of *Xist* was sufficient to overcome fetal losses seen during SCNT in mice [48]. It would be fair to say that since the discovery that an adult mammal can be cloned from a somatic cell in 1997, Ogura's findings represent the most significant advance in the field [48].

H3K9me perturbations resulting from SCNT

Histone methylation is another piece in the multistep process of epigenetic regulation during SCNT. Depending on the histone residue that is methylated, or demethylated, the region of the DNA associated with it will be either active (transcribing mRNA) or repressed (not transcribing mRNA), respectively. Paradoxically, some genes have H3K9 methylated regions interspersed with demethylated regions – so-called bivalent domains. Genes with such bivalent domains in their regulatory regions are thought to be poised for rapid activation during subsequent development. The first clear demonstration that SCNT embryos had a distinct pattern of histone methylation came from analyzing H3K9 levels in bovine SCNT embryos as compared to those in normally fertilized embryos. Significantly, H3K9 was hypermethylated in cloned embryos (showed high levels of H3K9 methylation), while fertilized embryos showed low levels. This reflects a demethylation process that takes place during the first three cell cycles of fertilized embryos that was absent in SCNT embryos [49]. Later studies indicated that the removal of H3K9me3 is required for DNA demethylation to take place in the heterochromatic regions of the genome [50]. Accordingly, there appears to be a causal correlation between the hypermethylation of H3K9 and DNA hypermethylation in SCNT embryos.

H3K4me perturbations

Recent studies using amphibian oocytes as host and mammalian cells as nuclear donors have shown that H3K4 methylation in certain key "pluripotency" genes (such as *Sox2* and *Oct4*) must be reactivated to obtain successful reprogramming and is directly correlated with their levels of expression. In these experiments, the H3K4me2 was observed in the regulatory regions of such pluripotency genes soon after the somatic cell was introduced into the oocyte cytosol. Genes that had H3K4me3 in the same regulatory regions were also more prone to activate these pluripotency genes.

Similar findings emerged when IVF mouse embryos were compared with SCNT embryos reconstructed with NIH3T3 cells. H3K4me2 levels at the time of embryonic genome activation – 2-cell stage in the mouse – were higher in fertilized embryos as compared to SCNT embryos [51]. Taken together these data point to a key role of H3K4 methylation during the early stages of reprogramming [52].

H3K27me perturbations

Histone 3 lysine 27 trimethylation (H3K27me3) is the chromatin hallmark that indicates gene silencing. It is required for primordial germ cell formation in both *Caenorhabditis elegans* and mice [53]. Mouse ESCs deficient for *Suz12*, which is responsible for methylating H3K27, are unable to differentiate properly [54]. It appears that pluripotency is maintained when H3K27me3 is located at the promoter region of genes responsible for early differentiation. There is a clear difference in the amounts of H3K27me3 between ICM and trophoblast cells in mouse IVF blastocysts, but not in cloned mouse embryos [55]. Cloned bovine embryos also show a clear difference in H3K27me3 distribution when compared with IVF embryos at the blastocyst stage [56]. It has recently been suggested that H3K27me3 is part of a larger group of epigenetic marks that will confer on the somatic cell its resistance to reprogramming [57]. Ross and co-workers found that in bovine fertilized embryos, H3K27me3 disappears at the morula stage and reappears at the blastocyst stage [58]. In further work our group showed that removal of the H3K27me3 mark is an active process mediated by JMD3 [59]. A better understanding of how H3K27me3 is maintained in preimplantation embryos during each cell cycle will provide an opportunity to explain not only the epigenetic memory observed in cloned embryos but also why some somatic cells are resistant to reprogramming.

Imprinting and SCNT

Work done in mice by Humpherys and collaborators showed for the first time a clear deregulation of imprinted genes in cloned embryos, at least for the genes analyzed. Such deregulation was independent of the cell type used as a nuclear donor [27, 60]. The expression of *H19, Snrpn, Peg1, Meg1,* and *Gbr10* was measured in the donor cell as well as in major organs in the cloned embryos and placenta. Great variation in the expression of these imprinted genes was observed among different cloned embryos, including those that originated from a single clonal ESC line. As some of these animals survived normally to adulthood, it appears that mammals are quite tolerant of some degree of variability in the epigenome. These results were independently confirmed by Ogawa and co-workers [61].

In summary, each of these epigenetic marks plays a key role in regulating embryonic gene expression, and indeed most of them work together to exert their function. Recent work in mESCs have shown an enrichment of H3K27me3, H3K4me3, and 5hMeC in genes that are poised to be reactivated, pointing to a multistep process of epigenetic regulation that is more complex than originally thought [62].

Evidence for epigenetic alterations in induced pluripotent stem cells (iPSCs)

Transcriptional consequences of reprogramming somatic cells to iPSCs

The transcriptional profiles of mouse and human iPSCs have been compared with their respective ESCs and found to differ in ways that suggest the retention of some characteristics of the somatic cells from which they were derived. Mouse iPSCs were found to differ from genetically identical ESCs by only a few genes, most notably those within the imprinted *Dlk1-Dio3* cluster, which were aberrantly silenced [63]. A comparison, by the same group, of mouse iPSCs generated from either fibroblasts, granulocytes, or skeletal muscle progenitors to ESCs revealed transcriptional differences between them, although these diminished with continuous passaging [64]. Studies comparing hiPSCs and ESCs also revealed transcriptional differences. Chin *et al.* reported nearly 4000 such differentially expressed genes, and they also recognized expression differences between early and late passage iPSCs [65]. They defined an enduring "iPSC epigenetic signature" in some 300 genes whose expression was perturbed at both early and late passage. Similarly, Ghosh *et al.* reported that hiPSCs derived from either fibroblasts, adipose cells, or keratinocytes were closer to their somatic cell of origin than they were to the other somatic cell types, and moreover that there was significant, residual donor-specific gene expression within each type of iPSC [66]. However, Guenther *et al.* contradicted these findings in human pluripotent cells, finding that no genes were significantly differentially expressed between hESCs and hiPSCs [67]. They also performed a meta-analysis on published findings and discounted other reports of differential gene expression between hESCs and hiPSCs on the basis that no shared genes were consistently perturbed between studies [67]. However, this would not rule out random perturbation of genes occurring during reprogramming to hiPSCs. A more recent study comparing transcription of hiPSCs derived from either hepatocytes, fibroblasts, or melanocytes found that the iPSCs preserved a transcriptional memory of their parent somatic cell type. In this study, fully half of the differentially expressed genes were among those whose expression distinguishes hESCs and the somatic cells [68]. Significantly, a quarter of the differentially expressed genes were not characteristic of the donor somatic cells, but instead appeared to represent random reprogramming aberrations with a transcriptional impact. In summary, a number of independent studies comparing either mouse or hiPSCs with their ESC counterparts have detected differences at the transcriptional level, and these deserve an epigenetic explanation.

DNA Methylation in iPSCs

As for SCNT-induced transcriptional perturbations, DNA methylation is the first "port of call" for explaining transcriptional perturbations induced by somatic cell reprogramming. As expected, the imprinted gene perturbations observed by Stadtfeld *et al.* [63] were accompanied by nearly 100% DNA methylation of their imprinting control regions. In contrast to this, a genome-wide, restriction enzyme-based analysis of DNA methylation did not distinguish between the granulocyte- and skeletal muscle progenitor-derived mouse iPSCs that were transcriptionally distinct [64]. Accordingly, these authors suggested that perturbations of DNA methylation induced by reprogramming are subtle and that transcriptional perturbations could arise at the level of chromatin modifications. Using a more comprehensive, array-based approach, Kim *et al.* indeed distinguished an abundance of genes (>5000) with DNA methylation differences between mESCs and iPSCs [69]. Intriguingly, there were fewer such differences between mESCs derived from fertilized embryos and those from SCNT-derived embryos. A similar genome-wide analysis of DNA methylation in hESCs and iPSCs readily distinguished cord blood-derived iPSCs from keratinocyte-derived iPSCs [70]. The variable differentially methylated regions (DMRs) were located in or near genes that distinguished between the two parent somatic cell types, leading the authors to conclude that the reprogramming process can leave residual DNA methylation marks that influence gene expression. Moreover, by this criterion, extended passaging did not bring the iPSCs closer to ESCs. By contrast, the aberrant DNA methylation observed by Nishino *et al.* [71] using a genome-wide approach was diminished by continuous passaging. Although these represented only a fraction of total methylated sites, the aberrantly methylated sites in hiPSCs were interesting because they were hypermethylated as compared to hESCs, the majority were located in promoters, and these varied between the iPSC lines analyzed [71]. A recent study similarly found perturbations of DNA methylation to be a regular feature of iPSCs, regardless of their somatic cell source [72]. This was confirmed by the first whole genome, single base resolution assessment of DNA methylation by Lister and co-workers [73], which found that while hESC and iPSC methylomes are very similar, every iPSC line shows significant reprogramming-based perturbations in DNA methylation as compared to ESCs, their parent somatic cell lines, and even other iPSCs. In contrast to the findings of Nishino *et al.* [71], however, the DMRs that distinguished iPSCs from hESCs as seen by Lister *et al.* [73] were predominantly hypomethylations of promoter regions (Figure 22.1). Taken together, these studies reveal that DNA methylation, rather

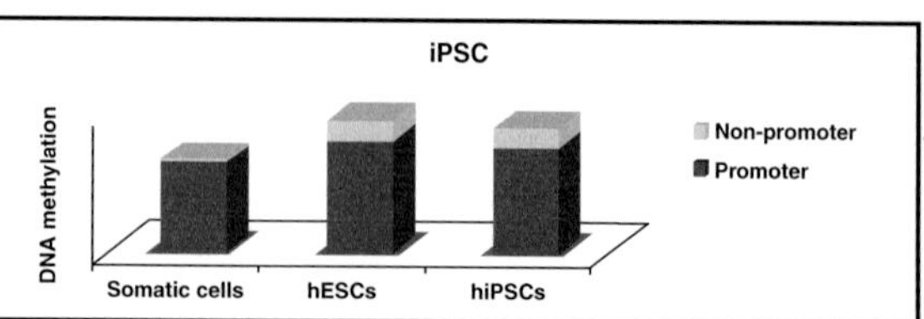

Figure 22.1 Charts depicting the DNA methylation of mouse SCNT embryos and hiPSCs. SCNT DNA methylation was measured in highly repetitive sequences (LINE, LTR, and SINE) and in promoters; values for each category are indicated at the same scale across cell types, but at different scales between categories. Notably, methylation of LINE and LTR repeats was higher in SCNT than in fertilized embryos (data adapted from Chan *et al.* [37]). DNA methylation in iPSCs was measured in non-promoter (MeCH, where H = A, T or G) or in promoter sequences (MeCG). Non-promoter and promoter methylation were higher in both hESCS and hiPSCs than in somatic cells, but promoter methylation was lower in hiPSCs than in hESCs (data adapted from Lister *et al.* [73]).

than being an insensitive indicator of epigenetic perturbation, is a sensitive and relevant one when analyzed on a genome-wide scale.

Histone modifications in iPSCs

The major alternative source of epigenetic perturbations in reprogrammed cells is modification of histones, particularly those known to affect transcription. Consistent with this, mouse iPSCs showed high levels of the transcription activity-associated H3K4me3 and low levels of the repression-associated H3K27me3 modification at promoters of expressed genes [64]. However, analysis of H3K27me3 distribution at the genome-wide level using ChIP-chip found hESCs and hiPSCs to be virtually indistinguishable, with the vast majority of genes similarly marked in both pluripotent cell types [65]. This suggests that perturbations in hiPSC transcription do not arise from faulty modifications of histone 3 at either H3K4 or H3K27. A similar conclusion arises from the study of Guenther *et al.* [67], who found highly similar distributions of H3K4me3 and H3K27me3 in hESCs and hiPSCs. In summary, the modifications of histone 3 appear to be correctly reset upon reprogramming of a somatic cell to a pluripotent cell phenotype.

Translational implications of epigenetic memory in hiPSCs

The generation of clinically relevant hiPSCs unlocks the potential for investigating human disease etiology in vitro, for toxicology studies using hiPSCs as a tool, and for generating an unlimited quantity of patient-specific cells for transplantation. Moreover, iPSCs lack ethical as well as immune rejection concerns associated with the utilization of hESCs in translational research.

As reported in the mouse [64, 69, 74] and in the human [75, 76], reprogramming parental somatic cells confers a tendency on iPSCs to retain an epigenetic memory of the starting cell type and thus acquire a capacity to redifferentiate to their parental cell origin. These recent studies show that epigenetic memory manifests at least in early-passage iPSCs as differential transcriptional profiles, epigenetic signatures, and in vitro differentiation capacity. This principle has recently been exemplified by Xu *et al.* who reported that murine ventricular cardiomyocyte-derived iPSCs (ViPSCs) exhibit a markedly higher propensity for spontaneous differentiation into beating cardiomyocytes as compared to genetically matched ESCs or iPSCs derived from tail-tip fibroblasts [74]. Linking residual methylation signatures in iPSCs to their tissue origin, Kim *et al.* similarly showed an increased propensity of blood-derived iPSC to form hematopoietic colonies when compared with fibroblast-derived iPSCs, ESCs, and SCNT-derived ESCs (ntESCs) [69]. Polo *et al.* were also able to correlate patterns of chromatin modification with a tendency to differentiate into the parent somatic cell type in early-passage murine iPSCs; in this case, however, continuous passaging of iPSCs largely abrogated the epigenetic memory observed at earlier passages [64].

Reprogramming of human somatic cells to iPSCs also demonstrates the effects of epigenetic memory [68, 73, 75, 76]. Among these studies, Bar-Nur *et al.* documented epigenetic memory in human pancreatic β-cell-derived iPSCs (BiPSCs), which maintained open chromatin structure at key β-cell genes [75]. Such epigenetic signatures appear to predispose BiPSCs to spontaneously differentiate more readily into insulin-producing cells expressing PDX1 during their expansion in vitro. Additionally, retinal pigment epithelial cell-derived iPSCs retained their epigenetic memory despite extensive passaging and exhibited spontaneous redifferentiation [76].

The higher efficiency of iPSC differentiation to their cell type of origin may be attributable to higher transcriptional similarity between closely related cell types, and the accessibility of essential transcription cofactors may account for such higher efficiency. This could in turn reflect incomplete reprogramming, resulting in the incomplete suppression of parental cell transcription and inadequate induction of ESC fate. These reports highlight that epigenetic memory, and thus the suitability of somatic cell-derived iPSCs for translational use, is highly influenced by stochastic variations associated with laboratory-specific biases in cell culture and iPSC derivation, passage number, and mode of molecular and epigenetic analysis. These data serve as a cautionary note for the suitability of iPSCs for translational use. If iPSC products are epigenetically distinct from hESCs, are functionally immature, and differ according to their cell origin, this may well deter their adoption for cell-based therapies.

Conversely, the observed tendency of early-passage iPSC lines to differentiate preferentially into the cell lineage of origin could potentially be exploited in translational settings to enhance differentiation into specific and potentially elusive cell types. With these cells, it is possible to determine the epigenetic or genetic regulation of tissue development by comparative studies of parental, iPSC, and ESC lines. Thus, the epigenetic landscape that emerges from reprogramming is likely to be a sensitive indicator of its past and current developmental state and may predict its future potential.

Conclusions

Looking at the process of SCNT from the time of donor cell fusion with the recipient oocyte through to the first differentiation event at the blastocyst stage offers a "bird's eye view" of the vast epigenetic changes taking place in the chromatin. However, this general perspective is of probably lesser value than zooming into the actual events that take place during the first few hours after the somatic cell is introduced into the cytosol of the MII oocyte. A mistake we might have made in the field as a whole is thinking that all MII oocytes are equally equipped to deal with somatic cells bearing a different epigenetic signature from that of a gamete. There is no doubt that some oocytes are thus capable; however, finding and carefully analyzing which oocytes (and of which species) are truly capable of remodeling the somatic cell chromatin at each specific gene locus is a more lofty goal. This may not be as difficult as it sounds. Paying special attention to the hotspots that are failing to be reprogrammed – like the X chromosome for example – is a good place to start.

As previously observed [10], the persistent lack of success in human SCNT has been a significant impediment to comparing the epigenetic consequences of SCNT and reprogramming to iPSCs. Despite isolated claims, there had been until very recently no convincing reports of successful human oocyte development after replacement of its genome by a somatic cell nucleus. While this impediment to human SCNT seemingly reflects primate-specific requirements for induction of zygote genome activation [77], all such requirements appear to be met by the oocyte's own nucleus, which is removed during standard SCNT procedures. This was clear from a study in which the human oocyte (with its own haploid nucleus) is left intact and a diploid human somatic nucleus is transferred to it, resulting in efficient blastocyst development; such an outcome is rarely observed following SCNT [78]. Using this approach, Noggle *et al.* generated two triploid, pluripotent stem cell lines and characterized their gene expression using a genome-wide method, finding no evidence for any epigenetic memory of fibroblast origin of the donor nucleus [78]. In this context, it is significant that Byrne *et al.* were able to derive two rhesus monkey pluripotent stem cell lines after SCNT; despite the low efficiency of their approach (<1%, starting with >300 oocytes), they nevertheless established proof of principle that combined SCNT and pluripotent stem cell derivation can be accomplished in a primate system [79]. To date, no epigenetic assessment of this material has been reported, so a systematic comparison to primate iPSCs remains for the future. In a recent human study, diploid SCNT pluripotent stem cells finally seem to have been derived [80]. By systematically improving the procedures for nuclear transfer, oocyte activation and by preventing premature oocyte maturation, Mitalipov and coworkers were able to generate six human SCNT-hESC lines [80]. While not yet experimentally confirmed by other laboratories, the properties of these reported

SCNT-derived hESCs are fully consistent with their derivation by nuclear transfer. Clearly, a thorough epigenetic assessment of these new human SCNT-hESC lines as compared to hiPSCS should provide penetrating insights into the relative merits of human SCNT-derived and iPSC-derived pluripotent stem cells for future therapeutic applications. In the meantime, hiPSCs remain promising starting materials for cell-based therapies, not only from the perspective of immune matching to the intended recipient but also because their epigenetic memory can potentially be exploited to enhance development into clinically useful cell types. Moreover, now that SCNT-hESCs seem finally to have been generated, these can be evaluated at the epigenetic level to determine whether they have the properties predicted from analysis of pluripotent mouse stem cells generated following SCNT.

References

1. Spemann H. Die Entwicklung seitlicher und dorso-ventraler Keimhalften bei verzogerter Kernversorgung. *Z wiss Zool* 1928; **132**: 105–34.
2. Briggs R, King TJ. Transplantation of living nuclei from blastula cells into enucleated frogs' eggs. *Proc Natl Acad Sci USA* 1952; **38**(5): 455–63.
3. King TJ, Briggs R. Changes in the nuclei of differentiating gastrula cells, as demonstrated by nulcear transplantation. *Proc Natl Acad Sci USA* 1955; 41(5): 321–5.
4. Gurdon JB. The developmental capacity of nuclei taken from intestinal epithelium cells of feeding tadpoles. *J Embryol Exp Morphol* 1962; **10**: 622–40.
5. Wilmut I, Schnieke AE, McWhir J, Kind AJ, Campbell KH. Viable offspring derived from fetal and adult mammalian cells. *Nature* 1997; **385**(6619): 810–13.
6. Takahashi K, Yamanaka S. Induction of pluripotent stem cells from mouse embryonic and adult fibroblast cultures by defined factors. *Cell* 2006; **126**(4): 663–76.
7. Yu J, Vodyanik MA, Smuga-Otto K, *et al.* Induced pluripotent stem cell lines derived from human somatic cells. *Science* 2007; **318**(5858): 1917–20.
8. Park I-H, Zhao R, West JA, *et al.* Reprogramming of human somatic cells to pluripotency with defined factors. *Nature* 2008; **451**(7175): 141–6.
9. Takahashi K, Tanabe K, Ohnuki M, *et al.* Induction of pluripotent stem cells from adult human fibroblasts by defined factors. *Cell* 2007; **131**(5): 861–72.
10. Grieshammer U, Shepard KA, Nigh EA, Trounson A. Finding the niche for human somatic cell nuclear transfer. *Nat Biotechnol* 2011; **29**(8): 701–5.
11. Meissner A. Epigenetic modifications in pluripotent and differentiated cells. *Nat Biotechnol* 2010; **28**(10): 1079–88.
12. Papp B, Plath K. Reprogramming to pluripotency: stepwise resetting of the epigenetic landscape. *Cell Res* 2011; **21**(3): 486–501.
13. Rada-Iglesias A, Wysocka J. Epigenomics of human embryonic stem cells and induced pluripotent stem cells: insights into pluripotency and implications for disease. *Genome Med* 2011; **3**(6): 36.
14. Orkin SH, Hochedlinger K. Chromatin connections to pluripotency and cellular reprogramming. *Cell* 2011; **145**(6): 835–50.
15. Watanabe A, Yamada Y, Yamanaka S. Epigenetic regulation in pluripotent stem cells: a key to breaking the epigenetic barrier. *Philos Trans R Soc Lond B Biol Sci* 2012; **368**(1609): 20120292.
16. Cibelli J. Developmental biology. A decade of cloning mystique. *Science* 2007; **316**(5827): 990–2.
17. Cibelli JB, Campbell KH, Seidel GE, West MD, Lanza RP. The health profile of cloned animals. *Nat Biotechnol* 2002; **20**(1): 13–14.
18. Evans MJ, Kaufman MH. Establishment in culture of pluripotential cells from mouse embryos. *Nature* 1981; **292**(5819): 154–6.
19. Brons IGM, Smithers LE, Trotter MWB, *et al.* Derivation of pluripotent epiblast stem cells from mammalian embryos. *Nature* 2007; **448**(7150): 191–5.
20. Tesar PJ, Chenoweth JG, Brook FA, *et al.* New cell lines from mouse epiblast share defining features with human embryonic stem cells. *Nature* 2007; **448**(7150): 196–9.
21. Brambrink T, Hochedlinger K, Bell G, Jaenisch R. ES cells derived from cloned and fertilized blastocysts are transcriptionally and functionally indistinguishable. *Proc Natl Acad Sci USA* 2006; **103**(4): 933–8.
22. Wakayama S, Jakt ML, Suzuki M, *et al.* Equivalency of nuclear transfer-derived embryonic stem cells to those derived from fertilized mouse blastocysts. *Stem Cells* 2006; **24**(9): 2023–33.
23. Ding J, Guo Y, Liu S, *et al.* Embryonic stem cells derived from somatic cloned and fertilized blastocysts are post-transcriptionally indistinguishable: a microRNA and protein profile comparison. *Proteomics* 2009; **9**(10): 2711–21.
24. Maruotti J, Dai XP, Brochard V, *et al.* Nuclear transfer derived epiblast stem cells are transcriptionally and epigenetically distinguishable

from their fertilized-derived counterparts. *Stem Cells* 2010; **28**(4): 743–52.

25. Sun B, Ito M, Mendjan S, *et al.* Status of genomic imprinting in epigenetically distinct pluripotent stem cells. *Stem Cells* 2012; **30**(2): 161–8.

26. Dean W, Santos F, Stojkovic M, *et al.* Conservation of methylation reprogramming in mammalian development: aberrant reprogramming in cloned embryos. *Proc Natl Acad Sci USA* 2001; **98**(24): 13734–8.

27. Humpherys D, Eggan K, Akutsu H, *et al.* Epigenetic instability in ES cells and cloned mice. *Science* 2001; **293**(5527): 95–7.

28. Rugg-Gunn PJ, Ferguson-Smith AC, Pedersen RA. Human embryonic stem cells as a model for studying epigenetic regulation during early development. *Cell Cycle* 2005; **4**(10): 1323–6.

29. International Stem Cell Initiative, Adewumi O, Aflatoonian B, Ahrlund-Richter L, *et al.* Characterization of human embryonic stem cell lines by the International Stem Cell Initiative. *Nat Biotechnol* 2007; **25**(7): 803–16.

30. Niemann H, Tian XC, King WA, Lee RSF. Epigenetic reprogramming in embryonic and foetal development upon somatic cell nuclear transfer cloning. *Reproduction* 2008; **135**(2): 151–63.

31. Yang X, Smith SL, Tian XC, *et al.* Nuclear reprogramming of cloned embryos and its implications for therapeutic cloning. *Nat Genet* 2007; **39**(3): 295–302.

32. Ohgane J, Wakayama T, Kogo Y, *et al.* DNA methylation variation in cloned mice. *Genesis* 2001; **30**(2): 45–50.

33. Golding MC, Williamson GL, Stroud TK, Westhusin ME, Long CR. Examination of DNA methyltransferase expression in cloned embryos reveals an essential role for Dnmt1 in bovine development. *Mol Reprod Dev* 2011; **78**(5): 306–17.

34. Kang Y-K, Koo D-B, Park J-S, *et al.* Aberrant methylation of donor genome in cloned bovine embryos. *Nat Genet* 2001; **28**(2): 173–7.

35. Ohgane J, Wakayama T, Senda S, *et al.* The Sall3 locus is an epigenetic hotspot of aberrant DNA methylation associated with placentomegaly of cloned mice. *Genes Cells* 2004; **9**(3): 253–60.

36. Gao F, Luo Y, Li S, *et al.* Comparison of gene expression and genome-wide DNA methylation profiling between phenotypically normal cloned pigs and conventionally bred controls. *PLoS One* 2011; **6**(10): e25901.

37. Chan MM, Smith ZD, Egli D, Regev A, Meissner A. Mouse ooplasm confers context-specific reprogramming capacity. *Nat Genet* 2012; **44**(9): 978–80.

38. Shimozawa N, Ono Y, Kimoto S, *et al.* Abnormalities in cloned mice are not transmitted to the progeny. *Genesis* 2002; **34**(3): 203–7.

39. Yamanaka K-I, Kaneda M, Inaba Y, *et al.* DNA methylation analysis on satellite I region in blastocysts obtained from somatic cell cloned cattle. *Anim Sci J* 2011; **82**(4): 523–30.

40. Iqbal K, Jin S-G, Pfeifer GP, Szabó PE. Reprogramming of the paternal genome upon fertilization involves genome-wide oxidation of 5-methylcytosine. *Proc Natl Acad Sci USA* 2011; 108(9): 3642–7.

41. Salvaing J, Aguirre-Lavin T, Boulesteix C, *et al.* 5-Methylcytosine and 5-hydroxymethylcytosine spatiotemporal profiles in the mouse zygote. *PLoS One* 2012; **7**(5): e38156.

42. Dawlaty MM, Ganz K, Powell BE, *et al.* Tet1 is dispensable for maintaining pluripotency and its loss is compatible with embryonic and postnatal development. *Cell Stem Cell* 2011; **9**(2): 166–75.

43. Nestor CE, Ottaviano R, Reddington J, *et al.* Tissue type is a major modifier of the 5-hydroxymethylcytosine content of human genes. *Genome Res* 2012; **22**(3): 467–77.

44. Gu T-P, Guo F, Yang H, *et al.* The role of Tet3 DNA dioxygenase in epigenetic reprogramming by oocytes. *Nature* 2011; **477**(7366): 606–10.

45. Kishigami S, Mizutani E, Ohta H, *et al.* Significant improvement of mouse cloning technique by treatment with trichostatin A after somatic nuclear transfer. *Biochem Biophys Res Commun* 2006; **340**(1): 183–9.

46. Dinnyes A, Dai Y, Levine H, Pereira LV, Yang X. Aberrant patterns of X chromosome inactivation in bovine clones. *Nat Genet* 2002; **31**(2): 216–20.

47. Inoue K, Kohda T, Sugimoto M, *et al.* Impeding Xist expression from the active X chromosome improves mouse somatic cell nuclear transfer. *Science* 2010; **330**(6003): 496–9.

48. Matoba S, Inoue K, Kohda T, *et al.* RNAi-mediated knockdown of Xist can rescue the impaired postimplantation development of cloned mouse embryos. *Proc Natl Acad Sci USA* 2011; **108**(51): 20621–6.

49. Santos F, Zakhartchenko V, Stojkovic M, *et al.* Epigenetic marking correlates with developmental potential in cloned bovine preimplantation embryos. *Curr Biol* 2003; **13**(13): 1116–21.

50. Mason K, Liu Z, Aguirre-Lavin T, Beaujean N. Chromatin and epigenetic modifications during early

mammalian development. *Anim Reprod Sci* 2012; 134(1–2): 45–55.

51. Shao G-B, Ding H-M, Gong A-H, Xiao D-S. Inheritance of histone H3 methylation in reprogramming of somatic nuclei following nuclear transfer. *J Reprod Dev* 2008; **54**(3): 233–8.

52. Murata K, Kouzarides T, Bannister AJ, Gurdon JB. Histone H3 lysine 4 methylation is associated with the transcriptional reprogramming efficiency of somatic nuclei by oocytes. *Epigenetics Chromatin* 2010; **3**(1): 4.

53. Seydoux G, Braun RE. Pathway to totipotency: lessons from germ cells. *Cell* 2006; **127**(5): 891–904.

54. Pasini D, Bracken AP, Hansen JB, Capillo M, Helin K. The polycomb group protein Suz12 is required for embryonic stem cell differentiation. *Mol Cell Biol* 2007; **27**(10): 3769–79.

55. Zhang M, Wang F, Kou Z, Zhang Y, Gao S. Defective chromatin structure in somatic cell cloned mouse embryos. *J Biol Chem* 2009; **284**(37): 24981–7.

56. Breton A, Le Bourhis D, Audouard C, Vignon X, Lelièvre J-M. Nuclear profiles of H3 histones trimethylated on Lys27 in bovine (*Bos taurus*) embryos obtained after in vitro fertilization or somatic cell nuclear transfer. *J Reprod Dev* 2010; **56**(4): 379–88.

57. Pasque V, Jullien J, Miyamoto K, Halley-Stott RP, Gurdon JB. Epigenetic factors influencing resistance to nuclear reprogramming. *Trends Genet* 2011; **27**(12): 516–25.

58. Ross PJ, Ragina NP, Rodriguez RM, *et al.* Polycomb gene expression and histone H3 lysine 27 trimethylation changes during bovine preimplantation development. *Reproduction* 2008; **136**(6): 777–85.

59. Canovas S, Cibelli JB, Ross PJ. Jumonji domain-containing protein 3 regulates histone 3 lysine 27 methylation during bovine preimplantation development. *Proc Natl Acad Sci USA* 2012; **109**(7): 2400–5.

60. Humpherys D. Abnormal gene expression in cloned mice derived from embryonic stem cell and cumulus cell nuclei. *Proc Natl Acad Sci USA* 2002; **99**(20): 12889–94.

61. Ogawa H, Ono Y, Shimozawa N, *et al.* Disruption of imprinting in cloned mouse fetuses from embryonic stem cells. *Reproduction* 2003; **126**(4): 549–57.

62. Pastor WA, Pape UJ, Huang Y, *et al.* Genome-wide mapping of 5-hydroxymethylcytosine in embryonic stem cells. *Nature* 2011; **473**(7347): 394–7.

63. Stadtfeld M, Apostolou E, Akutsu H, *et al.* Aberrant silencing of imprinted genes on chromosome 12qF1 in mouse induced pluripotent stem cells. *Nature* 2011; **465**(7295): 175–81.

64. Polo JM, Liu S, Figueroa ME, *et al.* Cell type of origin influences the molecular and functional properties of mouse induced pluripotent stem cells. *Nat Biotechnol* 2010; **28**(8): 848–55.

65. Chin MH, Mason MJ, Xie W, *et al.* Induced pluripotent stem cells and embryonic stem cells are distinguished by gene expression signatures. *Stem Cells* 2009; **5**(1): 111–23.

66. Ghosh Z, Wilson KD, Wu Y, *et al.* Persistent donor cell gene expression among human induced pluripotent stem cells contributes to differences with human embryonic stem cells. *PLoS One* 2010; **5**(2): e8975.

67. Guenther MG, Frampton GM, Soldner F, *et al.* Chromatin structure and gene expression programs of human embryonic and induced pluripotent stem cells. *Cell Stem Cell* 2010; **7**(2): 249–57.

68. Ohi Y, Qin H, Hong C, *et al.* Incomplete DNA methylation underlies a transcriptional memory of somatic cells in human iPS cells. *Nat Cell Biol* 2011; **13**(5):541–9.

69. Kim K, Doi A, Wen B, *et al.* Epigenetic memory in induced pluripotent stem cells. *Nature* 2010; **467**(7313): 285–90.

70. Kim K, Zhao R, Doi A, *et al.* Donor cell type can influence the epigenome and differentiation potential of human induced pluripotent stem cells. *Nat Biotechnol* 2011; **29**(12): 1117–19.

71. Nishino K, Toyoda M, Yamazaki-Inoue M, *et al.* DNA methylation dynamics in human induced pluripotent stem cells over time. *PLoS Genet* 2011; **7**(5): e1002085.

72. Ruiz S, Diep D, Gore A, *et al.* Identification of a specific reprogramming-associated epigenetic signature in human induced pluripotent stem cells. *Proc Natl Acad Sci USA* 2012; **109**(40): 16196–201.

73. Lister R, Pelizzola M, Kida YS, *et al.* Hotspots of aberrant epigenomic reprogramming in human induced pluripotent stem cells. *Nature* 2012; **471**(7336): 68–73.

74. Xu H, Yi BA, Wu H, *et al.* Highly efficient derivation of ventricular cardiomyocytes from induced pluripotent stem cells with a distinct epigenetic signature. *Cell Res* 2011; **22**(1): 142–54.

75. Bar-Nur O, Russ HA, Efrat S, Benvenisty N. Epigenetic memory and preferential lineage-specific differentiation in induced pluripotent stem cells derived from human pancreatic islet beta cells. *Cell Stem Cell* 2011; **9**(1): 17–23.

76. Hu Q, Friedrich AM, Johnson LV, Clegg DO. Memory in induced pluripotent stem cells: reprogrammed human retinal-pigmented epithelial cells show

tendency for spontaneous redifferentiation. *Stem Cells* 2010; **28**(11): 1981–91.

77. Egli D, Chen AE, Saphier G, *et al.* Reprogramming within hours following nuclear transfer into mouse but not human zygotes. *Nat Commun* 2011; **2**: 488–10.

78. Noggle S, Fung H-L, Gore A, *et al.* Human oocytes reprogram somatic cells to a pluripotent state. *Nature* 2012; **478**(7367): 70–5.

79. Byrne JA, Pedersen DA, Clepper LL, *et al.* Producing primate embryonic stem cells by somatic cell nuclear transfer. *Nature* 2007; **450**(7169): 497–502.

80. Tachibana M, Amato P, Sparman M, *et al.* Human embryonic stem cells derived by somatic cell nuclear transfer. *Cell* 2013; http://dx.doi.org/10.1016/j.cell.2013.05.006.

Chapter 23

Primate and human somatic cell nuclear transfer

Rita P. Cervera and Shoukhrat Mitalipov

Introduction

Non-human primates (NHPs) are an ideal model in preclinical research due to their remarkable genetic, physiological, and reproductive similarities to humans. NHPs are also critical in areas where basic discoveries in rodent or other animals were difficult to translate to clinical settings. Particularly, reprogramming of somatic cells to pluripotency by somatic cell nuclear transfer (SCNT) is a routine and efficient process in the mouse. However, these protocols were not applicable for human oocytes and embryos [1]. Reproductive cloning by SCNT would also be critical for replication of valuable genotypes or generation of genetically modified NHPs. In this chapter, we summarize the current state of SCNT in NHPs and the efforts to produce human pluripotent stem cells by SCNT-based reprogramming.

Milestones of somatic cell nuclear transfer

Nuclear transfer was originally proposed by Spemann (1938) as a method to "recycle" the nuclear genome from embryonic or somatic cells and evaluate its ability to support full-term development [2] (see also Chapters 1 and 22). The concept was first successfully tested by Briggs and King (1952) in amphibia by transplanting nuclei of embryonic blastomeres into enucleated eggs [3]. Later, Gurdon (1962) tested more advanced tadpole intestinal cells and produced viable *Xenopus* offspring [4]. Due to technical and biological limitations in manipulating oocytes, nuclear transfer experimentations in mammals were not reported until the early 1980s. Initial studies also used nuclei of blastomeres from cleaving preimplantation embryos and these studies demonstrated that enucleated zygotes have only limited utility as recipient cytoplasts [5, 6]. However, unfertilized, mature metaphase II (MII) oocytes provided better reprogramming capacity compatible with full-term development [5, 7]. The first offspring generated by SCNT using an adult somatic cell was Dolly the sheep [8]. Following similar SCNT techniques, researchers have now succeeded in producing live offspring or embryonic stem cells (ESCs) in a number of different mammals (Table 23.1).

A variety of nuclear donor somatic cell types were proven to support normal development, including cumulus cells, tail tip and skin fibroblasts, Sertoli cells, keratinocytes, and hematopoietic and neuronal stem cells [30]. Even terminally differentiated, mitotically inactive donor cells, such as mature B and T cells [31], muscle cells [32], post-mitotic granulocytes [33], and olfactory neurons [34], were able to produce normal live offspring following SCNT. Evidence also suggests that the lifespan and aging of cloned animals are normal and match that of IVF controls, but not the age of nuclear donor cells [35, 36]. Moreover, cloning of the same nuclear genome can be recycled many times with no signs of decline in cloning efficiency, of telomere shortening, or of premature aging. Thuan and colleagues reported successful "serial" cloning of mice for 15 generations (and still going!) using the same somatic cell nuclear genome [30]. These remarkable studies demonstrated the universal ability of oocytes to restore developmental totipotency in somatic cell nuclei regardless of the cell type or age.

As indicated above, cytoplasm of unfertilized, MII-arrested oocytes is routinely used for SCNT. More recently, mouse zygotic or even 2-cell embryo cytoplasts were used to reprogram somatic cells to ESCs. However, live offspring were only produced with

Biology and Pathology of the Oocyte, 2nd edn., ed. Alan Trounson, Roger Gosden, and Ursula Eichenlaub-Ritter.
Published by Cambridge University Press.

Table 23.1. Live offspring and embryonic stem cells produced by SCNT in mammals

Species	Date	Nuclear donor cell type	Live offspring or ESCs	Reference
Sheep	1997 1997	Fetal fibroblasts Adult mammary epithelial	Offspring Offspring	[8] [8]
Cattle	1998 1998	Fetal fibroblasts Adult oviduct epithelial	Offspring Offspring	[9] [10]
Mouse	1998 2001	Adult cumulus Adult cumulus/fibroblasts	Offspring ESCs	[11] [12]
Goat	1999	Fetal fibroblasts	Offspring	[13]
Pig	2000	Adult cumulus	Offspring	[14]
Gaur	2000	Adult fibroblasts	Offspring	[15]
Mouflon	2001	Adult granulosa	Offspring	[16]
Cat	2002	Adult cumulus	Offspring	[17]
Rabbit	2002	Adult cumulus	Offspring	[18]
Banteng	2003	Adult fibroblasts	Offspring	[19]
Rat	2003	Fetal fibroblasts	Offspring	[20]
Mule	2003	Fetal fibroblasts	Offspring	[21]
Horse	2003	Adult fibroblasts	Offspring	[22]
Deer	2003	Adult fibroblasts	Offspring	[23]
Dog	2005	Adult fibroblasts	Offspring	[24]
Ferret	2006	Fetal fibroblasts/Adult cumulus	Offspring	[25]
Buffalo	2007	Fetal fibroblasts/Adult granulosa	Offspring	[26]
Wolf	2007	Adult fibroblasts	Offspring	[27]
Rhesus macaque	2007	Adult fibroblasts	ESCs	[28]
Camel	2010	Adult fibroblasts	Offspring	[29]

zygotic cytoplasm when ESCs were used as donor nuclei (Figure 23.1) [1, 37, 38].

Despite this success, the overall efficiency of producing live SCNT offspring remained low, ranging from 1% to 5% [39]. This is mainly contributed to by high embryonic, fetal, or early postnatal loses following SCNT procedures. Interestingly, once SCNT offspring survive these critical stages, their subsequent postnatal development and aging is seemingly normal [40]. It is generally accepted that the observed low efficiencies are caused by "reprogramming errors" occurring soon after SCNT that subsequently result in abnormal gene expression in developing fetuses [41]. The cytoplasm of an enucleated oocyte (cytoplast) is expected to induce a series of epigenetic changes in the transplanted somatic nucleus that ideally would result in a complete erasure of the donor cell's "somatic memory" and establishment of the new zygotic chromatin program. Several studies have found abnormalities in DNA methylation or histone acetylation/methylation patterns in SCNT embryos [42–44].

However, since initial application of the SCNT for reproductive cloning, the efficiency of the procedure has been dramatically improved in many species. This was mainly achieved by incremental improvements and optimizations of standard SCNT protocols. Other protocol modifications include implementation of additional steps that aid in epigenetic reprogramming. For example, survival of mouse clones was increased up to fivefold using histone deacetylase inhibitors (HDACi) during the oocyte activation step [43, 45, 46]. HDACi were also shown to improve the overall cloning success rates in other species [47] including monkeys [48]. RNA interference (RNAi) against *Xist* was used to correct X chromosome inactivation and significantly increase the survival rate of cloned mouse offspring [49].

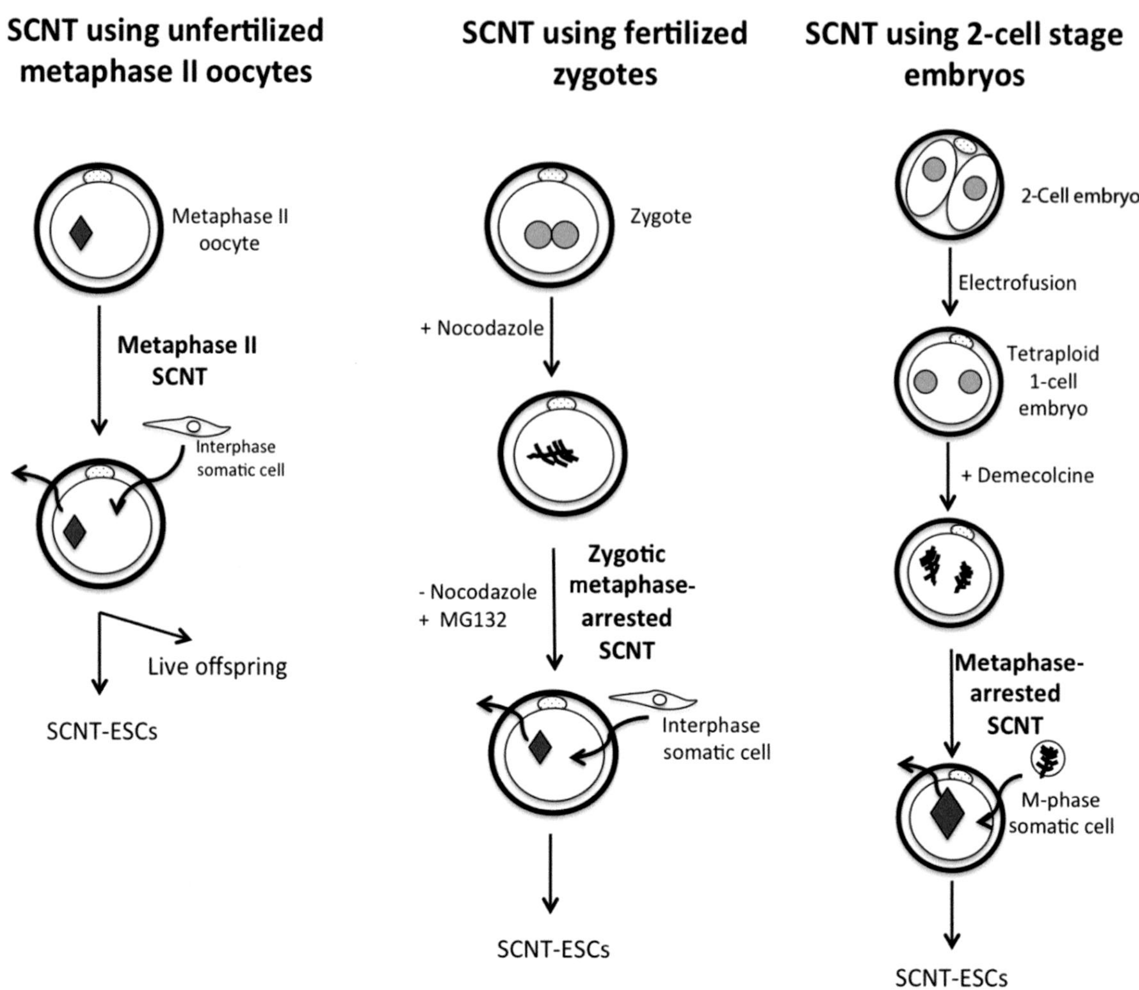

Figure 23.1 Schematic diagram of different cytoplast types capable of reprogramming somatic cell nuclei. Conventional SCNT approaches utilize enucleated metaphase II oocytes as recipient cytoplasm (cytoplast) for reprogramming of somatic cell nuclei. Continued SCNT success in numerous species demonstrated the universal capacity of unfertilized oocyte's cytoplasm to induce reprogramming [8]. In addition, fertilized mouse zygotic [1] or even 2-cell embryo cytoplasts [37, 38] arrested at M-phase were also capable of reprogramming somatic cells to functional ESCs.

Should SCNT efficiencies be compared with those of IVF?

It remains unclear whether the abnormalities and associated embryonic or fetal losses observed during reproductive cloning are inherent to SCNT due to a natural inability of the cytoplast to reprogram the somatic cell genome, or a result of suboptimal cloning protocols. SCNT efficiencies are often compared with in vitro fertilization (IVF) outcomes; however, SCNT and IVF procedures are entirely different. Compared with IVF, SCNT is associated with several additional and invasive steps that are likely detrimental and could be a primary cause of the abnormalities seen in cloned offspring.

During SCNT, the meiotic spindle apparatus that includes the oocyte's chromosomes must be removed and replaced with the somatic cell nucleus. In contrast to interphase nuclei, meiotic spindles cannot be identified inside MII oocytes using conventional light microscopes. Initial enucleation protocols utilized staining of chromosomes with fluorochromes (bisbenzimide Hoechst 33342) followed by UV light exposure to visualize and enucleate the oocytes. When this enucleation technique was applied to rhesus macaque oocytes, we reported that most SCNT embryos

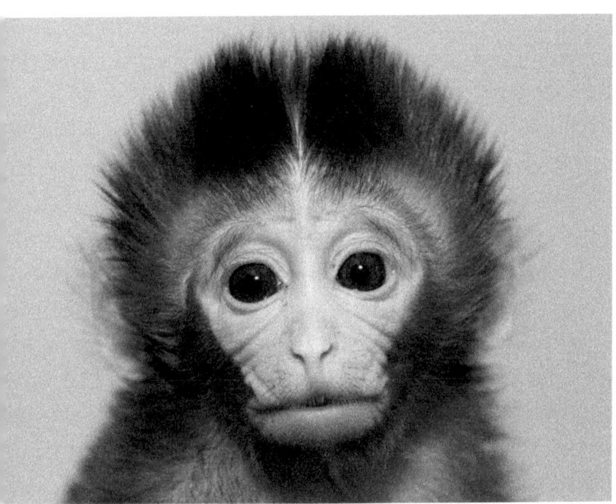

Figure 23.2 Crysta, a rhesus infant produced by metaphase spindle transfer. The meiotic spindle–chromosomal complex from vitrified–thawed rhesus oocyte was transplanted into a cytoplasm from another oocyte. After fertilization and in vitro culture to the blastocyst stage, the embryo was transferred into a recipient monkey. The pregnancy resulted in a birth of healthy female infant Crysta (unpublished data).

arrested during early cleavage stages, with only a few progressing to blastocysts [50]. We developed and introduced a non-invasive enucleation procedure that is based on the use of a polarized microscope for the spindle imaging and removal. This modification alone significantly increased monkey blastocyst formation after SCNT (from 1% to 16%) [28].

Another potentially harmful step is the introduction of the donor nucleus into the cytoplast. This is routinely achieved by whole cell fusion using electroporation. We tested the effect of electro fusion during nuclear transfer independently of SCNT, on the IVF platform, by transplanting MII spindle–chromosomal complexes between rhesus oocytes. We observed that exposure to the electrofusion regimen triggers premature cytoplast activation and subsequent meiotic resumption in MII spindles [51]. Following electrofusion, oocytes prematurely completed meiosis and extruded a second polar body, even prior to fertilization. Such oocytes were unable to support normal fertilization and development. To overcome this adverse effect, we tested an alternative fusion strategy between karyoplast/cytoplasts using an extract from Sendai virus. After reintroduction into cytoplasts, the MII spindle retained normal meiotic morphology and reconstructed oocytes were capable of normal fertilization and supported full-term development of healthy rhesus offspring (Figure 23.2) [51]. This study demonstrated that electrofusion, a routine approach for most SCNT protocols, is likely to be delivering a premature activation stimulus to cytoplasts. While somatic cell nuclei are introduced at the G0/G1-phase of the cell cycle, we demonstrated that successful integration and reprogramming is dependent on nuclear remodeling events associated with high levels of maturation-promoting factor (MPF) present in meiotic cytoplasts [50]. Since premature activation after electroporation induces MPF degradation and cytoplast activation, our current somatic cell fusion protocols are based on membrane fusion using Sendai envelope [48, 51].

Another SCNT protocol deficiency, that still remains to be resolved, is the cell-cycle mismatch between cytoplasts and somatic cell nuclei. While oocyte cytoplasm is naturally arrested at the metaphase, the somatic cell nucleus is introduced at the G0 or G1 of the cell cycle [52]. It is generally believed that cytoplasm/nucleus cell-cycle incompatibilities can cause abnormal DNA replication and subsequently aneuploidies [53]. Ideally, the somatic nucleus would need to be synchronized and introduced at the M-phase. This can be done by culturing nuclear donor cells with drugs that interfere with microtubule polymerization (colchicine, demecolcine, or nocodazole). However, even short exposure to these compounds is known to be toxic or irreversible and often incompatible with normal development [1].

Sperm entry during fertilization triggers the oocyte activation that is critical for resumption and completion of meiosis. Activation is also important for the oocyte's cytoplasm to acquire the reprogramming and metabolic activity necessary to support subsequent development [54]. Since fertilization by sperm is bypassed during SCNT, the activation stimulus is artificially induced. Artificial activation treatments mimicking natural sperm-induced biochemical processes were developed in the early 1980s for cattle oocytes [54]. Briefly, the protocol consists of chemical treatments that induce calcium oscillations, much like those detected following normal fertilization with sperm. However, this treatment alone does not always fully activate cytoplasts nor downregulate meiosis-associated protein kinases and MPF, and may result in the re-entry of cytoplasts into meiotic arrest. To overcome this, cytoplasts are additionally treated with kinase or protein synthesis inhibitors, such as 6-dimethylaminopurine [55, 56]. Presently, it is unclear how close these artificial protocols resemble natural, sperm activation-induced mechanisms. Ideally, the effect of artificial activation on subsequent development should be tested independently from other SCNT variables. For example, rescue of IVF embryos following intracytoplasmic sperm injection (ICSI) with sperm lacking activation capacity, but otherwise normal, would present an ideal platform for evaluation of activation procedures alone. Until then, it is reasonable to speculate that SCNT abnormalities are caused, in part, by suboptimal artificial activation.

Current status of SCNT in NHPs

Reproductive cloning has numerous applications for agricultural and laboratory animals, including replication of valuable genotypes and the generation of genetically modified animals [57]. The same reasons drive development of efficient SCNT approaches for NHPs. Production of genetically identical monkeys by SCNT would significantly reduce the number of animals utilized in biomedical research. Another application of SCNT in NHPs is generation of gene-targeted offspring for the study of gene function or modeling of human diseases. In the mouse model, this is routinely achieved by generating germline chimeras with genetically altered ESCs. Subsequent breeding of chimeric founders allows the production of heterozygous or homozygous offspring. This approach is currently not applicable in the rhesus macaque model for a couple of reasons. Firstly, available monkey ESCs do not seem capable of contributing to chimeras. We recently tested several rhesus ESCs by injection into blastocysts and subsequent transfer of these embryos to recipient females. Eight offspring were generated but none of them was confirmed to contain ESC progeny. However, chimeric monkey offspring were generated using non-cultured embryonic cells freshly isolated from preimplantation embryos [58]. It is likely that during derivation and culture, monkey ESCs lose their ability to contribute to chimeras. It is believed that more potent, so-called "naïve," primate ESCs could be established that should be chimera-competent [59]. However, even if primate ESC chimeras were ever produced, the disadvantage is that subsequent breeding of chimeric monkeys would require at least a decade of time, due to longer gestation, sexual maturity, and singleton pregnancies in rhesus macaques. In contrast, reproductive cloning with genetically altered donor cells would allow the generation of desirable animals in the first generation.

Despite success with SCNT in other mammals, reproductive cloning has not been achieved in NHPs yet. As pointed out above, direct application of standard SCNT techniques to rhesus monkeys initially resulted in limited development of cloned embryos. We tested independently several critical SCNT steps with monkey oocytes and introduced several modifications that currently allow the routine production of SCNT blastocysts [48]. On average, up to 20% of rhesus SCNT embryos reconstructed with fetal or adult skin fibroblasts reach the expanded blastocyst stage [48]. We were able consistently to derive ESCs from such SCNT embryos and their transcriptional and epigenetic profiles closely resemble IVF controls [28, 60]. Moreover, as few as 10 mature rhesus oocytes are needed to derive one ESC line using our current monkey SCNT procedures [60]. However, in vivo development of monkey SCNT embryos following transfer to recipients remains limited. Early pregnancies have been established with SCNT embryos at a reasonable rate. However, most pregnancies fail to progress beyond the first trimester and no live rhesus monkey offspring has been produced so far. It is possible that SCNT blastocysts are deficient in their ability to contribute to functional extraembryonic tissues, since SCNT-ESCs representing an embryo proper lineage seems to be normal. Our current efforts are focused on chimeric complementation of SCNT embryos with their IVF counterparts. As we recently reported, chimeric rhesus offspring can be efficiently produced by aggregation of cleaving IVF embryos [58]. Establishment of SCNT-IVF chimeric pregnancies and offspring would allow the determination of functional contributions of SCNT embryos to extraembryonic and embryo proper tissues.

Reprogramming of human somatic cells by SCNT

The ability to derive pluripotent cells using patients' cells holds tremendous potential in the understanding, prevention, and treatment of human diseases [61]. Currently, this can be achieved using transcription factor-mediated reprogramming of somatic cells into induced pluripotent stem cells (iPSCs) [62]. Studies on the derivation of human pluripotent cells by SCNT have resulted in early stage human SCNT embryos [63, 64] and more recently SCNT-ESCs [65].

One of the main roadblocks in experimenting with human SCNT has always been the availability of oocytes. This limitation is secondary to financial, regulatory, and ethical constraints surrounding procurement of human oocytes for research. For instance, in the United States, SCNT studies cannot be supported by federal funding because of the Dickey-Wicker Amendment, a bill passed by Congress in 1995. This bill prohibits the Department of Health and Human Services and the National Institutes of Health (NIH) from using appropriated funds for the creation of human embryos for research purposes or for research in which human embryos are destroyed.

Human SCNT studies aimed at deriving ESCs can be legally carried out in the USA using private or certain non-federal funding sources. However, human SCNT research is strictly regulated by local Institutional Review Boards (IRBs) and institutional assurances of compliance with ethical guidelines that have been issued by the US National Academy of Science (NAS), the International Society for Stem Cell Research (ISSCR), and the American Society for Reproductive Medicine (ASRM) [66].

Procurements of human oocytes for research can also depend on local state laws regulating oocyte donor compensation. For example, in California, research oocyte donors may only be reimbursed for out-of-pocket expenses, but cannot be compensated for "time, effort, and inconvenience" [66]. In contrast, in other jurisdictions (New York, Oregon) research oocyte donations can be compensated at the same level as oocyte donation for reproductive purposes [67].

Due to funding and/or ethical restrictions for compensating oocyte donations, several other alternative human oocyte sources for SCNT research have been explored. Particularly, a small number of immature oocytes are recovered and collected during conventional clinical IVF treatments. These oocytes are not suitable for fertilization and are therefore discarded. Since no additional clinical procedures are involved, patients readily donate this material for research. We recently investigated the possibility of rescuing such oocytes by in vitro maturation (IVM) and studied their potential to develop to blastocysts following IVF [68]. Our results suggest that up to 70% of immature human oocytes donated during IVF cycles can be matured and of those more than half can be fertilized. However, their subsequent developmental potential is significantly compromised as only 12% of fertilized embryos reached blastocysts. Given the current status of embryo development following human SCNT [69], we concluded that these compromised, in vitro matured oocytes are not suitable for optimization of SCNT protocols.

Another alternative approach is to recruit altruistic donors (without compensation) who would commit all their eggs for research. However, based on a study conducted at the Harvard University, women typically are not willing to endure ovarian stimulation and egg retrieval procedures without fair compensation [70].

When French and colleagues used premium quality human oocytes for SCNT, 23% of embryos developed to blastocysts [63]. However, derivation of ESCs from these blastocysts was not reported in this study. In contrast, in a more recent study, Noggle and colleagues concluded that even with high quality oocytes, SCNT embryos fail to develop to blastocysts [71]. Blastocysts were only derived when somatic cells were fused to intact, non-enucleated MII oocytes. Such blastocysts subsequently supported isolation of ESCs. These ESCs were partially parthenogenetic, but also contained chromosomes from the somatic cells. The authors speculated that the presence of the oocyte's chromosomes allows retention of molecules critical for reprogramming of the somatic cell nuclei. Apparently, these factors are removed during enucleation, rendering cytoplasts incapable of reprogramming following SCNT. Obviously, this assumption contradicts available SCNT evidence from other species suggesting that the oocyte's nuclear genome is not required for somatic cell nuclear reprogramming. It is more likely that spindle removal and somatic cell nuclear replacement procedures utilized in this particular study were incompatible with normal reprogramming and development. Early failures in development of monkey SCNT embryos were also thought to be linked to the removal of reprogramming factors bound to oocyte chromosomes [72]. However, subsequent studies proved that cytoplasts alone could provide successful reprogramming of primate somatic cells into ESCs [28]. Nonetheless, these studies suggest that each SCNT step must be rigorously tested on human oocytes and protocol optimizations and special adaptations will be required for success with human SCNT. Obviously, this will require a significant number of high quality human oocytes, a resource, as we discussed, that will remain limited.

A cybrid nature of SCNT progeny

One of the hallmarks of SCNT-based reprogramming is that all cloned ESCs and offspring are cybrids, that is, they contain a somatic cell nuclear genome and the oocyte's mitochondrial genome. This fundamental feature is generally under appreciated in understanding the basic mechanisms of oocyte-based reprogramming and the role of cytoplasmic factors responsible for complete reprogramming of somatic cells to totipotency. Is it just a coincidence that oocytes contribute their mitochondrial DNA (mtDNA) during SCNT? Or is it a prerequisite that cloned animals must have the oocyte's mitochondria and mtDNA for complete resetting of the full developmental potency of aged somatic cells?

Mitochondria are essential cytoplasmic organelles primarily responsible for providing most of the cellular energy for viability. Mitochondria possess their own genome (mtDNA) encoding critical components of oxidative phosphorylation (OXPHOS). The mtDNA genetics is markedly different from the nuclear DNA, including exclusively maternal intergenerational inheritance (from the oocyte) and the presence of thousands of mtDNA molecules per cell. It is believed that mtDNA has a very high mutation rate, up to 100-fold higher than nuclear DNA, in part due to the mtDNA's proximity to the mutagenic reactive oxygen species (ROS), the lack of histones, and limited mtDNA repair mechanisms. Mutations in mtDNA occur and accumulate in the somatic cell lineage during aging, and have been linked to many age-related diseases such as Parkinson's disease, cancer, and diabetes [73]. When mutations arise, normal and mutated mtDNA copies coexist within a cell, a state known as heteroplasmy. Often, these two mtDNA types are unevenly distributed to daughter cells during mitosis, resulting in a significant change in heteroplasmy levels. As a consequence, mtDNA type can drift toward homoplasmic mutant or wild type in certain tissues. Even in terminally differentiated post-mitotic cells, mtDNA replication continues, leading to a clonal amplification and change in heteroplasmy levels.

Presence of mutated mtDNA within a cell will further increase ROS production, which in turn induces more mtDNA damage, causing a positive feedback known as "a vicious cycle" [74]. As the proportion of mutant mtDNA reaches a certain threshold, the cell's ability to supply minimum energy for vital function is affected, leading to disease symptoms.

As pointed out above, a progressive decline in mitochondrial function and a gradual accumulation of mtDNA mutations over a lifetime have been linked to many age-related metabolic and degenerative diseases and aging itself [73]. A central role of the mitochondria and mtDNA as an "aging clock" was first proposed more than 30 years ago by Harman [75].

It is believed that the female germ line escapes mitochondrial aging, as offspring do not inherit the mother's somatic mitochondria with its reduced developmental competence. Female germ cells have relatively quiescent mitochondria that mainly rely on the glycolytic energy supply rather than on OXPHOS. It was postulated that oocyte mitochondria and mtDNA thereby evade mutagenesis from ROS, and the mitochondrial genome is preserved and replicated with minimal damage [76].

As pointed out earlier, the mitochondrial complement in cloned offspring or SCNT-ESCs is almost completely replaced by rejuvenated mitochondria and mtDNA derived from oocytes. This is likely one of the crucial components of SCNT-based reprogramming; ensuring that cloned offspring regain normal development and live normal lifespan, irrespective of somatic nuclear donor age.

Technically, a whole somatic cell is fused to a cytoplast, resulting in a small somatic cell/oocyte mtDNA heteroplasmy. However, due to significant copy number differences between somatic cells and MII oocytes (ratio $<$1:100), the donor cell mtDNA is diluted and practically undetectable in offspring [77]. In a few cases, a small contribution of somatic cell mtDNA in SCNT embryos or live offspring has been reported [77]; however, the significance of this phenomenon in survival of cloned offspring remains unknown.

The role of mitochondria and mtDNA in human ESCs is vitally important and the failure of stem cells to possess the full complement of functional mitochondria could limit their differentiation into energy-demanding cell types and diminish their therapeutic potential. This is particularly important for experimental pluripotent stem cells derived from a patient's somatic cells with dysfunctional mitochondria and accumulated mtDNA mutations. It is likely that SCNT offers more suitable reprogramming in such cases since somatic mtDNA is replaced with germline mitochondria. Genetically corrected SCNT-ESCs could also provide more potent and lifelong cell replacement therapies for patients with age-related disorders linked to mitochondrial dysfunctions (Figure 23.3).

Direct reprogramming into iPSCs could serve as a unique model to study the role of aged somatic cell mitochondria. Since mitochondria and mtDNA in

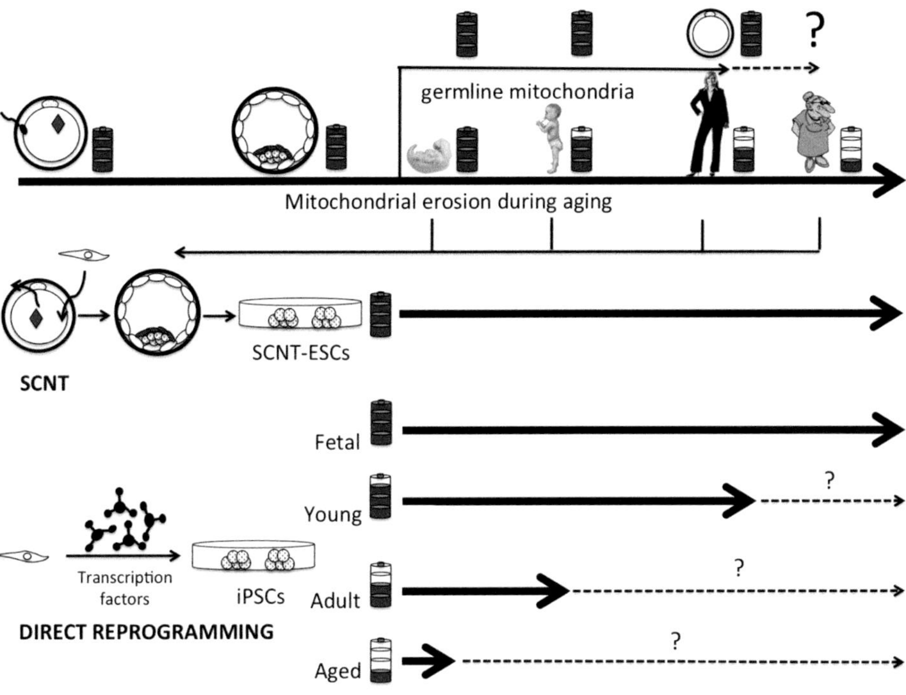

Figure 23.3 Mitochondrial aging during development and reprogramming. Mitochondria and mtDNA are inherited from the female germ line and remain intact during preimplantation embryo development, depicted as a fully charged battery. Upon implantation and differentiation into the somatic lineages, mitochondria turn on OXPHOS to support higher energy needs. This process induces ROS production, which, in turn, will inevitably cause a progressive mitochondrial deterioration and aging (represented by gradual depletion of the battery). However, the female germline lineage is set aside during early embryo development and maintains inactive but integral mitochondria regardless of aging in somatic cells. This ensures that next generation offspring inherit potent mitochondria. During SCNT-based reprogramming, the mitochondrial complement in somatic cells is completely replaced, reinstating full developmental competence regardless of the somatic cell age. In contrast, iPSCs retain dysfunctional mitochondria from aged somatic cells, leading to a compromised ability to differentiate and function. Thus, unlike SCNT-ESCs, the lifespan of iPSCs is limited by their "mitochondrial age."

iPSCs are exclusively derived from parental somatic cells, iPSCs can be derived from somatic cells with known mitochondrial dysfunctions and/or mtDNA mutations. Previous studies revealed that mtDNA mutations in somatic cells do not affect the actual reprogramming process and derivation of iPSCs [78, 79]. This is a somewhat expected outcome, since pluripotent cells rely little on aerobic mitochondrial OXPHOS. However, the effect of impaired mitochondria should be apparent upon in vitro or in vivo differentiation, once these cells acquire phenotypes with higher energy demands, which can be only resolved by mitochondrial respiration (Figure 23.3).

Mouse models could be particularly useful for studying the role of mitochondria, since we can derive live chimeric offspring using iPSCs. Specifically, the tetraploid complementation approach enables production of whole iPSC-derived mouse offspring. So far, available evidence suggests that mouse iPSCs from fetal fibroblasts or early postnatal parental cells with relatively young and unaffected mitochondria can support normal development of tetraploid chimeras [80–84]. However, questions remain as to whether iPSCs from aged and diseased tissues are developmentally competent to produce normal offspring.

Concluding remarks

The SCNT approach provides numerous biomedical applications in NHPs including generation of gene-targeted offspring and means to study early primate development and totipotency. In addition, SCNT offers the potential to discover mechanisms of oocyte-based reprogramming, including the role of mitochondria and mtDNA. Human SCNT-derived ESCs from patients with dysfunctional mitochondria would carry genetically corrected mtDNA, signifying the need to continue these studies.

References

1. Egli D, Chen AE, Saphier G, *et al.* Reprogramming within hours following nuclear transfer into mouse but not human zygotes. *Nat Commun* 2011; **2**: 488.
2. Spemann H, Mangold H. Induction of embryonic primordia by implantation of organizers from a different species. 1923. *Int J Dev Biol* 2001; **45**: 13–38.
3. Briggs R, King TJ. Transplantation of living nuclei from blastula cells into enucleated frogs' eggs. *Proc Natl Acad Sci USA* 1952; **38**: 455–63.
4. Gurdon JB. Adult frogs derived from the nuclei of single somatic cells. *Dev Biol* 1962; **4**: 256–73.
5. McGrath J, Solter D. Inability of mouse blastomere nuclei transferred to enucleated zygotes to support development in vitro. *Science* 1984; **226**: 1317–19.
6. Prather RS, Sims MM, First NL. Nuclear transplantation in early pig embryos. *Biol Reprod* 1989; **41**: 414–18.
7. Willadsen SM. Nuclear transplantation in sheep embryos. *Nature* 1986; **320**: 63–5.
8. Wilmut I, Schnieke AE, McWhir J, *et al.* Viable offspring derived from fetal and adult mammalian cells. *Nature* 1997; **385**: 810–13.
9. Cibelli JB, Stice SL, Golueke PJ, *et al.* Cloned transgenic calves produced from nonquiescent fetal fibroblasts. *Science* 1998; **280**: 1256–8.
10. Kato Y, Tani T, Sotomaru Y, *et al.* Eight calves cloned from somatic cells of a single adult. *Science* 1998; **282**: 2095–8.
11. Wakayama T, Perry AC, Zuccotti M, *et al.* Full-term development of mice from enucleated oocytes injected with cumulus cell nuclei. *Nature* 1998; **394**: 369–74.
12. Wakayama T, Tabar V, Rodriguez I, *et al.* Differentiation of embryonic stem cell lines generated from adult somatic cells by nuclear transfer. *Science* 2001; **292**: 740–3.
13. Baguisi A, Behboodi E, Melican DT, *et al.* Production of goats by somatic cell nuclear transfer. *Nat Biotechnol* 1999; **17**: 456–61.
14. Polejaeva IA, Chen SH, Vaught TD, *et al.* Cloned pigs produced by nuclear transfer from adult somatic cells. *Nature* 2000; **407**: 86–90.
15. Lanza RP, Cibelli JB, Moraes CT, *et al.* Cloning of an endangered species (*Bos gaurus*) using interspecies nuclear transfer. *Cloning* 2000; **2**: 79–90.
16. Loi P, Ptak G, Barboni B, *et al.* Genetic rescue of an endangered mammal by cross-species nuclear transfer using post-mortem somatic cells. *Nat Biotechnol* 2001; **19**: 962–4.
17. Shin T, Kraemer D, Pryor J, *et al.* A cat cloned by nuclear transplantation. *Nature* 2002; **415**: 859.
18. Chesne P, Adenot PG, Viglietta C, *et al.* Cloned rabbits produced by nuclear transfer from adult somatic cells. *Nat Biotechnol* 2002; **20**: 366–9.
19. BBC. Endangered animal clone produced. http://news.bbc.co.uk/2/hi/science/nature/2932225.stm, 2003 (accessed May 9, 2013).
20. Zhou Q, Renard JP, Le Friec G, *et al.* Generation of fertile cloned rats by regulating oocyte activation. *Science* 2003; **302**: 1179.
21. Woods GL, White KL, Vanderwall DK, *et al.* A mule cloned from fetal cells by nuclear transfer. *Science* 2003; **301**: 1063.
22. Galli C, Lagutina I, Crotti G, *et al.* Pregnancy: a cloned horse born to its dam twin. *Nature* 2003; **424**: 635.
23. Boyle A. White-tailed deer joins the clone parade. http://www.nbcnews.com/id/3785448/ns/health-cloning/t/white-tailed-deer-joins-clone-parade/#.UYu9SVT8SFo, 2003 (accessed May 9, 2013).
24. Lee BC, Kim MK, Jang G, *et al.* Dogs cloned from adult somatic cells. *Nature* 2005; **436**: 641.
25. Li Z, Sun X, Chen J, *et al.* Cloned ferrets produced by somatic cell nuclear transfer. *Dev Biol* 2006; **293**: 439–48.
26. Shi D, Wei F, Cui K, *et al.* Buffalos (*Bubalus bubalis*) cloned by nuclear transfer of somatic cells. *Biol Reprod* 2007; **77**: 285–91.
27. Kim MK, Jang G, Oh HJ, *et al.* Endangered wolves cloned from adult somatic cells. *Cloning Stem Cells* 2007; **9**: 130–7.
28. Byrne JA, Pedersen DA, Clepper LL, *et al.* Producing primate embryonic stem cells by somatic cell nuclear transfer. *Nature* 2007; **450**: 497–502.
29. Wani NA, Wernery U, Hassan FA, *et al.* Production of the first cloned camel by somatic cell nuclear transfer. *Biol Reprod* 2010; **82**: 373–9.
30. Thuan NV, Kishigami S, Wakayama T. How to improve the success rate of mouse cloning technology. *J Reprod Dev* 2010; **56**: 20–30.
31. Inoue K, Wakao H, Ogonuki N, *et al.* Generation of cloned mice by direct nuclear transfer from natural killer T cells. *Curr Biol* 2005; **15**: 1114–18.
32. Green AL, Wells DN, Oback B. Cattle cloned from increasingly differentiated muscle cells. *Biol Reprod* 2007; **77**: 395–406.
33. Sung LY, Gao S, Shen H, *et al.* Differentiated cells are more efficient than adult stem cells for cloning by somatic cell nuclear transfer. *Nat Genet* 2006; **38**: 1323–8.
34. Eggan K, Baldwin K, Tackett M, *et al.* Mice cloned from olfactory sensory neurons. *Nature* 2004; **428**: 44–9.

35. Kishigami S, Wakayama S, van Thuan N, *et al.* Cloned mice and embryonic stem cell establishment from adult somatic cells. *Hum Cell* 2006; **19**: 2–10.

36. Wakayama T. Production of cloned mice and ES cells from adult somatic cells by nuclear transfer: how to improve cloning efficiency? *J Reprod Dev* 2007; **53**: 13–26.

37. Egli D, Sandler VM, Shinohara ML, *et al.* Reprogramming after chromosome transfer into mouse blastomeres. *Curr Biol* 2009; **19**: 1403–9.

38. Riaz A, Zhao X, Dai X, *et al.* Mouse cloning and somatic cell reprogramming using electrofused blastomeres. *Cell Res* 2011; **21**: 770–8.

39. Oback B, Wells DN. Donor cell differentiation, reprogramming, and cloning efficiency: elusive or illusive correlation? *Mol Reprod Dev* 2007; **74**: 646–54.

40. Cibelli JB, Campbell KH, Seidel GE, *et al.* The health profile of cloned animals. *Nat Biotechnol* 2002; **20**: 13–14.

41. Wakayama S, Wakayama T. Improvement of mouse cloning using nuclear transfer-derived embryonic stem cells and/or histone deacetylase inhibitor. *Int J Dev Biol* 2010; **54**: 1641–8.

42. Dean W, Santos F, Stojkovic M, *et al.* Conservation of methylation reprogramming in mammalian development: aberrant reprogramming in cloned embryos. *Proc Natl Acad Sci USA* 2001; **98**: 13734–8.

43. Kishigami S, Mizutani E, Ohta H, *et al.* Significant improvement of mouse cloning technique by treatment with trichostatin A after somatic nuclear transfer. *Biochem Biophys Res Commun* 2006; **340**: 183–9.

44. Moreira PN, Robl JM, Collas P. Architectural defects in pronuclei of mouse nuclear transplant embryos. *J Cell Sci* 2003; **116**: 3713–20.

45. Dai X, Hao J, Hou XJ, *et al.* Somatic nucleus reprogramming is significantly improved by *m*-carboxycinnamic acid bishydroxamide, a histone deacetylase inhibitor. *J Biol Chem* 2010; **285**: 31002–10.

46. Ono T, Li C, Mizutani E, *et al.* Inhibition of class IIb histone deacetylase significantly improves cloning efficiency in mice. *Biol Reprod* 2010; **83**: 929–37.

47. Zhao J, Ross JW, Hao Y, *et al.* Significant improvement in cloning efficiency of an inbred miniature pig by histone deacetylase inhibitor treatment after somatic cell nuclear transfer. *Biol Reprod* 2009; **81**: 525–30.

48. Sparman ML, Tachibana M, Mitalipov SM. Cloning of non-human primates: the road "less traveled by". *Int J Dev Biol* 2010; **54**: 1671–8.

49. Matoba S, Inoue K, Kohda T, *et al.* RNAi-mediated knockdown of Xist can rescue the impaired postimplantation development of cloned mouse embryos. *Proc Natl Acad Sci USA* 2011; **108**: 20621–6.

50. Mitalipov SM, Zhou Q, Byrne JA, *et al.* Reprogramming following somatic cell nuclear transfer in primates is dependent upon nuclear remodeling. *Hum Reprod* 2007; **22**: 2232–42.

51. Tachibana M, Sparman M, Sritanaudomchai H, *et al.* Mitochondrial gene replacement in primate offspring and embryonic stem cells. *Nature* 2009; **461**: 367–72.

52. Campbell KH, McWhir J, Ritchie WA, *et al.* Sheep cloned by nuclear transfer from a cultured cell line. *Nature* 1996; **380**: 64–6.

53. Fulka J Jr., Notarianni E, Passoni L, *et al.* Early changes in embryonic nuclei fused to chemically enucleated mouse oocytes. *Int J Dev Biol* 1993; **37**: 433–9.

54. Susko-Parrish JL, Leibfried-Rutledge ML, Northey DL, *et al.* Inhibition of protein kinases after an induced calcium transient causes transition of bovine oocytes to embryonic cycles without meiotic completion. *Dev Biol* 1994; **166**: 729–39.

55. Alberio R, Zakhartchenko V, Motlik J, *et al.* Mammalian oocyte activation: lessons from the sperm and implications for nuclear transfer. *Int J Dev Biol* 2001; **45**: 797–809.

56. Nagai T. Parthenogenetic activation of cattle follicular oocytes in vitro with ethanol. *Gamete Res* 1987; **16**: 243–9.

57. Campbell KH, Alberio R, Choi I, *et al.* Cloning: eight years after Dolly. *Reprod Domest Anim* 2005; **40**: 256–68.

58. Tachibana M, Sparman M, Ramsey C, *et al.* Generation of chimeric rhesus monkeys. *Cell* 2012; **148**: 285–95.

59. Wang W, Yang J, Liu H, *et al.* Rapid and efficient reprogramming of somatic cells to induced pluripotent stem cells by retinoic acid receptor gamma and liver receptor homolog 1. *Proc Natl Acad Sci USA* 2011; **108**: 18283–8.

60. Sparman M, Dighe V, Sritanaudomchai H, *et al.* Epigenetic reprogramming by somatic cell nuclear transfer in primates. *Stem Cells* 2009; **27**: 1255–64.

61. Drukker M, Benvenisty N. The immunogenicity of human embryonic stem-derived cells. *Trends Biotechnol* 2004; **22**: 136–41.

62. Takahashi K, Tanabe K, Ohnuki M, *et al.* Induction of pluripotent stem cells from adult human fibroblasts by defined factors. *Cell* 2007; **131**: 861–72.

63. French AJ, Adams CA, Anderson LS, *et al.* Development of human cloned blastocysts following somatic cell nuclear transfer with adult fibroblasts. *Stem Cells* 2008; **26**: 485–93.

64. Li J, Liu X, Wang H, *et al.* Human embryos derived by somatic cell nuclear transfer using an alternative

enucleation approach. *Cloning Stem Cells* 2009; **11**: 39–50.

65. Tachibana M, Amato P, Sparman M, *et al.* Human embryonic stem cells derived by somatic cell nuclear transfer. *Cell* 2013; **153**: 1228–38.
66. Hyun I. Moving human SCNT research forward ethically. *Cell Stem Cell* 2011; **9**: 295–7.
67. Zacher A. Oocyte donor compensation for embryonic stem cell research: an analysis of New York's "payment for eggs program". *Albany Law School Journal* 2010; **21**(2): 323–58.
68. Tachibana M, Sparman M, Woodward J, *et al.* Derivation of human embryonic stem cells from discarded immature oocytes. International Society for Stem Cell Research (ISSCR), 10th Annual Meeting, June 13–16, 2012, Yokohama, Japan.
69. Heindryckx B, De Sutter P, Gerris J, *et al.* Embryo development after successful somatic cell nuclear transfer to in vitro matured human germinal vesicle oocytes. *Hum Reprod* 2007; **22**: 1982–90.
70. Egli D, Chen AE, Saphier G, *et al.* Impracticality of egg donor recruitment in the absence of compensation. *Cell Stem Cell* 2011; **9**: 293–4.
71. Noggle S, Fung HL, Gore A, *et al.* Human oocytes reprogram somatic cells to a pluripotent state. *Nature* 2011; **478**: 70–5.
72. Simerly C, Dominko T, Navara C, *et al.* Molecular correlates of primate nuclear transfer failures. *Science* 2003; **300**: 297
73. Wallace DC. A mitochondrial paradigm of metabolic and degenerative diseases, aging, and cancer: a dawn for evolutionary medicine. *Annu Rev Genet* 2005; **39**: 359–407.
74. Wallace DC. Mitochondrial diseases in man and mouse. *Science* 1999; **283**: 1482–8.
75. Harman D. The biologic clock: the mitochondria? *J Am Geriatr Soc* 1972; **20**: 145–7.
76. Allen JF. Separate sexes and the mitochondrial theory of ageing. *J Theor Biol* 1996; **180**: 135–40.
77. St John JC, Facucho-Oliveira J, Jiang Y, *et al.* Mitochondrial DNA transmission, replication and inheritance: a journey from the gamete through the embryo and into offspring and embryonic stem cells. *Hum Reprod Update* 2010; **16**: 488–509.
78. Prigione A, Fauler B, Lurz R, *et al.* The senescence-related mitochondrial/oxidative stress pathway is repressed in human induced pluripotent stem cells. *Stem Cells* 2010; **28**: 721–33.
79. Prigione A, Lichtner B, Kuhl H, *et al.* Human induced pluripotent stem cells harbor homoplasmic and heteroplasmic mitochondrial DNA mutations while maintaining human embryonic stem cell-like metabolic reprogramming. *Stem Cells* 2011; **29**: 1338–48.
80. Boland MJ, Hazen JL, Nazor KL, *et al.* Adult mice generated from induced pluripotent stem cells. *Nature* 2009; **461**: 91–4.
81. Kang L, Wu T, Tao Y, *et al.* Viable mice produced from three-factor induced pluripotent stem (iPS) cells through tetraploid complementation. *Cell Res* 2011; **21**: 546–9.
82. Wu G, Liu N, Rittelmeyer I, *et al.* Generation of healthy mice from gene-corrected disease-specific induced pluripotent stem cells. *PLoS Biol* 2011; **9**: e1001099.
83. Zhao XY, Li W, Lv Z, *et al.* iPS cells produce viable mice through tetraploid complementation. *Nature* 2009; 461: 86–90.
84. Zhao XY, Li W, Lv Z, *et al.* Viable fertile mice generated from fully pluripotent iPS cells derived from adult somatic cells. *Stem Cell Rev* 2010; **6**: 390–7.

Section 5 Pathology

Chapter 24

Gene expression in human oocytes

Gayle M. Jones and David S. Cram

Introduction

Early embryonic development of the human oocyte, as for the oocytes of all mammalian species, is under the control of the maternally inherited genome. It is not until the 4- to 8-cell stage of development in the human that the maternal genome is fully replaced by a transcriptionally active embryonic genome [1]. The maternal transcripts that control the events of mammalian oocyte growth, meiotic maturation, fertilization, and early embryonic development are transcribed and accumulated during oogenesis.

Transcription in primary human oocytes begins at a relatively high level during fetal life with levels falling in leptotene and zygotene and falling further, to almost undetectable levels, by early pachytene [2]. Transcription levels then rise again through mid-pachytene returning to levels similar to those observed in oogonia by the early diplotene stage [2]. Studies in the mouse suggest that transcription levels remain active, but low, in the mammalian oocytes in the resting pool within the ovary but increase significantly and dramatically when the oocyte enters the growth phase, peaking at the time that maximal oocyte diameter is attained and then falling from this point to very low levels a few hours before ovulation (Figure 24.1) [3–5]. During the growth phase there is no significant difference in the rates of accumulation of rRNA, tRNA, polyadenylated RNA, or specific mRNAs [6–8].

Messenger RNA is very stable and accumulates as a relatively constant proportion of total RNA with turnover of only the translated fraction [6, 9]. The stored message accumulated in the growth phase in the human oocyte must be progressively recruited and translated for the events of meiotic maturation, fertilization, and the first few embryonic cleavage divisions in a temporally sensitive and coordinated manner. Much of the stored message must therefore remain stable for a long period of time as it takes the human oocyte 80–90 days to complete the growth phase and meiotic maturation [10].

In order for the transcribed message to remain stable for long periods of time, the message undergoes post-transcriptional modifications, the most studied of which, in the oocyte, is the balance of polyadenylation and deadenylation. The length of the poly(A) tail at the 3′ end of the transcript is one of the most important regulators of transcript stability. Following transcription in the nucleus of mammalian cells, a 250–300 poly(A) tail is added to the 3′ end of the transcript prior to transport to the cytoplasm. Transport to the cytoplasm is associated with a characteristic shortening of the poly(A) tail. The majority of transcripts with a short poly(A) tail are not translated unless readenylated and poly(A) tail deletion is a prelude to mRNA degradation. In contrast, transcripts with a long poly(A) tail are destined for translation but further translational control can be achieved by 5′ end capping or the action of specific translational repressors (reviewed in [11, 12]).

According to mouse model studies, two major classes of mRNA have been described in the immature fully grown mammalian oocyte. The first class of mRNAs has a short poly(A) tail and is not available for translation in the immature oocyte but following polyadenylation during meiosis these messages are translated [13, 14]. The second class of mRNAs has a long poly(A) tail and these transcripts are actively translated in the immature oocyte. These transcripts follow a default pathway, becoming progressively more deadenylated and are either degraded or remain stable within the oocyte until readenylated when required

Biology and Pathology of the Oocyte, 2nd edn., ed. Alan Trounson, Roger Gosden, and Ursula Eichenlaub-Ritter.
Published by Cambridge University Press.

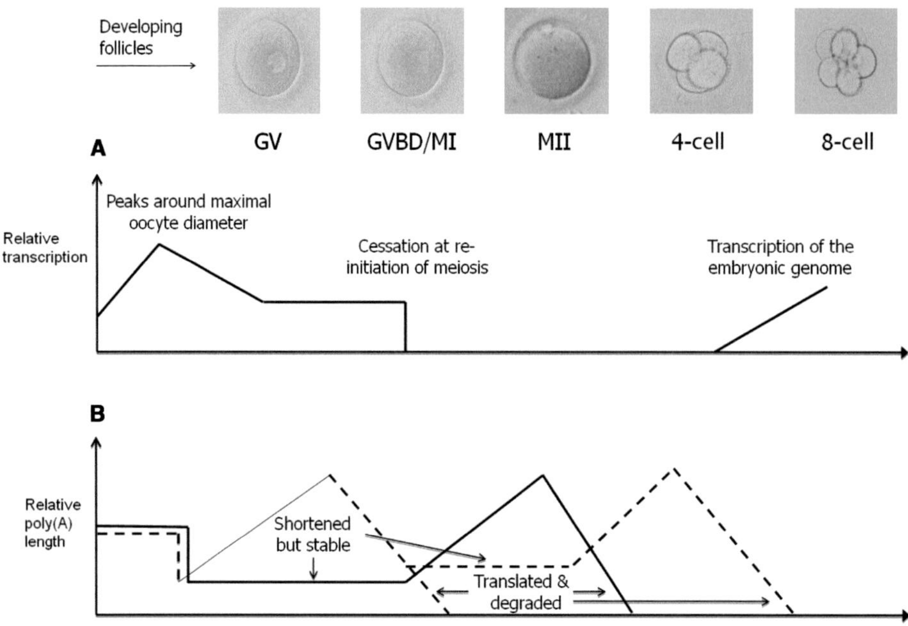

Figure 24.1 Cartoon of (A) relative transcription levels and (B) relative poly(A) length during early preimplantation development. Two different classes of mRNAs exist in the oocyte: the first class has a short poly(A) tail and is readenylated during meiosis and is translated and subsequently degraded (solid line); the second class has a long poly(A) tail and these transcripts are actively translated in the immature oocyte and then the transcripts follow a default pathway, becoming progressively more deadenylated and are either degraded or remain stable within the oocyte until readenylated when required at a later developmental stage (dotted line). GV, germinal vesicle; GVBD, germinal vesicle breakdown; MI, metaphase I; MII, metaphase II.

at a later developmental stage [13, 14] (Figure 24.1). Once the oocyte has attained full size, 18–20% of the accumulated RNA is polyadenylated, in contrast to somatic cells where only 1–2% of RNA is polyadenylated [15]. Following maturation, the percentage of polyadenylated RNA is halved, suggesting either deadenylation or degradation of half of the accumulated maternal mRNAs [7]. Destruction of transcripts following oocyte maturation is a selective process with the majority of the degraded transcripts being required to maintain meiotic arrest at the germinal vesicle (GV) stage and for progression of oocyte maturation [16]. Gene transcripts involved in oxidative phosphorylation, pyruvate metabolism, and the citrate cycle and those involved in protein synthesis and metabolism have been demonstrated to be degraded following maturation in the mouse oocyte whereas gene transcripts involved in signaling pathways, particularly the ERK/MAPK (mitogen-activated protein kinase) and phosphatidylinositol 3-kinase (PI3K)/AKT signaling pathways, important to the maintenance of metaphase II (MII) arrest, are maintained in a stable form [16].

Gene expression in the human oocyte

Due to the relatively limited availability of human oocytes for experimental purposes the detailed study of individual genes and their temporal expression patterns throughout development is lacking. Studies in laboratory and domestic animal species have revealed that some genes, such as those involved in the formation of the zona pellucida, are only synthesized and utilized during the life of the oocyte [17, 18], whereas the majority of genes transcribed during the growth phase are temporally translated and utilized during development [19]. Human oocytes that fail to complete the growth phase or grow in a pathological environment that could affect the accumulation and regulation of transcripts required for ongoing development would be expected to exhibit developmental delays or complete failure in progression through preimplantation development following fertilization [20].

A fully grown human GV stage oocyte has been estimated to contain approximately 100 pg poly(A) mRNA [21]. Early attempts to analyze gene expression in human oocytes utilized RT-PCR [22–24] or differential display [25] to identify only a few select genes. This was then followed by serial expression gene analysis (SAGE) [21, 26] and the creation of cDNA libraries, allowing the sequencing of SAGE tags and expressed sequence tags (ESTs) to gain a more comprehensive expression profile of human oocytes. These efforts have confirmed many of the qualitative and quantitative gene expression findings for the oocytes of other mammalian species as well as identifying oocyte-specific genes and a large number of known genes that were previously undocumented in oocytes. Interestingly, through the analysis and sequencing of oocyte cDNA libraries, in addition to genes, many retrotransposable elements have also been identified and appear to be abundantly expressed in the human oocyte [25, 27]. Recent advances in molecular biology such as highly sensitive RNA amplification systems and innovative microarray platforms now provide the opportunity to study mRNA and microRNA (miRNA) expression at a more global level in human oocytes that are available for research but are in short supply.

Determining global gene expression profiles of oocytes by microarray requires the pooling of a very large number of oocytes or an amplification step that does not significantly bias the true relative levels of mRNA expressed by the oocyte. Furthermore, it is important that the specific biological question to be answered is addressed in the design of the microarray experiment. For instance, failed fertilized oocytes should not be used to represent the mature MII oocyte as the prolonged in vitro culture alters both qualitative and quantitative gene expression profiles ([28], G. Jones and D. Cram, unpublished observations, 2003). In addition, amplification bias operates when only a small amount of RNA is present such as in single human oocytes [29]. Due to the variability in polyadenylation of transcripts in the GV and MII oocyte it has been recommended that both internal and 3′ poly(A) priming, rather than the usually adopted 3′ poly(A) priming, be used to amplify RNA prior to hybridization when making a comparison of gene expression between these two developmental stages in order to minimize any impact of variations in adenylation [16]. There is a significant degree of variability in gene expression particularly in MII oocytes, even from the same individual, and this may reflect differences in the progress of degradation of transcripts that follows maturation. For this reason caution is advised in interpreting any molecular profile using single oocytes, particularly if representative of pathological development.

Pathological gene expression in the human oocyte

Microarrays permit the profiling of global gene expression and relative quantitation of transcripts at any particular time in development. The first gene expression profile for human oocytes using microarray technology was reported by Bermúdez *et al.* [30]. They demonstrated that linear RNA amplification techniques could produce sufficient cRNA from a single failed fertilized MII oocyte to hybridize to a focused microarray representing 8793 expressed human sequences. The study identified 1361 transcripts that were consistently expressed by four single oocytes and two pools of five oocytes, of which 406 (30%) genes had previously been identified by conventional techniques to be expressed in the oocyte. Conversely, there were 7432 transcripts that were not expressed in any sample. There was a significant difference in the number of transcripts detected when pooled material was compared with single oocytes, which the authors interpreted as being a result of increased genetic complexity, as the pools of oocytes were obtained from several different patients. An alternate explanation is that there is an amplification bias when low template RNA is used as the starting material, which was demonstrated clearly by Jones *et al.* [29], who pooled 40 oocytes and then divided the lysis aliquot prior to amplification for micro-array hybridization into volume equivalents of single, 3, 5, 10, and 20 oocytes. The microarray results and principal components analysis showed a clear disparity in expression between the two single oocytes and the profile generated by pooled samples with little relative difference in expression between the volume equivalent pools of 5, 10, and 20 oocytes. There are no published data to suggest that other amplification and microarray methodologies are not similarly limited.

Several groups have since used microarrays to profile the transcriptome of the human oocyte [31–37]. Although much of the information is useful and concurs with previous findings in the oocytes of human and laboratory animal species, interpretation of gene expression patterns is nonetheless limited. Many of the studies have relied upon information derived from oocytes aged in vitro, that is, oocytes that failed to fertilize [30–32, 35], which are not representative of the fresh MII oocyte (G. Jones and D. Cram, unpublished observations, 2003). Others have utilized microarrays with only a limited coverage of the human transcriptome, which reveals only a portion of the global gene expression [30, 31, 34]. Importantly, for comparative microarray studies, sufficient biological replication is required to produce statistically meaningful results and this has not been performed in all published studies of the oocyte transcriptome [30–32, 34–37]. Furthermore, the majority of the studies of the oocyte transcriptome in the medical literature report on an isolated developmental stage and make comparisons to unrelated, or loosely related, biological material such as preimplantation embryos [31, 34, 37], cumulus cells [32], somatic tissues, and embryonic stem cells [33, 36] and as such, it is difficult to derive meaningful data about the true gene expression profile of a normal, developmentally competent human oocyte.

A recent study examined the gene expression profile of a single developmental stage (oocytes from primordial and primary follicles) and identified that the number of genes expressed was not dissimilar to the numbers expressed in mature MII oocytes [38]. There was, however, very high expression of three genes, *TMEFF2*, *ATPase6,* and *OPHNI*. The gene *TMEFF2* encodes a protein with both epidermal growth factor (EGF)-like and follistatin-like domains and is therefore likely to play an important role in early folliculogenesis [38]. Mutations in the gene *ATPase6* have recently been identified to be associated with primary ovarian insufficiency (POI) [39]. The gene *OPHNI* encodes a RHO-GTPase-activating protein and has not previously been identified with female reproduction [38]. This is the first time the gene expression of oocytes from an early developmental stage has been studied in the absence of the associated follicular cells and therefore forms an important reference sample for later stages of oocyte development. No comparison, however, was made to later stages of development so conclusions about genes essential to this stage of development only are limited.

The following sections introduce studies that have been conducted comparing the transcriptome of human oocytes derived from contrasting developmental or biological backgrounds and where the interpretation of the data presented is, in most instances, not limited by the experimental design.

In vivo versus in vitro maturation

The majority of oocytes recovered from infertile women following superovulation are mature MII oocytes and 70–80% of these are capable of fertilization, with approximately 50% of zygotes able to complete development to the blastocyst stage [40]. Approximately 35% of transferred embryos/blastocysts derived from these oocytes develop to term [41]. In contrast, when immature oocytes are recovered following superovulation and are matured in vitro, only 12% of the resulting zygotes develop to the blastocyst stage [42] and only 14% of these embryos when transferred develop to term [42–48], with the majority of these arising from in vitro maturation of partly mature metaphase I (MI) oocytes rather than the completely immature germinal vesicle (GV) stage oocyte. Furthermore, the majority of the pregnancies have been isolated case reports, resulting in under-reporting and a consequent artificial inflation of the actual competence of oocytes that are matured in vitro following superovulation ("rescue" in vitro maturation; rIVM).

Jones *et al.* [20] compared the gene expression profiles of oocytes with relatively high developmental competence (MII oocytes recovered following superovulation, that is, in vivo matured oocytes) to oocytes with very low developmental competence (rIVM of GV stage oocytes recovered following superovulation) in an attempt to identify a molecular basis for the significant difference in developmental competence between these two groups of oocytes.

Pools of five human oocytes were utilized for microarray profiling of each of the developmental groups recovered fresh from superovulated cycles: GV, MI, and MII oocytes [20]. In addition some GV oocytes were matured in vitro utilizing gonadotropin-supplemented medium and the resultant MII oocytes were pooled in groups of five for microarray profiling of rIVM oocytes. The number of genes routinely detected in human immature, GV and MI oocytes (10 962 and 12 329 genes, respectively) was significantly higher than the number of genes routinely detected in mature human oocytes regardless of the maturation conditions (7546 genes in in vivo matured oocytes compared to 9479 genes in rIVM oocytes) [20], which reflects the consistent findings of a selective reduction in the genes expressed during maturation of oocytes from laboratory and domestic animal species [16]. In addition, more than 2000 genes were identified as expressed at more than twofold higher levels in oocytes matured in vitro than those matured in vivo, with 162 of these genes expressed at tenfold or greater levels [20]. Many of the genes expressed at higher levels in rIVM oocytes are involved in transcription, the cell cycle, and its regulation, transport, and cellular protein metabolism [20].

It could be argued that the observed pathology in gene expression in oocytes matured in vitro originates in the GV oocyte that, for unknown reasons, has failed to mature in vivo despite exposure to the ovulatory dose of human chorionic gonadotropin (hCG), that is, a pre-existing pathology. A study by Zheng *et al.* demonstrated that GV oocytes recovered from the monkey following follicle-stimulating hormone (FSH)/hCG stimulation (hCG; high developmental competence), FSH alone (FSH; moderate developmental competence), or no hormonal stimulation (NS; low developmental competence) showed remarkably little difference in the expression levels of 23 maternal mRNAs that were selected on the basis of high expression levels in oocytes and preimplantation embryos [19]. What this study did show, however, was that these selected genes were expressed at significantly higher levels in oocytes matured in vitro than in oocytes matured in vivo, which is similar to the findings of Jones *et al.* [20] in the human, and suggests that the dysregulation in gene expression and mRNA homeostasis occurs during maturation and does not arise in the GV oocyte. FSH (from superovulated ovulatory cycles) oocytes and embryos showed a less severe alteration in gene expression than NS (non-stimulated ovulatory cycles) oocytes and embryos when compared to hCG (oocytes induced to mature by human chorionic gonadotropin injection) oocytes and embryos [19]. For most of the genes examined in oocytes with low developmental competence there was an overabundance initially in the metaphase II oocyte but this pattern was reversed with a substantial reduction in relative gene expression by the 2-cell stage [19]. For genes known to be required later in preimplantation development there was parity in expression at the oocyte stage with a significant increase in relative expression levels by the pronucleate stage of development, indicating that these genes were precociously up-regulated [19]. In most countries it is not ethically permissible to generate human embryos for the purpose of research so it is unlikely that these observations will be directly confirmed in the human. Zheng *et al.* suggested that the reduced developmental competence of non-human primate oocytes matured in vitro was a result of a failure of these oocytes to undergo the normal pattern of transcript silencing [19]. Jones *et al.* similarly proposed a failure in the normal post-transcriptional regulatory processes as an explanation for the relatively poor developmental competence of human oocytes matured in vitro [20].

"Rescue" IVM oocytes, unlike their in vivo matured counterparts, are matured in the absence of associated follicular cells. It is clear, from a vast number of publications, that the oocyte and its surrounding follicular cells undergo molecular "crosstalk" during development (reviewed in [49]). Although many important molecules have been identified that affect differentiation of either the oocyte or the associated follicular cells, it remains unclear whether the cumulus cell plays any direct role in transcriptional or post-transcriptional regulatory processes within the oocyte. A class of small silencing RNAs (ssRNAs), including small interfering RNAs (siRNAs or endo-siRNAs), Piwi-interacting RNAs (piRNAs), and miRNAs, has been implicated in the elimination of maternal transcripts [49–51] and it is certainly possible that some of these ssRNAs could be provided to the oocyte via the gap junctions between cumulus cells and the oocyte [52]. The relative amount of mRNA may not vary during oocyte growth but the amount of single miRNAs varies dynamically during oocyte growth [53]. When miRNAs have been transcribed they are translocated to the cytoplasm, processed by Dicer (an RNase III-like enzyme), and the resulting mature silencing form of the miRNA binds to the Argonaute protein to form an RNA-induced silencing protein (RISC) that binds to complementary RNAs and results in their degradation [49]. Dicer knockout mutant mouse oocytes show more than a 1.5-fold increase in expression levels for one-third of expressed genes compared to normal oocytes, supporting the important role miRNAs have in post-transcriptional regulation of gene expression [53]. Xu *et al.* reported that only 2% of miRNAs show differential expression in human oocytes from the GV stage to the MII stage following rIVM, that is, in the absence of follicular cells [54]. Comparative analysis of miRNA expression in oocytes matured in vivo versus in vitro has not been performed for the human to date; therefore, a definitive conclusion as to the role that supporting follicular cells play in influencing miRNA expression in the maturing oocyte cannot be made.

An explanation for the transcript abundance observed in human oocytes matured in vitro may be a failure of the default deadenylation pathway that usually occurs in oocytes matured in vivo and this would lead to precocious translation and subsequent degradation of transcripts that may be required downstream in development, resulting in the, often observed, delays or failure in progression of embryo development from rIVM oocytes. To this end, G. Jones and D. Cram (unpublished observations, 2008) selected several genes involved in the cell cycle and its regulation for studies of poly(A) tail length determination in GV, rIVM, and in vivo matured oocytes. Four genes, *BUB1B, CENPE, MAD2L1,* and *AURKA,* were expressed at more than fivefold higher levels in comparative microarrays of rIVM versus in vivo matured oocytes, whereas two genes, *CCNK* and *AURKB,* showed no significant difference in expression. Three of the four genes, *BUB1B, CENPE,* and *MAD2L1,* determined to be expressed at higher levels in rIVM oocytes also showed a significantly longer mean poly(A) tail length than for in vivo matured oocytes or GV oocytes (Figure 24.2) indicating that polyadenylation of these genes had occurred during in vitro maturation. The fourth gene, *AURKA,* showed a significantly longer poly(A) tail length than for in vivo matured oocytes but there was no significant difference in length compared to GV oocytes (Figure 24.2) indicating that this gene is normally deadenylated when maturation occurs in vivo and this does not occur when maturation occurs in vitro. The two genes, *CCNK* and *AURKB,* that were demonstrated to show no significant difference in expression levels in rIVM oocytes compared to in vivo matured oocytes, did not show a significant difference in poly(A) tail length in mature oocytes regardless of the maturation conditions (Figure 24.2). GV oocytes, however, showed a significantly longer poly(A) tail length for *CCNK* and *AURKB* than mature oocytes independent of the maturation conditions, indicating that these are examples of genes that undergo default deadenylation following maturation (Figure 24.2). Taken together, these data demonstrate a significant dysregulation in adenylation/deadenylation of transcripts in rIVM oocytes that would have an impact on the temporal utilization of affected genes and may provide an explanation as to the severe reduction in developmental competence observed for embryos derived from rIVM oocytes.

Fertilization failure

The maturation and developmental potential of oocytes is prescribed by the maternal message accumulated prior to the initiation of maturation. The maternal message is responsible for all events from maturation to the activation of the embryonic genome at the 4- to 8-cell stage and includes the processes associated with fertilization. Gasca *et al.* compared the microarray expression profile of a single pool of failed fertilized oocytes from a patient that had presented with total fertilization failure (TFF) following both IVF and ICSI using sperm with normal parameters to two pools of failed fertilized oocytes harvested from patients that had achieved better than 60% fertilization in their remaining cohort of oocytes (controls) [55]. The TFF oocytes showed higher RNA content than control oocytes and large sets of genes that showed aberrant expression, the majority of which were over- rather than under-expressed. The majority of the more than 1000 genes uniquely expressed in TFF compared to control oocytes were also found to be expressed in immature human oocytes [55]. The genes whose expression was altered included: biological processes relevant to oocyte maturation and viability such as meiosis, cell growth, and apoptosis. This study revealed that despite morphological confirmation that the oocytes had undergone nuclear maturation, the TFF oocytes carried molecular abnormalities at the gene expression level associated with failure of complete maturation and MII activation [55].

Polycystic ovary syndrome

Polycystic ovary syndrome (PCOS) is a common endocrine/metabolic condition characterized by anovulatory infertility, increased circulating androgen levels, and frequently insulin resistance and hyperinsulinemia. Although the anovulatory infertility can be overcome with interventions such as ovulation induction or assisted reproductive technology, many women with PCOS are at risk of pregnancy loss. The question arises as to whether the severely altered intrafollicular microenvironment has an effect on the oocyte that may have long-term consequences on embryo viability. Oocytes retrieved from nine women with PCOS and ten normal ovulatory women were subjected to microarray comparison in an attempt to

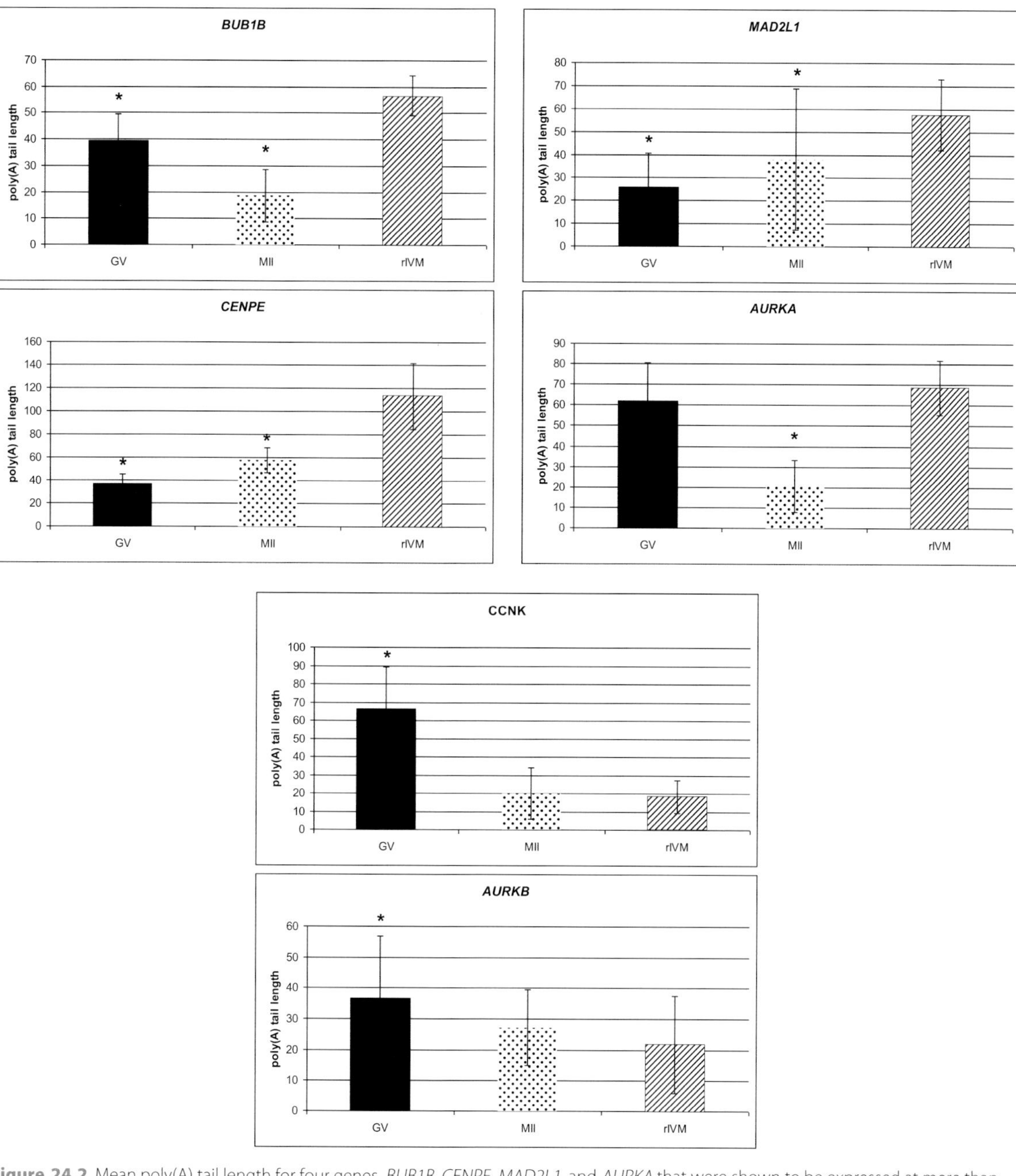

Figure 24.2 Mean poly(A) tail length for four genes, *BUB1B*, *CENPE*, *MAD2L1*, and *AURKA* that were shown to be expressed at more than fivefold higher levels and two genes, *CCNK* and *AURKB*, that were shown to be expressed at levels that were not significantly different in microarray experiments comparing global gene expression in "rescue" in vitro matured MII oocytes (rIVM) and *in vivo* matured MII oocytes (MII). Results are graphed as mean length ± SD for GV (solid black bars), MII (vertical line bars), and rIVM oocytes (hatched bars). Asterisks indicate poly(A) tail lengths significantly different to the poly(A) tail length in rIVM oocytes.

identify whether perturbations in follicular growth and the intrafollicular environment associated with PCOS alters the oocyte gene expression profile [56]. Of the 8123 transcripts expressed in the MII oocytes, 374 (4.6%) genes showed a significant difference in abundance in PCOS oocytes [56]. Two major themes were identified in the 374 genes showing altered mRNA abundance, namely, maternal-effect genes and genes associated with the meiotic/mitotic cell cycle [56]. The maternal-effect gene *Mater/NALP5*, which is essential for embryonic progression beyond the 2-cell stage in mice [57], was shown to be increased threefold in PCOS oocytes [56]. Similarly the maternal-effect genes *BNC1*, which has been shown to regulate transcription of rRNA during oogenesis [58], and *FMN2*, which has been shown to regulate spindle dynamics during meiosis [59], were up-regulated fourfold in PCOS oocytes [56]. Eight genes, involved in chromosome alignment (*ATRX, EME1,* and *NBN*), spindle dynamics (*ECT2, EML1, DIAPH2,* and *FMN2*), and cell-cycle checkpoint (*BUB3*), showed altered mRNA abundance in PCOS oocytes [56]. In addition, seven centrosome-associated genes (*CEP70, FGFR1OP2, NEK2, NEK4, PCM1, SPAST,* and *TACC1*) had increased mRNA abundance in PCOS oocytes [56]. Promoter analysis of the differentially expressed genes identified binding sites for the androgen receptor and/or peroxisome proliferating receptor gamma, suggesting that the altered intrafollicular milieu in PCOS women, in particular the elevated androgen level, alters the gene expression profile in these women and may negatively affect the meiotic or first few mitotic cell cycles [56].

Maternal age and aneuploidy

The reproductive capacity of women declines rapidly in their mid thirties with not only a decline in the numbers of ovarian follicles available for recruitment to the growth phase but also a decline in oocyte quality. This age-related decline in oocyte quality has been associated with an increased incidence of aneuploidy in the oocytes of older women (reviewed in [60, 61]). Mitochondrial dysfunction has also been implicated as a cause of the age-related decline in oocyte developmental competence (reviewed in [62]). Both the accumulation of mitochondrial mutations with age and alterations in metabolic activity of these organelles could contribute to reduced developmental competence.

Microarray expression profiling of human oocytes using slightly different experimental designs has been undertaken in an attempt to identify whether there is a major shift in gene expression with advancing maternal age. Steuerwald *et al.* compared two pools of ten MII oocytes that had failed to fertilize from women <32 years and women <40 years, whereas Grøndahl *et al.* compared single fresh MII oocytes from superovulated women ≤35 years (10 oocytes) versus 37–39 years (5 oocytes) [63, 64]. In our recent studies (G. Jones and D. Cram, unpublished observations, 2008) we compared pools of 5 fresh MII oocytes from superovulated women 28–37 years (9 pools) and women 38–43 years (12 pools) (Figure 24.3). Cluster analysis or principal components analysis of the microarray data from all three studies revealed a clear distinction in the gene expression profiles of oocytes from young women compared to the oocytes from older women. Steuerwald *et al.* found 181 genes differentially expressed at fold change values of greater than or equal to two [63]. Grøndahl *et al.* identified 102 genes differentially expressed at fold change values of greater than or equal to two [64]. G. Jones and D. Cram (unpublished observations, 2008) found over 2000 genes up-regulated at fold change values of greater than or equal to two in the oocytes from older women and 49 genes that were down-regulated. The reason for the disparity in the number of genes determined to be significantly expressed differentially may be due to several differences in the methodologies employed by the three studies. Steuerwald *et al.* used in vitro aged oocytes, which have been shown to be unrepresentative of fresh oocytes (see previous discussion of this point) [63]. Grondahl *et al.* utilized single oocytes for their microarray studies, which may have under-represented the ability to detect genes present at low levels and this effect would further be confounded by the fact that these workers required genes to be detected as present in 80% of

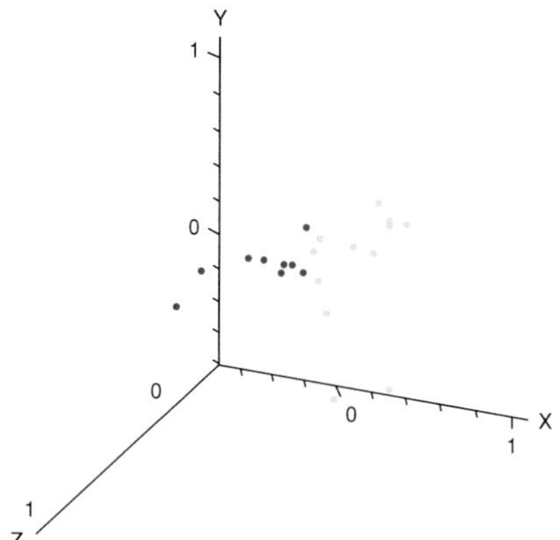

Figure 24.3 Principal components analysis of the microarray results for 9 pools of human oocytes from women 28–37 years of age (red circles) and 12 pools of human oocytes from women 38–43 years of age (yellow circles) showing a relatively clear distinction in oocyte gene expression between the two age groups.

the samples for each of the comparative groups, further reducing the number of genes available for comparative analysis [64]. G. Jones and D. Cram (unpublished observations, 2008), on the other hand, utilized pooled oocytes, large numbers of replicates and required genes to be detected as present in 5 of 9 of the samples representative of oocytes from younger women and 7 of 12 samples representative of oocytes from older women. Apart from methodological differences in the three studies, biological heterogeneity among individual MII oocytes, including aneuploidy, may also explain some of the non-overlapping gene data.

Nevertheless, there were some consistent findings from all three studies. Steuerwald *et al.* [63] confirmed previous findings in the mouse [65] that age-related changes are found in the expression of genes involved in regulation and control of the cell cycle, DNA damage response and repair, energy pathways, cytoskeletal structure, and transcription. Specifically, the cell-cycle checkpoint genes *BUB1B* and *BUB3* were identified to be down-regulated in oocytes from older women, confirming previous studies undertaken using PCR-based technologies [66]. These findings may provide further evidence that a defective cell-cycle checkpoint in the oocytes of older women may contribute to the observed increased incidence in aneuploidy in these oocytes [63]. In contrast, genes involved in the mitochondrial electron transport chain were up-regulated whereas those related to ATP binding, oxidoreductase, and the mitochondrial membrane were down-regulated in the oocytes from older women. These findings are consistent with the results of decreased mitochondrial membrane potential [67] and decreased ATP content [68] in the oocytes of older women. Grøndahl *et al.* found age-related changes in the expression of genes involved in cell-cycle regulation, chromosome alignment, sister chromatid separation, oxidative stress, and ubiquitination [63]. G. Jones and D. Cram (unpublished observations, 2008) found that for genes up-regulated in the oocytes of older women, the major biological pathways that were over-represented were for genes involved in mitochondrial function and energy production and genes involved in translation and RNA processing (Table 24.1).

Aneuploidy is implicated as a major cause of the age-related decline in reproductive function in women. G. Jones and D. Cram (unpublished observations, 2008) compared the gene expression profiles of pools of aneuploid oocytes from young (six pools)

Table 24.1. The top ten most significant functional biological processes identified as being over-represented, relative to all genes represented on the microarray, among transcripts expressed more that twofold higher in oocytes from older women (38–43 years) compared to younger women (28–37 years)

Biological process	Number of overlapping genes	Significance
Translation	82	3.48E^{-19}
RNA splicing	46	3.72E^{-4}
Mitochondrial electron transport, NADH to ubiquinone	13	0.000888
Aerobic respiration	5	0.00147
Methionyl-tRNA aminoacylation	3	0.00219
Retrograde vesicle-mediated transport, Golgi to endoplasmic reticulum	7	0.00243
Protein folding	47	0.00255
Amyloid precursor protein catabolic process	4	0.00343
Cytokinesis	10	0.00343
Regulation of progression through cell cycle	50	0.00357

versus older women (ten pools) and found that there were still more than 2000 genes expressed at greater than or equal to twofold higher levels in the oocytes from older women, indicating that aneuploidy is not the only, and perhaps not even the major, cause of the age-related decline in female fertility. A recent study has demonstrated that 327 genes are statistically different in comparative microarray analysis of four aneuploid versus three normal oocytes derived from the same patient who was 30 years of age [69]. This study revealed that as many as 44 different biological pathways may be malfunctioning or abnormally activated or repressed in aneuploid oocytes. Examples of the pathways affected were glycolysis and pyruvate metabolism, DNA replication, and apoptosis. Among the biological processes showing the greatest disturbance in transcript abundance were spindle assembly, and chromosome alignment and segregation. It was also generally found that aneuploid oocytes contained less mRNA than normal oocytes and it was concluded that aneuploid oocytes are either poorly resourced with mRNA or that transcripts are prematurely degraded or have reduced polyadenylation making mRNA difficult to detect using the methodologies employed [69].

Summary

It has only been in recent times that it has been possible to efficiently mine the human oocyte transcriptome. The oocyte accumulates all the transcripts required for maturation, fertilization, and development until the 4- to 8-cell stage during its growth phase and prior to the re-initiation of the meiotic cycle. The transcripts accumulated during this time undergo many post-transcriptional regulatory mechanisms and modifications that are to this day poorly understood in the oocyte. Pathology to any of these elements can be caused in vivo or in vitro and can have major consequences to downstream development. All the studies highlighted in this chapter have contributed significantly to our understanding of the molecular basis for oocyte developmental competence but there is still much more to be discovered. A consistent finding in the majority of highlighted comparative microarray studies of developmentally competent and developmentally incompetent oocytes is that developmentally incompetent oocytes show up-regulation rather than down-regulation for the majority of genes found to be differentially expressed. This probably means that there is dysregulation in the post-transcriptional regulation or modification of transcripts acquired during oocyte growth that manifests as incorrect temporal translation and a concomitant decrease in availability of transcripts when required during later preimplantation development. Further studies similar to those outlined in this chapter may reveal the molecular basis of the dysregulation.

References

1. Braude P, Bolton V, Moore S. Human gene expression first occurs between the four- and eight-cell stages of preimplantation development. *Nature* 1988; **332**: 459–61.
2. Hartung M, Stahl A. Autoradiographic study of RNA synthesis during meiotic prophase in the human oocyte. *Cytogenet Cell Genet* 1978; **20**: 51–8.
3. Moore GP, Lintern-Moore S, Peters H, Faber M. RNA synthesis in the mouse oocyte. *J Cell Biol* 1974; **60**: 416–22.
4. Jahn CL, Baran MM, Bachvarova R. Stability of RNA synthesized by the mouse oocyte during its major growth phase. *J Exp Zool* 1976; **197**: 161–71.
5. Moore GP, Lintern-Moore S. Transcription of the mouse oocyte genome. *Biol Reprod* 1978; **18**: 865–70.
6. Sternlicht AL, Schultz RM. Biochemical studies of mammalian oogenesis: kinetics of accumulation of total and poly(A)-containing RNA during growth of the mouse oocyte. *J Exp Zool* 1981; **215**: 191–200.
7. De Leon V, Johnson A, Bachvarova R. Half-lives and relative amounts of stored and polysomal ribosomes and poly(A) + RNA in mouse oocytes. *Dev Biol* 1983; **98**: 400–8.
8. Bachvarova R. Gene expression during oogenesis and oocyte development in mammals. *Dev Biol* 1985; **1**: 453–524.
9. Pikó L, Clegg KB. Quantitative changes in total RNA, total poly(A), and ribosomes in early mouse embryos. *Dev Biol* 1982; **89**: 362–78.
10. Gougeon A. Dynamics of follicular growth in the human: a model from preliminary results. *Hum Reprod* 1986; **1**: 81–7.
11. Eichenlaub-Ritter U, Peschke M. Expression in in-vivo and in-vitro growing and maturing oocytes: focus on regulation of expression at the translational level. *Hum Reprod Update* 2002; **8**: 21–41.
12. Kang MK, Han SJ. Post-transcriptional and post-translational regulation during mouse oocyte maturation. *BMB Rep* 2011; **44**: 147–57.
13. Bachvarova RF. A maternal tail of poly(A): the long and the short of it. *Cell* 1992; **69**: 895–7.
14. Paynton BV, Bachvarova R. Polyadenylatiion and deadenylation of maternal mRNAs during oocyte growth and maturation in the mouse. *Mol Reprod Dev* 1994; **37**: 172–80.
15. Bachvarova R, De Leon V. Polyadenylated RNA of mouse ova and loss of maternal RNA in early development. *Dev Biol* 1980; **74**: 1–8.
16. Su YQ, Sugiura K, Woo Y, *et al.* Selective degradation of transcripts during meiotic maturation of mouse oocytes. *Dev Biol* 2007; **302**: 104–17.
17. Kinloch RA, Wassarman PM. Profile of a mammalian sperm receptor gene. *New Biol* 1989; **1**: 232–8.
18. Roller RJ, Kinloch RA, Hiraoka BY, Li SS, Wassarman PM. Gene expression during mammalian oogenesis and early embryogenesis: quantification of three messenger RNAs abundant in fully grown mouse oocytes. *Development* 1989; **106**: 251–61.

19. Zheng P, Patel B, McMenamin M, *et al.* Effects of follicle size and oocyte maturation conditions on maternal messenger RNA regulation and gene expression in rhesus monkey oocytes and embryos. *Biol Reprod* 2005; **72**: 890–97.

20. Jones GM, Cram DS, Song B, *et al.* Gene expression profiling of human oocytes following in vivo or in vitro maturation. *Hum Reprod* 2008; **23**: 1138–44.

21. Neilson L, Andalibi A, Kang D, *et al.* Molecular phenotype of the human oocyte by PCR-SAGE. *Genomics* 2000; **63**: 13–24.

22. Steuerwald N, Cohen J, Herrera RJ, Brenner CA. Analysis of gene expression in single oocytes and embryos by real-time rapid cycle fluorescence monitored RT-PCR. *Mol Hum Reprod* 1999; **5**: 1034–9.

23. Steuerwald N, Cohen J, Herrera RJ, Brenner CA. Quantification of mRNA in single oocytes and embryos by real-time rapid cycle fluorescence monitored RT-PCR. *Mol Hum Reprod* 2000; **6**: 448–53.

24. Wells D, Bermudez MG, Steuerwald N, *et al.* Expression of genes regulating chromosome segregation, the cell cycle and apoptosis during human preimplantation development. *Hum Reprod* 2005; **20**: 1339–48.

25. Goto T, Jones GM, Lolatgis N, *et al.* Identification and characterisation of known and novel transcripts expressed during the final stages of human oocyte maturation. *Mol Reprod Dev* 2002; **62**: 13–28.

26. Stanton JL, Bascand M, Fisher L, *et al.* Gene expression profiling of human GV oocytes: an analysis of a profile obtained by Serial Analysis of Gene Expression (SAGE). *J Reprod Immunol* 2002; **53**: 193–201.

27. Serafica MD, Goto T, Trounson AO. Transcripts from a human primordial follicle cDNA library. *Hum Reprod* 2005; **20**: 2074–91.

28. Metcalfe AD, Bloor DJ, Lieberman BA, Kimber SJ, Brison DR. Amplification of representative cDNA pools from single human oocytes and pronucleate embryos. *Mol Reprod Dev* 2003; **65**: 1–8.

29. Jones GM, Song B, Cram DS, Trounson AO. Optimization of a microarray based approach for deriving representative gene expression profiles from human oocytes. *Mol Reprod Dev* 2007; **74**: 8–17.

30. Bermúdez MG, Wells D, Malter H, *et al.* Expression profiles of individual human oocytes using microarray technology. *Reprod Biomed Online* 2004; **8**: 325–37.

31. Dobson AT, Raja R, Abeyta MJ, *et al.* The unique transcriptome through day 3 of human preimplantation development. *Hum Mol Genet* 2004; **13**: 1461–70.

32. Assou S, Anahory T, Pantesco V, *et al.* The human cumulus-oocyte complex gene-expression profile. *Hum Reprod* 2006; **21**: 1705–19.

33. Kocabas AM, Crosby J, Ross PJ, *et al.* (2006) The transcriptome of human oocytes. *Proc Natl Acad Sci USA* 2006; **103**: 14027–32.

34. Li SS-L, Liu Y-H, Tseng C-N, Singh S. Analysis of gene expression in single human oocytes and preimplantation embryos. *Biochem Biophys Res Comm* 2006; **340**: 48–53.

35. Gasca S, Pellestor F, Assou S, *et al.* Identifying new human oocyte marker genes: a microarray approach. *Reprod BioMed Online* 2007; **14**: 175–83.

36. Zhang P, Kerkela E, Skottman H, *et al.* Distinct sets of developmentally regulated genes that are expressed by human oocytes and human embryonic stem cells. *Fertil Steril* 2007; **87**: 677–90.

37. Zhang P, Zucchelli M, Bruce S, *et al.* Transcriptome profiling of human pre-implantation development. *PLoS One* 2009; **4**: e7844.

38. Markholt S, Grøndahl ML, Ernst EH, *et al.* Global gene analysis of oocytes from early stages in human folliculogenesis shows high expression of novel genes in reproduction. *Mol Hum Reprod* 2012; **18**: 96–110.

39. Venkatcsh S, Dada R. An evolutionary insight into mutation of ATPase6 gene in primary ovarian insufficiency. *Arch Gynecol Obstet* 2011; **284**: 251–2.

40. Jones GM. Growth and viability of human blastocysts in vitro. *Reprod Med Rev* 2000; **8**: 241–87.

41. Blake D, Procton M, Johnson N, Olive D. Cleavage stage versus blastocyst stage embryo transfer in assisted conception. *Cochrane Database Syst Rev* 2005; **4**: CD002118.

42. Chen SU, Chen HF, Lien YR, *et al.* Schedule to inject in vitro matured oocytes may increase pregnancy after intracytoplasmic sperm injection. *Arch Androl* 2000; **44**: 197–205.

43. Veeck LL, Wortham JWE, Jr., Witmyer J, *et al.* Maturation and fertilization of morphologically immature human oocytes in a program of in vitro fertilization. *Fertil Steril* 1983; **39**: 594–602.

44. Nagy ZP, Cecile J, Liu J, *et al.* Pregnancy and birth after intracytoplasmic sperm injection of in vitro matured germinal-vesicle stage oocytes: case report. *Fertil Steril* 1996; **65**: 1047–50.

45. Edirisinghe WR, Junk SM, Matson PL, Yovich JL. Birth from cryopreserved embryos following in-vitro maturation of oocytes and intracytoplasmic sperm injection. *Hum Reprod* 1997; **12**: 1056–58.

46. Tucker MJ, Wright G, Morton PC, Massey JB. Birth after cryopreservation of immature oocytes with subsequent in vitro maturation. *Fertil Steril* 1998; **70**: 578–79.
47. De Vos A, Van de Velde H, Joris H, Van Steirteghem A. In-vitro matured metaphase-I oocytes have a lower fertilization rate but similar embryo quality as mature metaphase-II oocytes after intracytoplasmic sperm injection. *Hum Reprod* 1999; **14**: 1859–63.
48. Vanhoutte L, De Sutter P, Van der Elst J, Dhont M. Clinical benefit of metaphase I oocytes. *Reprod Biol Endocrinol* 2005; **3**: 71–6.
49. Zuccotti M, Merico V, Cecconi S, Redi CA, Garagna S. What does it take to make a developmentally competent mammalian egg? *Hum Reprod Update* 2011; **17**: 525–40.
50. Tam OH, Aravin AA, Stein P, *et al.* Pseudogene-derived small interfering RNAs regulate gene expression in mouse oocytes. *Nature* 2008; **453**: 534–8.
51. Watanabe T, Imai H, Minami N. Identification and expression analysis of small RNAs during development. *Methods Mol Biol* 2008; **442**: 173–85.
52. Kizana E, Cingolani E, Marbán E. Non-cell-autonomous effects of vector-expressed regulatory RNAs in mammalian heart cells. *Gene Ther* 2009; **16**: 1163–8.
53. Tang F, Kaneda M, O'Carroll D, *et al.* Maternal microRNAs are essential for mouse zygotic development. *Genes Dev* 2007; **21**: 644–8.
54. Xu YW, Wang B, Ding CH, *et al.* Differentially expressed micoRNAs in human oocytes. *J Assist Reprod Genet* 2011; **28**: 559–66.
55. Gasca S, Reyftmann L, Pellestor F, *et al.* Total fertilization failure and molecular abnormalities in metaphase II oocytes. *Reprod Biomed Online* 2008; **17**: 772–81.
56. Wood JR, Dumesic DA, Abbott DH, Strauss JF, 3rd. Molecular abnormalities in oocytes from women with polycystic ovary syndrome revealed by microarray analysis. *J Clin Endocrinol Metab* 2007; **92**: 705–13.
57. Tong ZB, Gold L, Pfeifer KE, *et al.* Mater, a maternal effect gene required for early embryonic development in mice. *Nat Genet* 2000; **26**: 267–8.
58. Tian Q, Kopf GS, Brown RS, Tseng H. Function of basonuclin in increasing transcription of the ribosomal RNA genes during mouse oogenesis. *Development* 2001; **128**: 407–16.
59. Leader B, Lim H, Carabatsos MJ, *et al.* Formin-2, polyploidy, hypofertility and positioning of the meiotic spindle in mouse oocytes. *Nat Cell Biol* 2002; **4**: 921–8.
60. Pellestor F, Anahory T, Hamamah S. Effect of maternal age on the frequency of cytogenetic abnormalities in human oocytes. *Cytogenet Genome Res* 2005; **111**: 206–12.
61. Fragouli E, Wells D, Delhanty JD. Chromosome abnormalities in the human oocyte. *Cytogenet Genome Res* 2011; **133**: 107–18.
62. Eichenlaub-Ritter U, Vogt E, Yin H, Gosden R. Spindles, mitochondria and redox potential in ageing oocytes. *Reprod Biomed Online* 2004; **8**: 45–58.
63. Steuerwald NM, Bermúdez MG, Wells D, Munné S, Cohen J. Maternal age-related differential global expression profiles observed in human oocytes. *Reprod Biomed Online* 2007; **14**: 700–8.
64. Grøndahl ML, Yding Andersen C, Bogstad J, *et al.* Gene expression profiles of single human mature oocytes in relation to age. *Hum Reprod* 2010; **25**: 957–68.
65. Hamatani T, Falco G, Carter MG, *et al.* Age-associated alteration of gene expression patterns in mouse oocytes. *Hum Mol Genet* 2004; **13**: 2263–78.
66. Steuerwald N, Cohen J, Herrera RJ, Sandalinas M, Brenner CA. Association between spindle assembly checkpoint expression and maternal age in human oocytes. *Mol Hum Reprod* 2001; **7**: 49–55.
67. Wilding M, Dale B, Marino M, *et al.* Mitochondrial aggregation patterns and activity in human oocytes and preimplantation embryos. *Hum Reprod* 2001; **16**: 909–17.
68. Van Blerkom J, Davis PW, Lee J. ATP content of human oocytes and developmental potential and outcome after in-vitro fertilization and embryo transfer. *Hum Reprod* 1995; **10**: 415–24.
69. Fragouli E, Bianchi V, Patrizio P, *et al.* Transcriptomic profiling of human oocytes: association of meiotic aneuploidy and altered oocyte gene expression. *Mol Hum Reprod* 2010; 16: 570–82

Chapter 25 Omics as tools for oocyte selection

Marc-André Sirard and Isabelle Gilbert

Introduction

The neologism "omics" encompasses several new disciplines, such as genomics, transcriptomics, proteomics, metabolomics, and epigenomics, associated with the molecular analysis of biological events (Figure 25.1). Recently, a combination of whole genome sequencing; to RNA sequencing; and to proteomic, metabolomic, and autoantibody profiling has been realized from an individual to obtain an "integrative personal omics profile" (iPOP) [1]. This individual profile offers the perspective of a personal medicine and predicts future health and disease possibilities. For fertility comprehension, omics offers all the tools required for an in-depth study of the different steps required for a successful reproductive process. Since about 15% of couples have fertility problems, omics offers also diagnostic possibilities for assisted reproduction. For example, follicular cells (as well as cumulus cells) transcriptomes can help to predict which oocyte has the best potential to develop into an embryo or to determine the embryo(s) most likely to result in a pregnancy.

Omics include all high-throughput techniques of every cellular metabolic component. At the DNA level, genomics refers to whole genome sequencing, DNA polymorphisms (such as single-nucleotide polymorphism [SNP]) or sequence variation (such as insertion, deletion, duplication, and copy number variants), etc. For RNA, transcriptomics studies the transcribed genome including mainly messenger RNA (mRNA) but also the ribosomal RNA (rRNA), transfer RNA (tRNA), and other non-coding RNA. When mRNAs have been translated, proteomics studies proteins, especially their structures and functions. Metabolomics involves the study of cellular activities with small-molecule metabolites profiles. Finally, epigenetics refers to the comprehension of different events (such as DNA methylation and histone modification) which influence gene expression without altering the DNA sequence. Taken together, integration of all these omics fields in a systems biology perspective is the ultimate research goal in order to give the complete picture of a cell. However, achieving this concept remains a big challenge.

In the field of assisted reproductive technology (ART), the fact that oocytes or embryos or even cumulus–granulosa cells contain a small amount of material has triggered the investigations using genomic tools where methods of signal amplification partially resolve the problem. Transcriptomics analyses are a method of choice for the study of tissue with a minute amount of material since various techniques allow the amplification of the RNA starting material (such as PCR and in vitro RNA amplification) [2]. However, the different metabolomic and proteomic methods (like mass spectrometry) are slowly getting sensitive enough to analyze follicular cells, oocytes, and embryos.

It is important to realize that omics represents the most sensitive tool available ever made to assess global cell physiology and status. In the oocyte selection context, omics can be extremely useful to study various tissues to extract information relevant to potential pregnancy rates. Therefore, this review will expose the advantages and the limitations of the different omics tools in the context of oocyte selection.

Genomics

Testing oocytes for aneuploidy

Aneuploidy is the most common chromosome abnormality and it is characterized by a missing (monosomy) or supplementary (trisomy) chromosome.

Biology and Pathology of the Oocyte, 2nd edn., ed. Alan Trounson, Roger Gosden, and Ursula Eichenlaub-Ritter.
Published by Cambridge University Press.

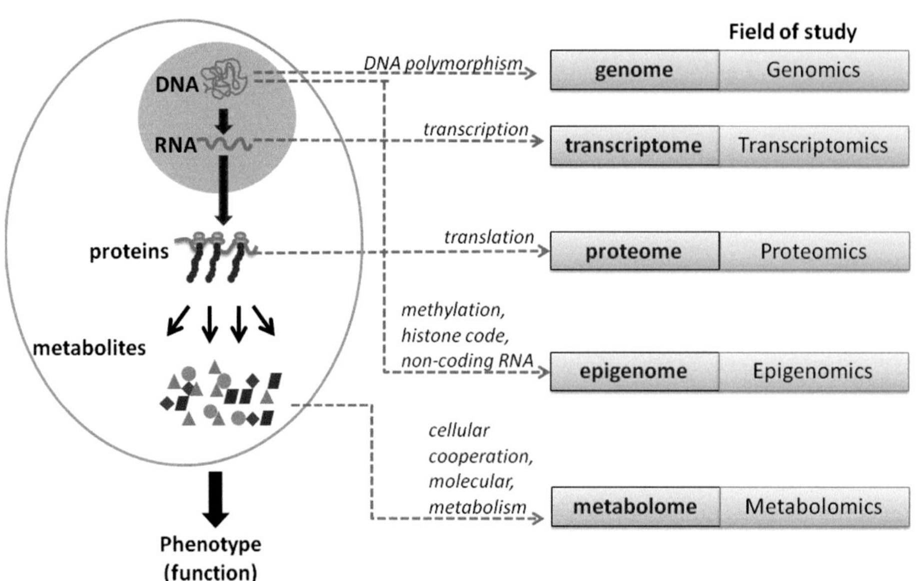

Figure 25.1 Schematic description of the different omics fields. Genomics is the study of DNA and DNA polymorphism. DNA sequences containing genes can be transcribed into RNA (trancriptomics) and translated into proteins (proteomics). Epigenetic modifications (epigenomics) are control by DNA methylation, histone code, and non-coding RNA (microRNA, siRNA, lncRNA, etc.). Metabolites (small molecules such as sugar, lipids, amino acids, etc.) are implicated in metabolism such as cellular cooperation, molecular processes, and metabolism.

Moreover, the increasing demand in ART has been associated with a higher number of chromosome abnormalities (such as aneuploidy or trisomy). For these reasons, great efforts were made to develop tools for embryo chromosome analyses in order to increase in vitro fertilization (IVF) success with techniques allowing the identification or elimination of an aneuploid embryo. This type of analysis is also called preimplantation genetic screening (PGS). In theory, this test can be achieved at all preimplantation stages, but only three are currently used: (1) the polar bodies from non-fertilized or fertilized oocytes, (2) the blastomere from a cleaved embryo at day 3, or (3) a group of cells from the trophectoderm at the blastocyste stage. Considering the topic of this review, we will focus on the tools available for oocyte screening.

Fluorescence *in situ* hybridization

Fluorescence *in situ* hybridization (FISH) was for some time the most commonly used method for PGS. Compared to karyotyping, it offers the possibility of probing interphase chromosomes and could therefore be used on polar bodies, blastomere, and trophectoderm cells. Hybridization malfunction and overlap of the fluorescence signal of two chromosomes are the main inconveniences of the FISH method. Briefly, the biopsied cell is fixed on a glass slide and probes for 9–12 chromosomes to be tested are labeled with different fluorophores (colors) and hybridized to the slide in successive hybridizations. The most commonly screened chromosomes are 13, 15, 16, 17, 18, 21, 22, X, and Y [3]. More recently, several reviews have indicated the poor predictive value of this analysis compared to the potential harm done to the embryo [4–6]. Finally, recent randomized controlled trials not only showed no improvement with FISH but instead a decrease in implantation and pregnancy rates and it was concluded that aneuploidy screening with PGS using FISH in IVF practice cannot be justified [7].

Comparative genomic hybridization

Comparative genomic hybridization (CGH) allows comparison between a sample and a reference (normal cells) differentially labeled and simultaneously analyzed on a microscope slide. In comparison to the FISH method, CGH permits the verification of the copy number and the entire length of all chromosomes. However the main disadvantage of CGH is that it requires around 1 μg of DNA, which is too large when working with single cells which contain around 5–10 pg. Thus prior to CGH analysis, an amplification step is needed, lengthening the procedure, which requires approximately 4 days to perform. The use of CGH on polar bodies is even more challenging as the cell is very small and the amount of DNA is one or 2 N. Also, this approach will fail to detect abnormal segregation that may occur during meiosis II, and that of paternal origin [8].

Microarray-CGH involves the competitive hybridization of the targeted amplified genome with a reference DNA sample. In this case, the patient's DNAs are hybridized to a microscope slide where oligomers of DNA have been printed instead of metaphase chromosomes. Each probe on the slide is specific to a different chromosomal region and all chromosomes are fully represented. The benefit of using microarrays instead of chromosomes is that the evaluation is simpler, easily automated and faster (less than 2 days [8].

Transcriptomics

Compared to the genome, which is relatively stable (except for mutation events), the transcriptome shows tissue-specific profiles as well as huge flexibility, depending on the environmental conditions.

A multitude of transcriptome analyses and contrasts can be performed with follicular cells, oocytes, and embryos. The complete coverage of the exome (coding sequence of the genome) on a microarray slide offers the possibility to measure the expression level of more than 35 000 genes or isoforms. Since a typical microarray experiment allows the profiling of between 10 000 and 15 000 active genes simultaneously in any given tissue, including the oocyte, microarray offers the possibility of significantly speeding up many research studies. Although this method is very informative, the physiology behind transcription is far from being completely understood as thousands of genes have no real defined functions yet. Therefore, the use of transcriptomics relies on the physiological contrasts that are used or the phenotypes to be compared to be very informative. On the other hand, the quest for a biomarker can rapidly result in predictive gene expression levels associated with a given phenotype. For example we may find that when a given gene is overexpressed in the follicle, the pregnancy rate is better. This link does not explain the phenotype (why better pregnancy rates occur) but predicts the phenotype.

Using the follicular transcriptome to predict oocyte quality

The first question to be addressed is: what is the evidence that the follicular status at oocyte collection indicates the potential developmental competence of this oocyte?

In humans, many studies examine the follicular sizes and try to correlate them with the oocyte developmental potential. The majority of these reports agree that a follicle of medium size, corresponding to about 12 mm or more (equivalent to a volume of 1 ml or more), possesses an oocyte with a higher developmental competence [9–11]. However, large (>23 mm, volume >6 ml) or small follicles (<16 mm, volume <2 ml) may have an oocyte with an inferior competence [12]. Pregnancy rates are also positively correlated with increased follicular sizes and volumes [13–15].

On the other hand, it was observed that oocytes from follicles with an aspirated volume ≤1 ml resulted in a significantly lower fertilization rate but cleave at the same rate as oocytes obtained from larger follicles, resulting in embryos of comparable quality [16]. More recently, using intracytoplasmic sperm injection (ICSI) as a background to reduce fertilization failure, Lee *et al.* re-examined the effect of follicular size on embryonic development and found that the rates of good quality embryos from the large, medium, and small groups on days 2 and 3 were 76.85% and 66.20%, 74.00% and 61.33%, and 69.81% and 58.49%, respectively [17]. There were no significant differences in the rates of good quality embryos between the three follicular volume groups even though fewer oocytes completed maturation in the small follicle group than in the other two groups [17].

Another study involving ovarian stimulation in human IVF has further explored the relationship between follicle size and pregnancy rates [15]. The aim of this study was first to verify the relationship between follicular steroid content, follicular size, oocyte maturity, and fertilization outcome in women with normal ovaries following recombinant human follicle-stimulating hormone administration (rhFSH). Follicular diameter was classified as small (8–13 mm) or large (>14 mm) and sex steroid content was analyzed for each group. In ovulation groups, estradiol and progesterone concentrations were significantly higher in large follicles with meiotically competent oocytes compared with those containing meiotically incompetent oocytes. The relationship between follicle size and embryo development indicated that 14 mm could be a threshold value following rhFSH induction in normal women. This follicular size correlates with the appearance of luteinizing hormone (LH) receptors in human granulosa cells [18].

A different perspective comes from the treatment of polycystic ovary syndrome (PCOS) patients with clomiphene and looking at the follicular size at induction in relation to pregnancy rates. Pregnancy rates were highest (13.6–18.6%) when human chorionic gonadotropin (hCG) was administered in the presence of an 18–22 mm follicle, and lowest with 17 mm, 23 mm, and 24 mm follicles (8.8%, 8.8%, and 5.7%, respectively), indicating that too early and too late triggering could be less efficient [19]. However, when oocytes from PCOS are used for in vitro maturation, even follicles as small as 9 mm can translate into pregnancies [20].

Data from unstimulated human follicles are indicative of a rather different relationship between follicle size and developmental competence [21]. In clomiphene-treated or natural ovulatory cycles, where hCG was given (one to three growing follicles of 7 mm to 26 mm in diameter – as measured by vaginal ultrasound) oocytes produced blastocysts from the full range of follicle sizes. Offspring were produced following embryo transfer of the blastocysts from follicles as small as 9 mm in diameter. This indicates a potential independence of follicle size and developmental competence, at least above 9 mm diameter but in potentially various differentiation statuses. If size is used strictly as an indicator, the level of maturation might vary between stimulated and non-stimulated cycles. Furthermore, developmental competence is probably not acquired in a linear fashion but more likely through some thresholds. The example of the appearance of LH receptors is potentially one of these thresholds. The other critical aspect in follicular maturation is the health of the follicle. Our original hypothesis was that the healthier the follicle at any given size, the better the developmental competence of the oocyte would be.

In IVF patients, a number of parameters were measured in the follicular fluid aspirated at the same time as oocytes following stimulation and ovulation induction. Although a number of measurements were found to be associated with fertilization rates, embryo morphology, or pregnancy outcome, there is very little information on the physiological value of these measurements since they represent "after the fact evidence". Only a few of the reported experiments will be listed to highlight the variation in terms of the predictive value of the different variables.

Andersen found a correlation between the pregnancy potential of oocytes and the ratio of estradiol 17β (E_2) to androgens in follicular fluid but no difference was found when pregnancy-associated follicles and follicles not associated with pregnancy were compared with respect to the levels of free and total E_2, progesterone (P_4), testosterone (T), androstenedione (A), immunoreactive inhibin, insulin-like growth factor-binding protein-1, α1-antitrypsin, placental protein-14, and the E_2/P_4 ratio [22].

In a similar analysis Artini *et al.* found that follicular fluid concentrations of growth hormone (GH), insulin-like growth factor-I (IGF-I), epidermal growth factor (EGF), and E_2 were related to differences in oocyte maturation and fertilization rates among oocytes obtained for IVF [23]. Follicular fluid GH, IGF-I, and E_2 concentrations were significantly correlated with increasing follicular size. Follicles with immature oocytes had concentrations of estradiol that were significantly lower than those in follicles with intermediate and mature oocytes. Follicular fluid EGF concentration was similar for all oocyte maturational stages. In follicular fluids with mature oocytes, IGF-I and GH concentrations were significantly higher compared to those of follicular fluids with atretic oocytes. Follicular fluids with immature and intermediate oocytes had similar concentrations of GH and IGF-I to follicular fluid containing mature oocytes and higher concentrations than follicular fluid with atretic oocytes. They concluded that maturation of oocytes is associated with higher concentrations of GH, IGF-I, and E_2, but follicular fluid IGF-I and GH concentrations cannot serve as a predictor for IVF.

Premature ovarian failure is a medical condition affecting women's fertility. Recently, a microarray analysis was performed on granulosa cells of young women with a diagnosis of diminished ovarian reserve and undergoing IVF and those of women with a normal reserve [24]. The results obtained show a down-regulation of the IGF gene family in granulosa cells from women with diminished ovarian reserve, suggesting that IGF system deregulation decreases reproductive capacity [24].

At the beginning of the in vitro maturation story, hCG bolus injection was given to patients 36 hours before oocyte recovery, but at a stage where the follicles had not yet reached the size at which they have LH receptors [25]. The recovered oocytes were then matured and fertilized in vitro, leading to pregnancies. In this case, the LH might have affected the theca cells, where LH receptors are present, and caused an early atretic signal, leading to early differentiation of the oocyte (reviewed recently by Sirard [26]). The same hCG priming 36 hours before immature oocyte retrieval in patients with PCOS followed by an oocyte culture for 24–48 hours resulted in a higher rate of oocytes achieving maturation than in the non-hCG-primed group. There were five clinical pregnancies (38.5%) in the hCG-primed group, and three pregnancies (27.3%) in the non-hCG-primed group [27]. Since then results obtained around the world support the early atresia hypothesis as the maximum size of the dominant follicle at the time of hCG injection remains below 13 mm [26].

As mentioned above, the follicle clearly has an influence on oocyte quality. Are such physiological characteristics visible in the complete transcriptome? Surely. Can we find powerful biomarkers reflective of such status? Probably. Finding relevant biomarkers to predict oocyte quality is therefore of primary interest to offer efficient approaches to improve pregnancy outcome, especially for infertile couples. The transfer of multiple embryos and its heavy consequences on both women's and babies' health has made this biomarkers research more important [28–29].

Transcriptomics and granulosa cells

Transcriptome analysis of the granulosa cells has shown a powerful capacity to distinguish between follicular conditions. Already some genomic studies have reported an increase in differentially expressed genes associated with apoptosis in subordinate versus dominant follicles [30–33]. These candidate genes were suggested as possible markers of the dominant follicle in animals. For example, LH was shown to induce an early effect (6 hours after the LH surge) marked by the transcription of ovulation-related genes and a late LH effect (22 hours after LH surge), where the transcriptome was characterized by the up-regulation of luteinization-related genes [34]. Some reports have also analyzed the gene expression patterns associated with ovarian stimulation in human or bovine [34, 35].

One of the goals of transcriptomic analysis of granulosa cells is to identify quantitative and non-invasive gene markers that could predict oocyte competence and reinforce the morphological criteria already used. Several studies performed in many mammalian species including cattle [34, 36–38] and human [39–41] have revealed key gene markers that could increase the efficiency and the safety of ART. This technology can therefore be applied to individual follicles and even individual cumulus complexes.

One of the challenges associated with the analysis of competence markers is the individual assessment of follicles performed by analyzing separately the gene expression of follicular cells and recording the pregnancy output of the oocyte. Our laboratory is the only one so far that has used a human individual follicle aspiration scheme associated with individual oocyte culture and follow-up [42]. This first analysis comparing inter-patient results (patient group with successful pregnancy vs. the non-pregnant group) has generated a list of ten potential biomarkers with five of them reaching a high significance in the PCR validation performed in additional patients. A second study where intra-patient (follicle leading to pregnancy vs. follicle leading to pregnancy failure) analysis approaches were used resulted in three more significant biomarkers of oocyte developmental competence [43]. Following the intra-patient analysis and gene candidate validation on separate samples, seven confirmed biomarkers were found: phosphoglycerate kinase 1 (PGK1), regulator of G-protein signaling 2 (RGS2), regulator of G-protein signaling 3 (RGS3), aromatase (CYP19a), cell division cycle 42 (CDC42), UDP-glucose pyrophosphorylase-2 (UGP2), and pleckstrin homology-like domain, family A, member 1 (PHLDA1) [43, 44]. Functional analysis of these markers supports their involvement in specific cell signaling pathways and some are associated with early follicular cell luteinization.

Our most recent study in the bovine examined the emergence and the retraction of oocyte competence in bovine follicles that were harvested early, at the right time or late after FSH withdrawal [45]. The blastocyst rate goes up and then down, illustrating the importance of the proper follicular timing before oocyte aspiration. One of the surprising observations is that despite FSH support cessation, the follicles continue to grow for at least 4 days under basal LH context (luteal phase) but the oocyte competence increases only up to the third day and then decreases. This is the first controlled experiment where larger follicles can contain oocytes of decreased value.

Transcriptomics and cumulus cells

The cumulus cells are specialized follicular cells maintaining close cell–cell connections with the oocyte. Their removal or the inhibition of their metabolic, transcriptional, and/or translational activities reduces the oocyte developmental potential [46–51]. The cumulus cells are therefore considered an important factor in oocyte quality.

Because the cumulus cells are physically attached to the oocyte, they are easier to obtain as individualized samples. Indeed all the follicles can be aspirated at once and, during oocyte recovery and selection, a sample of the cells can be obtained and associated with a specific oocyte. Consequently, cumulus cells are the target of increasing genomic studies in mammalian species to establish possible correlations between the cumulus cell transcriptome and oocyte developmental competence.

A proteomic analysis of cumulus cells and oocyte identified 811 and 1247 proteins in each cell type, respectively and of those, 371 proteins were differently expressed [52]. Some of these proteins are implicated in cell-to-cell signaling, suggesting their implication in oocyte maturation and competence [52].

In our laboratory, several gene markers of bovine oocyte competence expressed in cumulus cells were suggested to be important in the preovulatory stage, following a superovulation program or after in vitro FSH treatment [53]. These gene candidates have provided precious and meaningful data about cumulus cell behavior during follicular growth and differentiation, and offer objective and quantitative parameters of high quality oocyte selection.

Hamamah's group has particularly focused on this concept through the analysis of human cumulus cell gene expression profile and suggested interesting markers that are awaiting further validation [54, 55]. These biomarkers associated with both pregnancy success and failure should improved our understanding of the cumulus involvement in the competence process although they are measured at some 34 hours post LH when their influence on oocytes has disappeared [40, 56–58]. The use of these markers has clear clinical applications but they also represent downstream events of changes that could be associated with follicular and oocyte differentiation which happen upstream.

Transcriptomics and the polar body

The increasing power or amplification strategies even allow the introspection of polar body (PB) RNA content. The first PB is extruded from the oocyte before fertilization and can be biopsied without damaging the oocyte. Reich *et al.* tested the hypothesis that the PB transcriptome is representative of that of the oocyte [59]. PB biopsy was performed on metaphase II (MII) oocytes followed by single-cell transcriptome analysis of the oocyte and its sibling PB. Over 12 700 unique mRNAs and miRNAs from the oocyte samples were compared with the 5431 mRNAs recovered from the sibling PBs (5256 [or 97%] shared mRNAs, including miRNAs). The results show that human PBs reflect the oocyte transcript profile and suggest that mRNA detection and quantification through high-throughput quantitative PCR could result in the first molecular diagnostic for gene expression in MII oocytes. This could allow for both oocyte ranking and embryo preferences in IVF applications. Although preliminary and technically challenging, this approach could be added to the list of minimally invasive techniques for assessing oocyte quality.

Proteomics and follicular fluid

Given the impossibility of amplifying protein, proteomic studies are less abundant in the literature since they require a huge amount of starting material. However, for this type of analysis, follicular fluid accumulated in the follicle antrum is often chosen since proteins accumulated in the fluid can originate from blood and the surrounding somatic cells. In women, different proteomic analyses have been performed. For example, differential protein profiles from mature and immature follicles were examined [60]. A study on the follicular fluid protein profiles of women undergoing IVF due to male infertility have found several proteins implicated in the acute-phase response and various antioxidant enzymes, suggesting that the follicle is protected from oxidative stress injuries [61]. Another report on follicular fluid from women undergoing IVF has discovered many proteins associated with a successful pregnancy. Some of the proteins found were associated with immune function but many of them remain unknown for their implications in follicular development or oocyte maturation [62].

Conclusion

For both scientists and clinicians, understanding the signaling pathways from the follicle to the cumulus and from the cumulus to the oocyte remains the ultimate key to act on oocyte competence through different in vitro or in vivo treatments. Functional analysis of the gene candidates and their matching with what is already known about follicular physiology is the way to unravel the competence enigma. Several morphological, ultrastructural, and metabolic criteria have been used to predict oocyte competence. Despite some improvements in pregnancy outcomes, these morphological criteria remain subjective, in some cases invasive, and/or poorly correlated with oocyte competence. Therefore, the identification of other relevant biomarkers to predict accurately oocyte quality is of primary interest. In this context, the new potential offered by genomic tools allows the exploration of gene expression level in very small samples. This can therefore be applied to individual follicles and even individual cumulus complexes or polar bodies. The final test remains clinical evaluation using predictive clinical trials and hopefully such testing will come soon.

References

1. Chen R, Mias GI, Li-Pook-Than J, *et al.* Personal omics profiling reveals dynamic molecular and medical phenotypes. *Cell* 2012; **148**(6): 1293–307.
2. Gilbert I, Scantland S, Sylvestre EL, *et al.* Providing a stable methodological basis for comparing transcript abundance of developing embryos using microarrays. *Mol Hum Reprod* 2010; **16**(8): 601–16.
3. Lalioti MD. Can preimplantation genetic diagnosis overcome recurrent pregnancy failure? *Curr Opin Obstet Gynecol* 2008; **20**(3): 199–204.
4. Harper JC, Sengupta SB. Preimplantation genetic diagnosis: state of the art 2011. *Hum Genet* 2012; **131**(2): 175–86.
5. Ly KD, Agarwal A, Nagy ZP. Preimplantation genetic screening: does it help or hinder IVF treatment and what is the role of the embryo? *J Assist Reprod Genet* 2011; **28**(9): 833–49.
6. Basille C, Frydman R, El Aly A, *et al.* Preimplantation genetic diagnosis: state of the art. *Eur J Obstet Gynecol Reprod Biol* 2009; **145**(1): 9–13.
7. Checa MA, Alonso-Coello P, Sola I, *et al.* IVF/ICSI with or without preimplantation genetic screening for aneuploidy in couples without genetic disorders: a systematic review and meta-analysis. *J Assist Reprod Genet* 2009; **26**(5): 273–83.
8. Wells D, Escudero T, Levy B, *et al.* First clinical application of comparative genomic hybridization and polar body testing for preimplantation genetic diagnosis of aneuploidy. *Fertil Steril* 2002; **78**(3): 543–9.
9. Dubey AK, Wang HA, Duffy P, Penzias AS. The correlation between follicular measurements, oocyte morphology, and fertilization rates in an in vitro fertilization program. *Fertil Steril* 1995; **64**(4): 787–90.
10. Nataprawira DS, Harada T, Sekijima A, Mio Y, Terakawa N. Assessment of follicular maturity by follicular diameter and fluid volume in a program of in vitro fertilization and embryo transfer. *Asia Oceania J Obstet Gynaecol* 1992; **18**(3): 225–30.
11. Wittmaack FM, Kreger DO, Blasco L, *et al.* Effect of follicular size on oocyte retrieval, fertilization, cleavage, and embryo quality in in vitro fertilization cycles: a 6-year data collection. *Fertil Steril* 1994; **62**(6): 1205–10.
12. Ectors FJ, Vanderzwalmen P, Van Hoeck J, *et al.* Relationship of human follicular diameter with oocyte fertilization and development after in-vitro fertilization or intracytoplasmic sperm injection. *Hum Reprod* 1997; **12**(9): 2002–5.
13. Arnot AM, Vandekerckhove P, DeBono MA, Rutherford AJ. Follicular volume and number during in-vitro fertilization: association with oocyte developmental capacity and pregnancy rate. *Hum Reprod* 1995; **10**(2): 256–61.
14. Bergh C, Broden H, Lundin K, Hamberger L. Comparison of fertilization, cleavage and pregnancy rates of oocytes from large and small follicles. *Hum Reprod* 1998; **13**(7): 1912–15.
15. Teissier MP, Chable H, Paulhac S, Aubard Y. Comparison of follicle steroidogenesis from normal and polycystic ovaries in women undergoing IVF: relationship between steroid concentrations, follicle size, oocyte quality and fecundability. *Hum Reprod* 2000; **15**(12): 2471–7.
16. Salha O, Nugent D, Dada T, *et al.* The relationship between follicular fluid aspirate volume and oocyte maturity in in-vitro fertilization cycles. *Hum Reprod* 1998; **13**(7): 1901–6.
17. Lee TF, Lee RK, Hwu YM, *et al.* Relationship of follicular size to the development of intracytoplasmic sperm injection-derived human embryos. *Taiwan J Obstet Gynecol* 2010; **49**(3): 302–5.
18. Shima K, Kitayama S, Nakano R. Gonadotropin binding sites in human ovarian follicles and corpora

lutea during the menstrual cycle. *Obstet Gynecol* 1987; **69**(5): 800–6.

19. Farhi J, Orvieto R, Homburg R. Administration of clomiphene citrate in patients with polycystic ovary syndrome, without inducing withdrawal bleeding, achieves comparable treatment characteristics and outcome. *Fertil Steril* 2010; **93**(6): 2077–9.
20. Guzman L, Ortega-Hrepich C, Albuz FK, *et al.* Developmental capacity of in vitro-matured human oocytes retrieved from polycystic ovary syndrome ovaries containing no follicles larger than 6 mm. *Fertil Steril* 2012; **98**(2): 503-7.e1–2.
21. Trounson A, Anderiesz C, Jones G. Maturation of human oocytes in vitro and their developmental competence. *Reproduction* 2001; **121**(1): 51–75.
22. Andersen CY. Characteristics of human follicular fluid associated with successful conception after in vitro fertilization. *J Clin Endocrinol Metab* 1993; **77**(5): 1227–34.
23. Artini PG, Battaglia C, D'Ambrogio G, *et al.* Relationship between human oocyte maturity, fertilization and follicular fluid growth factors. *Hum Reprod* 1994; **9**(5): 902–6.
24. Greenseid K, Jindal S, Hurwitz J, Santoro N, Pal L. Differential granulosa cell gene expression in young women with diminished ovarian reserve. *Reprod Sci* 2011; **18**(9): 892–9.
25. Chian RC, Buckett WM, Too LL, Tan SL. Pregnancies resulting from in vitro matured oocytes retrieved from patients with polycystic ovary syndrome after priming with human chorionic gonadotropin. *Fertil Steril* 1999; **72**(4): 639–42.
26. Sirard MA. Follicle environment and quality of in vitro matured oocytes. *J Assist Reprod Genet* 2011; **28**(6): 483–8.
27. Chian RC, Buckett WM, Tulandi T, Tan SL. Prospective randomized study of human chorionic gonadotrophin priming before immature oocyte retrieval from unstimulated women with polycystic ovarian syndrome. *Hum Reprod* 2000; **15**(1): 165–70.
28. Gelbaya TA, Tsoumpou I, Nardo LG. The likelihood of live birth and multiple birth after single versus double embryo transfer at the cleavage stage: a systematic review and meta-analysis. *Fertil Steril* 2009; **94**(3): 936–45.
29. Felberbaum RE. Multiple pregnancies after assisted reproduction – international comparison. *Reprod Biomed Online* 2007; **15** Suppl 3: 53–60.
30. Bedard J, Brule S, Price CA, Silversides DW, Lussier JG. Serine protease inhibitor-E2 (SERPINE2) is differentially expressed in granulosa cells of dominant follicle in cattle. *Mol Reprod Dev* 2003; **64**(2): 152–65.
31. Evans AC, Ireland JL, Winn ME, *et al.* Identification of genes involved in apoptosis and dominant follicle development during follicular waves in cattle. *Biol Reprod* 2004; **70**(5): 1475–84.
32. Mihm M, Baker PJ, Ireland JL, *et al.* Molecular evidence that growth of dominant follicles involves a reduction in follicle-stimulating hormone dependence and an increase in luteinizing hormone dependence in cattle. *Biol Reprod* 2006; **74**(6): 1051–9.
33. Wells D, Patrizio P. Gene expression profiling of human oocytes at different maturational stages and after in vitro maturation. *Am J Obstet Gynecol* 2008; **198**(4): 455.e1–9; discussion 455.e9–11.
34. Gilbert I, Robert C, Dieleman S, Blondin P, Sirard MA. Transcriptional effect of the LH surge in bovine granulosa cells during the peri-ovulation period. *Reproduction* 2011; **141**(2): 193–205.
35. Grondahl ML, Borup R, Lee YB, *et al.* Differences in gene expression of granulosa cells from women undergoing controlled ovarian hyperstimulation with either recombinant follicle-stimulating hormone or highly purified human menopausal gonadotropin. *Fertil Steril* 2009; **91**(5): 1820–30.
36. Bettegowda A, Patel OV, Lee KB, *et al.* Identification of novel bovine cumulus cell molecular markers predictive of oocyte competence: functional and diagnostic implications. *Biol Reprod* 2008; **79**(2): 301–9.
37. Burns KH, Owens GE, Ogbonna SC, Nilson JH, Matzuk MM. Expression profiling analyses of gonadotropin responses and tumor development in the absence of inhibins. *Endocrinology* 2003; **144**(10): 4492–507.
38. Fayad T, Levesque V, Sirois J, Silversides DW, Lussier JG. Gene expression profiling of differentially expressed genes in granulosa cells of bovine dominant follicles using suppression subtractive hybridization. *Biol Reprod* 2004; **70**(2): 523–33.
39. Ferrari S, Lattuada D, Paffoni A, *et al.* Procedure for rapid oocyte selection based on quantitative analysis of cumulus cell gene expression. *J Assist Reprod Genet* 2010; **27**(7): 429–34.
40. Feuerstein P, Cadoret V, Dalbies-Tran R, *et al.* Gene expression in human cumulus cells: one approach to oocyte competence. *Hum Reprod* 2007; **22**(12): 3069–77.
41. Koks S, Velthut A, Sarapik A, *et al.* The differential transcriptome and ontology profiles of floating and cumulus granulosa cells in stimulated human antral follicles. *Mol Hum Reprod* 2010; **16**(4): 229–40.
42. Hamel M, Dufort I, Robert C, *et al.* Identification of differentially expressed markers in human follicular

cells associated with competent oocytes. *Hum Reprod* 2008; **23**(5): 1118–27.

43. Hamel M, Dufort I, Robert C, *et al.* Genomic assessment of follicular marker genes as pregnancy predictors for human IVF. *Mol Hum Reprod* 2010; **16**(2): 87–96.

44. Hamel M, Dufort I, Robert C, *et al.* Identification of follicular marker genes as pregnancy predictors for human IVF: new evidence for the involvement of luteinization process. *Mol Hum Reprod* 2010; **16**(8): 548–56.

45. Nivet AL, Bunel A Labrecque R, *et al.* FSH withdrawal improves developmental competence of oocytes in the bovine model. *Reproduction* 2012; **143**(2): 165–71.

46. Tatemoto H, Terada T. Time-dependent effects of cycloheximide and alpha-amanitin on meiotic resumption and progression in bovine follicular oocytes. *Theriogenology* 1995; **43**(6): 1107–13.

47. Tanghe S, Van Soom A, Nauwynck H, Coryn M, de Kruif A. Minireview: Functions of the cumulus oophorus during oocyte maturation, ovulation, and fertilization. *Mol Reprod Dev* 2002; **61**(3): 414–24.

48. Tanghe S, Van Soom A, Mehrzad J, *et al.* Cumulus contributions during bovine fertilization in vitro. *Theriogenology* 2003; **60**(1): 135–49.

49. Sutton ML, Gilchrist RB, Thompson JG. Effects of in-vivo and in-vitro environments on the metabolism of the cumulus-oocyte complex and its influence on oocyte developmental capacity. *Hum Reprod Update* 2003; **9**(1): 35–48.

50. Matzuk MM, Burns KH, Viveiros MM, Eppig JJ. Intercellular communication in the mammalian ovary: oocytes carry the conversation. *Science* 2002; **296**(5576): 2178–80.

51. Atef A, Francois P, Christian V, Marc-Andre S. The potential role of gap junction communication between cumulus cells and bovine oocytes during in vitro maturation. *Mol Reprod Dev* 2005; **71**(3): 358–67.

52. Peddinti D, Memili E, Burgess SC. Proteomics-based systems biology modeling of bovine germinal vesicle stage oocyte and cumulus cell interaction. *PLoS One* 2010; **5**(6): e11240.

53. Assidi M, Dufort I, Ali A, *et al.* Identification of potential markers of oocyte competence expressed in bovine cumulus cells matured with follicle-stimulating hormone and/or phorbol myristate acetate in vitro. *Biol Reprod* 2008; **79**(2): 209–22.

54. Assou S, Haouzi D, Mahmoud K, *et al.* A non-invasive test for assessing embryo potential by gene expression profiles of human cumulus cells: a proof of concept study. *Mol Hum Reprod* 2008; **14**(12): 711–19.

55. Assou S, Haouzi D, De Vos J, Hamamah S. Human cumulus cells as biomarkers for embryo and pregnancy outcomes. *Mol Hum Reprod* 2010; **16**(8): 531–8.

56. Assou S, Anahory T, Pantesco V, *et al.* The human cumulus–oocyte complex gene-expression profile. *Hum Reprod* 2006; **21**(7): 1705–19.

57. Assidi M, Montag M, Van Der Ven K, Sirard MA. Biomarkers of human oocyte developmental competence expressed in cumulus cells before ICSI: a preliminary study. *J Assist Reprod Genet* 2011; **28**(2): 173–81.

58. Huang Z, Wells D. The human oocyte and cumulus cells relationship: new insights from the cumulus cell transcriptome. *Mol Hum Reprod* 2010; **16**(10): 715–25.

59. Reich A, Klatsky P, Carson S, Wessel G. The transcriptome of a human polar body accurately reflects its sibling oocyte. *J Biol Chem* 2011; **286**(47):40743–9.

60. Spitzer D, Murach KF, Lottspeich F, Staudach A, Illmensee K. Different protein patterns derived from follicular fluid of mature and immature human follicles. *Hum Reprod* 1996;**11**(4): 798–807.

61. Angelucci S, Ciavardelli D, Di Giuseppe F, *et al.* Proteome analysis of human follicular fluid. *Biochim Biophys Acta* 2006; **1764**(11): 1775–85.

62. Jarkovska K, Martinkova J, Liskova L, *et al.* Proteome mining of human follicular fluid reveals a crucial role of complement cascade and key biological pathways in women undergoing in vitro fertilization. *J Proteome Res* 2010; **9**(3): 1289–301.

Section 5 Pathology

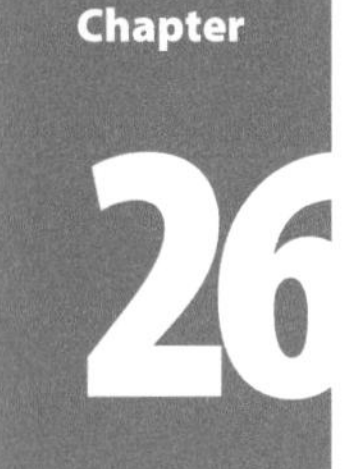

The legacy of mitochondrial DNA

Helen A. L. Tuppen, Mary Herbert, and Doug M. Turnbull

Introduction

Present in all nucleated cells, mitochondria are essential subcellular organelles that play a crucial role in several different biochemical processes, including energy production. Mitochondria are believed to be evolutionary relics of ancient bacterial symbionts [1], and an important legacy of this history is the persistence within these organelles of a small genome, termed mitochondrial DNA (mtDNA). MtDNA is the only extranuclear source of DNA in the cell and it follows a different mode of inheritance from nuclear DNA. We highlight the important role of mitochondria in reproduction and why this small molecule of DNA presents so many interesting and important challenges particularly in reproductive biology.

Mitochondrial function

Mitochondria are double-membraned structures which are central to a multitude of biological functions in all nucleated mammalian cells, including the regulation of apoptotic cell death, the control of cytosolic calcium concentration, and the biogenesis of iron–sulfur clusters. Mitochondria are also the primary source of endogenous reactive oxygen species and they house several critical biochemical pathways, including the tricarboxylic acid cycle and part of the urea cycle. However, arguably the most important function of mitochondria is the production of ATP, the energy carrier of the cell, via oxidative phosphorylation (OXPHOS). OXPHOS requires the coordinated activity of five multi-subunit enzyme complexes located in the inner mitochondrial membrane. Electrons, resulting from the oxidation of fat and carbohydrates, are transported along complexes I–IV, thus creating an electrochemical gradient for protons across the inner mitochondrial membrane that drives the synthesis of ATP by complex V (ATP synthase).

Mitochondrial DNA

Mitochondrial DNA is a circular, double-stranded DNA molecule, present in multiple copies in all nucleated cells (Figure 26.1). The complete sequence of the human mitochondrial genome was elucidated in 1981 [2, 3] and contains 16 569 base pairs. It encodes 37 genes, located on both its heavy (H; guanine-rich) and light (L; cytosine-rich) strands. Thirteen of these genes encode subunits of the respiratory chain enzyme complexes, while the remainder encode the 22 transfer RNAs (tRNA) and 2 ribosomal RNAs (rRNA) necessary for the translation of these polypeptides. All other proteins required for mitochondrial structure, maintenance, and metabolism are encoded by the nuclear genome and are specifically targeted, sorted, and imported to their correct mitochondrial location from the cytosol [4].

The mitochondrial genome is extremely compact. It contains no introns, there are a number of overlapping coding regions (namely *MT-ATP6* and *MT-ATP8*, and *MT-ND4* and *MT-ND4L*), and several transcripts lack a complete termination codon, which is added post-transcriptionally by polyadenylation [5]. Furthermore, there are merely two intergenic noncoding regions in the genome, the origin of light chain replication (O_L) and the 1.1 kb-long displacement loop (D-loop), so called as it is formed by the displacement of the two genomic strands by a third single-stranded DNA molecule. The D-loop harbors the transcriptional promoters for both the H- and L-strands and one of the proposed origins of replication (O_H).

Biology and Pathology of the Oocyte, 2nd edn., ed. Alan Trounson, Roger Gosden, and Ursula Eichenlaub-Ritter. Published by Cambridge University Press.

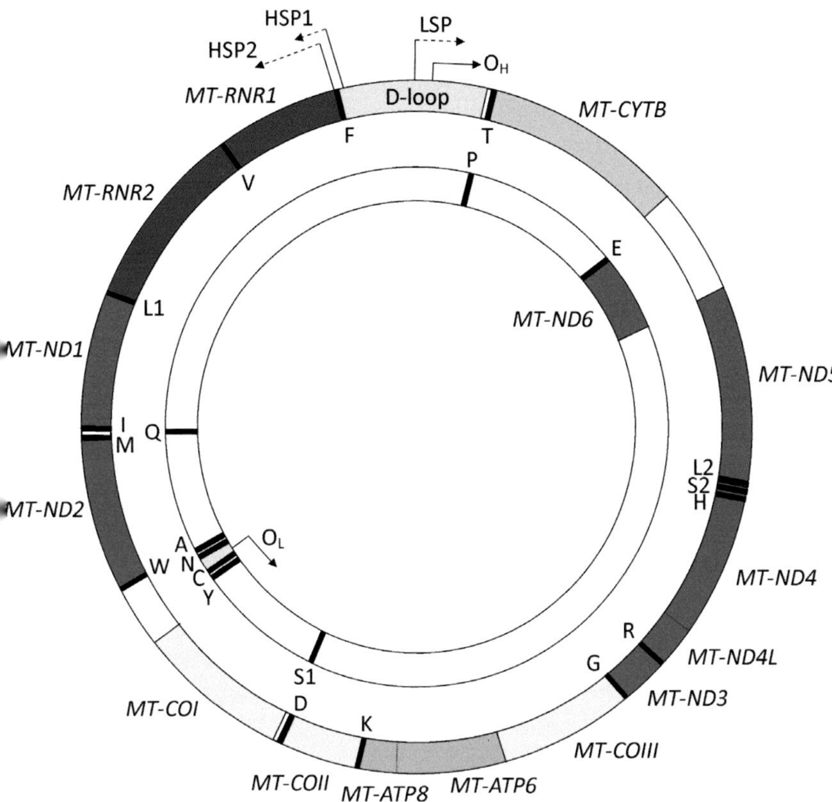

Figure 26.1 The human mitochondrial genome. Schematic diagram of the ~16.6 kb circular, double-stranded human mitochondrial genome. The human mtDNA encodes 37 genes, which are indicated on the strand, heavy (H; outer circle) or light (L; inner circle), containing the coding sequence. The two mt-rRNA genes are represented in red and the 22 mt-tRNA genes are depicted as black bars, denoted by their single-letter abbreviation. The genes encoding seven subunits of respiratory chain complex I are shown in blue, the complex III gene *MT-CYTB* in orange, the three catalytic subunits of complex IV in yellow, and the two subunits of complex V in green. Non-coding regions of the genome, represented in gray, include the origin of L-strand replication (O_L) and the 1.1 kb D-loop. The latter contains several regulatory sequences, namely the origin of H-strand replication (O_H) and the transcription initiation sites for both strands (HSP1, HSP2, and LSP). Transcription from HSP1 generates a short transcript that terminates at the MT-RNR2/MT-TL1 boundary; HSP2 transcription produces a polycistronic transcript of almost the entire H-strand.

It is commonly accepted that mtDNA is continually turned over in the cell, independently of the nuclear genome and the cell cycle [6]. However, the mechanism of mtDNA replication has been debated over the last decade (reviewed in [7]). A traditional strand-asynchronous method proposes that mtDNA replication initiates on the H-strand at O_H. After two-thirds of the H-strand has been replicated, the O_L is uncovered, at which point replication of the displaced L-strand can commence in the opposite direction. A second, more conventional strand-synchronous replication mechanism postulates that bidirectional replication of the H- and L-strands is launched from a zone of replication (OriZ) located near O_H and proceeds via conventional coupled leading- and lagging-strand synthesis, probably involving the synthesis of short Okazaki fragments. It is currently thought that both models likely exist and their occurrence is cell type dependent, with the original strand-displacement method more prevalent in cells in a steady state and the leading–lagging-strand model more predominant in cells requiring rapid mtDNA synthesis [8].

In both models, mtDNA replication is performed by a single mtDNA polymerase, POLG, which also mediates mtDNA recombination and repair [9]. Two additional nuclear-encoded factors are key components of the mtDNA replisome: the helicase Twinkle and the single-stranded binding protein mt-SSB [10].

mtDNA transcription occurs from one of two promoters on the H-strand (HSP1, situated upstream of the *MT-TF* gene, and HSP2, at the 5′ end of the

MT-RNR1 gene) and from a single promoter on the L-strand (LSP, located in the D-loop). Transcription from HSP2 and LSP generates almost genome-length polycistronic transcripts, whereas HSP1 produces a shorter transcript consisting only of the two mt-rRNAs (12S and 16S) and mt-tRNA^{Phe} and mt-tRNA^{Val}. MtDNA transcription is performed by various nuclear-encoded factors including a single-subunit RNA polymerase (POLRMT), the transcriptional activator TFAM, the transcription factor TFB2M, and the termination factor mTERF. Maturation of the polycistronic mitochondrial transcripts relies upon 5′ (RNase P) and 3′ (RNase Z) endonuclease recognition and cleavage of mt-tRNAs, indirectly releasing processed mRNAs and rRNAs as a consequence [11]. Further post-transcriptional modifications of the RNAs are necessary (e.g., mt-tRNA CCA addition, mt-mRNA polyadenylation) to obtain fully functional molecules ready for translation.

Like nuclear DNA, mtDNA molecules are assembled into stable protein–DNA aggregates. These nucleoids are approximately 70 nm in diameter and in somatic cells contain on average six copies of mtDNA [12]. Key proteins involved in mtDNA replication, maintenance, repair, and recombination (e.g., POLG, mt-SSB, and TFAM) are just some of the major constituent proteins associated with these macrocomplexes. Nucleoids are tethered to the inner mitochondrial membrane, in close proximity to the mitochondrial respiratory chain, a potent source of reactive oxygen species.

Oocyte mitochondria

Mature oocyte mitochondria possess several distinguishing features. Firstly, they are generally discrete, small, immature, spherical structures, less than 1 μm in diameter, with few cristae and an electron dense matrix, quite distinct from their fully differentiated somatic cell counterparts, which are highly dynamic organelles that constantly fuse and divide, creating large interconnected networks [13]. By contrast, mitochondrial fission and fusion cycles are believed to be quite rare in growing oocytes [14]. Secondly, mature oocyte mitochondria are traditionally considered to harbor only one or two mtDNA molecules [15, 16], unlike somatic organelles, which generally contain between two and ten. This assumption of mtDNA genomic distribution has frequently been used along with measurements of mtDNA copy number to determine the number of mitochondria in the mature ooplasm. With mtDNA copy number estimates ranging from 2×10^4 to 10^7 (reviewed in [17]), average mature human oocytes are thought to harbor several hundred thousand mitochondria, and numbers of mitochondria between oocytes from a same cohort can potentially differ by over an order of magnitude. It must be noted here, however, that whilst this statistic of one to two genomes/organelle has been frequently reported in the literature, it has not yet been directly measured in human oocytes and current estimates of mitochondrial numbers in the mature ooplasm are considered to be a gross overestimation [18].

Thirdly, with the exception of the porcine oocyte, it is widely accepted that mtDNA replication and transcription are suspended in the mature mammalian oocyte, and that these processes are not re-established until after fertilization [19]. Active transcription of the mitochondrial genome appears to recommence in a species-specific manner, around the time of embryonic genome activation. In mice, mtDNA transcription begins at the late 2-cell stage, whereas it occurs in the 4- to 8-cell stage in humans and in the 8- to 16-cell stage in cattle (reviewed in [20]). mtDNA replication does not take place during early embryogenesis and the number of mtDNA molecules per blastomere progressively decreases in conjunction with cytoplasmic volume with each embryonic cell division. It is only at the blastocyst stage that the expression of mtDNA replication factors is up-regulated and mtDNA replication resumes, initially in the trophectodermal cells. Mitochondrial ultrastructure also changes at this time; the organelles become more elongated, with swollen cristae and increased OXPHOS activity [21]. During oogenesis, mtDNA copy number steadily increases in parallel with cytoplasmic volume, from approximately 200 molecules in primordial germ cells (PGCs) [22–24] to an estimated 10 000 in primordial follicle oocytes (reviewed in [25]). Morphologically, the organelles become more rounded and oval-shaped (Figure 26.2).

Mitochondrial DNA inheritance

In contrast to nuclear DNA, mtDNA is only transmitted down the female line [26]. Mature mammalian sperm possess fewer than 100 mitochondria (reviewed

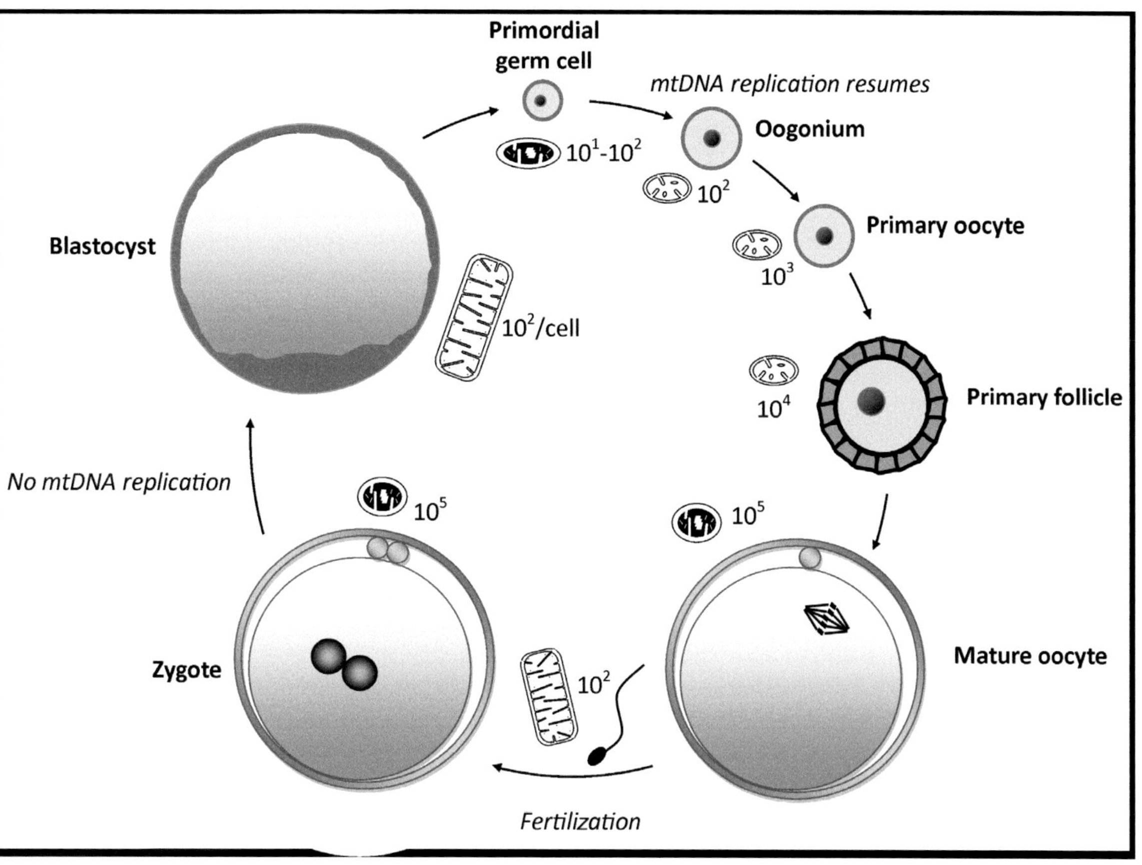

Figure 26.2 Mitochondrial DNA copy number during development of the female germ line. Mitochondrial morphology and an estimate of the number of mtDNA molecules at each stage of development are indicated.

in [27]). Furthermore, there is an active degradation of sperm mitochondria after fertilization. In early primate and bovine embryos, sperm mitochondria are ubiquitinated, likely targeting the organelles for destruction by the ubiquitin proteasome system [28]. In fish, paternal mtDNA is thought to be enzymatically digested [29]. Recently, the removal of sperm mitochondria in fertilized *Caenorhabditis elegans* and mouse oocytes has been shown to occur by autophagy [30, 31]. Post-fertilization degradation of paternal mitochondria must also occur in humans. Mature human sperm have been shown to contain mtDNA [32] and, while there has been a reported case of paternal mtDNA inheritance in a single patient [33], subsequent population-based studies have uncovered no further evidence of paternal transmission through the human germ line [34, 35]. In addition, concerns over increased risks of paternal mtDNA inheritance following intracytoplasmic sperm injection, a procedure which bypasses various stages of natural fertilization and may bypass the as yet undetermined mechanism by which paternal mitochondria are degraded in the human embryo, have so far proven unfounded [36]. The strict maternal inheritance of mtDNA has been used to map the evolution of species for many years and analyzing mtDNA has been crucial in proposing that modern humans are all descended from a single woman from Africa about 200 000 years ago ("Mitochondrial Eve")[37].

Mitochondrial DNA diseases

Without protective histones and only rudimentary DNA repair mechanisms, the mitochondrial genome is highly susceptible to mutations. Pathogenic mtDNA mutations were first identified in the late 1980s [38, 39] and currently more than 250 have been reported, associated with a group of clinically heterogeneous disorders, commonly defined by a lack of ATP production [40]. Mutations of the mitochondrial genome are either large-scale rearrangements (mostly mtDNA deletions) or point mutations.

mtDNA diseases are often severe and progressive, and tend to involve tissues heavily dependent upon oxidative metabolism such as the brain, heart, and skeletal muscles. However, the clinical features are very variable and patients may present at any age. For specific mutations there are some characteristic clinical features; for example large-scale single mtDNA deletions cause Kearns–Sayre syndrome, the m.3243A>G mutation is associated with MELAS (mitochondrial encephalomyopathy, lactic acidosis, and stroke-like episodes), and the m.8344A>G mutation results in MERRF (myoclonic epilepsy with ragged red fibers). However, even with specific mutations there can be a marked variation in phenotype. Patients who harbor the m.3243A>G mutation might develop severe symptoms with stroke-like episodes, seizures, and cognitive impairment whilst others remain asymptomatic or only present with diabetes and deafness.

The prevalence of clinically manifest mtDNA disease in the North East of England has been estimated to be at least 1 in 10 000 with a further 1 in 6000 at risk [41]. However, recent birth prevalence studies have reported m.3243A>G mutation frequencies of 0.14–0.2%, suggesting the perceived incidence of mtDNA disease is most likely an underestimation [42, 43].

Due to the multicopy nature of mtDNA, mtDNA mutations may be either homoplasmic (all mtDNA molecules are mutated) or heteroplasmic (both mutated and wild-type mtDNA molecules coexist in a cell). The vast majority of mtDNA mutations are functionally recessive and in the presence of heteroplasmy a biochemical defect will only develop when levels of mutated mtDNA accumulate above a critical threshold, specific for each mtDNA mutation, but typically ranging from 60% to 90% of mutated mtDNA. In each cell, including post-mitotic cells, mtDNA replicates autonomously. This leads to a marked variation in levels of heteroplasmy among different cells in the same tissue, often resulting in a mosaic pattern of respiratory chain deficiency.

Levels of heteroplasmy are also crucial to determining the clinical phenotype in patients. As discussed above, the same mtDNA mutation may present with very different clinical features in different patients. For example, an individual with only a 5% m.3243A>G mutation load will not develop symptoms whereas someone with a 90% mutation load is likely to have very severe disease.

Transmission of mitochondrial DNA mutations

In view of the maternal pattern of transmission of mtDNA, patients carrying mtDNA mutations are at risk of transmitting mtDNA disease to their offspring. For patients with homoplasmic mtDNA mutations all offspring will inherit the mutation at homoplasmic levels. However, with heteroplasmic mtDNA mutations the situation is more complicated. Pedigree analyses of heteroplasmic cattle and humans have shown that mtDNA genotypes shift rapidly between generations with a return to homoplasmy in some progeny (reviewed in [44]). These observations suggest the existence during development of an evolutionary mechanism to prevent mutational meltdown of the mitochondrial genome by Muller's ratchet, that is, a genetic bottleneck to decrease the mutation load in the presence of uniparental inheritance. The precise mechanism by which this genetic bottleneck occurs is still under intense debate. One hypothesis proposes that a marked reduction in mtDNA copy number immediately prior to PGC expansion may be the basis of the mtDNA bottleneck [23]. Conversely, the bottleneck may be generated through the unequal partitioning of nucleoids between PGCs, without a reduction in mtDNA content [22]. Alternatively, the mtDNA bottleneck had been suggested to occur during postnatal folliculogenesis and not during embryonic oogenesis, as a result of the replication of a subpopulation of mitochondrial genomes during oocyte maturation in postnatal life (Figure 26.3) [24]. However, a recent report by Freyer and colleagues, which examined the transmission in mice of a heteroplasmic single base pair deletion in the mitochondrial tRNA^{Met} gene, provides further compelling evidence for a prenatal timing for the mtDNA bottleneck, during the development of the female germ line [45]. The transmission of mtDNA mutations has been studied in mice expressing error-prone mtDNA polymerase (POLG). These mice accumulate a large number of different mtDNA mutations which are present in the oocytes and thus provide an excellent model for studying the genomic changes able to pass through the bottleneck. The studies revealed a very strong selection against mutations in the protein-encoding genes of mtDNA but not for mt-tRNA mutations [46].

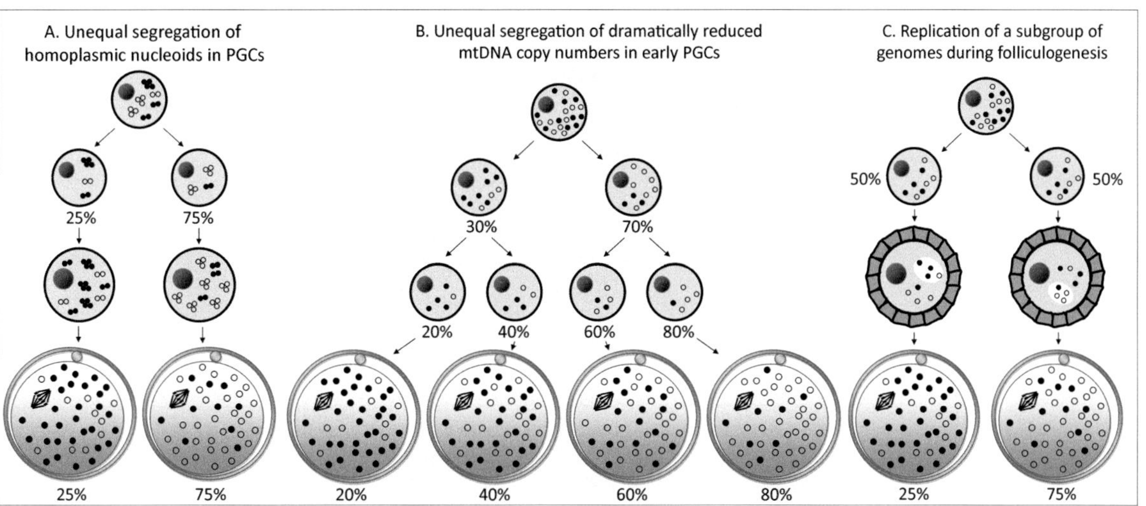

Figure 26.3 Models for the mtDNA genetic bottleneck. Three different mechanisms have been proposed to explain rapid variations in heteroplasmy between single generations. (A) Unequal segregation of homoplasmic nucleoids, each containing multiple copies of mtDNA, in primordial germ cells (PGCs) [22]. (B) Unequal segregation of dramatically reduced mtDNA copy numbers in early PGCs [23]. (C) Replication of a subgroup of mitochondrial genomes during folliculogenesis in postnatal life [24]. White ellipses highlight the molecules selected for replication.

The consequences of this genetic bottleneck are seen in mothers with mtDNA mutations. Some mtDNA mutations such as large-scale single mtDNA deletions or some protein-encoding mtDNA point mutations are only rarely transmitted through to offspring, presumably due to the strong selection which was also seen in mice. For other heteroplasmic mtDNA mutations, particularly those involving mt-tRNA genes, transmission through the germ line occurs but there is often marked variation in the level of heteroplasmy between offspring. Since the level of heteroplasmy is the main determinant of the phenotype in individual patients, the genetic bottleneck can lead to offspring with very different clinical features and clinical outcomes.

Current reproductive options for women carrying an mtDNA mutation

There are very limited treatment options for patients with mtDNA disease. These treatments tend to be supportive, for example management of diabetes and epilepsy. At present there is no curative therapy and for families with mtDNA mutations trying to prevent severe disease in offspring is a priority. Genetic counseling is important to explain the risks involved, but must be given carefully, taking account of the specific mutation and the number of affected family members. In some countries oocyte donation is an option, but oocytes tend to be in short supply and do not provide the option for an affected woman to have a genetically related child.

For women with heteroplasmic mtDNA mutations other options might be appropriate. Recent studies have shown that the level of heteroplasmic mtDNA mutations does not vary between different tissues and cells in the early embryo and developing fetus [47]. Consequently, for some mtDNA mutations both prenatal and preimplantation genetic diagnosis (PGD) are options. There are now several examples of successful pregnancies using these techniques, with offspring with low levels of a pathogenic mtDNA mutation [48].

For women harboring high levels of heteroplasmic or homoplasmic mutations, PGD and prenatal genetic diagnosis are not an option. New techniques to prevent transmission of mtDNA defects are being explored. One approach involves transplanting the nuclear genome from an oocyte or zygote from an affected woman to those from a healthy donor [49]. This has the potential to enable women to have a genetically related child without transmitting mutated mtDNA.

There are two main approaches to the prevention – pronuclear transfer and metaphase II spindle transfer (Figure 26.4). Pronuclear transfer has been used in

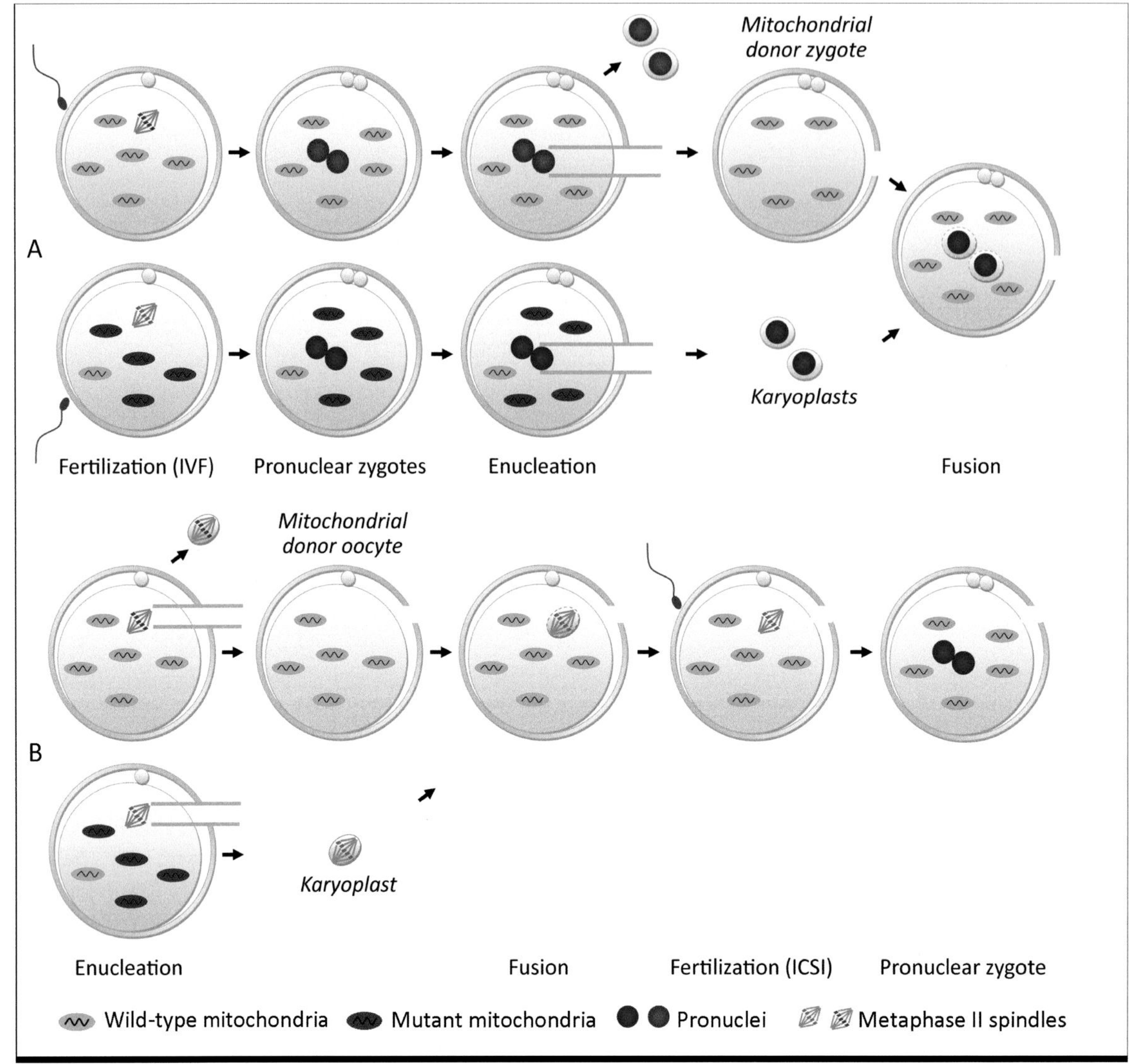

Figure 26.4 Nuclear transfer techniques to prevent the transmission of mtDNA disease. (A) Pronuclear transfer between human zygotes. Pronuclei are removed in small volumes of membrane-bound cytoplasm (karyoplasts) from an in vitro fertilized (IVF) mitochondrial donor zygote and replaced with the pronuclei from a nuclear donor zygote. (B) Metaphase II spindle transfer between human oocytes. The metaphase II spindle is removed in a karyoplast from a mitochondrial donor oocyte and replaced with the spindle from a spindle donor oocyte. The oocyte is then fertilized by intracytoplasmic sperm injection (ICSI).

mice for some years and has been shown to be compatible with onward development and birth of normal offspring [50]. It was later demonstrated that pronuclear transfer is effective in preventing transmission of an mtDNA rearrangement in a mouse model of mtDNA disease [51]. More recently, proof of principle experiments have been conducted using abnormally fertilized human zygotes [52]. These later experiments showed that the approach is feasible in humans and the carryover of mtDNA from the donor zygote was either undetectable or around 2%. From studies in patients we are aware that this level of heteroplasmy would not lead to mtDNA disease (for most mtDNA mutations the threshold for disease is >60%). A related technique involving transplantation of the metaphase II spindle between unfertilized oocytes followed by ICSI has resulted in live-born primates [53].

These techniques raise a number of ethical and legal issues. In the UK there is permission under the Human Fertilisation and Embryology (HFE) Act 2008 to carry out this research in the laboratory, but the Act prohibits an embryo which has undergone these manipulations from being implanted into a woman. However, if an acceptably safe and effective technique does become possible, then the HFE Act enables secondary legislation to be passed by Parliament to permit its use. Recently the Nuffield Council on Bioethics, an influential independent body that examines and reports on ethical issues in biology and medicine, issued a report examining whether such techniques would be ethical. Its report, entitled *Novel techniques for the prevention of mitochondrial DNA disorders*, concludes: "Due to the health and social benefits to individuals and families of living free from mitochondrial disorders, and where potential parents express a preference to have genetically-related children, on balance we believe that if these novel techniques are adequately proven to be acceptably safe and effective as treatments, it would be ethical for families to use them, if they wish to do so and have been offered an appropriate level of information and support."

Mitochondrial DNA and mammalian fertility

Relative to other mammalian cells, oocytes possess an abundant reserve of mtDNA molecules, a fact that has prompted much interest in establishing and understanding the importance of mitochondria and their genomes to fertility. OXPHOS is believed to be active throughout the reproductive process, from oogenesis through oocyte maturation and early embryogenesis to blastocyst development and implantation (reviewed in [17]). During the early stages of oocyte development, when the mitochondrial population is rapidly increasing, the metabolic requirements of the immature oocyte are mostly supported by the surrounding cumulus cells, with higher levels of ATP being recorded in oocytes enclosed in cumulus cells than those lacking these cells [54]. Cumulus cells supply substrates such as pyruvate and lactate to the glycolytic enzyme-deficient oocytes (reviewed in [55]). They may even compensate for metabolic impairments in growing oocytes; despite the conditional knockout of *Pdha1*, a gene encoding an enzymatic subunit of the pyruvate dehydrogenase complex, which catalyzes the first step in the oxidative metabolism of pyruvate, mouse oocyte development is still maintained until ovulation [56]. At oocyte maturation, cytoplasmic connections with the follicle cells are disrupted and mitochondrial biogenesis and mtDNA replication are suspended. Presumably the mitochondrial content in the fully grown oocyte is sufficient to support fertilization and maintain embryonic development until mtDNA replication resumes at the blastocyst stage [19, 20]. It is therefore only at the onset of oocyte maturation that mitochondrial dysfunction is likely to be expressed in the oocyte [56]. In view of the high energy demands of oogenesis and embryogenesis, it is not surprising that there is active debate to determine if any structural or numerical defects of the mitochondria and their genomes will impact adversely on the ability of the fertilized oocyte to develop.

mtDNA copy number, ATP production, and embryo developmental competence have thus been a subject of study for many years. It has been found that mammalian meiotic maturation can occur over a wide range of ATP contents [57], although mature human oocytes with ATP levels $\geq$2 pmol have a much higher potential for continued embryogenesis and implantation. mtDNA copy numbers in mature human oocytes can also vary considerably, even in oocytes from the same individual. Estimates currently range from approximately 2×10^4 to 10^7 copies per oocyte (reviewed in [17]). A low mtDNA copy number appears to adversely affect the ability of the oocyte to become fertilized [58]. A positive association between infertility and mtDNA depletion, arising as a result of a mutation in the *POLG* gene, has been established (reviewed in [59]). Furthermore, oocytes of women with ovarian insufficiency have been found to contain, on average, threefold fewer copies of mtDNA [60]. Conversely, high mitochondrial and ATP content are reported to increase the quality and competence of mature mammalian oocytes [61]. Wai and colleagues recently established the critical threshold of mtDNA molecules required for normal embryonic development [62]. Using a heterozygous *Tfam* knockout mouse model, with an average 90% reduction in mtDNA content relative to controls, they showed that oocytes with as few as 4000 mtDNA copies can be fertilized and develop to the blastocyst stage. However, a minimum of 40 000–50 000 molecules were required for post-implantation development to proceed.

The importance of mitochondria in fertility has been further extended with the suggestion of their involvement in age-related female infertility. Most women are infertile by their mid-to-late forties and the oocyte is considered the main locus for reproductive senescence [63], characterized by aneuploidy and a depletion of molecular stores, specifically transcripts of loci involved in cell-cycle regulation, oxidative stress, and mitochondrial functions [64]. Mitochondria play a central role in the aging of somatic tissues; as a major site of reactive oxygen species production, mitochondria are prime targets for the progressive accumulation of oxidative damage, ultimately leading to a decline in their function (reviewed in [65]). Primordial oocytes may remain in a resting phase for over 40 years, maintaining a low level of OXPHOS. The constant exposure of the mitochondria and their DNA to free radical attack has led many to believe that mitochondrial aging may underlie the meiotic aberrations and failed embryonic development that are associated with advanced maternal age. In support of this theory, mitochondria in human oocytes from aged women have been shown to present ultrastructural features similar to their somatic counterparts in aged tissues and organs, such as swelling and vacuolization [66]. Furthermore, in vitro maturation of mouse oocytes cultured with the oxidizing agent tertiary butyl hydroperoxide induces an increase in the incidence of aneuploidy [67], and the exposure of MII oocytes from young mice to hydrogen peroxide leads to a decrease in ATP content and a disruption of meiotic spindles [68]. If mitochondrial dysfunction were indeed the cause of age-related infertility then a deficiency in ATP content in oocytes from older women might be expected. To date, there is however no evidence that ATP levels in older oocytes differ significantly from those in younger gametes. Furthermore, while increases in levels of mtDNA mutations and large-scale rearrangements are commonly observed with age in somatic tissues, including in cumulus cells [69, 70], where age-dependent increases in the levels of the common 4977 base pair mitochondrial deletion have been negatively correlated with pregnancy rates [70], there are conflicting reports on whether similar age-associated mtDNA defects accumulate in human oocytes (reviewed in [71]). Nevertheless, some functional consequences of age have been observed; mitochondrial membrane potential reportedly decreases with age [21], and chromosome scattering and decondensation have been linked to mitochondrial clustering in the ooplasm of older female mice [72]. Further investigations are necessary to uncover exactly if and how mitochondrial dysfunction may be involved in oocyte senescence.

It is becoming increasingly apparent that while OXPHOS is important for oocyte developmental competence, it certainly does not support oogenesis, embryogenesis, and fetal development alone. Indeed, early embryonic development and implantation can persist in the absence of OXPHOS in mice [19] and the occurrence of individuals with severely deleterious mtDNA mutations indicates that the presence of dysfunctional mitochondria per se is not a barrier for fertilization or gestation to term. Wilding *et al.* have proposed that, whilst OXPHOS is continually active during embryo development, additional requirements for energy are supplied through the less-efficient process of anaerobic respiration [17].

Conclusion

Mitochondrial biology and genetics in reproductive biology remains an area of major research activity. Mitochondria are numerous in the oocyte but have different characteristics to those in most somatic cells. The maternal pattern of inheritance of mtDNA has also increased interest in this area because of the importance of mtDNA disease. There are many challenges ahead, not least in trying to prevent transmission of mtDNA disease. However, with new approaches for exploring mitochondrial physiology using live-cell imaging and the development of new IVF-related techniques such as pronuclear transfer and metaphase II spindle transfer, it is likely that we will be able to better understand and perhaps mitigate some of the potential harmful effects of the legacy of mitochondria.

References

1. Margulis L. Symbiosis and evolution. *Sci Am* 1971; **225**(2): 48–57.
2. Anderson S, Bankier AT, Barrell BG, *et al.* Sequence and organization of the human mitochondrial genome. *Nature* 1981; **290**(5806): 457–65.
3. Andrews RM, Kubacka I, Chinnery PF, *et al.* Reanalysis and revision of the Cambridge reference sequence for human mitochondrial DNA. *Nat Genet* 1999; **23**(2): 147.
4. Mokranjac D, Neupert W. Protein import into mitochondria. *Biochem Soc Trans* 2005; **33**(Pt 5): 1019–23.
5. Ojala D, Montoya J, Attardi G. tRNA punctuation model of RNA processing in human mitochondria. *Nature* 1981; **290**(5806): 470–4.

6. Bogenhagen D, Clayton DA. Mouse L cell mitochondrial DNA molecules are selected randomly for replication throughout the cell cycle. *Cell* 1977; **11**(4): 719–27.
7. Holt IJ. Mitochondrial DNA replication and repair: all a flap. *Trends Biochem Sci* 2009; **34**(7): 358–65.
8. Fish J, Raule N, Attardi G. Discovery of a major D-loop replication origin reveals two modes of human mtDNA synthesis. *Science* 2004; **306**(5704): 2098–101.
9. Graziewicz MA, Longley MJ, Copeland WC. DNA polymerase gamma in mitochondrial DNA replication and repair. *Chem Rev* 2006; **106**(2): 383–405.
10. Korhonen JA, Pham XH, Pellegrini M, *et al.* Reconstitution of a minimal mtDNA replisome in vitro. *EMBO J* 2004; **23**(12): 2423–9.
11. Rossmanith W. Of P and Z: mitochondrial tRNA processing enzymes. *Biochim Biophys Acta* 2012; **1819**(9–10): 1017–26.
12. Holt IJ, He J, Mao CC, *et al.* Mammalian mitochondrial nucleoids: organizing an independently minded genome. *Mitochondrion* 2007; **7**(5): 311–21.
13. Bereiter-Hahn J. Behavior of mitochondria in the living cell. *Int Rev Cytol* 1990; **122**: 1–63.
14. Sathananthan AH, Trounson AO. Mitochondrial morphology during preimplantational human embryogenesis. *Hum Reprod* 2000; **15** Suppl 2: 148–59.
15. Jansen RP. Germline passage of mitochondria: quantitative considerations and possible embryological sequelae. *Hum Reprod* 2000; **15** Suppl 2: 112–28.
16. Piko L, Matsumoto L. Number of mitochondria and some properties of mitochondrial DNA in the mouse egg. *Dev Biol* 1976; **49**(1): 1–10.
17. Wilding M, Coppola G, Dale B, *et al.* Mitochondria and human preimplantation embryo development. *Reproduction* 2009; **137**(4): 619–24.
18. Van Blerkom J. Mitochondrial function in the human oocyte and embryo and their role in developmental competence. *Mitochondrion* 2011; **11**(5): 797–813.
19. Larsson NG, Wang J, Wilhelmsson H, *et al.* Mitochondrial transcription factor A is necessary for mtDNA maintenance and embryogenesis in mice. *Nat Genet* 1998; **18**(3): 231–6.
20. St John JC, Facucho-Oliveira J, Jiang Y, *et al.* Mitochondrial DNA transmission, replication and inheritance: a journey from the gamete through the embryo and into offspring and embryonic stem cells. *Hum Reprod Update* 2010; **16**(5): 488–509.
21. Wilding M, Dale B, Marino M, *et al.* Mitochondrial aggregation patterns and activity in human oocytes and preimplantation embryos. *Hum Reprod* 2001; **16**(5): 909–17.
22. Cao L, Shitara H, Horii T, *et al.* The mitochondrial bottleneck occurs without reduction of mtDNA content in female mouse germ cells. *Nat Genet* 2007; **39**(3): 386–90.
23. Cree LM, Samuels DC, de Sousa Lopes SC, *et al.* A reduction of mitochondrial DNA molecules during embryogenesis explains the rapid segregation of genotypes. *Nat Genet* 2008; **40**(2): 249–54.
24. Wai T, Teoli D, Shoubridge EA. The mitochondrial DNA genetic bottleneck results from replication of a subpopulation of genomes. *Nat Genet* 2008; **40**(12): 1484–8.
25. Bogenhagen DF. Does mtDNA nucleoid organization impact aging? *Exp Gerontol* 2010; **45**(7–8): 473–7.
26. Giles RE, Blanc H, Cann HM, *et al.* Maternal inheritance of human mitochondrial DNA. *Proc Natl Acad Sci USA* 1980; **77**(11): 6715–19.
27. Ramalho-Santos J, Varum S, Amaral S, *et al.* Mitochondrial functionality in reproduction: from gonads and gametes to embryos and embryonic stem cells. *Hum Reprod Update* 2009; **15**(5): 553–72.
28. Sutovsky P, Moreno RD, Ramalho-Santos J, *et al.* Ubiquitin tag for sperm mitochondria. *Nature* 1999; **402**(6760): 371–2.
29. Nishimura Y, Yoshinari T, Naruse K, *et al.* Active digestion of sperm mitochondrial DNA in single living sperm revealed by optical tweezers. *Proc Natl Acad Sci USA* 2006; **103**(5): 1382–7.
30. Al Rawi S, Louvet-Vallee S, Djeddi A, *et al.* Postfertilization autophagy of sperm organelles prevents paternal mitochondrial DNA transmission. *Science* 2011; **334**(6059): 1144–7.
31. Sato M, Sato K. Degradation of paternal mitochondria by fertilization-triggered autophagy in *C. elegans* embryos. *Science* 2011; **334**(6059): 1141–4.
32. Manfredi G, Thyagarajan D, Papadopoulou LC, *et al.* The fate of human sperm-derived mtDNA in somatic cells. *Am J Hum Genet* 1997; **61**(4): 953–60.
33. Schwartz M, Vissing J. Paternal inheritance of mitochondrial DNA. *N Engl J Med* 2002; **347**(8): 576–80.
34. Taylor RW, McDonnell MT, Blakely EL, *et al.* Genotypes from patients indicate no paternal mitochondrial DNA contribution. *Ann Neurol* 2003; **54**(4): 521–4.
35. Filosto M, Mancuso M, Vives-Bauza C, *et al.* Lack of paternal inheritance of muscle mitochondrial DNA in sporadic mitochondrial myopathies. *Ann Neurol* 2003; **54**(4): 524–6.
36. Sutovsky P, Van Leyen K, McCauley T, *et al.* Degradation of paternal mitochondria after

fertilization: implications for heteroplasmy, assisted reproductive technologies and mtDNA inheritance. *Reprod Biomed Online* 2004; **8**(1): 24–33.

37. Lewin R. The unmasking of mitochondrial Eve. *Science* 1987; **238**(4823): 24–6.
38. Holt IJ, Harding AE, Morgan-Hughes JA. Deletions of muscle mitochondrial DNA in patients with mitochondrial myopathies. *Nature* 1988; **331**(6158): 717–19.
39. Wallace DC, Singh G, Lott MT, *et al.* Mitochondrial DNA mutation associated with Leber's hereditary optic neuropathy. *Science* 1988; **242**(4884): 1427–30.
40. Tuppen HA, Blakely EL, Turnbull DM, *et al.* Mitochondrial DNA mutations and human disease. *Biochim Biophys Acta* 2010; **1797**(2): 113–28.
41. Schaefer AM, McFarland R, Blakely EL, *et al.* Prevalence of mitochondrial DNA disease in adults. *Ann Neurol* 2008; **63**(1): 35–9.
42. Manwaring N, Jones MM, Wang JJ, *et al.* Population prevalence of the MELAS A3243G mutation. *Mitochondrion* 2007; **7**(3): 230–3.
43. Elliott HR, Samuels DC, Eden JA, *et al.* Pathogenic mitochondrial DNA mutations are common in the general population. *Am J Hum Genet* 2008; **83**(2): 254–60.
44. Carling PJ, Cree LM, Chinnery PF. The implications of mitochondrial DNA copy number regulation during embryogenesis. *Mitochondrion* 2011; **11**(5): 686–92.
45. Freyer C, Cree LM, Mourier A, *et al.* Variation in germline mtDNA heteroplasmy is determined prenatally but modified during subsequent transmission. *Nat Genet* 2012; **44**(11): 1282–5.
46. Stewart JB, Freyer C, Elson JL, *et al.* Strong purifying selection in transmission of mammalian mitochondrial DNA. *PLoS Biol* 2008; **6**(1): e10.
47. Monnot S, Gigarel N, Samuels DC, *et al.* Segregation of mtDNA throughout human embryofetal development: m.3243A>G as a model system. *Hum Mutat* 2011; **32**(1): 116–25.
48. Steffann J, Frydman N, Gigarel N, *et al.* Analysis of mtDNA variant segregation during early human embryonic development: a tool for successful NARP preimplantation diagnosis. *J Med Genet* 2006; **43**(3): 244–7.
49. Craven L, Elson JL, Irving L, *et al.* Mitochondrial DNA disease: new options for prevention. *Hum Mol Genet* 2011; **20**(R2): R168–74.
50. McGrath J, Solter D. Nuclear transplantation in the mouse embryo by microsurgery and cell fusion. *Science* 1983; **220**(4603): 1300–2.
51. Sato A, Kono T, Nakada K, *et al.* Gene therapy for progeny of mito-mice carrying pathogenic mtDNA by nuclear transplantation. *Proc Natl Acad Sci USA* 2005; **102**(46): 16765–70.
52. Craven L, Tuppen HA, Greggains GD, *et al.* Pronuclear transfer in human embryos to prevent transmission of mitochondrial DNA disease. *Nature* 2010; **465**(7294): 82–5.
53. Tachibana M, Sparman M, Sritanaudomchai H, *et al.* Mitochondrial gene replacement in primate offspring and embryonic stem cells. *Nature* 2009; **461**(7262): 367–72.
54. Downs SM. The influence of glucose, cumulus cells, and metabolic coupling on ATP levels and meiotic control in the isolated mouse oocyte. *Dev Biol* 1995; **167**(2): 502–12.
55. Sutton-McDowall ML, Gilchrist RB, Thompson JG. The pivotal role of glucose metabolism in determining oocyte developmental competence. *Reproduction* 2010; **139**(4): 685–95.
56. Johnson MT, Freeman EA, Gardner DK, *et al.* Oxidative metabolism of pyruvate is required for meiotic maturation of murine oocytes in vivo. *Biol Reprod* 2007; **77**(1): 2–8.
57. Van Blerkom J, Davis PW, Lee J. ATP content of human oocytes and developmental potential and outcome after in-vitro fertilization and embryo transfer. *Hum Reprod* 1995; **10**(2): 415–24.
58. Reynier P, May-Panloup P, Chretien MF, *et al.* Mitochondrial DNA content affects the fertilizability of human oocytes. *Mol Hum Reprod* 2001; **7**(5): 425–9.
59. Copeland WC. Inherited mitochondrial diseases of DNA replication. *Ann Rev Med* 2008; **59**: 131–46.
60. May-Panloup P, Chretien MF, Jacques C, *et al.* Low oocyte mitochondrial DNA content in ovarian insufficiency. *Hum Reprod* 2005; **20**(3): 593–7.
61. Zeng HT, Ren Z, Yeung WS, *et al.* Low mitochondrial DNA and ATP contents contribute to the absence of birefringent spindle imaged with PolScope in in vitro matured human oocytes. *Hum Reprod* 2007; **22**(6): 1681–6.
62. Wai T, Ao A, Zhang X, *et al.* The role of mitochondrial DNA copy number in mammalian fertility. *Biol Reprod* 2010; **83**(1): 52–62.
63. Sauer MV, Paulson RJ, Lobo RA. A preliminary report on oocyte donation extending reproductive potential to women over 40. *N Engl J Med* 1990; **323**(17): 1157–60.
64. Steuerwald NM, Bermudez MG, Wells D, *et al.* Maternal age-related differential global expression

profiles observed in human oocytes. *Reprod Biomed Online* 2007; **14**(6): 700–8.

65. Trifunovic A, Larsson NG. Mitochondrial dysfunction as a cause of ageing. *J Intern Med* 2008; **263**(2): 167–78.

66. Muller-Hocker J, Schafer S, Weis S, *et al.* Morphological-cytochemical and molecular genetic analyses of mitochondria in isolated human oocytes in the reproductive age. *Mol Hum Reprod* 1996; **2**(12): 951–8.

67. Tarin JJ, Vendrell FJ, Ten J, *et al.* The oxidizing agent tertiary butyl hydroperoxide induces disturbances in spindle organization, c-meiosis, and aneuploidy in mouse oocytes. *Mol Hum Reprod* 1996; **2**(12): 895–901.

68. Zhang X, Wu XQ, Lu S, Guo YL, Ma X. Deficit of mitochondria-derived ATP during oxidative stress impairs mouse MII oocyte spindles. *Cell Res* 2006; **16**: 841–50. doi: 10.1038/sj.cr.7310095.

69. Seifer DB, DeJesus V, Hubbard K. Mitochondrial deletions in luteinized granulosa cells as a function of age in women undergoing in vitro fertilization. *Fertil Steril* 2002; **78**(5): 1046– 8.

70. Tsai HD, Hsieh YY, Hsieh JN, *et al.* Mitochondria DNA deletion and copy numbers of cumulus cells associated with in vitro fertilization outcomes. *J Reprod Med* 2010; **55**(11–12): 491–7.

71. St John JC. Transmission, inheritance and replication of mitochondrial DNA in mammals: implications for reproductive processes and infertility. *Cell Tissue Res* 2012; **349**(3): 795–808.

72. Tarin JJ, Perez-Albala S, Cano A. Cellular and morphological traits of oocytes retrieved from aging mice after exogenous ovarian stimulation. *Biol Reprod* 2001; **65**(1): 141–50.

Chapter 27

Relative contribution of advanced age and reduced follicle pool size on reproductive success

The quantity–quality enigma

Frank Broekmans and Madeleine Dólleman

Introduction to reproductive aging

It is a well-known phenomenon that as a woman becomes older, her chances of reproductive success decrease. This is largely attributed to ovarian aging, the age-related decline in the quantity and quality of oocytes in the ovaries. At birth every woman has a certain endowment of oocytes. This number of oocytes decreases at various rates during life until the ovarian reserve is exhausted and menopause is reached [1]. Renewal of the oocyte pool from pluripotent stem cells has so far been denied, but recent studies have elicited possible new insights into this field [2]. The gradual decline in oocyte quantity with age is accompanied by a decrease in oocyte quality. This is substantiated by decreased pregnancy rates, increased miscarriage rates, and an increase in the rate of aneuploidy leading to offspring with trisomic karyotypes [3, 4]. Also, a growing incidence of unexplained infertility is apparent in women trying to achieve a pregnancy at a more advanced age [5]. The age related decrease in female fertility has direct repercussions in Western societies, as the trend to delayed childbearing continues.

The introduction of effective contraceptive methods in the 1960s and the growing participation of women in the labor force has resulted in a major change in reproductive behavior [6]. The average age at the birth of the first child has increased from approximately 24 years of age in 1970 to the age of 30 or over in recent years [7, 8]. In addition, the completed fertility rate (number of children born per woman) has decreased considerably and a growing proportion of women seek the help of assisted reproductive technology (ART) to conceive. As modern infertility treatments can only help around 50% of these women, a considerable proportion of women will remain childless involuntarily, with increased levels of personal distress and grave effects on relationship stability [9, 10]. The continuing trend to delay childbearing does not only have a large impact on population demographics; the annual costs for society from infertility treatments and ART-related complications, such as multiple pregnancies, are also high [11, 12].

In this chapter we will discuss factors that influence the quantitative and qualitative depletion of the ovarian reserve and how this affects cyclic ovarian function as well as the chances for reproductive success. The way in which quantity and quality decline are interrelated will be extensively reviewed. Furthermore, we will address available methods for assessing a woman's individual reproductive age status and how this information can be used to predict her current and future fertility potential.

Follicle quantity and cyclic ovarian function

During the fourth month of fetal development the ovaries contain between six and seven million oocytes. These oocytes are surrounded by a layer of flat granulosa cells and together they are referred to as the primordial follicle pool [13–15]. In the second half of fetal life, the number of oocytes decreases rapidly due to a process of apoptosis. Consequently only one to two million oocytes are left in the ovaries at

Biology and Pathology of the Oocyte, 2nd edn., ed. Alan Trounson, Roger Gosden, and Ursula Eichenlaub-Ritter. Published by Cambridge University Press.

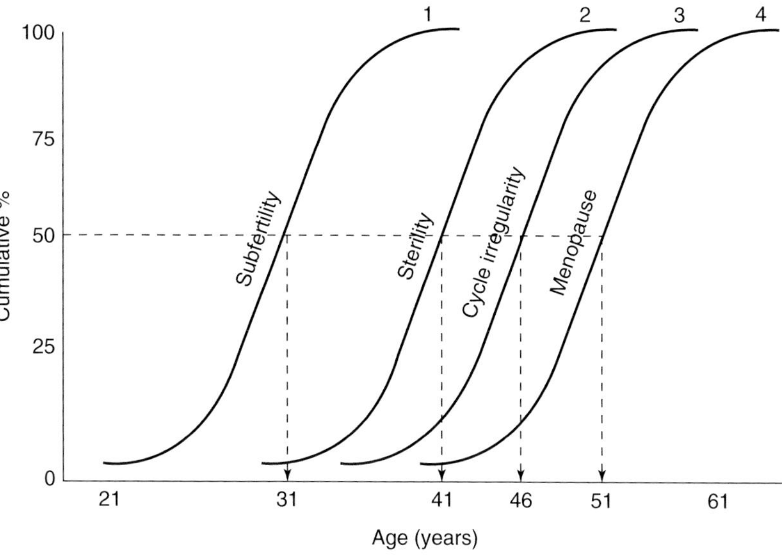

Figure 27.1 Graphical representation of the variation in the ages at the four reproductive milestones. Curve 1 represents variation in onset of subfertility and is supported by data from Eijkemans *et al.* [84]. Curve 2 shows variation in the end of natural fertility and is based on data from Bouchard [31]. Curve 3 represents individual variability in occurrence of cycle irregularity from den Tonkelaar *et al.* [39]. The variation in menopausal age has been derived from data by Treloar and Broekmans [37, 85]. The average age at which the event occurs in the general population is shown on the x-axis. This figure represents the notion that the occurrence of reduced fertility occurs approximately ten years before sterility and that the menopausal transition precedes the onset of menopause by approximately five years. Reproduced from Broekmans *et al.* Female reproductive ageing: current knowledge and future trends, *Trends in Endocrinology & Metabolism*, 18(2), p59, by permission of Oxford University Press [33].

birth [16]. The process of apoptosis continues after birth, but at a slower rate so that at menarche approximately 300 000 to 400 000 primordial follicles remain. In a woman's reproductive years, the gradual decline in follicle quantity is responsible for the occurrence of two reproductive milestones, menopause and the onset of overt cycle irregularity, being the two final events of the quantitative ovarian aging process [1].

Throughout the period in which follicle numbers decline, the number of continuously present antral follicles remains sufficient to ensure the monthly process of single dominant follicle development and ovulation. It is not until only a few thousand follicles remain in the ovaries that the reduced negative feedback from the ovaries to the hypothalamo-pituitary unit leads to elevated gonadotropin levels, resulting in dysregulated folliculogenesis. Soon thereafter, the availability of sufficient antral follicles for cyclic follicle development cannot always be ensured, causing the menstrual cycle to become irregular [17, 18]. The years before the final menstrual period, when variability in the menstrual cycle is increased, are referred to as the menopausal transition [17]. During this period exhaustion of primordial follicles occurs at an accelerated pace. Eventually, the cycle stops completely, the event known as menopause, which marks the last reproductive milestone [18–21]. Menopause is defined as a period of amenorrhea of at least 12 months. The average age at which menopause occurs is 51 years, with a range from 40 to 60 years [7]. Mathematical models that have been designed to portray the age-related depletion of the follicle pool show that the pool has been exhausted when menopause occurs.

A fixed temporal relationship between the last two reproductive milestones is thought to be present (Figure 27.1). Prospective recordings of mean cycle duration and variation around the mean age at menopause have made it possible to assess the onset of the menopausal transition. It was subsequently demonstrated that age at menopause was directly related to age at which cycle irregularity was initiated, with a reasonably fixed interval of approximately 5 years [7, 22].

Quality decline and fertility

The age-related decline in follicle numbers is accompanied by a diminishing oocyte quality. Oocyte quality is not uniformly defined. It can be assessed through

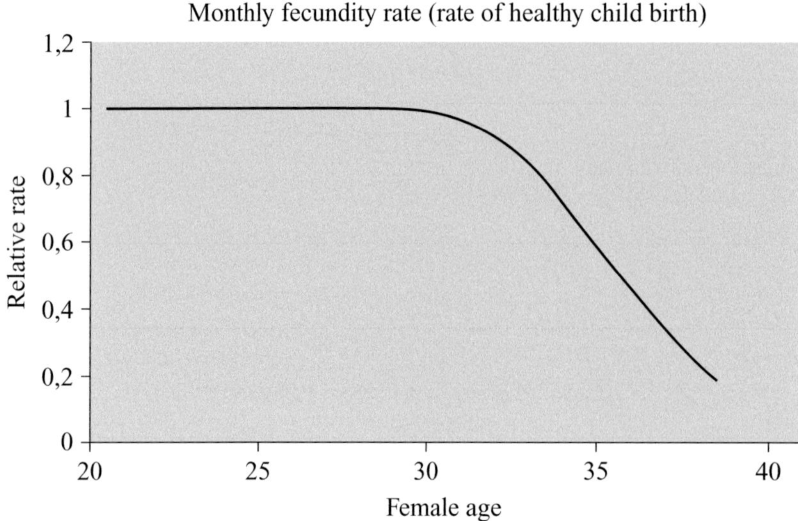

Figure 27.2 Graphical representation of decreased monthly fecundity rates with increasing age. It demonstrates that after the age of 31 years there is a rapid decrease in the monthly fecundity rate. Reproduced from Broekmans *et al.* Female reproductive ageing: current knowledge and future trends, *Trends in Endocrinology & Metabolism*, 18(2), p60, by permission of Oxford University Press [33].

the ability of achieving an ongoing pregnancy or by assessing the occurrence of aneuploidy or miscarriage. The declining ability to give birth to a healthy child and the increasing time to pregnancy with increasing female age have been documented from numerous sources. With increasing female age, the risk of a pregnancy resulting in early pregnancy loss or the birth of a child with a numerical chromosome abnormality will become more and more substantial [3, 4]. An increase in the occurrence of meiotic non-disjunction is accepted to lie at the heart of the decreasing oocyte quality. Meiotic non-disjunction leads to frequent aneuploidy in oocytes and the early embryo at more-advanced female ages. In women approaching the age of 40, the majority of oocytes and embryos are chromosomally abnormal as confirmed by research on chromosome numbers in embryos derived from in vitro fertilization (IVF) programs [23–25] (see discussion in Chapters 28 and 35).

Several mechanisms are associated with a decline in oocyte quality, including a life-long accumulation of damage to the oocyte and changes in the granulosa cells that surround the oocyte. It is also theorized that there may be inherent differences in the quality of germ cells from which oocytes are formed [7]. A two-hit model exists which suggests that there is a first hit due to an inherent reduction in the frequency and pattern of recombination in a fraction of oocytes from the beginning. The second hit encompasses the accumulation of damage to the oocyte and damage to the follicle. This damage results from oxidative stress, lifestyle factors, and microenvironmental factors such as a decreased circulation around the leading follicle or impaired functionality of the granulosa cells [26–28]. Moreover, accumulation of damage with age results in inadequate reserves of energy due to mitochondrial dysfunction which may lead to chaotic mosaicism in human preimplantation embryos [29]. Furthermore, gene expression patterns appear altered, as implied by transcriptome analysis of young and aged metaphase II oocytes from human and mouse suggesting that an abundance of factors in chromosome, cell cycle, spindle regulation, and other cellular processes change. The exact cellular basis of oocyte aneuploidy in reproductive aging is complex and will be explained in detail in Chapter 28.

Much like the decline in follicle quantity, the waning oocyte quality will also be reflected in reproductive milestones, although these are not as noticeable as the menopausal transition and menopause.

The first reproductive milestone is the onset of declining fertility at a mean age of 31 years (Figure 27.1). The best notion of this declining natural fertility stems from semen donation studies where the male factor was controlled for (Figure 27.2) [5, 30]. Next is the advent of natural sterility, defined as the loss of the ability to conceive and give birth to viable offspring, even if well-timed exposure is attempted for several years. Knowledge on the advent of natural sterility stems from a nineteenth-century population study, in which the highly religious nature of the cohort prohibited the use of contraception and therefore procreation until natural sterility had been reached was ensured. It could be shown that age at last child birth, as a proxy for the loss of natural fertility, was on average at the age of 41 years [31]. The gradual decline in fertility during the fourth decade of life passes largely unnoticed from the individual's perspective. Monthly ovulations are believed to ensure that prospects for pregnancy occur, while in fact fecundity rates will distinctly decline after the age of 30.

A total of four reproductive milestones are thus believed to be present, namely decreasing natural fertility, sterility, menopausal transition, and menopause. The fixed time interval, as demonstrated by the relationship between the onset of menopausal transition and menopause, may also be true for the milestones of quality decline. The above-mentioned nineteenth-century population study also demonstrated that a reduced birth rate in the early stages of marriage (between age 20 and 30 years) was associated with an early age at last child birth (approximately at age of 35 years). This suggests that early sterility is preceded by a decrease in natural fertility from before the age of 30 years [31].

The concept of a fixed temporal relationship between the quantity and quality milestones, though plausible, has not been substantiated by a vast amount of clinical and experimental observations. However, a study in women who had both reduced pregnancy chances and obviously reduced numbers of antral follicles for their age group has indicated that these women will enter menopause earlier than women without these characteristics [32]. The same line of evidence has been shown from smaller studies relating either poor response in IVF or elevated basal follicle-stimulating hormone (FSH) levels with subsequent occurrence of menopause [33]. It is important to realize, however, that ultimate proof for this concept is impossible to obtain, as it would require highly refined assessment of fecundity in a population not applying contraceptive measures and challenging fertility until the age at which natural sterility is reached. Availability of such a cohort in the current era is elusive [32, 34].

From the relationship between the reproductive events it is clear that the end of natural fertility occurs approximately 10 years before menopause is established. During these 10 years, ovulated oocytes may get fertilized, but due to a high frequency of chromosomal abnormalities either implantation may fail or, if implantation is successful, the implanted embryo may produce a pregnancy that terminates at an early stage [35]. The increase in female infertility with increasing age is thus twofold. First of all, monthly chances of conception are lower and secondly there is a higher probability that the pregnancy will terminate around conception or implantation [7]. The former could be due either to depletion of the number of follicles or the demise of quality while the latter can be interpreted predominantly as a problem of oocyte quality. It could be argued that other factors leading to increased miscarriage rates in women of higher chronological age may also play a role. However, in oocyte donation programs, where oocytes from young fertile women are placed in older non-fertile women, both pregnancy and miscarriage rates have been very satisfactory, maintaining the view that it is largely an ovarian factor, and not a uterine or other factor [36].

Variability in reproductive aging

The individual variability of ovarian aging between women of the same chronological age is large. The range for the age at menopause extends from 40 to 60 years with a mean age of 51 years [37]. Variation of age at menopause has a Gaussian distribution in which there are fewer cases at the extremes of age. This does not include women diagnosed with premature ovarian insufficiency (women who reach menopause before the age of 40) because they are not thought to represent natural variation in age at menopause [38]. Similarly, the age at which women start to notice menstrual cycle irregularity (associated with ovarian reserve exhaustion) ranges from 35 to 54 years with an average age of 46 years [39]. The mean age at which a woman reaches natural sterility is difficult to establish. One study assessed the age at which women gave birth to their last child in 1040 women born in Canada in the second half of the nineteenth century. The maternal age at the birth of the last child was used as a proxy for calculating age at the end of natural fertility, and was shown to occur on average at the age of 41 years with a spread from 23 to 51 years [31].

The fact that it is not uncommon for women to reach the end of natural fertility at a young age sparked the realization that chronological aging (i.e., a woman's age in years) and biological aging (i.e., the functional age of the ovaries) do not always coincide. From studies performed in IVF populations we have learnt that ovarian response to controlled ovarian hyperstimulation (COH) during IVF treatment, as measured by the number of oocytes retrieved, reflects the quantitative aspect of the ovarian reserve. Young women with a repeated poor response to COH (defined as the retrieval of a small number of oocytes) tend to enter menopause earlier than women with a normal response [32]. Such a poor responder is thus seen to have advanced biological aging for her chronological age and is predisposed to go through all four reproductive milestones earlier than someone of similar age with a normal response to COH. In such women with a young chronological age but an old biological age, other factors must be implicated that have an important influence on the ovarian aging process.

The quantity–quality enigma

The decline in both quantity and quality have been addressed separately, but neither process alone can really explain the severely decreased fecundity at the point where a woman may first experience cycle changes due to exhaustion of her ovarian reserve. At this point a woman still has approximately 25 000 oocytes [1]. This is considerably less than her endowment of six to seven million oocytes during fetal life, but it seems like more than enough to maintain fertility as regular ovulation cycles occur until then. There must then be a complicated interrelationship between oocyte quantity and quality. In a mouse study it was shown that after the removal of one ovary in newborn mice, thus halving the ovarian reserve, the quality of the oocytes in the other ovary was considerably worse. The unilaterally ovariectomized mice had not only an early onset of cycle irregularity, but also a much earlier rise in the rate of aneuploidy in the offspring [40]. Another mouse study revealed an increase in the number of metaphase II oocytes with unaligned chromosomes from depleted mouse ovaries, while spindle size decreased with advancing age, irrespective of pool size [41].

In humans it has been suggested that women with a reduced ovarian reserve due to ovarian surgery have an increased rate of trisomy-21 offspring [42, 43]. This is in line with two other studies that have suggested that women who have an aneuploid conception are often found to have higher levels of FSH [44, 45]. A third study suggests that women with a history of a trisomy 21 pregnancy at a young age had subtle signs of limited ovarian reserve as measured by slightly higher FSH and slightly lower anti-Müllerian hormone (AMH) values [46, 47]. The increased level of FSH was suggested to represent early depletion of the primordial follicle pool independently from age. All this would support the idea of a close relation between quantity and quality in the ovarian aging process. However, there are various observations that contradict this one-to-one relation between quantitative and qualitative demise. Follow-up studies on the value of basal FSH levels in predicting aneuploidy failed to clearly confirm this obvious relation after correcting for female age [45, 48].

The hypothesis that there is a direct relationship between oocyte quantity and oocyte quality has become known as the limited oocyte pool hypothesis and was introduced by Warburton in 1989 [26]. It is based on the idea that in a young woman an oocyte of suboptimal condition would not become the dominant follicle because of an abundance of better quality oocytes. On the contrary, in an older woman with a small ovarian reserve a faulty oocyte would be more likely to become the dominant follicle and be more likely to exhibit chromosome non-disjunction [26]. Although feasible, this hypothesis does not address the issue of age-related damage accumulation, and merely assumes a hierarchy in oocyte quality present from the prenatal life phase onwards.

The possible inconsistency in the relationship between quantity and quality in the ovarian aging process has been underlined by several studies from ART programs. Young women with a low ovarian reserve, as represented by a poor response to COH during IVF, have higher pregnancy rates than older women with a similar poor response [49–51]. Similarly, women in whom a higher number of oocytes are retrieved after COH have higher pregnancy chances than women with a lower number of oocytes retrieved. A combination of young age and a high number of oocytes retrieved is a good measure of reproductive success. However, a young female with a low number of retrieved oocytes still has a higher chance of achieving a pregnancy than an older female with a higher number of retrieved oocytes, as shown in Figure 27.3 [52]. This demonstrates that there is not a one-to-one ratio in quantity versus quality decline and suggests a

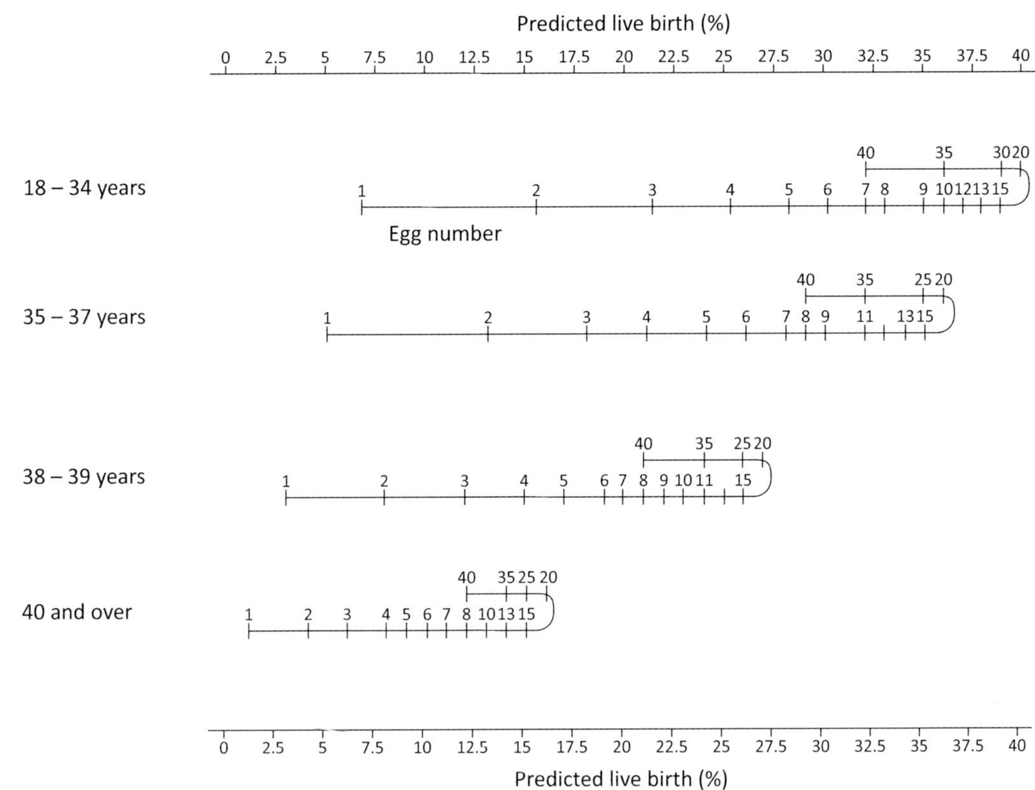

Figure 27.3 Nomogram of predicted live birth rates according to female age and the number of oocytes retrieved after controlled ovarian hyperstimulation during IVF. It demonstrates three things. Firstly, that live birth rates are influenced by age. Younger women have a better prognosis than older women. Secondly, it shows that a higher number of oocytes is associated with a higher live birth rate, with 15 oocytes being the optimal number. Lastly it shows that the effect between live birth rate and the number of oocytes retrieved is age-modulated, where young poor responders have a reasonably good prognosis. Reproduced from Sunkara *et al.*, Association between the number of eggs and live birth in IVF treatment: an analysis of 400 135 treatment cycles, *Human Reproduction*, 26(7) p1773, by permission of Oxford University Press [52].

complex interplay of factors still poorly understood today. For now, the available data seem to point towards the relationship between quantity and quality being female age-modulated, where low quantity leads to poor quality but with either protective or augmenting effects of female age. This is portrayed in Figure 27.4. Supportive evidence comes from a study performed in women with a reduced ovarian reserve, as measured by extremely low anti-Müllerian hormone values, where reasonable chances of pregnancy were observed, especially in those women of a younger age [53]. Moreover, in women with a low ovarian reserve (as represented by a poor response to COH) the proportion of miscarriages and trisomic pregnancies appeared to become more clearly increased in women at more adanced age [43, 54]. A possible explanation may be that quantity in young women is much more variable, so that an observed low quantity in young women is far less consistent and thus less indicative of poor ovarian reserve than a low quantity at advanced age. The consequences attached to it (i.e., loss in quality) may thus also be less evident. The young poor responder may therefore more often be based on a chance finding [51]. To further understand the complex interaction between quantity and quality, genetic factors and environmental influences on reproductive aging may also need to be considered.

Determinants of reproductive aging

The variability of age at menopause together with the observation that age at menopause is highly heritable (estimates of heritability range from 30% to 85%) has led to the search for a gene or set of genes that determines at what age a woman enters menopause [55–61]. It is thought that the identification of such

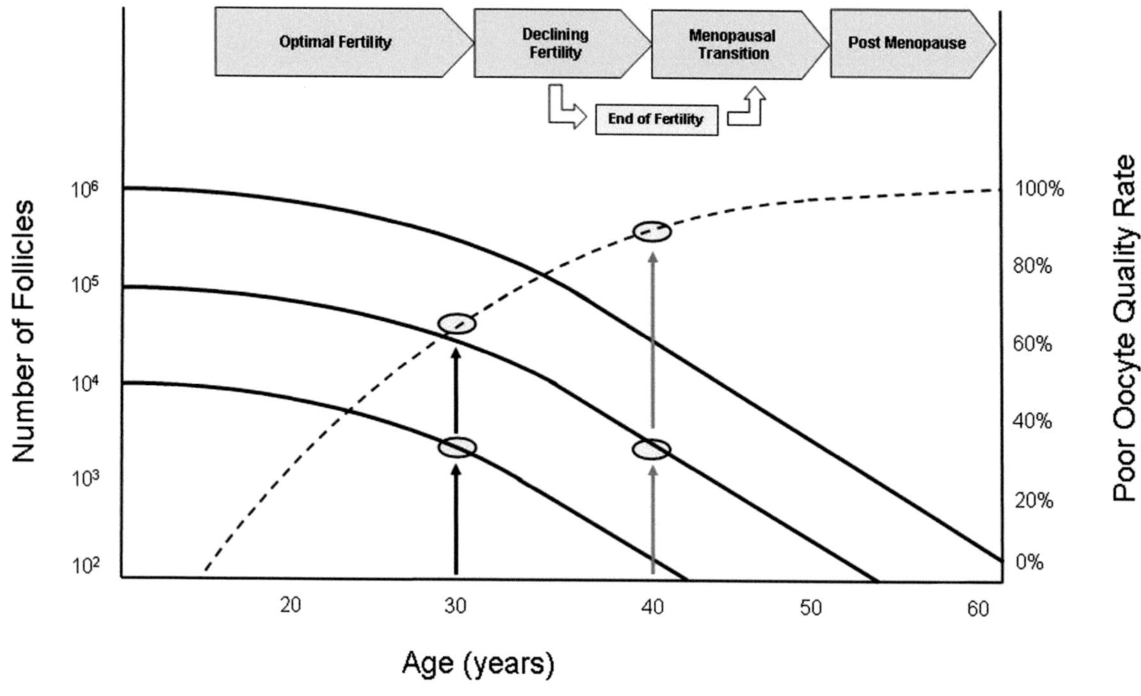

Figure 27.4 Solid lines represent variability in quantitative decline of oocytes based on different endowments at birth. The dotted line represents the increasing proportion of poor quality oocytes with increasing age based on the theory that damage accumulates with increasing age. It furthermore explains why young women with a low quantity can still have reasonable pregnancy prospects due to relatively good oocyte quality. Reproduced with permission from Broer *et al.* 2011 [74].

a gene would not only determine menopause but all preceding reproductive milestones as well. For a long time proposed candidate genes included those with a role in fetal ovarian development, primordial follicle maturation, follicular apoptosis, ovarian vascularization as well as genes associated with premature ovarian insufficiency [33]. Currently, the paradigm seems to be shifting towards a search for genes that influence general health and aging and not only ovarian function. Genome-wide association studies (GWAS) have demonstrated that genes involved in DNA repair and function, autoimmunity, and neuroendocrine pathways, and genes associated with ovarian function all play a role in regulating age at menopause [62]. Other studies have indicated a role for genes associated with vascular support. Both an increase in cardiovascular risk factors like hypertension, obesity, atherosclerosis, and hypercholesterolemia and mutations in factor V Leiden, clotting factor VII, as well as genes involved in atherosclerosis have been associated with earlier menopause [63–67]. The hunt for genes associated with age at menopause has thus far focused on identifying variation in the decline of oocyte quantity and not yet on oocyte quality.

The functional lifespan of a woman's ovaries may also be influenced by environmental factors. Of such factors the effect of smoking has been documented most thoroughly. Smoking has been reported to be associated with lower pregnancy rates and earlier onset of menopause and an increased risk for second meiotic non-disjunction causing trisomy 21 may be present in women who smoke and take contraceptives [68, 69]. Polycyclic aromatic hydrocarbons, found in cigarette smoke and air pollution, interact with the aryl hydrocarbon receptor to cause reproductive defects [70]. Smoking accelerates follicle damage and can induce ovarian failure. Furthermore, the identification of DNA repair, as one of the candidate genes involved in menopausal age, could also explain the association between menopausal age and smoking. The damage that results from cigarette smoke activates DNA repair mechanisms that may be associated with age at menopause [62]. Women with extreme malnutrition are known to enter menopause earlier.

showing that nutritional status influences the rate of reproductive aging as well, but this has not been elaborately studied [7]. In conclusion the rate of follicle depletion and oocyte quality is an interactive puzzle of inherent and environmental factors.

Assessment of ovarian age

The demand for a critical assessment of ovarian age is increasing as more older women seek infertility treatment. Adequate evaluation of reproductive age could open doors to individualized patient counseling, personalized treatment protocols (what stimulation dosage to administer for achieving an optimal response), and potentially to abstaining from further treatment in a null-prognosis group of patients. Several markers have been identified that can predict the current ovarian reserve. Ovarian reserve tests (ORTs) reflect the numbers of follicles that are left in the ovaries, therefore these markers are suggested to reflect the quantitative aspect of ovarian age. It is not possible to measure ovarian reserve directly, but it has been shown by measuring the number of antral follicles in the ovaries (the antral follicle count or AFC) that it is proportionally related to the remaining number of primordial follicles [71, 72]. There are some endocrine markers that have been shown to do the same. AMH, FSH, and inhibin are endocrine markers that are released from antral follicles. Studies assessing the predictive capacity of these tests show that most tests have an adequate capacity to identify the ovarian reserve [73] and they are therefore used as representatives of the quantitative aspect of ovarian aging. Through this, AMH has also been suggested as an adequate predictor of age at menopause [74, 75].

Oocyte quality has proven to be more difficult to measure. This is partly due to the absence of a clear definition of oocyte quality. One definition is the ability of an oocyte to produce an ongoing pregnancy. Unfortunately, the capacity of any ORT to predict pregnancy, both after one IVF cycle and cumulative cycles, has proven to be limited [76]. This is probably due to the fact that ORTs relate fully to quantity aspects of the ovarian aging process and due to the ambiguous relationship between oocyte quantity and quality. In studies assessing the accuracy of ongoing pregnancy prediction, only small proportions of non-pregnant women were correctly identified, with a high occurrence of false-positively predicted cases even when extreme cut-off values were applied [38, 71, 73, 77, 78]. This makes the test unsuitable for the identification of women who should abstain from further ART treatment due to unfavorable pregnancy prospects. The clinical applicability is limited to the identification of chance categories as depicted in Table 27.1. The limited clinical applicability is evidenced by the large and overlapping confidence intervals, but a trend towards a higher ongoing pregnancy rate with higher values of the ORTs is evident across age categories.

Table 27.1. Prognostic categories of achieving an ongoing pregnancy using AMH, AFC and age as predictors. The trend towards higher ongoing pregnancy rates is shown amongst young women with high ovarian reserves, as measured by either AMH or AFC

	Percentage of ongoing pregnancies across AMH categories				
Age	**Anti-Müllerian hormone (ng/ml)**				
(years)	**<0.4**	**0.4–0.8**	**0.8–1.6**	**1.6–2.8**	**>2.8**
<31	17.80%	19.90%	30.30%	25.60%	40.20%
(95% CI)	*6–44%*	*7–44%*	*12–58%*	*7–62%*	*15–73%*
31–36	13.80%	15.40%	24%	20.20%	33%
(95% CI)	*5–34%*	*6–34%*	*12–43%*	*6–49%*	*11–65%*
36–38	8.10%	9.2%	15%	12.3%	22%
(95% CI)	*2–24%*	*3–24%*	*6–35%*	*3–39%*	*6–54%*
38–40	15.8%	17.7%	27.3%	22.9%	36.7%
(95% CI)	*5–41%*	*6–41%*	*11–53%*	*6–59%*	*10–75%*
>40	8%	9.1%	15%	12.2%	21.3%
(95% CI)	*2–23%*	*3–27%*	*5–37%*	*3–43%*	*5–57%*
	Percentage of ongoing pregnancies across AFC categories				
Age	**Antral follicle count (2–10 mm follicles)**				
(years)	**<4**	**4–8**	**8–10**	**10–15**	**>15**
<31	13.00%	16.2%	25.3%	17.3%	26.3%
(95% CI)	*4–39%*	*5–45%*	*7–61%*	*4–50%*	*5–70%*
31–36	7.85%	9.93%	15.9%	10.4%	16.6%
(95% CI)	*3–21%*	*4–23%*	*6–36%*	*3–28%*	*4–52%*
36–38	9.75%	12.3%	19.4%	12.9%	20.2%
(95% CI)	*4–23%*	*5–28%*	*7–43%*	*4–33%*	*5–57%*
38–40	13.5%	16.8%	25.8%	17.6%	26.8%
(95% CI)	*5–31%*	*7–37%*	*9–54%*	*5–46%*	*5–70%*
>40	7.7%	9.7%	15.6%	10.3%	16.3%
(95% CI)	*3–18%*	*4–23%*	*5–39%*	*3–31%*	*3–56%*

Unpublished data from the IPD-EXPORT collaboration project.

Other aspects of quality assessment could include morphological evaluation of oocytes or analysis of polar bodies with fluorescence *in situ* hybridization [79]. Alternatively, the developmental potential of oocytes has been linked to the appearance and number of cumulus cells around the oocyte [80] as well as to their gene expression [81]. These measures, however, are invasive and can only be used post hoc during ART treatment where oocytes are aspirated from a stimulated ovary. Furthermore, in this scenario the chance of ongoing pregnancy is also dependent on embryo quality, endometrial receptivity, and transfer technique [82, 83]. Ideally, a different assessment of ovarian quality is needed. As elective single embryo transfer becomes more applied globally there will be an even higher demand for new biomarkers of oocyte competence. To this date the most reliable marker for oocyte quality still seems to be age. However, to improve the accuracy of identifying women with a reduced ovarian reserve for their age it may be necessary to combine endocrine markers, ultrasound imaging, and genetic tests. If a genetic marker is found, this may improve the accuracy of such a multivariate model even further [33].

Conclusions

Ovarian aging is a multifactorial process in which genetic factors, other physiological factors, and environmental factors all play a role. The way in which these factors interact to cause both a quantitative and qualitative depletion of the ovarian reserve remains largely unknown. Elucidation of these pathways of interaction will create more understanding about the individual variation that exists in women of the same chronological age. ORTs can be seen as an expression of this individual constitution. If such tests can adequately predict the ovarian reserve, in the future it may be possible to identify those women who are at risk of early infertility or those at risk of early menopause. This will open doors to primary prevention of infertility by counseling women to conceive early. However, it has been argued that quantity and quality decline do not happen in a one-to-one ratio; therefore it is also necessary that future research aims to identify markers that adequately reflect oocyte quality and not only quantitative aspects of the reproductive aging process. The ultimate goal is thus to clarify the processes that influence ovarian aging and to design treatments towards ameliorating pregnancy outcomes in patients with advanced ovarian age.

Acknowledgments

We would like to thank the IPD-EXPORT group (Individual Patient Data Meta-Analysis of Excessive Response Prediction using Ovarian Reserve Tests) for collaborating with our center to make available the data on the prediction of ongoing pregnancy using ovarian reserve tests. Thanks to S. L. Broer, J. van Disseldorp, K. A. Broeze, B. C. Opmeer, A. Aflatoonian, R. A. Anderson, M. Ashrafi, L. Bancsi, E. Caroppo, A. B. Copperman, T. Ebner, T. Eldar-Geva, M. Erdem, T. Freour, C. Gnoth, E. M. Greenblatt, K. Jayaprakasan, N. Raine-Fenning, E. Klinkert, J. Kwee, C. B. Lambalk, A. La Marca, M. McIlveen, L. Mohiyiddeen, L. T. Merce, S. Muttukrishna, L. G. Nardo, S. M. Nelson, H. Y. Ng, B. Popovic-Todorovic, J. M. J. Smeenk, C. Tomás, P. J. Q. van der Linden, I. K. Vladimirov, P. Bossuyt, M. J. C. Eijkemans, and B. W. Mol.

References

1. Faddy MJ, Gosden RG. A model conforming the decline in follicle numbers to the age of menopause in women. *Hum Reprod* 1996; **11**(7): 1484–86.
2. White YA, Woods DC, Takai Y, *et al.* Oocyte formation by mitotically active germ cells purified from ovaries of reproductive-age women. *Nat Med* 2012; **18**(3): 413–21.
3. Nybo Andersen AM, Wohlfahrt J, Christens P, Olsen J, Melbye M. Maternal age and fetal loss: population based register linkage study. *BMJ* 2000; **320**(7251): 1708–12.
4. Nicolaidis P, Petersen MB. Origin and mechanisms of non-disjunction in human autosomal trisomies. *Hum Reprod* 1998; **13**(2): 313–19.
5. van Noord-Zaadstra BM, Looman CW, Alsbach H, *et al.* Delaying childbearing: effect of age on fecundity and outcome of pregnancy. *BMJ* 1991; **302**(6789): 1361–5.
6. Leridon H. Demographic effects of the introduction of steroid contraception in developed countries. *Hum Reprod Update* 2006; **12**(5): 603–16.
7. te Velde ER, Pearson PL. The variability of female reproductive ageing. *Hum Reprod Update* 2002; **8**(2): 141–54.
8. OECD. OECD Family Database. 2011. http://www.oecd.org/els/soc/oecdfamilydatabase.htm
9. Leridon H. Can assisted reproduction technology compensate for the natural decline in fertility with age? A model assessment. *Hum Reprod* 2004; **19**(7): 1548–53.

10. Habbema JD, Eijkemans MJ, Nargund G, *et al.* The effect of in vitro fertilization on birth rates in western countries. *Hum Reprod* 2009; **24**(6): 1414–19.

11. Fauser BC, Devroey P, Macklon NS. Multiple birth resulting from ovarian stimulation for subfertility treatment. *Lancet* 2005; **365**(9473): 1807–16.

12. Lutz W, O'Neill BC, Scherbov S. Demographics. Europe's population at a turning point. *Science* 2003; **299**(5615): 1991–2.

13. Block E. A quantitative morphological investigation of the follicular system in newborn female infants. *Acta Anat (Basel)* 1953; **17**(3): 201–6.

14. Block E. Quantitative morphological investigations of the follicular system in women; variations at different ages. *Acta Anat (Basel)* 1952; **14**(1–2): 108–23.

15. Baker TG. A quantitative and cytological study of germ cells in human ovaries. *Proc R Soc Lond B Biol Sci* 1963; **158**: 417–33.

16. Markström, E, Svensson ECh, Shao R, Svanberg B, Billig H. Survival factors regulating ovarian apoptosis – dependence on follicle differentiation. *Reproduction* 2002; **123**(1): 23–30.

17. Santoro N, Randolph JF, Jr. Reproductive hormones and the menopause transition. *Obstet Gynecol Clin North Am* 2011; **38**(3): 455–66.

18. Richardson SJ, Senikas V, Nelson JF. Follicular depletion during the menopausal transition: evidence for accelerated loss and ultimate exhaustion. *J Clin Endocrinol Metab* 1987; **65**(6): 1231–7.

19. Leidy LE, Godfrey LR, Sutherland MR. Is follicular atresia biphasic? *Fertil Steril* 1998; **70**(5): 851–9.

20. Hansen KR, Knowlton NS, Thyer AC, *et al.* A new model of reproductive aging: the decline in ovarian non-growing follicle number from birth to menopause. *Hum Reprod* 2008; **23**(3): 699–708.

21. Faddy MJ, Gosden RG, Gougeon A, Richardson SJ, Nelson JF. Accelerated disappearance of ovarian follicles in mid-life: implications for forecasting menopause. *Hum Reprod* 1992; **7**(10): 1342–6.

22. Lisabeth L, Harlow S, Qaqish B. A new statistical approach demonstrated menstrual patterns during the menopausal transition did not vary by age at menopause. *J Clin Epidemiol* 2004; **57**(5): 484–96.

23. Gianaroli L, Magli MC, Ferraretti AP, Munné S. Preimplantation diagnosis for aneuploidies in patients undergoing in vitro fertilization with a poor prognosis: identification of the categories for which it should be proposed. *Fertil Steril* 1999; **72**(5): 837–44.

24. Wells D, Delhanty JD. Comprehensive chromosomal analysis of human preimplantation embryos using whole genome amplification and single cell comparative genomic hybridization. *Mol Hum Reprod* 2000; **6**(11): 1055–62.

25. Handyside AH, Montag M, Magli MC, *et al.* Multiple meiotic errors caused by predivision of chromatids in women of advanced maternal age undergoing in vitro fertilisation. *Eur J Hum Genet* 2012; **20**(7): 742–7.

26. Warburton D. The effect of maternal age on the frequency of trisomy: change in meiosis or in utero selection? *Prog Clin Biol Res* 1989; **311**: 165–81.

27. Lamb NE, Yu K, Shaffer J, Feingold E, Sherman SL. Association between maternal age and meiotic recombination for trisomy 21. *Am J Hum Genet* 2005; **76**(1): 91–9.

28. Tarin JJ. Aetiology of age-associated aneuploidy: a mechanism based on the 'free radical theory of ageing'. *Hum Reprod* 1995; **10**(6): 1563–5.

29. Wilding M, De Placido G, De Matteo L, *et al.* Chaotic mosaicism in human preimplantation embryos is correlated with a low mitochondrial membrane potential. *Fertil Steril* 2003; **79**(2): 340–6.

30. Schwartz D, Mayaux MJ. Female fecundity as a function of age: results of artificial insemination in 2193 nulliparous women with azoospermic husbands. Federation CECOS. *N Engl J Med* 1982; **306**(7): 404–6.

31. Bouchard G. Population studies and genetic epidemiology in northeast Quebec. *Can Stud Popul* 1989; **16**(1): 61–86.

32. de Boer EJ, den Tonkelaar I, te Velde ER, *et al.* A low number of retrieved oocytes at in vitro fertilization treatment is predictive of early menopause. *Fertil Steril* 2002; **77**(5): 978–85.

33. Broekmans FJ, Knauffe EA, te Velde ER, Macklon NS, Fauser BC. Female reproductive ageing: current knowledge and future trends. *Trends Endocrinol Metab* 2007; **18**(2): 58–65.

34. te Velde ER, Eijkemans R, Habbema HD. Variation in couple fecundity and time to pregnancy, an essential concept in human reproduction. *Lancet* 2000; **355**(9219): 1928–9.

35. O'Connor KA, Holman DJ, Wood JW. Declining fecundity and ovarian ageing in natural fertility populations. *Maturitas* 1998; **30**(2): 127–36.

36. Sauer MV, Kavic SM. Oocyte and embryo donation 2006: reviewing two decades of innovation and controversy. *Reprod Biomed Online* 2006; **12**(2): 153–62.

37. Treloar AE, Boynton RE, Behn BG, Brown BW. Variation of the human menstrual cycle through reproductive life. *Int J Fertil* 1967; **12**(1 Pt 2): 77–126.

38. Broekmans FJ, Soules MR, Fauser BC. Ovarian aging: mechanisms and clinical consequences. *Endocr Rev* 2009; **30**(5): 465–93.

39. den Tonkelaar I, te Velde ER, Looman CW. Menstrual cycle length preceding menopause in relation to age at menopause. *Maturitas* 1998; **29**(2): 115–23.

40. Brook JD, Gosden RG, Chandley AC. Maternal ageing and aneuploid embryos – evidence from the mouse that biological and not chronological age is the important influence. *Hum Genet* 1984; **66**(1): 41–5.

41. Eichenlaub-Ritter U, Chandley AC, Gosden RG. The CBA mouse as a model for age-related aneuploidy in man: studies of oocyte maturation, spindle formation and chromosome alignment during meiosis. *Chromosoma* 1988; **96**(3): 220–6.

42. Freeman SB, Yang Q, Allran K, Taft LF, Sherman SL. Women with a reduced ovarian complement may have an increased risk for a child with Down syndrome. *Am J Hum Genet* 2000; **66**(5): 1680–3.

43. Haadsma ML, Mooij TM, Groen H, *et al.* A reduced size of the ovarian follicle pool is associated with an increased risk of a trisomic pregnancy in IVF-treated women. *Hum Reprod* 2010; **25**(2): 552–8.

44. Nasseri A, Mukherjee T, Grifo JA, *et al.* Elevated day 3 serum follicle stimulating hormone and/or estradiol may predict fetal aneuploidy. *Fertil Steril* 1999; **71**(4): 715–18.

45. van Montfrans JM, Dorland M, Oosterhuis GJ, *et al.* Increased concentrations of follicle-stimulating hormone in mothers of children with Down's syndrome. *Lancet* 1999; **353**(9167): 1853–54.

46. van der Stroom EM, König T, van Dulmen-den Broeder E, *et al.* Early menopause in mothers of children with Down syndrome? *Fertil Steril* 2011; **96**(4): 985–90.

47. Kline JK, Kinney AM, Levin B, *et al.* Trisomic pregnancy and elevated FSH: implications for the oocyte pool hypothesis. *Hum Reprod* 2011; **26**(6): 1537–50.

48. Thum MY, Kalu E, Abdalla H. Elevated basal FSH and embryo quality: lessons from extended culture embryos: raised FSH and blastocyst quality. *J Assist Reprod Genet* 2009; **26**(6): 313–18.

49. Biljan MM, Buckett WM, Dean N, Phillips SJ, Tan SL. The outcome of IVF-embryo transfer treatment in patients who develop three follicles or less. *Hum Reprod* 2000; **15**(10): 2140–4.

50. Hanoch J, Law J, Holzer H, *et al.* Young low responders protected from untoward effects of reduced ovarian response [see comments]. *Fertil Steril* 1998; **69**(6): 1001–4.

51. Oudendijk JF, Yarde F, Eikjemans MJ, Broekmans FJ, Broer SL. The poor responder in IVF: is the prognosis always poor?: A systematic review. *Hum Reprod Update* 2012; **18**(1): 1–11.

52. Sunkara SK, Rittenberg V, Raine-Fenning N, *et al.* Association between the number of eggs and live birth in IVF treatment: an analysis of 400 135 treatment cycles. *Hum Reprod* 2011; **26**(7): 1768–74.

53. Weghofer A, Dietrich W, Barad DH, Gleicher N. Live birth chances in women with extremely low-serum anti-Mullerian hormone levels. *Hum Reprod* 2011; **26**(7): 1905–9.

54. Haadsma ML, Groen H, Mooij TM, *et al.* Miscarriage risk for IVF pregnancies in poor responders to ovarian hyperstimulation. *Reprod Biomed Online* 2010; **20**(2): 191–200.

55. Voorhuis M, Onland-Moret NC, van der Schouw YT, Fauser BC, Broekmans FJ. Human studies on genetics of the age at natural menopause: a systematic review. *Hum Reprod Update* 2010; **16**(4): 364–77.

56. Morris DH, Jones ME, Schoemaker MJ, Ashworth A, Swerdlow AJ. Familial concordance for age at natural menopause: results from the Breakthrough Generations Study. *Menopause* 2011; **18**(9): 956–61.

57. Torgerson DJ, Thomas RE, Reid DM. Mothers and daughters menopausal ages: is there a link? *Eur J Obstet Gynecol Reprod Biol* 1997; **74**(1): 63–6.

58. Snieder H, MacGregor AJ, Spector TD. Genes control the cessation of a woman's reproductive life: a twin study of hysterectomy and age at menopause. *J Clin Endocrinol Metab* 1998; **83**(6): 1875–80.

59. de Bruin JP, Bovenhuis H, van Noord PA, *et al.* The role of genetic factors in age at natural menopause. *Hum Reprod* 2001; **16**(9): 2014–18.

60. Murabito JM, Yang Q, Fox C, Wilson PW, Cupples LA. Heritability of age at natural menopause in the Framingham Heart Study. *J Clin Endocrinol Metab* 2005; **90**(6): 3427–30.

61. van Asselt KM, Kok HS, Pearson PL, *et al.* Heritability of menopausal age in mothers and daughters. *Fertil Steril* 2004; **82**(5): 1348–51.

62. Stolk L, Perry JR, Chasman DI, *et al.* Meta-analyses identify 13 loci associated with age at menopause and highlight DNA repair and immune pathways. *Nat Genet* 2012; **44**(3): 260–8.

63. Kok HS, van Asselt KM, van der Schouw YT, *et al.* Heart disease risk determines menopausal age rather than the reverse. *J Am Coll Cardiol* 2006; **47**(10): 1976–83.

64. Koochmeshgi J, Hosseini-Mazinani SM, Morteza Seifati S, Hosein-Pur-Nobari N, Teimoori-Toolabi L.

Apolipoprotein E genotype and age at menopause. 2004; *Ann NY Acad Sci* **1019**: 564–7.

65. Bonomini F, Filippini F, Hayek T, *et al.* Apolipoprotein E and its role in aging and survival. *Exp Gerontol* 2010; **45**(2): 149–57.

66. van Disseldorp J, Broekmans FJ, Peeters PH, Fauser BC, van der Schouw YT. The association between vascular function-related genes and age at natural menopause. *Menopause* 2008; **15**(3): 511–16.

67. van Asselt KM, Kok HS, Peeters PH, *et al.* Factor V Leiden mutation accelerates the onset of natural menopause. *Menopause* 2003; **10**(5): 477–81.

68. Midgette AS, Baron JA. Cigarette smoking and the risk of natural menopause. *Epidemiology* 1990; **1**(6): 474–80.

69. Yang Q, Sherman SL, Hassold TJ, *et al.* Risk factors for trisomy 21: maternal cigarette smoking and oral contraceptive use in a population-based case-control study. *Genet Med* 1999; **1**(3): 80–8.

70. Matzuk MM. Eggs in the balance. *Nat Genet* 2001; **28**(4): 300–1.

71. Broer SL, Mol B, Dólleman M, Fauser BC, Broekmans FJ. The role of anti-Mullerian hormone assessment in assisted reproductive technology outcome. *Curr Opin Obstet Gynecol* 2010; **22**(3): 193–201.

72. Gougeon A, Ecochard R, Thalabard JC. Age-related changes of the population of human ovarian follicles: increase in the disappearance rate of non-growing and early-growing follicles in aging women. *Biol Reprod* 1994; **50**(3): 653–63.

73. Broekmans FJ, Kwee J, Hendriks DJ, Mol BW, Lambalk CB. A systematic review of tests predicting ovarian reserve and IVF outcome. *Hum Reprod Update* 2006; **12**(6): 685–718.

74. Broer SL, Eijkemans MJ, Scheffer GJ, *et al.* Anti-mullerian hormone predicts menopause: a long-term follow-up study in normoovulatory women. *J Clin Endocrinol Metab* 2011; **96**(8): 2532–39.

75. Tehrani FR, Shakeri N, Solaymani-Dodaran M, Azizi F. Predicting age at menopause from serum antimullerian hormone concentration. *Menopause* 2011; **18**(7): 766–70.

76. Hendriks DJ, te Velde ER, Looman CW, *et al.* The role of a poor response in the prediction of the cumulative ongoing pregancy rate in in vitro fertilisation. In: Dynamic and basal ovarian reserve tests for outcome prediction in IVF: comparisons and meta-analyses. Academic Thesis, Utrecht. 2005; 162–79.

77. Hendriks DJ, Kwee J, Mol BW, te Velde ER, Broekmans FJ. Ultrasonography as a tool for the prediction of outcome in IVF patients: a comparative meta-analysis of ovarian volume and antral follicle count. *Fertil Steril* 2007; **87**(4): 764–75.

78. Scott RT, Jr., Elkind-Hirsch KE, Styne-Gross A, Miller KA, Frattarelli JL. The predictive value for in vitro fertility delivery rates is greatly impacted by the method used to select the threshold between normal and elevated basal follicle-stimulating hormone. *Fertil Steril* 2008; **89**(4): 868–78.

79. Patrizio P, Fragouli E, Bianchi V, Borini A, Wells D. Molecular methods for selection of the ideal oocyte. *Reprod Biomed Online* 2007;**15**(3): 346–53.

80. Tanghe S, Van Soome A, Nauwynck H, Coryn M, de Kruif A. Minireview: Functions of the cumulus oophorus during oocyte maturation, ovulation, and fertilization. *Mol Reprod Dev* 2002; **61**(3): 414–24.

81. Adriaenssens T, Segers I, Wathlet S, Smitz J. The cumulus cell gene expression profile of oocytes with different nuclear maturity and potential for blastocyst formation. *J Assist Reprod Genet* 2011; **28**(1): 31–40.

82. Boomsma CM, Macklon NS. What can the clinician do to improve implantation? *Reprod Biomed Online* 2006; **13**(6): 845–55.

83. Broer SL. *Assessment of Current and Future Ovarian Reserve Status.* Enschede, the Netherlands: Gildeprint Drukkerijen, 2011.

84. Eijkemans MJ, Habbema JDF, te Velde ER. Age at last childbirth and fertility at young age. In: Eijkemans MJ, Fertility in populations and in patients. Academic Thesis, Erasmus Medical Center Rotterdam: the Netherlands. 2005; 23–34.

85. Broekmans FJ, Faddy MJ, Scheffer G, te Velde ER. Antral follicle counts are related to age at natural fertility loss and age at menopause. *Menopause* 2004; **11**(6 Pt 1): 607–14.

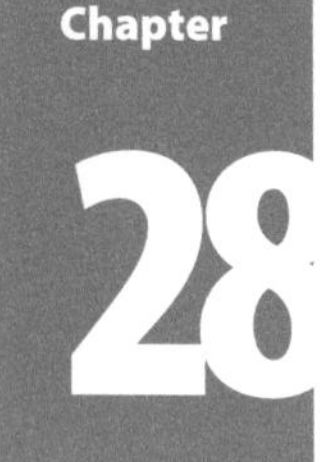

Cellular origin of age-related aneuploidy in mammalian oocytes

Ursula Eichenlaub-Ritter and Roger Gosden

Introduction

Separation of chromosomes in meiosis is a well-guarded process such that errors in chromosome segregation are rare events. For instance, only 1 in every 100 000 divisions in yeast is associated with non-disjunction. Aneuploidy in germ cells of mammals like the mouse is generally much higher, in the range 0.5–1% [1]. Furthermore, there is a gender-specific difference in susceptibility to meiotic errors during germ cell formation in mammals, particularly in humans. On average, only 1–4% of sperm in healthy men have numerical chromosomal aberrations, while on average about 20% of all human meiosis II oocytes are aneuploid [1–4]. The correlation between the incidence of the birth of a trisomic child with Down's syndrome and maternal age was first recognized in 1933 by Penrose [5], confirmed by chromosomal analysis of spontaneous abortions and live births and, since the introduction of assisted reproduction, by evidence from polar bodies, oocytes, and embryos (e.g., [3, 6–8]). However, the cause(s) of the extraordinary susceptibility of aging oocytes to meiotic errors was obscure until recently.

Intrinsic susceptibility and age-related contributions to non-disjunction

Meiotic stages at which errors may occur

In typical mitosis there is division of sister chromatids derived from replication of each chromosome, and each pair therefore carries the same alleles along their arms (Figure 28.1A). In contrast, in meiosis I the two originally paternally and maternally derived homologs, each containing two sister chromatids, separate during first meiotic division (termed reductional division, Figure 28.1B, Ciii). They are normally physically attached to each other by at least one chiasma from recombination between sister chromatids of parental homologs (indicated by X in Figure 28.1B, Ci, Ciii). Chiasmata are held in place by cohesion between sister chromatid arms and centromeres (Figure 28.1Ci–Ciii) placed on chromatids before S-phase (Figure 28.1Ci), which is maintained until anaphase I (Figure 28.1Ciii, B) (reviewed in [9]). The paternal and maternal alleles along chromatid arms of recombined chromosomes switch left and right of a chiasma or exchange (indicated by different coloring in Figure 28.1B, Ci, E–J). Hence, the distribution of polymorphisms can be used to trace the origin and recombinational history of a chromosome in a zygote or child.

Separation of chromosomes at anaphase I of meiosis is mediated by resolution of cohesion along the chromatid arms – except for the centromeres – by the activity of separase, a proteolytic enzyme that recognizes the phosphorylated Rec8 protein in the meiotic cohesion complexes (Figure 28.1B) [9–11]. Proteins like shugoshins, Aurora kinase B or C (AURB/C), and phosphatase PP2A play essential roles to prevent cohesin Rec8 protein phosphorylation at centromeres and thereby protect centromeres from precocious sister chromatid separation. AURB/C promotes recruitment and regulation of a microtubule depolymerase, MCAK (mitotic centromere-associated kinase), that is also involved in resolving attachment errors and chromosome congression [12, 13]. After completion of meiosis I, the MII oocyte and its first polar body (PB) should contain one set of homologous chromosomes, each comprising two sister chromatids (termed dyads), which may or may not be recombinant and are

Biology and Pathology of the Oocyte, 2nd edn., ed. Alan Trounson, Roger Gosden, and Ursula Eichenlaub-Ritter.

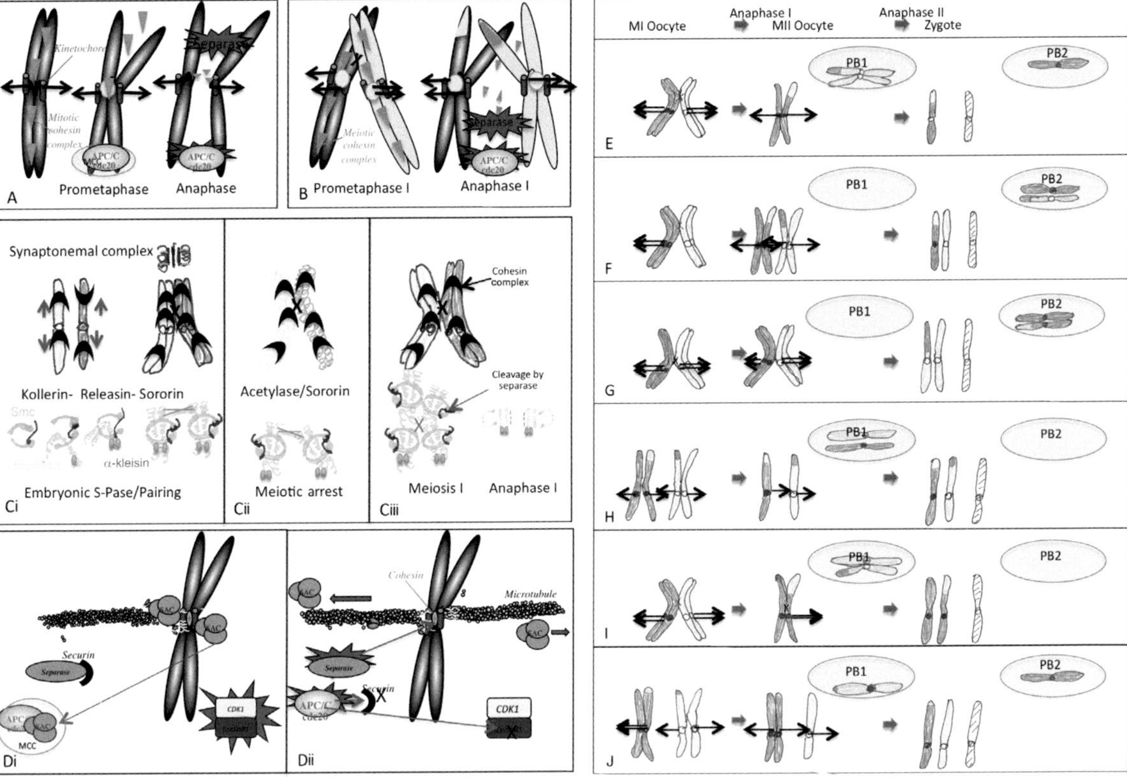

Figure 28.1 (A–J) Acquisition and loss of chromosome cohesion (A–Ciii), timing of loss of cohesion by the spindle assembly checkpoint (SAC) (D, Dii) and segregation of chromosomes at meiosis I and meiosis II in oocytes (E–J). For further explanation, see text.

still attached at their centromeres (Figure 28.1B, E). Resumption of meiosis II is triggered by fertilization and mediated by proteolytic cleavage of separase and loss of cohesion between sister centromeres, similar to mitosis (Figure 28.1A, E). This division results in formation of a second PB with one set of recombinant or non-recombinant chromatids (also termed monads, Figure 28.1E). The euploid 1-cell embryo therefore contains one copy of each chromosome from the oocyte and one from the sperm (Figure 28.1E, colored and striped chromatids, respectively). The haploid set of chromatids in the oocyte is transformed into the female pronucleus, while sperm chromatin is remodeled and, after acquiring a new nuclear membrane, constitutes the male pronucleus.

Errors in chromosome segregation (termed nondisjunction) at meiosis I typically derive from failure to separate and/or segregate the two homologs (Figure 28.1F). One homolog may fail to attach properly, but especially the presence of univalents (e.g., from failures to recombine) increases risks of random segregation, for example when homologs attach randomly and by chance to the same instead of opposite spindle poles. There is evidence from yeast that loss of cohesion between the core centromeres of sister chromatids predisposes them on the same parental chromosome (or of an achiasmatic univalent) to attach to opposite poles (bi-orientation or amphitelic orientation) instead of to one spindle pole (monopolar or syntelic attachment), as is normal in meiosis I (Figure 28.1H, J). They therefore undergo an equatorial rather than a reductional separation at meiosis I [14] which, on separation at anaphase I, results in one (Figure 28.1J) or two chromatids (Figure 28.1H) instead of homologs (dyads) in the first PB and the oocyte, thereby predisposing to random segregation at meiosis II (Figure 28.1H).

Typical meiotic II errors may occur when the sister chromatids of a homolog derived from a normal first meiotic reduction division attach and segregate to the same pole (syntelic) at meiosis II (Figure 28.1I). This may be related to failure to resolve cohesion between

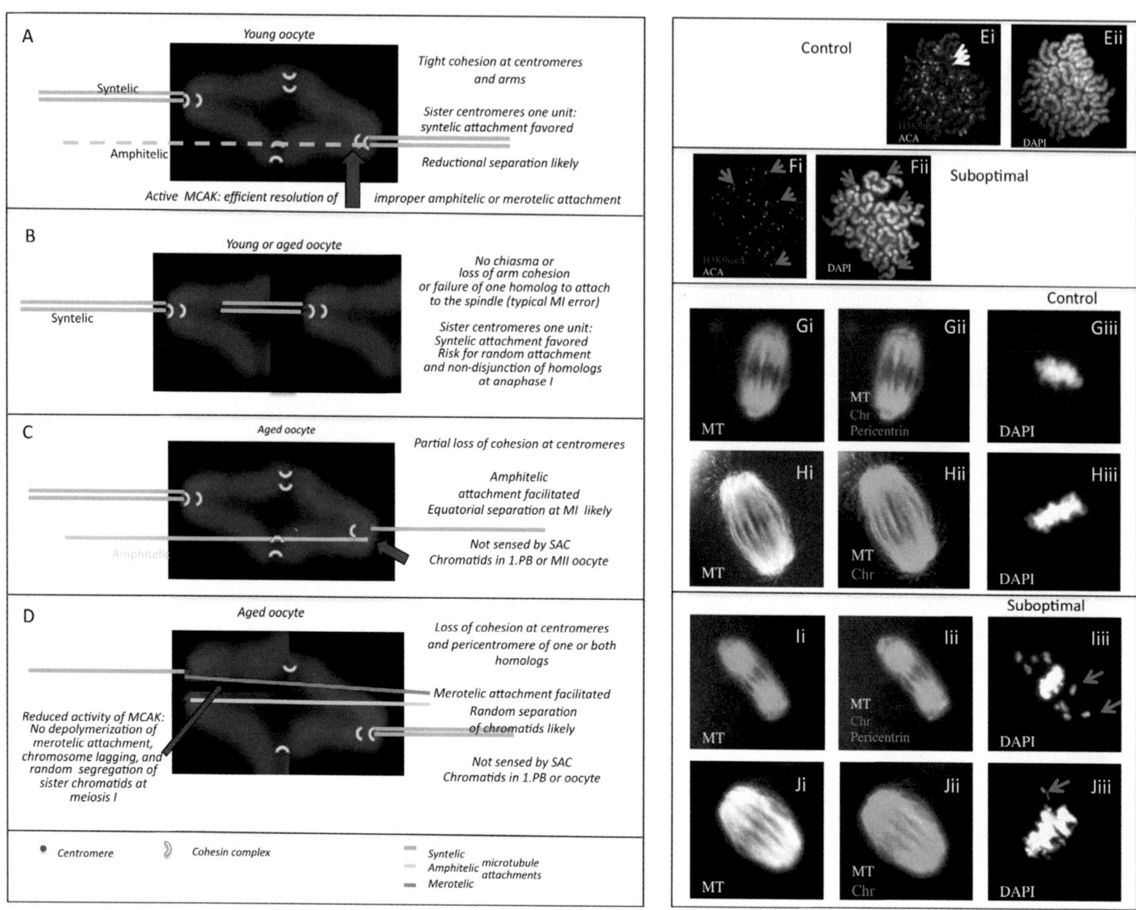

Figure 28.2 (A–Jiii) Attachment of centromeres to spindle microtubules (A–D) and normal chromatid cohesion at centromeres and chromosome congression on the metaphase II spindle in a control group of mouse oocytes undergoing in vitro maturation (Ei, Eii, Gi–Hiii), compared to loss of centromere cohesion and failure to align at the spindle equator in oocytes cultured to MII in suboptimal medium (Fi, Fii, Ii–Jiii). White arrows in Ei, Eii: normal attachment of sister centromeres; blue arrows in Fi, Fii predivision and in Iiii and Kiii unaligned chromatids at metaphase II. Staining of chromosomes in A–D by DAPI (blue) and centromeres by anticentromere antibody (red). Staining in Ei–Jiii as indicated. H3K9me3, antibody to trimethylated histone H3 lysine 9; ACA, anticentromere antibody; DAPI: chromosomes stained by 4′,6-diamidino-2-phenylindole; MT, spindle microtubules; Chr, chromosomes. For further explanation, see text.

centromeres at anaphase II, but can also be caused by a loss of cohesion, or failure to attach to spindle fibers with random segregation (as in Figure 28.1H, J). Furthermore, failure to separate from each other can also occur when sister chromatids are lagging, as occurs for instance when a single centromere attaches to both spindle poles instead of one (termed merotelic attachment, indicated by green and orange coloring of microtubules in Figure 28.2D). Such chromatids may become trapped in the interpolar region of the spindle, thus becoming incorporated into the same daughter cell as their sister. Loss of cohesion in the core centromere and pericentromeric chromatin (indicated in Figure 28.2D) appears to predispose to errors in chromosome segregation at meiosis I or II, particularly when enzymes for resolving erroneous attachments are deficient (discussed in [14, 15]).

When sister chromatids of truly non-disjoined homologs from a first meiotic error separate equatorially at meiosis II instead of meiosis I (Figure 28.1F), the embryo is expected to contain three copies of a chromosome, one from the sperm and two from the oocyte, each of which carries centromeres and alleles of corresponding homologs of the oocyte, except for sites that were subject to recombination (Figure 28.1F). It is different for a typical second meiotic error, such that meiosis I is normal (Figure 28.1I), and the two centromeres and sister chromatids of one homologous chromosome fail to separate at meiosis II. In this case, the embryo should carry the two copies of one homolog with the same alleles, except for sites where recombination occurred (for typical meiosis II error, see Figure 28.1I). In cases where non-disjunction occurs in meiosis I (Figure 28.1G) and is followed by a reductional separation (as in Figure 28.1B) rather than an equatorial separation of the two homologs at meiosis II, the presence of two maternal sister chromatids (blue or yellow) and centromeres from the same parental chromosome (open or dark circle) plus the one derived from the sperm (striped) cannot be distinguished retrospectively from a typical second meiotic error (Figure 28.1I). Similiarly, separation of sister chromatids and not homologs at meiosis I (Figure 28.1H) followed by a non-disjunction of the two non-homologous sister chromatids at meiosis II cannot be distinguished retrospectively from a first meiotic error, although the failure to separate the chromatids actually occured at meiosis II. The single or multiple chromatids in the first PB (Figure 28.1H, J) recognized in cytogenetic analysis indicate that the sequential separation of chromatids is aberrant and cohesion was resolved precociously (predivision). Array technologies identifying DNA content might predict normal chromosomal constitution with twice the haploid amount of the chromosome-specific DNA in the oocyte or its first PB, although two chromatids are present and predivision occurred.

Secondary non-disjunction, in which a first meiotic error is followed by another at meiosis II (e.g., when both homologs remain in the oocyte but one homolog plus one chromatid segregate to the second PB at anaphase II) may restore euploidy in the oocyte. This can be detected by analysis of ploidy in the first and second PB and in the zygote (e.g., [7]). Second meiotic errors may also compensate for a first non-disjunction event when the two physically unattached chromatids from predivision (Figure 28.1H) segregate from each other, such that one chromatid segregates into the second PB and one into the oocyte, respectively.

Mitotic non-disjunction events should always lead to the presence of two chromatids with the same parental alleles and polymorphisms from either the oocyte- or sperm-derived set of chromatids/chromosomes that fail to separate from each other. When mitotic non-disjunction occurs in one or several cells during early embryogenesis, the zygote/embryo becomes mosaic for the aneuploidy.

Polymorphic centromere markers and polymorphisms have been used to analyze retrospectively the origin of an extra chromosome in trisomy to identify: (1) the parental origin (maternal or paternal meiosis); (2) the stage of the meiotic error (meiosis I or meiosis II); and (3) the recombinational history with respect to presence and position of exchanges and maternal age. In such analyses the presence of two centromeres from both parental homologs are typically assigned as first meiotic errors (Figure 28.1F), and those with the centromeres of only one parental chromosome as second meiotic errors (Figure 28.1I), although this might be misleading (Figure 28.1G, see above). In cases of no recombination (achiasmatic chromosomes) it may be impossible to distinguish between a meiotic and a mitotic error, when cells analyzed from the embryos are not mosaic for the aneuploidy and contain achiasmatic chromosomes.

Recombinational history, chromosome shape, and the "production line"

Recognizing an increase in chromosomes with apparently few, distal chiasmata and what appeared to be "univalent chromosomes" in aged mouse oocytes led Henderson and Edwards in 1968 [16] to suggest that there is a "production line" for oogenesis in the ovary. According to this hypothesis, oocytes entering meiosis late in the embryonic ovary would have reduced recombination. When primordial follicles and oocytes become recruited in the order they are formed (i.e., according to the "production line") this would lead to increased numbers of oocytes with chromosomes lacking an exchange that are at risk of random segregation at meiosis I in aging ovaries. To test this hypothesis, the origin and recombinational history of extra chromosomes has been traced in trisomies and revealed that most errors giving rise to trisomies originate from maternal meiosis I, while some trisomies involve mainly chromatids, for example trisomy 18 [3, 17–19]. Failure to recombine poses a risk for random segregation of chromosomes 21 at meiosis I in an estimated 40% of all cases, irrespective of maternal age. A single exchange in the distal part of the chromosomes predisposes younger oocytes to non-disjunction of chromosome 21 at meiosis I. However, the overall distribution of exchanges does not appear to differ between a normally segregating chromosome 21 and that giving rise to trisomy 21 in an aged oocyte, challenging the prediction by the production line [19]. Unexpectedly, trisomy 21 involving a second meiotic error and advanced maternal age frequently involves chromosomes that possess a chiasma in the pericentromeric region. Therefore, the origin of the error must be related to events in first meiosis. For instance, when bivalents with pericentromeric exchange fail to segregate at meiosis I in an aged oocyte, but separate reductionally instead of equatorially at meiosis II (Figure 28.1G), zygotes contain centromeres from one maternal homolog recognized as a meiosis II error. Further analysis of the recombinational history of extra chromosomes in other trisomies revealed chromosome-specific patterns of exchanges for each trisomy and gonosomal aneuploidies that were associated with aneuploidy derived from oocytes of young and advanced aged women. Therefore, the presence and localization of chiasmata affects the risk of meiotic errors in a chromosome-specific fashion in aged oocytes (see [3]). For instance, a single distal chiasma may not be sufficient to mediate correct segregation of a small, acrocentric chromosome in a young oocyte, while all types of exchanges are susceptible to meiotic errors in an aged oocyte, including those that permit normal segregation in a young oocyte. Accordingly, it was proposed that more than one event ("hit") is associated with age-related increases in oocyte aneuploidy in a general fashion (absence of exchanges) as well as in a chromosome-specific fashion. Array analysis of ploidy in first and second PBs and human embryos confirms earlier observations that chromosomes of all sizes are susceptible to meiotic errors in aged oocytes [7], although the relative risks are differentially correlated with age. For instance, errors of small acrocentrics are particularly frequent in aged oocytes [7, 8], while gains and losses involving exchange chromosomes are especially common and increase linearly rather than exponentially with advanced maternal age for trisomy 16 [3, 4, 8].

Concerning the existence of a production line, a recent analysis of recombination events along all chromosomes of euploid children from younger or aged mothers in a Canadian population found a slightly reduced frequency overall up to the age of 32 years, but not afterwards [20]. In this Canadian pedigree there was a tendency for a reduction in the frequency of recombination events in the distal and in intermediate portions of chromosomes of euploid children of mothers of advanced reproductive age, but paternal age had no effect. Thus, a general alteration in recombination rate may not exist, as predicted by the production line hypothesis, but there is a selective mechanism protecting oocytes against non-disjunction when they possess chiasmata that are more proximal as opposed to peritelomeric. In contrast, earlier studies in a different population and with fewer polymorphisms suggested an increase in recombination gives rise to euploid children in aged mothers, implying that increased recombination protects aged oocytes from segregation errors [21]. Methodological differences or the genetic background might have influenced the outcomes. Although unlikely, a production line of oocytes with differences in recombination may exist in human ovaries, and we cannot exclude the possibility that recombination differs in cohorts of oocytes in the embryonic ovary becoming ovulated either early or late in adult life.

The Hultén group detected mosaicism for trisomy 21 in primary oocytes of all eight fetal ovaries examined [22]. They suggested that aneuploid oogonia and oocytes become recruited late in the reproductive period, preferentially contributing to trisomy 21 in children of older mothers. However, this hypothesis cannot explain the relative patterns of chromosome distribution as deduced from analyses of first and second PBs and zygotes by comparative genomic hybridization [8]. Interestingly, the mechanisms leading to non-disjunction appear distinct in certain pathologies. There was more predivision in oocytes of patients of advanced maternal age compared to a group with repeat implantation failures (RIF), but more first meiotic errors in the RIF group [23].

Knockout of genes involved in recombination, DNA repair, or meiotic chromosome cohesion in mice can induce subfertility or sterility. Oocytes may die at early stages thereby protecting them from non-disjunction, while a moderately reduced survival of primary oocytes with asynapsed chromosomes can lead to premature ovarian insufficiency as well as a dramatic increase in meiotic errors in ovulated oocytes, irrespective of age [24, 25]. Sex-specific differences in the stage at which meiotic arrest occurs in mice deficient in specific recombination proteins suggest that female meiosis is more permissive to disturbances in pairing and recombination, because oocytes survive to more advanced stages in animals with induced deficiencies in chromosome cohesion compared to

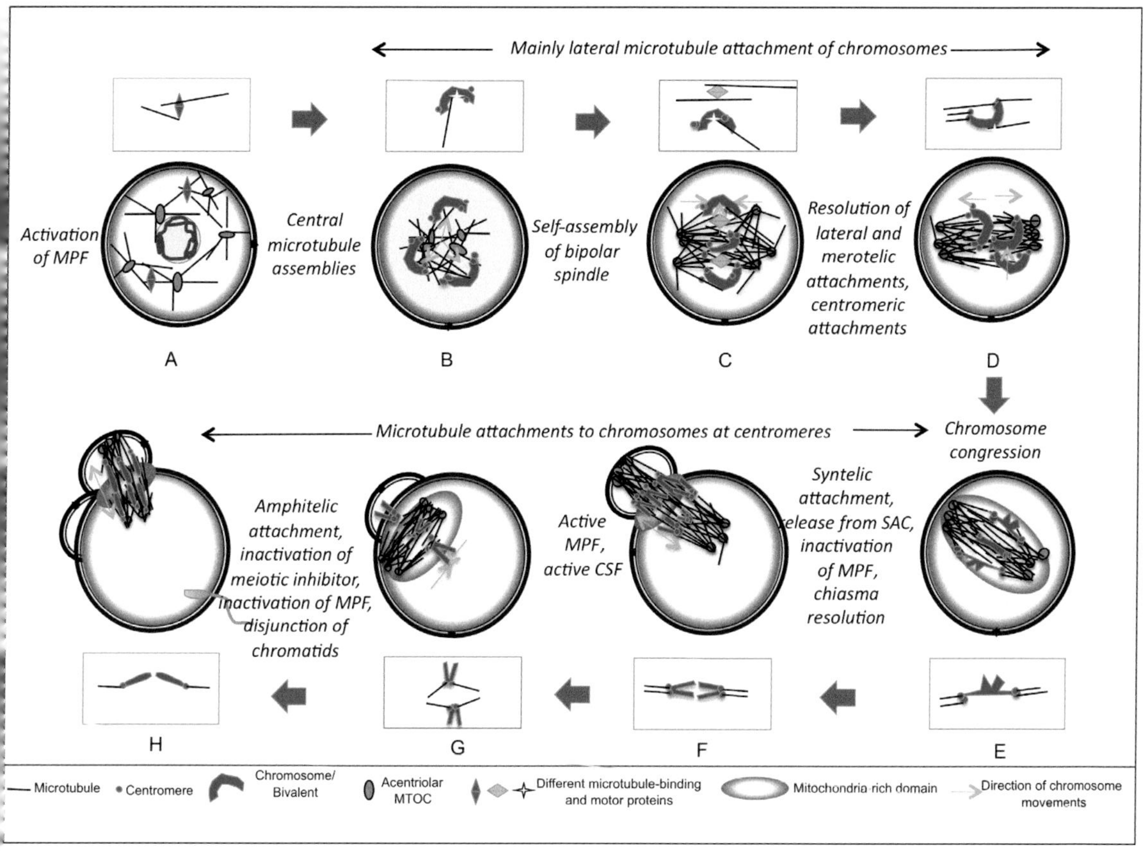

Figure 28.3 (A–H) Schematic processes of microtubule polymerization, spindle formation, chromosome attachment, and cell-cycle progression during mouse oocyte maturation, at resumption of maturation (A), at germinal vesicle breakdown and circular bivalent stage (B), at early prophase I with formation of a pre-prophase belt (C), at prometaphase I (D), at metaphase I (E), at anaphase I (F), at metaphase II after activation of maturation-promoting factor/Cdk1 (MPF) and cytostatic factor (CSF) maintaining metaphase II arrest (G), and at anaphase II after fertilization (H). Blue boxes above or below stages indicate interactions between microtubules and spindle microtubule attachments at chromosome arms (A–D) and centromeres (D–H). Based on Kitajima *et al.* [41]. For further explanation, see text.

males with the same mutation in which meiosis is blocked at an early stage [24–26]. In humans, some mutations of genes coding for components of the synaptonemal complex (an organelle formed in the prophase I oocytes involved in pairing and recombination) can increase the risk of recurrent spontaneous abortion, presumably from disturbed recombination, non-disjunction, and aneuploidy in the oocyte, irrespective of maternal age [27, 28]. Disturbances in recombination and chromosome cohesion in mice [29] may also raise the risk of aneuploidy at young maternal ages [30]. This could be a synergistic effect of reduced numbers of chiasmata and age-related loss of cohesion (see below), but may also reflect correlations between susceptibility to meiotic errors and follicular pool size/hormonal homeostasis.

Spindle formation and chromosome attachment in aging oocytes

Unlike spermatocytes, oocytes do not possess pairs of centrioles for organizing a bipolar spindle. Instead, they possess multiple microtubule-organizing centers (MTOCs), which have to become recruited to the spindle poles of the acentriolar spindle (Figure 28.3A) (see Chapter 12). Polymerization dynamics, microtubule and actin cytoskeletal organization, and bundling of microtubules at the poles (Figure 28.3B–D) involve a number of motor proteins, kinases, and gradients of nucleotide exchange factors driven by ATP and GTP in a self-assembly process [31, 32]. Thus, they require local mitochondria and high energy substrates (see Chapters 12 and 26 and [15, 33]). Integration of signaling and coordination of actin-based and microtubule-mediated processess in spindle function and positioning at the cell cortex for unequal division is complex (see Chapter 12) and potentially vulnerable to age changes, including gene expression which becomes altered and unbalanced (Chapters 13, 24 and 29), or insufficient high energy substrates (Chapter 26). Hence, aberrant spindles are a hallmark of aged human oocytes [34]. Altered abundance of mRNAs of cell cycle and spindle-regulating proteins were noted in transcriptome analyses of aged rodent and human MII oocytes [35–40] (see Chapter 29).

High susceptibility to meiotic errors is correlated with unique characteristics of spindle formation. Confocal imaging of mouse oocyte maturation showed that multiple asters are formed from cytoplasmic MTOCs (Figure 28.3A), and bivalents initially attach laterally all along the chromosome arms to microtubules after germinal vesicle breakdown [41]. Bivalents are pushed out of the centrally located mass of asters assembling in the ooplasm (Figure 28.3B) to align on the surface of the large microtubular ball (so-called circular bivalent stage). This is followed by formation of a short bipolar spindle which has broad poles in the mouse (Figure 28.3C). On this still unfocused bipolar spindle bivalents align equatorially in a hollow ring, called a "pre-prophase belt" (Figure 28.3C) [41]. Only later in prometaphase I do the centromeres of the chromosomes establish firm connections to the spindle microtubules (Figure 28.3E). This period up to metaphase I is characterized by chromosome invasion into the spindle and a very dynamic repolymerization/depolymerization of microtubules, as well as by cycles involving bipolar attachment of sister centromeres or a single centromere to both instead of only one spindle pole (amphitelic or merotelic rather than syntelic attachment, Figures 28.1H and 28.2A–D). At a late stage of prometaphase I (ProMI)/MI bivalents finally congress at the equator (Figure 28.3E). Kinetochores (the specific structures and molecules regulating spindle attachment at metaphase) are thus not involved in initial spindle formation, but control the activity of the spindle assembly checkpoint (SAC), sensing microtubule attachment. The SAC determines the timing of anaphase I progression [42] (Chapter 11). The process of bi-orientation appears therefore to be initially highly error-prone, requiring resolution of erroneous chromosome attachments by AURB/C [43], and MCAK and other microtubule depolymerases (e.g., [44–46]; Figure 28.3A, D). Resolution of merotelic attachments is mandatory to ensure fidelity of chromosome separation. Compared to young mice, mRNA of MCAK depolymerase is reduced in aging mouse oocytes at metaphase II [38], possibly compromising the efficient resolution of merotelic attachments [15].

Tension and the relative cohesion between sister chromatid arms, pericentromeric regions, and the centromeres appear to influence the probability that sister centromeres of a meiotic chromosome will attach to one spindle pole (syntelic attachment, Figure 28.2A), or both poles (amphitelic, Figure 28.2C) or singly to both spindle poles (merotelic, Figure 28.2D). Loss of regulation of proper attachment/cohesion between sister chromatids in yeast contributes to untimely and aberrant chromosome behavior [14], as discussed below.

The spindle assembly checkpoint (SAC) and cell-cycle control

The SAC monitors chromosome attachment to the spindle [47] (Figure 28.1Di; Chapter 11), such that when there is no full attachment it causes meiotic arrest. In this circumstance, SAC proteins (Mad2, BubR1, Msp1) are retained at the centromeres. The release of checkpoint proteins like Mad2 and its conformational change contributes to a blocked state that initiates an inhibitory signal [48], leading to formation of a complex termed "mitotic checkpoint complex" (MCC) (Figure 28.1Di) (reviewed in [47]). The MCC consists of checkpoint components and the Cdc20 (cell division cycle 20) protein, the latter being an activator of the anaphase-promoting complex/cyclosome (APC/C) (Figure 28.1Di). APC/C^{cdc20} activity is required to mark proteins like cyclin B and securin for degradation by polyubiquitination, thus targetting them for degradation by the proteasome (see Chapter 11). Upon anaphase progression, this leads to inactivation of Cdk1/cyclin B1, and degradation of securin with release of separase, a proteolytic enzyme (Chapter 11). The formation of the MCC renders APC/C^{cdc20} inactive, causing cell-cycle arrest (Figure 28.1Di). The current model suggests that SAC proteins become transported away from centromeres when chromosomes are fully attached such that no MCC is formed and cells can enter anaphase with active APC/C^{cdc20} (Figure 28.1B, Dii). Upon degradation of cyclin B1 and securin, separase is released and cleaves cohesin proteins, thereby causing loss of cohesion (Figure 28.1Ciii, Dii), (reviewed in [9]; see below) and separation of chromosomes (Figure 28.1B, Dii).

Initial studies suggested that cell-cycle control in aged oocytes is disturbed. Anaphase I occurs precociously and is error-prone in some strains of mice [49]. In contrast, aged human oocytes undergoing in vitro maturation appear to have delayed emission of the first PB compared to those of younger women [50]. Analysis of the transcriptome and gene ontology in oocytes of both species showed that transcripts in pathways involving spindle formation and function and cell-cycle control were altered, although there were differences in the up- or down-regulated transcripts between species and studies [35–40] (Chapters 24 and 29). Furthermore, gene ontology indicated that transcripts related to DNA damage, metabolism, mitochondria, oxidative stress, and some that are essential for preimplantation development are either less or more abundant in aged compared to young oocytes. The origin of the altered transcriptome is still unclear. Such data need to be interpreted cautiously since different protocols for mRNA isolation and types of mRNA extracted (e.g., + or – poly(A) tail, splice variants, polysome-associated or negative) can affect results [51, 52] (Chapter 13). Whether increases or decreases in transcript abundance correspond to differences in the proteome or disturbances in RNA metabolism/turnover is currently unknown. However, modeling alterations in transcript abundance in rodent oocytes, for example by targeted knockout, knockdown, or overexpression, provided information on increased aneuploidy after mimicking changes in transcriptome as in aged oocytes [53–55].

Mammalian oocytes were initially suspected to have poor checkpoint control since they undergo anaphase I in the presence of one or several univalents, unlike spermatogenesis [56, 57]. However, depletion of SAC components induces susceptibility to meiotic errors, particularly when oocyte spindle formation is compromised by exposure to chemicals affecting microtubule polymerization and turnover (see [58, 59]). On the other hand, checkpoint control may be rather permissive in oocytes, irrespective of age, because recent studies in the mouse indicated that one bivalent, but possibly not a single chromosome (dyad) or chromatid (monard), is sufficient to trigger meiotic arrest [60]. Within the voluminous ooplasm the signals released from a single unattached centromere might be too weak after diffusion to cause arrest at meiotic M-phase to efficiently prolong the SAC (Figure 28.1Di). Furthermore, the loss of the Mad2 checkpoint protein upon centromeric attachment of chromosomes at late prometaphase I does not monitor positional information within the spindle, thereby permitting oocytes with bivalents away from the equator to enter anaphase I [42]. Similarly, oocytes can enter anaphase and exhibit silenced SAC without interkinetochore tension and when chromosomes are still unaligned [61]. This relative insensitivity of checkpoint control may contribute to the gender-specific risks of aneuploidy in mammalian oogenesis, particularly in the presence of univalents and a threshold number of incompletely attached and merotelically attached chromosomes [62]. This also explains why in some strains of mice aged oocytes have normal cell cycles [63], become arrested after exposure to a microtubule depolymerizing agent, and do not necessarily exhibit a correlation between a delayed cell cycle and aneuploidy [63]. In contrast to mitosis, young oocytes are not irreversibly blocked at prometaphase I in the presence of unaligned chromosomes, as revealed also in those possessing multiple univalents and reduced numbers and altered distribution of chiasmata, for example in *Mlh1* knockout oocytes [62]. This finding might also be related to the relative abundance and turnover of SAC proteins and blocking versus activating signals in the ooplasm, since oocytes can enter anaphase I after an initial delay. Increases in non-disjunction, predivision, and chromosome lagging were observed [62]. Since human oocytes have a much larger volume but a comparatively smaller spindle apparatus than mouse oocytes, they may be more susceptible to minor disturbances. A stronger signal may be needed to form the MCC to prevent APC/C activation efficiently [47, 60]. Synergistic effects of incomplete attachments, slightly aberrant spindles, and deficiencies in checkpoint control might therefore act synergistically, putting aging human oocytes at higher risk for meiotic errors [15]. In particular, when the supply of high energy substrates such as ATP is inadequate the mechanisms for spindle formation, monitoring chromosome attachment, and cell-cycle regulation can contribute to meiotic errors [15, 64] (Chapters 11, 12, 26, and 29). Aging may affect the localization and function of mitochondria within the oocyte, as well as within granulosa cells thus indirectly compromising bidirectional signaling in the follicle (see below).

Chromosome cohesion

Regulation of sister chromatid cohesion is a fundamental processs mediating stage-specific behavior of chromosomes in mitosis and meiosis that is not only essential for normal chromosome segregation [9] but also for DNA repair and control of gene expression [65]. Furthermore, condensin and cohesin protein complexes are important for the regulation of chromatin conformation at different stages of the cell cycle and for meiotic pairing and recombination [9]. Cohesion between chromosomes is mediated by the highly conserved, tripartite cohesin protein complexes that embrace chromatid DNA like a ring according to current models (green rods and pink line in Figure 28.1Ci). A V-shaped part of the cohesin complex comprises two proteins of the "structural maintenance of chromosomes (SMC)" family of proteins, Smc1 and Smc3 (green in Figure 28.1Ci). Each Smc forms a rod-shaped coiled-coil structure with a looped dimerization domain at the tip of the V, while the C- and N-terminal portions of the Smc proteins form lobes with a nucleotide-binding domain at the open side of the V-shaped complex. The lobes are kept close together in the tripartite ring structure of the cohesin complex by interaction with a protein of the conserved α-kleisin family of proteins (typically, Scc1 in mitosis and Rec8 in meiosis, pink line in Figure 28.1Ci–Ciii). Other proteins binding to the α-kleisin protein present in mitosis or meiosis modulate stability of the complex (see [9]). The interaction/dimerization domain between the Smc1 and Smc3 proteins acts as a "hinge" region, which according to the current model may be involved in loading and opening the ring structure before and upon replication. According to current concepts, the cohesin ring becomes loaded at the centromeres prior to S-phase and glides along the chromosomes towards the pericentromeric region, and possibly to more distal parts of the chromosome (Figure 28.1Ci, red arrows). The initially loaded complex appears to be unstable, which can be promoted by binding proteins and/or sororin (termed releasins) [9]. ATP hydrolysis at the nucleotide binding lobes of the Smc protein, and the activity of so-called "kollerin loading proteins" plus acetylation of residues in Smc3 stabilize the cohesin complex at the chromatin after initial recruitment (Figure 28.1Cii). These "static" cohesin complexes remain stably embracing sister chromatids until prometaphase in mitosis or anaphase I or II in meiosis (Figure 28.1B, Cii, Ciii).

In mitosis, there is a non-proteolytic loss of cohesion on chromatid arms at late prometaphase (green triangles, Figure 28.1A), involving releasin protein and phosphorylation of cohesin proteins by polo-like kinase and AURB kinase activity. This opens the cohesin complexes at the sister chromatid arms, but not at the centromeres (Figure 28.1A). At anaphase of mitosis, the opening of the ring at the centromeres of sister chromatids occurs by proteolytic cleavage of the α-kleisin Scc1 protein by separase (Figure 28.1A). Through activity of APC/C^{cdc20}, securin is degraded and separase released. Separase then cleaves the Scc1 α-kleisin protein, thus causing release of cohesion at sister centromeres and chromosome segregation [9].

In contrast, in prometaphase of meiosis I sister chromatid arm cohesion is maintained until anaphase I (Figure 28.1B). At anaphase I, arm cohesion is lost by separase proteolytic cleavage of the phosphorylated meiotic Rec8 α-kleisin protein (Figure 28.1B and Ciii). This causes opening of the cohesin complex, separation of sister chromatid arms, and chiasma resolution. The centromeres appear protected by proteins like shugoshin 2, a phosphatase PP2A, and AURB/C (indicated by yellow circles in Figure 28.1B) preventing Rec8 phosphorylation. Sister chromatids therefore stay attached to each other until anaphase II. After fertilization, degradation of the meiotic inhibitor Emi2 (early mitotic inhibitor 2) causes release from cytostatic arrest, and activation of APC/C^{cdc20} degrades securin and releases separase. Separase then cleaves the phosphorylated Rec8 cohesin at sister chromatid centromeres, similiar to mitotic anaphase (see Figure 28.1A).

Some years ago, studies in mice with an XO karyotype or after knocking out the synaptonemal complex gene, *Sycp3*, suggested that univalency may predispose homologs to amphitelic rather than syntelic attachment of sister chromatids at meiosis I in oocytes (Figures 28.1H and 28.2B). This appears to influence loss of cohesion of centromeres at anaphase I, thereby raising the risk of first and second meiotic errors [56, 57]. This suggests that behavior and loss of cohesion is chromosome- rather than stage-specifically regulated. Furthermore, experimentally overexpressing a hyperactive separase in mouse oocytes causes gradual loss of centromere cohesion and increased distance between centromeres of sister chromatids at prometaphase I, followed by loss of arm cohesion and precocious separation of chromatids at anaphase I [66].

Overexpression of separase has more severe effects on aged than young mouse oocytes, implying there are fewer cohesion complexes [66]. This confirms studies that suggested a reduced concentration of cohesin complexes at sister chromatid arms and centromeres in aged oocytes [29, 67–69]. An increased distance between centromeres of sister chromatids occurs in aged oocytes (although not in the most advanced age group), suggesting that loss of chromosome cohesion may be the primary cause of meiotic errors in mice [69]. Cohesins thus appear not to be replaced during meiotic arrest, as implied in germinal vesicle stage oocytes with targeted proteolysis of Rec8 [70]. Even overexpression of human REC8 cohesin could not restore cohesion in these oocytes. Therefore, it has been hypothesised that prolonged meiotic arrest leads to loss of cohesion, as a primary lesion responsible for higher risks of meiotic errors in aged oocytes [66, 67].

Since separase transcripts are increased in aged human oocytes this might possibly lead to imbalance between securin and separase and loss of cohesion [39]. Although separase is also inhibited after phosphorylation by Cdk1 kinase, this is not activated in germinal vesicle-arrested oocytes prior to resumption of maturation. Therefore, free separase might contribute to "hyperactivity" and predivision, as observed in mice [70]. However, there is no evidence so far that REC8, STAG3, SMC1 β, and SMC3 cohesin proteins are reduced in abundance in human MII oocytes up to 37 years [71], and the link between loss of cohesion and maternal age has still to be confirmed. Furthermore, there is no increase in aneuploidy in aged pig oocytes, challenging a general correlation between loss of cohesion due to prolonged meiotic arrest, chronological age, and non-disjunction in oocytes [72]. However, it is feasible that loss of cohesion over time can cause formation of "functional" univalents resembling achiasmatic univalents inducing predivision in human and rodent oocytes (Figure 28.1H, J) [73]. Furthermore, loss of cohesion at centromeres or pericentromeric chromatin can favor amphitelic and merotelic attachments that are not recognized by the SAC (Figure 28.2C, D). Additionally, when depolymerases, like MCAK, are less abundant, resolution of erroneous attachments might lead to chromosome lagging at anaphase and random chromosome segregation (Figure 28.1H). A reduction in shugoshin 2 activity [68] can also be critical because of its role in preventing protection of centromeres from Rec8 phosphorylation before anaphase II and predisposing them to equatorial rather than reductional separation at meiosis I.

It appears that the non-proteolytic release of cohesin proteins in prometaphase of mitosis is influenced by neutralization of releasin protein, and possibly by acetylation of Smc3 cohesin (Figure 28.1Cii) [9]. Alterations in the activities of the respective acetylases, deacetylases, phosphorylation of cohesins by kinases, availability of ATP, and importantly, defects in condensin and cohesin metabolism might all contribute to age-associated alterations in gene expression in meiotic oocytes as well as to susceptibility to meiotic errors from predivision. In fact, there is evidence that post-translational modification of histones and epigenetically controlled chromatin conformation are altered in aged human oocytes [74]. Whether loss of cohesion might be influenced by the size of the follicle pool, the length of meiotic arrest, and oocyte age, as opposed to ovarian stimulation protocols, lifestyle, and metabolic disturbances is still unknown (see Chapters 27, 31 and 32). However, we found that maturation of cumulus-denuded young mouse oocytes in a suboptimal culture medium affecting metabolism, redox regulation, and mitochondrial distribution induced predivision (Figure 28.2Fi, Fii, Ii–Jiii) [75]. Trimethylation of histone H3K9 appeared normal (Figure 28.2Fi, Gi), without evidence of changes in abundance of centromeric proteins. However, predivision also caused chromosome congression failure at MII, thus predisposing cells to second meiotic errors (Figure 28.2Ii, Iiii, Ji, Jiii). This model offers hope that predivision errors in aged oocytes might be reduced if they mature in an environment that is optimal for bidirectional signaling and mitochondrial function in cumulus–oocyte complexes (see below).

Further evidence showing that age and ovarian stimulation affect chromosome cohesion comes from conventional chromosome spreading and staining techniques and from array comparative genomic hybridization (CGH). Aneuploidy in PB1 and PB2 of aged human oocytes from stimulated cycles frequently involves chromatids rather than whole chromosomes [6] (compare Figure 28.1J). The multitude of chromatid-type errors in these PBs and zygotes detected by array-CGH [8] does not parallel the predominance of first meiotic errors in most human trisomies. Hence, the possibility remains that stimulation protocols for harvesting multiple oocytes in assisted reproductive technology (ART) might affect chromosome cohesion, enhancing susceptibility to meiotic errors involving chromatids. Indeed, superovulation in the mouse is known to increase sister centromere distance, which is indicative of reduced cohesion [69].

Mitochondria, metabolism, and advanced glycation end products

The distribution of mitochondria in oocytes is dynamic. Thus, mitochondria with a high inner membrane potential ($\Delta\Psi$m) were preferentially detected in the subcortical domain of MII mouse and human oocytes by J-aggregate formation after staining with the mitochondria-specific dye JC-1 [76]. In resting and maturing oocytes, contacts with cumulus cells via transzonal projections and possibly cumulus-derived nitric oxide prevent precocious "hyperactivation" of mitochondria in the subcortical cytoplasm (Figure 28.3) [76], somewhat protecting them from highly reactive oxygen species (ROS). Functional compartmentalization of relatively quiescent mitochondria may be vital for providing high energy substrates at dynamic sites of the cytoskeleton and for turnover/translation of mRNAs, and concomitantly to minimize exposure of DNA and organelles to damaging ROS. Oocyte maturation in mice is accompanied by changes in the mitochondrial distribution and stage-specific bursts in ATP production [77]. Claims from mtDNA copy number that mitochondria in older oocytes are less abundant, more often functionally compromised (see Chapter 26 and [78, 79]), and impaired in sustaining metabolic support from cumulus cells [63, 80] require further investigation. Interestingly, damage by advanced glycation end products (AGEs) may affect mitochondrial function and alter their distribution [80], potentially affecting spindle regulation, chromosome attachment, chromosome congression, and separation. Notably, mouse oocytes maturing in suboptimal media were not only predisposed to precocious loss of chromatid cohesion prior to anaphase II (Figure 28.2Ii), but the stage-specific association of mitochondria with the spindle was also affected (Figure 28.3E, G) [75]. Exposure to methylglyoxal, a highly reactive metabolite of glycolysis that can form AGEs and adducts with membrane proteins, induces DNA breaks and reduces the inner mitochondrial GSH-dependent redox potential, leading to spindle aberrations, chromosome congression failures, and delayed anaphase I in young mouse oocytes [80]. Oocytes of senescence accelerated mice (SAM) characterized by mitochondrial mutations exhibited accelerated aging and contained reduced levels of Rec8 protein [81].

Furthermore, aged mice fed with either a moderately calorie-restricted diet [82] or the antioxidant, *N*-acetyl-*L*-cysteine [83], exhibited improved oocyte quality, fewer meiotic errors, and an extended reproductive lifespan [82]. Whether the improvement in oocyte health resulted from prevention of ROS-related damage with maternal age or from the side-effects of reducing obesity is unclear (Chapter 31). Oocytes of mice fed *ad libitum* may suffer from the metabolic disturbances of obesity rather than age-related changes per se. In fact, recent evidence shows that diabetes, obesity, and high dietary fat reduces fertility in animal models, in which spindle aberrations were implicated [84]. Glucose metabolism of cumulus appeared to be protective during postovulatory aging [85]. The impact of deficiencies in bidirectional signaling, hormonal homeostasis, and the supply of nutrients and oxygen on oocyte quality are discussed in detail in other chapters.

Since serum follicle-stimulating hormone (FSH) levels gradually rise during the premenopausal decade in women, it is interesting to note that elevated FSH was associated with failure of chromosome congression in mouse oocytes and a higher incidence of aneuploidy in human oocytes after in vitro maturation [86, 87]. Excessive stimulation is considered a risk factor for non-disjunction in ART cycles, irrespective of maternal age, encouraging the practice of milder stimulation protocols [88]. The relative impact of follicle pool size, reflected by levels of anti-Müllerian hormone (AMH) and FSH, on cellular processes affecting chromosome segregation in oocytes still needs to be determined at the cellular level because there are contradictory reports about correlations between trisomies in offspring and hormone levels [89, 90]. Prospective randomized studies and approaches using "omics" as well as array technologies may all be useful for identifying signaling cascades and chromosomal constitution in oocytes at risk of aneuploidy [91–93]. Unfortunately, human oocytes and embryos are scarce, their use in research is limited by ethical and legal considerations, and animal models are far from ideal. However, CGH analyses of PBs promise new insights into the cause(s) of chromosome segregation errors in oocytes from older women and other groups at risk (Chapter 35). Links between metabolism, aging, and chromosome non-disjunction in oocytes need to be addressed in robust experimental models and by studies of cumulus and oocyte gene expression. Some data give hope of halting the vicious cycle of age-related deterioration and release of ROS by mitochondria in aged oocytes, and a healthy diet, avoidance of tobacco products, and regular exercise can undoubtedly help to preserve these cells at all ages.

Conclusions

For some time, it has been known that aging affects mitochondrial morphology in resting human oocytes and aging is accompanied by an increased incidence of spindle aberrations and chromosome congression failures. Evidence from animal models also suggests that the transcriptome and presumably protein expression are influenced by age and/or follicle pool size. Furthermore, experimental studies and analysis of recombination patterns provide compelling evidence that chromatid exchanges already determined in early prophase I in the embryonic ovary influence the fidelity of chromosome segregation later in life, even decades after meiosis was initiated. Although the question remains whether pairing disturbances are the primary cause of age-related non-disjunction, animal studies suggest that the in utero environment may upset pairing and recombination, with impact on oocyte health later in life [94]. Presently, it appears that loss of cohesion, possibly associated with age-related deterioration of cohesin complexes or perhaps more complex alterations in metabolism, might significantly contribute to aneuploidy by disturbing the sequential segregation of homologs and chromatids. By influencing steric constraints favoring correct attachments or rather predisposing to merotelic attachments of chromosomes such disturbances cannot be sensed by checkpoints. This appears to be particularly critical in cells as large as mammalian oocytes which have a small spindle and a relatively permissive checkpoint, aggravated by any age-related alterations in spindle and chromosome-associated proteins. It will be interesting to determine why oocytes of some species, such as pigs, are resistant to age-related non-disjunction. Perhaps differential susceptibility to non-disjunction between women will be discovered and found to be predicted by their genetic background and/or lifestyle. Even more challenging is the goal of defining conditions that protect cohesion or prevent critical changes in auto- and paracrine signaling that affect spindle self-assembly, chromosome attachment, and cell-cycle control that might eventually enable treatment of defective oocytes. Even though a healthy lifestyle cannot halt the aging process, it might delay age-effects, and so there is a take-home message for young women. The health of their future children, and even grandchildren, is likely to depend on the environment to which they expose their irreplaceable store of germ cells. Since it is likely that not every type of deterioration can be slowed or reversed, preservation technologies will be needed while oocytes are still young and healthy (Chapters 36 and 37). Perhaps one day this need will be rendered redundant by the development of stem cell-based technologies to manufacture new oocytes (see Preface). Until that time it is important to refine methods for detecting aneuploidies (Chapter 35) and continue the ongoing process of optimizing treatment protocols in ART for generating oocytes that can give rise to healthy babies for women of all reproductive ages.

Acknowledgment

We apologize to those whose studies could not be cited due to space limitations. The work has been supported by DFG (FOR 1401).

References

1. Pacchierotti F, Adler ID, Eichenlaub-Ritter U, *et al.* Gender effects on the incidence of aneuploidy in mammalian germ cells. *Environ Res* 2007; **104**: 46–69.
2. Templado C, Vidal F, Estop A. Aneuploidy in human spermatozoa. *Cytogenet Genome Res* 2011; **133**: 91–9.
3. Hassold T, Hall H, Hunt P. The origin of human aneuploidy: where we have been, where we are going. *Hum Mol Genet* 2007; **16**(Spec No. 2): R203–8.
4. Hassold T, Hunt P. Maternal age and chromosomally abnormal pregnancies: what we know and what we wish we knew. *Curr Opin Pediatr* 2009; **21**(6): 703–8.
5. Penrose LS. The relative effects of paternal and maternal age in mongolism. *J Genet* 1933; **27**: 219–24.
6. Pellestor F, Andréo B, Arnal F, *et al.* Maternal aging and chromosomal abnormalities: new data drawn from *in vitro* unfertilized human oocytes. *Hum Genet* 2003; **112**: 195–203.
7. Handyside AH, Montag M, Magli MC, *et al.* Multiple meiotic errors caused by predivision of chromatids in

women of advanced maternal age undergoing *in vitro* fertilisation. *Eur J Hum Genet* 2012; **349**: 795–808. doi: 10.1038/ejhg.2011.272.

8. Gabriel AS, Thornhill AR, Ottolini CS, *et al.* Array comparative genomic hybridisation on first polar bodies suggests that non-disjunction is not the predominant mechanism leading to aneuploidy in humans. *J Med Genet* 2011; **48**: 433–7.
9. Nasmyth K. Cohesin: a catenase with separate entry and exit gates? *Nat Cell Biol* 2011; **13**: 1170–7.
10. Kudo NR, Anger M, Peters AH, *et al.* Role of cleavage by separase of the Rec8 kleisin subunit of cohesin during mammalian meiosis I. *J Cell Sci* 2009; **122**: 2686–98.
11. Ishiguro T, Tanaka K, Sakuno T, *et al.* Shugoshin-PP2A counteracts casein-kinase-1-dependent cleavage of Rec8 by separase. *Nat Cell Biol* 2010; **12**: 500–6.
12. Tanno Y, Kitajima TS, Honda T, *et al.* Phosphorylation of mammalian Sgo2 by Aurora B recruits PP2A and MCAK to centromeres. *Genes Dev* 2010; **24**: 2169–79.
13. Xu Z, Cetin B, Anger M, *et al.* Structure and function of the PP2A-shugoshin interaction. *Mol Cell* 2009; **35**: 426–41.
14. Sakuno T, Tada K, Watanabe Y. Kinetochore geometry defined by cohesion within the centromere. *Nature* 2009; **458**: 852–8.
15. Eichenlaub-Ritter U, Staubach N, Trapphoff T. Chromosomal and cytoplasmic context determines predisposition to maternal age-related aneuploidy: brief overview and update on MCAK in mammalian oocytes. *Biochem Soc Trans* 2010; **38**: 1681–6.
16. Henderson SA, Edwards RG. Chiasma frequency and maternal age in mammals. *Nature* 1968; **218**: 22–8.
17. Nicolaidis P, Petersen MB. Origin and mechanisms of non-disjunction in human autosomal trisomies. *Hum Reprod* 1998; **13**: 313–19.
18. Bugge M, Collins A, Hertz JM, *et al.* Non-disjunction of chromosome 13. *Hum Mol Genet* 2007; **16**: 2004–10.
19. Oliver TR, Feingold E, Yu K, *et al.* New insights into human nondisjunction of chromosome 21 in oocytes. *PLoS Genet* 2008; **4**: e1000033.
20. Hussin J, Roy-Gagnon MH, Gendron R, *et al.* Age-dependent recombination rates in human pedigrees. *PLoS Genet* 2011; **7**: e1002251.
21. Kong A, Barnard J, Gudbjartsson DF, *et al.* Recombination rate and reproductive success in humans. *Nat Genet* 2004; **36**: 1203–6.
22. Hultén MA, Patel S, Jonasson J, *et al.* On the origin of the maternal age effect in trisomy 21 Down syndrome: the Oocyte Mosaicism Selection model. *Reproduction* 2010; **139**: 1–9.
23. Vialard F, Lombroso R, Bergere M, *et al.* Oocyte aneuploidy mechanisms are different in two situations of increased chromosomal risk: older patients and patients with recurrent implantation failure after *in vitro* fertilization. *Fertil Steril* 2007; **87**: 1333–9.
24. Morelli MA, Cohen PE. Not all germ cells are created equal: aspects of sexual dimorphism in mammalian meiosis. *Reproduction* 2005; **130**: 761–81.
25. Hunt PA, Hassold TJ. Sex matters in meiosis. *Science* 2002; **296**: 2181–3.
26. Yuan L, Liu JG, Hoja MR, *et al.* Female germ cell aneuploidy and embryo death in mice lacking the meiosis-specific protein SCP3. *Science* 2002; **296**: 1115–18.
27. Bolor H, Mori T, Nishiyama S, *et al.* Mutations of the SYCP3 gene in women with recurrent pregnancy loss. *Am J Hum Genet* 2009; **84**: 14–20.
28. Mizutani E, Suzumori N, Ozaki Y, *et al.* SYCP3 mutation may not be associated with recurrent miscarriage caused by aneuploidy. *Hum Reprod* 2011; **26**: 1259–66.
29. Revenkova E, Herrmann K, Adelfalk C, *et al.* Oocyte cohesin expression restricted to predictyate stages provides full fertility and prevents aneuploidy. *Curr Biol* 2010; **20**: 1529–33.
30. Hodges CA, Revenkova E, Jessberger R, *et al.* SMC1beta-deficient female mice provide evidence that cohesins are a missing link in age-related nondisjunction. *Nat Genet* 2005; **37**: 1351–5.
31. Brunet S, Dumont J, Lee KW, *et al.* Meiotic regulation of TPX2 protein levels governs cell cycle progression in mouse oocytes. *PLoS One* 2008; **3**: 3338.
32. Breuer M, Kolano A, Kwon M, *et al.* HURP permits MTOC sorting for robust meiotic spindle bipolarity, similar to extra centrosome clustering in cancer cells. *J Cell Biol* 2010; **191**: 1251–60.
33. Eichenlaub-Ritter U, Vogt E, Yin H, *et al.* Spindles, mitochondria and redox potential in ageing oocytes. *Reprod Biomed Online* 2004; **8**: 45–58.
34. Battaglia DE, Goodwin P, Klein A, *et al.* Influence of maternal age on meiotic spindle assembly in oocytes from naturally cycling women. *Hum Reprod* 1996; **11**: 2217–22.
35. Hamatani T, Falco G, Carter MG, *et al.* Age-associated alteration of gene expression patterns in mouse oocytes. *Hum Mol Genet* 2004; **13**: 2263–78.
36. Steuerwald N, Cohen J, Herrera RJ, *et al.* Association between spindle assembly checkpoint expression and maternal age in human oocytes. *Mol Hum Reprod* 2001; **7**: 49–55.

37. Steuerwald NM, Bermúdez MG, Wells D, *et al.* Maternal age-related differential global expression profiles observed in human oocytes. *Reprod Biomed Online* 2007; **14**: 700–8.

38. Pan H, O'Brien MJ, Wigglesworth K, *et al.* Transcript profiling during mouse oocyte development and the effect of gonadotropin priming and development *in vitro*. *Dev Biol* 2005; **286**: 493–506.

39. Grøndahl ML, Yding Andersen C, Bogstad J, *et al.* Gene expression profiles of single human mature oocytes in relation to age. *Hum Reprod* 2010; **25**: 957–68.

40. Fragouli E, Bianchi V, Patrizio P, *et al.* Transcriptomic profiling of human oocytes: association of meiotic aneuploidy and altered oocyte gene expression. *Mol Hum Reprod* 2010; **16**: 570–82.

41. Kitajima TS, Ohsugi M, Ellenberg J. Complete kinetochore tracking reveals error-prone homologous chromosome biorientation in mammalian oocytes. *Cell* 2011; **146**: 568–81.

42. Lane SI, Yun Y, Jones KT. Timing of anaphase-promoting complex activation in mouse oocytes is predicted by microtubule-kinetochore attachment but not by bivalent alignment or tension. *Development* 2012; **139**: 1947–55.

43. Avo Santos M, van de Werken C, de Vries M, *et al.* A role for Aurora C in the chromosomal passenger complex during human preimplantation embryo development. *Hum Reprod* 2011; **26**: 1868–81.

44. Vogt E, Kipp A, Eichenlaub-Ritter U. Aurora kinase B, epigenetic state of centromeric heterochromatin and chiasma resolution in oocytes. *Reprod Biomed Online* 2009; **19**: 352–68.

45. Vogt E, Sanhaji M, Klein W, *et al.* MCAK is present at centromeres, midspindle and chiasmata and involved in silencing of the spindle assembly checkpoint in mammalian oocytes. *Mol Hum Reprod* 2010; **16**: 665–84.

46. Illingworth C, Pirmadjid N, Serhal P, *et al.* MCAK regulates chromosome alignment but is not necessary for preventing aneuploidy in mouse oocyte meiosis I. *Development* 2010; **137**: 2133–8.

47. Musacchio A. Spindle assembly checkpoint: the third decade. *Philos Trans R Soc Lond B Biol Sci* 2011; **366**: 3595–604.

48. Homer HA, McDougall A, Levasseur M, *et al.* Mad2 prevents aneuploidy and premature proteolysis of cyclin B and securin during meiosis I in mouse oocytes. *Genes Dev* 2005; **19**: 202–7.

49. Eichenlaub-Ritter U, Boll I. Nocodazole sensitivity, age-related aneuploidy, and alterations in the cell cycle during maturation of mouse oocytes. *Cytogenet Cell Genet* 1989; **52**: 170–6.

50. Volarcik K, Sheean L, Goldfarb J, *et al.* The meiotic competence of in-vitro matured human oocytes is influenced by donor age: evidence that folliculogenesis is compromised in the reproductively aged ovary. *Hum Reprod* 1998; **13**: 154–60.

51. Seli E, Robert C, Sirard MA. OMICS in assisted reproduction: possibilities and pitfalls. *Mol Hum Reprod* 2010; **16**: 513–30.

52. Salisbury J, Hutchison KW, Wigglesworth K, *et al.* Probe-level analysis of expression microarrays characterizes isoform-specific degradation during mouse oocyte maturation. *PLoS One* 2009; **4**: e7479.

53. Baker DJ, Jeganathan KB, Cameron JD, *et al.* BubR1 insufficiency causes early onset of aging-associated phenotypes and infertility in mice. *Nat Genet* 2004; **36**: 744–9.

54. Li M, Li S, Yuan J, *et al.* Bub3 is a spindle assembly checkpoint protein regulating chromosome segregation during mouse oocyte meiosis. *PLoS One* 2009; **4**: e7701.

55. Hached K, Xie SZ, Buffin E, *et al.* Mps1 at kinetochores is essential for female mouse meiosis I. *Development* 2011; **138**: 2261–71.

56. LeMaire-Adkins R, Radke K, Hunt PA. Lack of checkpoint control at the metaphase/anaphase transition: a mechanism of meiotic nondisjunction in mammalian females. *J Cell Biol* 1997; **139**:1611–19.

57. Kouznetsova A, Lister L, Nordenskjold M, *et al.* Bi-orientation of achiasmatic chromosomes in meiosis I oocytes contributes to aneuploidy in mice. *Nat Genet* 2007; **39**: 966–8.

58. Vogt E, Kirsch-Volders M, Parry J, *et al.* Spindle formation, chromosome segregation and the spindle checkpoint in mammalian oocytes and susceptibility to meiotic error. *Mutat Res* 2008; **651**: 14–29.

59. Pacchierotti F, Eichenlaub-Ritter U. Environmental hazard in the aetiology of somatic and germ cell aneuploidy. *Cytogenet Genome Res* 2011; **133**: 254–68.

60. Hoffmann S, Maro B, Kubiak JZ, *et al.* A single bivalent efficiently inhibits cyclin B1 degradation and polar body extrusion in mouse oocytes indicating robust SAC during female meiosis I. *PLoS One* 2011; **6**: e27143.

61. Kolano A, Brunet S, Silk AD, *et al.* Error-prone mammalian female meiosis from silencing the spindle assembly checkpoint without normal interkinetochore tension. *Proc Natl Acad Sci USA* 2012: **109**: E1858–67. doi/10.1073/pnas.1204686109.

62. Nagaoka SI, Hodges CA, Albertini DF, *et al.* Oocyte-specific differences in cell-cycle control create an innate susceptibility to meiotic errors. *Curr Biol* 2011; **21**: 651–7.

63. Duncan FE, Chiang T, Schultz RM, *et al.* Evidence that a defective spindle assembly checkpoint is not the primary cause of maternal age-associated aneuploidy in mouse eggs. *Biol Reprod* 2009; **81**: 768–76.

64. Eichenlaub-Ritter U, Wieczorek M, Lüke S, *et al.* Age related changes in mitochondrial function and new approaches to study redox regulation in mammalian oocytes in response to age or maturation conditions. *Mitochondrion* 2011; **11**: 783–96.

65. Feeney KM, Wasson CW, Parish JL. Cohesin: a regulator of genome integrity and gene expression. *Biochem J* 2010; **428**: 147–61.

66. Chiang T, Schultz RM, Lampson MA. Age-dependent susceptibility of chromosome cohesion to premature separase activation in mouse oocytes. *Biol Reprod* 2011; **85**: 1279–83.

67. Chiang T, Duncan FE, Schindler K, *et al.* Evidence that weakened centromere cohesion is a leading cause of age-related aneuploidy in oocytes. *Curr Biol* 2010; **20**: 1522–8.

68. Lister LM, Kouznetsova A, Hyslop LA, *et al.* Age-related meiotic segregation errors in mammalian oocytes are preceded by depletion of cohesin and Sgo2. *Curr Biol* 2010; **20**: 1511–21.

69. Merriman JA, Jennings PC, McLaughlin EA, *et al.* Effect of aging on superovulation efficiency, aneuploidy rates, and sister chromatid cohesion in mice aged up to 15 months. *Biol Reprod* 2012; **86**: 49.

70. Tachibana-Konwalski K, Godwin J, van der Weyden L, *et al.* Rec8-containing cohesin maintains bivalents without turnover during the growing phase of mouse oocytes. *Genes Dev* 2010 **24**: 2505–16.

71. Garcia-Cruz R, Brieno MA, Roig I, *et al.* Dynamics of cohesin proteins REC8, STAG3, SMC1 beta and SMC3 are consistent with a role in sister chromatid cohesion during meiosis in human oocytes. *Hum Reprod* 2010; **25**: 2316–27.

72. Hornak M, Jeseta M, Musilova P, *et al.* Frequency of aneuploidy related to age in porcine oocytes. *PLoS One* 2011; **6**: e18892.

73. Angell R. First-meiotic-division nondisjunction in human oocytes. *Am J Hum Genet* 1997; **61**: 23–32.

74. van den Berg IM, Eleveld C, van der Hoeven M, *et al.* Defective deacetylation of histone 4 K12 in human oocytes is associated with advanced maternal age and chromosome misalignment. *Hum Reprod* 2011; **26**: 1181–90.

75. Cukurcam S, Betzendahl I, Michel G, *et al.* Influence of follicular fluid meiosis-activating sterol on aneuploidy rate and precocious chromatid segregation in aged mouse oocytes. *Hum Reprod* 2007; **22**: 815–28.

76. Van Blerkom J, Davis P, Thalhammer V. Regulation of mitochondrial polarity in mouse and human oocytes: the influence of cumulus derived nitric oxide. *Mol Hum Reprod* 2008; **14**: 431–44.

77. Yu Y, Dumollard R, Rossbach A, *et al.* Redistribution of mitochondria leads to bursts of ATP production during spontaneous mouse oocyte maturation. *J Cell Physiol* 2010; **224**: 672–80.

78. de Bruin JP, Dorland M, Spek ER, *et al.* Age-related changes in the ultrastructure of the resting follicle pool in human ovaries. *Biol Reprod* 2004; **70**: 419–24.

79. Thouas GA, Trounson AO, Jones GM. Effect of female age on mouse oocyte developmental competence following mitochondrial injury. *Biol Reprod* 2005; **73**: 366–73.

80. Tatone C, Heizenrieder T, Di Emidio G, *et al.* Evidence that carbonyl stress by methylglyoxal exposure induces DNA damage and spindle aberrations, affects mitochondrial integrity in mammalian oocytes and contributes to oocyte ageing. *Hum Reprod* 2011; **26**: 1843–59.

81. Liu L, Keefe DL. Defective cohesin is associated with age-dependent misaligned chromosomes in oocytes. *Reprod Biomed Online* 2008; **1 6**: 103–12.

82. Selesniemi K, Lee HJ, Tilly JL. Moderate caloric restriction initiated in rodents during adulthood sustains function of the female reproductive axis into advanced chronological age. *Aging Cell* 2008; **7**: 622–9.

83. Liu J, Liu M, Ye X, *et al.* Delay in oocyte aging in mice by the antioxidant N-acetyl-L-cysteine (NAC). *Hum Reprod* 2012; **27**: 1411–20.

84. Wang Q, Ratchford AM, Chi MM, *et al.* Maternal diabetes causes mitochondrial dysfunction and meiotic defects in murine oocytes. *Mol Endocrinol* 2009; **23**: 1603–12.

85. Li Q, Miao DQ, Zhou P, *et al.* Glucose metabolism in mouse cumulus cells prevents oocyte aging by maintaining both energy supply and the intracellular redox potential. *Biol Reprod* 2011; **84**: 1111–8.

86. Roberts R, Iatropoulou A, Ciantar D, *et al.* Follicle-stimulating hormone affects metaphase I chromosome alignment and increases aneuploidy in mouse oocytes matured *in vitro*. *Biol Reprod* 2005; **72**: 107–18.

87. Xu YW, Peng YT, Wang B, *et al.* High follicle-stimulating hormone increases aneuploidy in human oocytes matured *in vitro*. *Fertil Steril* 2011; **95**: 99–104.

88. Baart EB, Martini E, Eijkemans MJ, *et al.* Milder ovarian stimulation for in-vitro fertilization reduces aneuploidy in the human preimplantation embryo: a randomized controlled trial. *Hum Reprod* 2007; **22**: 980–8.

89. Kline JK, Kinney AM, Levin B, *et al.* Trisomic pregnancy and elevated FSH: implications for the oocyte pool hypothesis. *Hum Reprod* 2011; **26**: 1537–50.

90. Haadsma ML, Mooij TM, Groen H, *et al.* A reduced size of the ovarian follicle pool is associated with an increased risk of a trisomic pregnancy in IVF-treated women. *Hum Reprod* 2010; **25**: 552–8.

91. Fragouli E, Bianchi V, Patrizio P, *et al.* Transcriptomic profiling of human oocytes: association of meiotic aneuploidy and altered oocyte gene expression. *Mol Hum Reprod* 2010; **16**: 570–82.

92. Guglielmino MR, Santonocito M, Vento M, *et al.* TAp73 is downregulated in oocytes from women of advanced reproductive age. *Cell Cycle* 2011; **10**: 3253–6.

93. Demant M, Trapphoff T, Fröhlich T, *et al.* Vitrification at the pre-antral stage transiently alters inner mitochondrial membrane potential but proteome of *in vitro* grown and matured mouse oocytes appears unaffected. *Hum Reprod* 2012; **27**: 1096–111.

94. Susiarjo M, Hassold TJ, Freeman E, *et al.* Bisphenol A exposure in utero disrupts early oogenesis in the mouse. *PLoS Genet* 2007; **3**: e5.

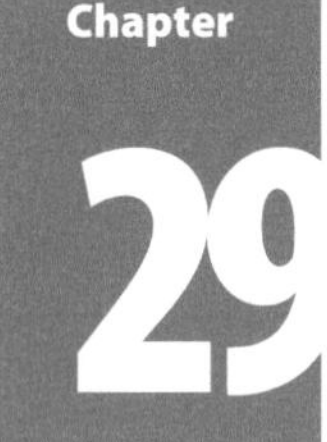

Chapter 29

Alterations in the gene expression of aneuploid oocytes and associated cumulus cells

Dagan Wells

The importance of aneuploidy in human reproductive failure

Human reproduction is a remarkably inefficient process. On average, fertile couples attempting to conceive only succeed in achieving a clinical pregnancy one month out of every five. For infertile patients undergoing in vitro fertilization (IVF) pregnancy rates are similarly low. More than 80% of the embryos transferred to the uterus during IVF treatment fail to implant and two-thirds of cycles do not produce a child [1]. As a result, most IVF patients require two or more rounds of treatment to achieve a pregnancy. There are many potential reasons why an embryo might not establish a pregnancy; however, it is clear that one of the most important is chromosome abnormality. This is particularly true for embryos derived from women of advanced reproductive age. While it is not unusual for half of the blastocyst stage embryos produced by women in their early thirties to be chromosomally abnormal, this figure increases dramatically with age, such that an aneuploidy rate exceeding 75% is typical for blastocysts from women over the age of 40 [2]. The high prevalence of aneuploidy, coupled with its detrimental impact on development, explains the majority of embryo implantation failures and miscarriages. Evidence for the lethality of aneuploidy comes from the detection of chromosome imbalances in the majority of miscarriages [3, 4] and from blinded studies where embryos, later revealed to be chromosomally abnormal, had been transferred to patients [5].

Aneuploidy detected in human preimplantation embryos can be derived from sperm or arise due to errors occurring in the mitotic divisions following fertilization. However, the vast majority of such anomalies originate in the oocyte. In recent years, the introduction of molecular cytogenetic techniques that permit a comprehensive assessment of the chromosomes in human oocytes and their associated polar bodies has provided an unparalleled insight into the frequency and spectrum of aneuploidies occurring during the female meiotic divisions (at least those that occur during assisted reproductive cycles) [6–9]. These studies have also revealed information concerning the mechanisms of chromosome malsegregation that produce aneuploidy. For example, it is now clear that errors caused by premature separation of chromatids during meiosis I are at least ten times more common than those resulting from nondisjunction of whole chromosomes (composed of two chromatids) [6–8, 10]. It is also apparent that in young women the first meiotic division is the source of most oocyte aneuploidies, whereas for women over 40 years of age meiosis II is the division where most errors occur [6, 7]. While both meiotic divisions become increasingly error-prone with advancing female age, this deterioration appears to be more pronounced for meiosis II.

Preimplantation genetic screening for the selection of chromosomally normal oocytes

The role of oocyte aneuploidy in many failed IVF cycles has led to suggestions that oocytes used for infertility treatments should be screened for chromosome imbalance, with the aim of only transferring embryos produced from oocytes found to be normal haploid. This approach, known as preimplantation genetic screening (PGS), involves biopsy of the polar bodies followed by their genetic analysis using methods such as microarray comparative

Biology and Pathology of the Oocyte, 2nd edn., ed. Alan Trounson, Roger Gosden, and Ursula Eichenlaub-Ritter.

genomic hybridization (array-CGH) [6, 7, 9, 11, 12]. Ideally, the first polar body is removed from mature meiosis II oocytes after oocyte retrieval and the oocyte is then fertilized using intracytoplasmic sperm injection (ICSI). The second polar body is biopsied the next day, following completion of meiosis II. The two polar bodies are each analyzed, providing an overview of the chromosomal status of the oocyte after each of the meiotic divisions. While the process of polar body removal and array-CGH provides an accurate and clinically valuable insight into the cytogenetics of the oocyte, it is an expensive procedure and the biopsy entails a risk, albeit relatively small, to the viability of the oocyte. If less invasive methods of oocyte aneuploidy detection could be developed, this would represent a significant advance (as discussed in more detail below).

Differences between the transcriptomes of chromosomally normal and aneuploid oocytes

Despite the biological and clinical importance of oocyte-derived aneuploidy, the genesis of such abnormalities remains relatively poorly understood. In recent years, this deficiency has prompted research into gene expression both in oocytes and also in the cumulus cells that surround them. Virtually every process that occurs within a cell is regulated, to a greater or lesser extent, by adjusting the production of new mRNA transcripts or by altering their availability, utilization, or rate of degradation. Consequently, characterization of the mRNA levels for individual genes can reveal a great deal of information regarding the cellular pathways and processes that are active or repressed within cells at a given moment in time.

Several studies have sought to investigate gene expression in individual oocytes or small groups of oocytes, a technically challenging aim, requiring the development of extremely sensitive methods of mRNA assessment [13–16]. These studies have shed light on the processes governing the latter stages of oocyte maturation (germinal vesicle to meiosis II oocyte) and the impact of different pathologies on cellular function. A single study has defined the pattern of mRNA transcripts in chromosomally normal oocytes and then compared this with results obtained from aneuploid oocytes [14]. The investigation involved removal of the first polar body from oocytes donated for research. The polar bodies were subjected to comparative genomic hybridization, revealing whether any chromosome or chromatid segregation errors had occurred during the first meiotic division. RNA was extracted from the corresponding oocytes, amplified using an in vitro transcription technique, and analyzed via gene expression microarray. This provided data on approximately 30 000 distinct transcripts for each cytogenetically characterized oocyte. The vast majority of genes were found to have similar levels of expression in all oocytes and were unaffected by aneuploidy. However, a subset of 327 genes displayed significant differences in their number of transcripts in all of the chromosomally abnormal oocytes. These differences were consistent across all abnormal oocytes, regardless of the specific chromosome(s) found to be aneuploid, suggesting they are related to oocyte aneuploidy in general.

Interestingly, 40% of the genes showing different mRNA transcript numbers between chromosomally normal and aneuploid oocytes are currently of unknown function, highlighting the unique, highly specialized, and poorly characterized nature of oogenesis. The genes with defined biological functions have roles in a wide variety of cellular processes, some of which have obvious links to chromosome segregation. For example, there are genes with altered mRNA levels in aneuploid oocytes that play a part in spindle assembly and chromosome alignment, while others are known to influence chromatin remodeling and the cell cycle. These genes have been reviewed in detail by Fragouli *et al.* [14].

Among the genes displaying altered quantities of mRNA transcripts were several involved in the cytoskeleton. One such gene showing decreased transcript abundance was *ASPM* (abnormal spindle-like microcephaly-associated), whose protein is an important regulator of meiotic spindle organization and rotation, also responsible for the localization of dynein at the spindle poles [17]. Another gene of potential relevance to chromosome segregation, which had increased mRNA levels in aneuploid oocytes, was *KIF2B* (kinesin 2B), which encodes a microtubule depolymerase thought to be involved in spindle assembly and chromosome movement [18, 19]. Copy number variants (duplication) of KIF2B were recently shown to be associated with childhood obesity [20]. The abnormal expression of these genes, along with others that had atypical transcript levels, including some that produce tubulins and motor proteins, might conceivably lead to aneuploidy by disrupting spindle function or indirectly by affecting metabolism. In fact, a number of genes involved in cellular metabolism and energy production were also found to have abnormal mRNA transcript numbers in chromosomally abnormal oocytes, raising the question of whether energetic cellular processes (including chromosome segregation) could have been compromised. A reduced number of transcripts from the PDHB (pyruvate dehydrogenase [lipoamide] beta) gene was detected in abnormal oocytes. PDHB has a role in ATP generation, interacting with the products of other pyruvate dehydrogenase genes in a multi-enzyme complex [21]. Reduced levels of PDHB are likely to affect the quantity of active pyruvate dehydrogenase, impairing mitochondrial metabolism and ATP generation. Disruption of *PDHA1* (another pyruvate dehydrogenase gene) has been shown to induce meiotic defects, affecting chromatin condensation, chromosome movement, and microtubule assembly [22].

Mitochondrial function and energy production could also be affected by reduced production of phosphatidylethanolamine, an important mitochondrial phospholipid [23]. Decreases in the number of transcripts from two genes involved in phosphatidylethanolamine production, *PISD* (phosphatidylserine decarboxylase) and *AGPAT7* (1-acylglycerol-3-phosphate *O*-acyltransferase 7 [lysophosphatidic acid acyltransferase, eta]), were detected in oocytes from older women. As well as having a role in the mitochondria, phosphatidylethanolamine also functions in autophagy, a process used by cells to clear and recycle defective or unwanted organelles and macromolecules. It is a component of a scaffold protein responsible for determining the size of the autophagosome, the cytoplasmic vacuole that encloses cellular components targeted for degradation and contains enzymes for their digestion. This may be relevant to oocyte aneuploidy since there have been reports suggesting that failure of autophagy could be associated with increased aneuploidy risk [24]. Another challenge to the correct functioning of autophagy in aneuploid oocytes is the reduced expression seen for the ATG7 (autophagy-related 7 homolog) gene. This gene is one of a large group of autophagy-related genes and also functions in the ubiquitin proteasome pathway. The ATG7 protein interacts with phosphatidylethanolamine during autophagosome formation [25].

Earlier studies have also reported alterations in gene transcript number in the oocytes of reproductively older women. Since aneuploidy and age are so closely associated it is possible that some of the changes described are of relevance to chromosome abnormality. One report suggested that the levels of MAD2 and BUB1 gene transcripts are reduced with age [26]. This is of potential importance given that both genes are involved in the regulation of the metaphase–anaphase (spindle assembly) checkpoint, a cellular mechanism which protects against aneuploidy by preventing cell-cycle progression if chromosomes are not correctly connected to a bipolar spindle. Another study, using a microarray approach to look at a large number of genes, concluded that multiple cellular processes are abnormally expressed in oocytes from women of advanced reproductive age [15]. Some of the processes identified overlap with those that were seen when aneuploid oocytes were assessed by microarray [14]. These may be of particular relevance when considering the phenomenon of age-related aneuploidy.

While a plausible link to the formation of aneuploidy can be envisaged for some of the genes identified following transcriptomic analysis of human oocytes, for many no clear functional association is apparent. The diversity of genes displaying altered transcript quantities suggests that oocytes that become chromosomally abnormal may be flawed on multiple levels. It is possible that aneuploidy is just the most obvious manifestation of a more generalized problem affecting oocytes predisposed to chromosome malsegregation. However, given that most aneuploid oocytes appear to be fertilization-competent, capable of supporting embryonic development to the cleavage stage, and, in some cases, forming pregnancies, it is clear that if these deficiencies genuinely exist they do not usually have a catastrophic impact on oocyte function.

Identifying new biomarkers of oocyte aneuploidy

One possible outcome of research into the oocyte transcriptome is that novel biomarkers of oocyte competence, and more specifically aneuploidy, might be identified [27]. Several of the genes displaying altered quantities of transcripts in chromosomally abnormal oocytes produce proteins that are expressed on the cell surface or are secreted by the cell [14]. The externalization of these elements increases their accessibility, making them potential targets for aneuploidy detection assays that avoid the use of polar body biopsy. Another attractive possibility for the non-invasive evaluation of oocyte chromosomes is assessment of follicular cells. Appropriate interactions between the oocyte, somatic cells within the follicle, and endocrine systems are essential if the oocyte is to achieve competence [28–31]. The analysis of follicular cells may therefore be valuable both diagnostically and scientifically.

Research into the transcriptome of cumulus cells associated with chromosomally abnormal oocytes

Two distinct types of somatic cell can be found in ovarian follicles, the mural granulosa cells, which line the follicle wall, and the cumulus cells, which surround the oocyte. Cumulus cells have a number of unique biological features that allow them to fulfill vital roles in the support of oocyte maturation. They are able to receive and transmit endocrine signals to the oocyte and provide it with essential resources (the oocyte lacking gonadotropin receptors and relying on cumulus cells to provide it with a range of molecules). Cumulus cells satisfy many of the oocyte's energy requirements, metabolizing glucose and supplying it with pyruvate [32]. Additionally, they also provide many other macromolecules, including nucleotides, amino acids and RNA (reviewed in [33]; see also Chapter 8). These molecules are transferred to the oocyte via transporters or through gap junctions. The cumulus cells in contact with the zona pellucida, the glycoprotein membrane that encapsulates the oocyte, have cytoplasmic projections that pierce through it and form gap junctions where they come into contact with the plasma membrane of the oocyte. These gap junctions help to facilitate a bidirectional communication, the adherent cumulus cells relaying signals from the external environment and the oocyte regulating the metabolism and biosynthesis occurring within the cumulus cells [34, 35]. The intimate connections between the oocyte and its surrounding cumulus cells, their communication and exchange of molecules, and the fact that they share the same follicular microenvironment have led to the suggestion that analysis of these somatic cells could reveal much concerning the quality of the oocyte with which they are associated [27].

The possibility that cumulus cells could be used for oocyte evaluation is attractive, not least because the cells are readily accessible during IVF treatment and can be sampled without risk to the oocyte. Several studies have sought to characterize the cumulus cell transcriptome and search for differences in gene expression related to oocyte quality [36–39]. Essentially, the underlying theory is that changes in gene transcription could be induced by the presence of a compromised oocyte or by a suboptimal follicular environment shared by the oocyte and cumulus cells. The transcriptional footprint left behind by these factors could then be detected in the cumulus cells. Various outcomes have been measured, ranging from fertilization rate and embryo morphology to the frequencies of blastocyst formation and pregnancy, revealing several candidate genes that may be relevant to oocyte quality.

It has also been speculated that oocyte aneuploidy might have an impact on cumulus cell gene expression, or that a poor follicular environment could produce a characteristic change in cumulus cell gene expression as well as increasing the risk that aneuploidy will arise. To date, a single study addressing this question has been reported. This involved the classification of oocytes into normal or aneuploid groups based upon analysis of the first polar body using comparative genomic hybridization, followed by characterization of gene expression in the associated cumulus cells using microarrays and real-time PCR [40]. Approximately 700 genes were found to be differentially expressed in cumulus cells surrounding oocytes that had an abnormal first polar body (i.e., oocytes that were aneuploid after completion of meiosis I) and a generalized reduction in RNA levels was observed. The reduced levels of RNA echo findings in studies that had investigated cumulus cell gene expression in relation to clinical outcome and found reduce expression of most genes in cells associated with oocytes that failed to produce pregnancies [36]. It may be the case that less transcriptionally active cumulus cells are unable to provide sufficient resources to the oocyte, reducing its ability to sustain the embryo through early preimplantation development and possibly predisposing to chromosome segregation errors during meiosis.

A number of genes that function in metabolic processes, hypoxia, and apoptosis were found to be abnormally expressed in cumulus cells enclosing aneuploid oocytes [40]. Although not conclusive, these findings provide some support for the notion that a suboptimal follicular microenvironment might contribute to aneuploidy risk. Reduced metabolic and synthetic processes in cumulus cells and low oxygen concentrations might act together to limit the quantity of energy substrates and other molecules transported to the oocyte. This is likely to have a detrimental impact on many cellular processes of which chromosome segregation could be one. It is also possible that perturbations of the follicular environment, affecting cumulus cell gene expression, could be caused by the oocyte itself. The oocyte can exert a significant level of control over the surrounding cumulus cells and consequently it can be envisaged that inappropriate signaling by a defective oocyte could lead to alterations in cumulus cell gene expression. However, whether aneuploidy is associated with any derangement of normal oocyte communications is not known.

Of the many candidate genes identified in cumulus cells associated with aneuploid oocytes, two yielded particularly interesting results and were analyzed in greater detail than the others. The first gene, *SPSB2*, produces an adapter protein in the E3 ubiquitin ligase complex, which is responsible for the targeted degradation of the inducible form of nitric oxide synthase (iNOS) [41]. Reduced expression of SPSB2 was observed in cumulus cells encapsulating aneuploid oocytes, potentially leading to a reduction in proteosomal degradation activity, which in turn could result in persistence and accumulation of abnormal or redundant proteins, interfering with many cellular processes. Another negative consequence of reduced SPSB2 expression could be excessive levels of iNOS, producing increased quantities of nitric oxide and, as a result, elevated levels of reactive oxygen species.

The second candidate to receive a detailed evaluation was *TP53I3*, a gene which produces a protein acting downstream of p53 (a protein with multiple functions in DNA damage repair, determination of cell fate, and apoptosis). TP53I3 is involved in activation of cell-cycle checkpoints in response to DNA damage [42]. Cumulus cells associated with chromosomally abnormal oocytes displayed lower levels of TP53I3 transcripts, suggesting that cellular responses to DNA damage, such as apoptosis, might be impaired. This could lead to an accumulation of dysfunctional cumulus cells, ill-equipped to transmit signals and/or provide resources to the oocyte. The possibility of an effect on apoptosis is particularly interesting given that previous studies have suggested a link between cumulus cell apoptosis rates and oocyte quality [43].

As well as being tested for an association with aneuploidy, the expression of SBSB2 and TP53I3 was also examined in relation to pregnancy rates. In theory, if reduced expression of these genes was indicative of aneuploidy then it should also be correlated with a lower chance of a pregnancy. A preliminary study, undertaken using 38 oocytes and corresponding cumulus cell samples, revealed a strong trend linking reduced expression of both genes and oocytes that did not produce a pregnancy [40].

Further work is needed before firm conclusions can be drawn concerning the significance of gene expression differences in chromosomally abnormal oocytes and their surrounding cumulus cells. It is important to verify that protein levels are affected by the altered levels of mRNA and that there is an impact on the activity of the associated cellular pathways. This is especially important for research involving the oocyte transcriptome, as oocytes frequently employ post-transcriptional methods for controlling pathway activity (e.g., alteration of mRNA stability and translation). Nevertheless, the transcriptomic studies carried out thus far have revealed potentially valuable targets for future research, show promise for the development of improved methods of clinical oocyte evaluation and offer new perspectives on the environmental and intrinsic factors that predispose to aneuploidy.

References

1. Kovalevsky G, Patrizio P. High rates of embryo wastage with the use of assisted reproductive technology: trends between 1995 and 2001 in the United States. *Fertil Steril* 2005; **84**: 325–30.
2. Fragouli E, Wells D. Aneuploidy in the human blastocyst. *Cytogenet Genome Res* 2011; **133**(2–4): 149–59.
3. Menasha J, Levy B, Hirschhorn K, *et al.* Incidence and spectrum of chromosome abnormalities in spontaneous abortions: new insights from a 12-year study. *Genet Med* 2005; **7**: 251–63.
4. Hassold T, Chen N, Funkhouser J, *et al.* A cytogenetic study of 1000 spontaneous abortions. *Ann Hum Genet* 1980; **44**(Pt 2): 151–78.
5. Scott RT Jr, Ferry K, Su J, *et al.* Comprehensive chromosome screening is highly predictive of the reproductive potential of human embryos: a prospective, blinded, nonselection study. *Fertil Steril* 2012; **97**: 870–5.

6. Fragouli E, Wells D, Delhanty JD. Chromosome abnormalities in the human oocyte. *Cytogenet Genome Res* 2011; **133**(2–4): 107–18.

7. Fragouli E, Alfarawati S, Goodall NN, *et al.* The cytogenetics of polar bodies: insights into female meiosis and the diagnosis of aneuploidy. *Mol Hum Reprod.* 2011; **17**(5): 286–95.

8. Handyside AH, Montag M, Magli MC, *et al.* Multiple meiotic errors caused by predivision of chromatids in women of advanced maternal age undergoing in vitro fertilisation. *Eur J Hum Genet* 2012; **20**: 742–7.

9. Fishel S, Gordon A, Lynch C, *et al.* Live birth after polar body array comparative genomic hybridization prediction of embryo ploidy-the future of IVF? *Fertil Steril* 2010; **93**: 1006.e7–10.

10. Gabriel AS, Thornhill AR, Ottolini CS, *et al.* Array comparative genomic hybridisation on first polar bodies suggests that non-disjunction is not the predominant mechanism leading to aneuploidy in humans. *J Med Genet* 2011; **48**: 433–7.

11. Fragouli E, Katz-Jaffe M, Alfarawati S, *et al.* Comprehensive chromosome screening of polar bodies and blastocysts from couples experiencing repeated implantation failure. *Fertil Steril* 2010; **94**: 875–87.

12. Geraedts J, Montag M, Magli MC, *et al.* Polar body array CGH for prediction of the status of the corresponding oocyte. Part I: clinical results. *Hum Reprod* 2011; **26**: 3173–80.

13. Jones GM, Cram DS, Song B, *et al.* Gene expression profiling of human oocytes following in vivo or in vitro maturation. *Hum Reprod* 2008; **23**: 1138–44.

14. Fragouli E, Bianchi V, Patrizio P, *et al.* Transcriptomic profiling of human oocytes: association of meiotic aneuploidy and altered oocyte gene expression. *Mol Hum Reprod* 2010; **16**: 570–82.

15. Grøndahl ML, Yding Andersen C, Bogstad J, *et al.* Gene expression profiles of single human mature oocytes in relation to age. *Hum Reprod* 2010; **25**: 957–68.

16. Wood JR, Dumesic DA, Abbott DH, *et al.* Molecular abnormalities in oocytes from women with polycystic ovary syndrome revealed by microarray analysis. *J Clin Endocrinol Metab* 2007; **92**: 705–13.

17. Voet M, Berends CWH, Perreault A, *et al.* NuMA-related LIN-5, ASPM-1, calmodulin and dynein promote meiotic spindle rotation independently of cortical LIN-5/GPR/Ga. *Nat Cell Biol* 2009; **11**: 269–77.

18. Manning AL, Ganem N, Bakhoum SF, *et al.* The kinesin-13 proteins Kif2a, Kif2b, and Kif2c/MCAK have distinct roles during mitosis in human cells. *Mol Biol Cell* 2007; **18**: 2970–9.

19. Bakhoum SF, Thompson SL, Manning AL, *et al.* Genome stability is ensured by temporal control of kinetochore-microtubule dynamics. *Nat Cell Biol* 2009; **11**: 27–35.

20. Glessner Bradfield JP, Wang K, *et al.* A genome-wide study reveals copy number variants exclusive to childhood obesity cases. *Am J Hum Genet* 2010; **87**(5): 661–6.

21. Johnson F, Kaplitt MG. Novel mitochondrial substrates of OMI indicate a new regulatory role in neurodegenerative disorders. *PLoS One* 2009; **18**: e7100.

22. Johnson MT, Freeman EA, Gardner DK, *et al.* Oxidative metabolism of pyruvate is required for meiotic maturation of murine oocytes in vivo. *Biol Reprod* 2007; **77**: 2–8.

23. Gohil VM, Greenberg ML. Mitochondrial membrane biogenesis: phospholipids and proteins go hand in hand. *J Cell Biol* 2009; **184**: 469–72.

24. Mathew R, Kongara S, Beaudoin B, *et al.* Autophagy suppresses tumour progression by limiting chromosomal instability. *Genes Dev* 2007; **21**: 1367–81.

25. Geng J, Klionsky DJ. The Atg8 and Atg12 ubiquitin-like conjugation systems in macroautophagy. *EMBO Rep* 2008; **9**: 859–64.

26. Steuerwald N, Cohen J, Herrera RJ, *et al.* Association between spindle assembly checkpoint expression and maternal age in human oocytes. *Mol Hum Reprod* 2001; **7**: 49–55.

27. Patrizio P, Fragouli E, Bianchi V, *et al.* Molecular methods for selection of the ideal oocyte. *Reprod Biomed Online* 2007; **15**: 346–53.

28. Eppig JJ, Chesnel F, Hirao Y, *et al.* Oocyte control of granulosa cell development: how and why. *Hum Reprod* 1997; **12**: 127–32.

29. Eppig JJ,Wigglesworth K, Pendola FL. The mammalian oocyte orchestrates the rate of ovarian follicular development. *Proc Natl Acad Sci USA* 2002; **99**: 2890–4.

30. Assou S, Anahory T, Pantesco V, *et al.* The human cumulus–oocyte complex gene-expression profile. *Hum Reprod* 2006; **21**: 1705–19.

31. Feuerstein P, Cadoret V, Dalbies-Tran R, *et al.* Gene expression in human cumulus cells: one approach to oocyte competence. *Hum Reprod* 2007; **22**: 3069–77.

32. Sutton-McDowall ML, Gilchrist RB, Thompson JG. The pivotal role of glucose metabolism in determining oocyte developmental competence. *Reproduction* 2010; **139**: 685–95.

33. Huang Z, Wells D. The human oocyte and cumulus cells relationship: new insights from the cumulus cell transcriptome. *Mol Hum Reprod* 2010; **16**: 715–25.

34. Gilchrist RB, Lane M, Thompson JG. Oocyte-secreted factors: regulators of cumulus cell function and oocyte quality. *Hum Reprod Update* 2008; **14**: 159–77.

35. Su YQ, Sugiura K, Wigglesworth K, *et al.* Oocyte regulation of metabolic cooperativity between mouse cumulus cells and oocytes: BMP15 and GDF9 control cholesterol biosynthesis in cumulus cells. *Development* 2008; **135**: 111–21.

36. Assou S, Haouzi D, Mahmoud K, *et al.* A non-invasive test for assessing embryo potential by gene expression profiles of human cumulus cells: a proof of concept study. *Mol Hum Reprod* 2008; **14**(12): 711–19.

37. Assou S, Haouzi D, De Vos J, *et al.* Human cumulus cells as biomarkers for embryo and pregnancy outcomes. *Mol Hum Reprod* 2010; **16**(8): 531–8.

38. Gebhardt KM, Feil DK, Dunning KR, *et al.* Human cumulus cell gene expression as a biomarker of pregnancy outcome after single embryo transfer. *Fertil Steril* 2011; **96**: 47–52.e2.

39. Ouandaogo ZG, Haouzi D, Assou S, *et al.* Human cumulus cells molecular signature in relation to oocyte nuclear maturity stage. *PLoS One* 2011; **6**: e27179.

40. Fragouli E, Wells D, Iager AE, *et al.* Alteration of gene expression in human cumulus cells as a potential indicator of oocyte aneuploidy. *Hum Reprod* 2012; **27**: 2559–68.

41. Kuang Z, Lewis RS, Curtis JM, *et al.* The SPRY domain-containing SOCS box protein SPSB2 targets iNOS for proteasomal degradation. *J Cell Biol* 2010; **190**: 129–41.

42. Lee JH, Kang Y, Khare V, *et al.* The p53-inducible gene 3 (PIG3) contributes to early cellular response to DNA damage. *Oncogene* 2010; **29**: 1431–50.

43. Høst E, Gabrielsen A, Lindenberg S, *et al.* Apoptosis in human cumulus cells in relation to zona pellucida thickness variation, maturation stage, and cleavage of the corresponding oocyte after intracytoplasmic sperm injection. *Fertil Steril* 2002; 77: 511–15.

Chapter 30

Transgenerational risks by exposure in utero

Miguel A. Velazquez and Tom P. Fleming

Introduction

A significant proportion of human deaths worldwide are caused by non-communicable diseases (NCDs) and it has been estimated that by 2030 NCDs will account for over 60% of human mortality in both economically developed and developing countries [1]. Experimental trials in animals and epidemiological and clinical studies in humans have revealed that development of NCDs in adult life can be programmed during the prenatal period [2–8]. This adverse programming is the basis of the developmental origins of health and disease (DOHaD) concept [7]. Several lines of evidence indicate that this detrimental programming can be induced not only during fetal development but also during the preimplantation period [3, 4, 6, 7, 9]. However, this unfavorable programming can also be exerted before conception. In mammals, events occurring during primordial germ cell generation, oogonia differentiation, primordial oocyte formation, and folliculogenesis can have an impact on oocyte developmental competence (Figure 30.1). Accordingly, it has long been recognized that mammalian oocytes rely on unperturbed maternal mRNA stored during oogenesis to reach proper cytoplasmic and nuclear maturation, which is essential for successful fertilization and the first cell divisions of the newly formed embryo [10]. Likewise, successive developmental stages such as blastocyst formation, implantation, and fetal development can also be influenced by oocyte quality [7, 9, 11]. Growing evidence also indicates that oocyte developmental competence acquired during folliculogenesis can critically affect the development of NCDs in adulthood [9, 11]. Of further significance is the transgenerational non-genomic transmission of phenotypes caused by adverse uterine environments beyond the F1 generation [2, 12, 13], suggesting a possible effect on events involved in oocyte formation during fetal development. This chapter will focus on the available evidence supporting the notion that maternal challenges affecting folliculogenesis in postnatal life or oogenesis during fetal development can program the development of NCDs in offspring adult life across generations.

Preconception maternal challenges may increase the risk of developing disease in the postnatal life of F1 offspring

Ovarian follicular development takes place during childhood, but the small antral follicles formed [14] do not achieve ovulation due to the immaturity of the hypothalamo-pituitary axis [15]. Once puberty is reached, ovarian folliculogenesis can be completed in the presence of the preovulatory gonadotropin surge, resulting in the production of a mature oocyte ready for fertilization [16]. Cellular and molecular changes taking place in the oocyte during ovarian folliculogenesis are controlled by endocrine (e.g., gonadotropins) and paracrine/autocrine (e.g., growth factors) pathways [17]. The resultant ovarian follicular microenvironment from these interactive pathways determines the developmental competence of the oocyte. Oocyte developmental competence can be defined as the ability of the oocyte to achieve maturation, fertilization, embryonic and fetal development, and ultimately give rise to healthy and fertile offspring [18].

One of the most investigated maternal challenges affecting oocyte developmental competence is malnutrition (i.e., overnutrition and undernutrition). Overnutrition is a form of malnutrition in which

Biology and Pathology of the Oocyte, 2nd edn., ed. Alan Trounson, Roger Gosden, and Ursula Eichenlaub-Ritter. Published by Cambridge University Press.

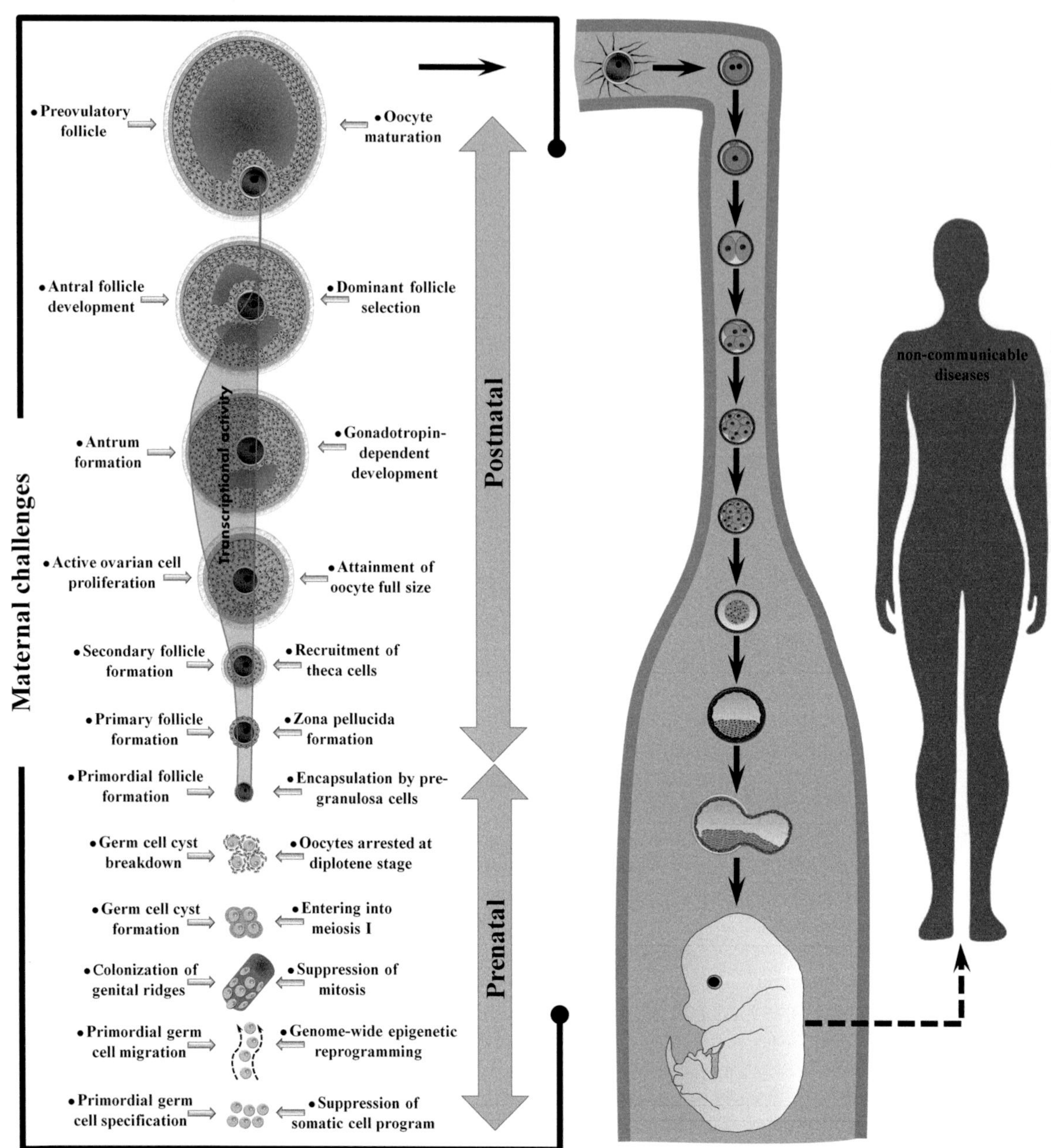

Figure 30.1 Maternal challenges taking place during primordial germ cell generation, oogonia differentiation and primordial oocyte formation in the prenatal life (in mice primordial oocyte formation takes place shortly after birth), and during critical steps of folliculogenesis in the postnatal life can have an impact on oocyte developmental competence and offspring health.

bioavailability of one or more macro- and micronutrients exceeds the amounts necessary for normal physiological activity and metabolism, which usually results in overweight or obesity [11]. On the other hand, undernutrition is the result of deficient bioavailability of one or more macro- and micronutrients caused by decreased dietary intake, increased nutritional requirements or losses, or impaired ability to absorb or utilize nutrients [11]. It is known that oocytes that develop under a microenvironment of malnutrition in vivo can impair the establishment of pregnancy [11, 19]. However, pregnancies can be achieved with oocytes subjected to malnutrition and successful delivery to term is usually possible, even in extreme cases of undernutrition and overnutrition [11]. Still, several studies have indicated that malnutrition during folliculogenesis can compromise offspring health. For example, female mice fed with an isocaloric low protein diet exclusively during the later stages of ovarian folliculogenesis, when oocyte maturation takes place, produced offspring with increased systolic blood pressure detected in both sexes at 21 weeks post-partum [20]. In this nutritional model an attenuated in vitro vasoreactivity of mesenteric arteries to vasodilators was detected in male offspring from underfed mothers, along with positive correlations between systolic blood pressure and morphological variables such as kidney:body weight ratio and heart:body weight ratio not observed in male offspring from well-fed mothers [20]. The study also revealed that female offspring from mice fed with the low protein diet exhibited a lower kidney weight with increased number of glomeruli. This compensatory response induced by maternal undernutrition was associated with a negative correlation between systolic blood pressure and glomerular number [20]. This experimental model has recently been replicated and the increased systolic blood pressure was again detected in both sexes at 52 weeks post-partum in offspring from mothers subjected to protein restriction during the period of oocyte maturation [21]. All these changes were observed without changes in postnatal growth [20, 21]. A similar scenario has been found in sheep, where female offspring from ewes fed half of their maintenance nutritional requirements for 30 days before conception showed attenuated vasodilatation in the left descending coronary artery, left internal thoracic artery, and third-order femoral artery [22].

On the other hand, overnutrition during folliculogenesis can also affect offspring health. In a study in which obesity was induced in female mice with a high fat diet before conception for 3 months, 6-month-old male offspring from obese mothers displayed high blood concentrations of insulin, triglycerides, free fatty acids, adiponectin, and C-reactive protein (CRP), whereas female obese offspring did not have high levels of insulin, adiponectin, and CRP, but showed increased concentrations of cholesterol, leptin, triglycerides, free fatty acids, and soluble intercellular adhesion molecular-1 (sICAM-1) [23]. Furthermore, offspring of both sexes from obese mothers were heavier and had greater visceral adipose tissue and increased adipose tissue:body mass ratio compared to non-obese controls [23]. Since in this latter study obesity was maintained during pregnancy, an effect via the uterus cannot be ruled out. Nevertheless, a recent embryo transfer study reported similar results. Accordingly, female lambs from dams fed with a high energy diet prior to conception displayed increased total fat mass at 4 months of age [24]. In this study, superovulated ewes with a high body condition score were fed *ad libitum* with a diet containing 170–190% of maintenance energy requirements (MER) for 4 months before conception, and preimplantation embryos produced on day 6–7 after artificial insemination were transferred to recipients fed with a control diet (100% MER) [24]. These animal studies of overnutrition have provided partial support to the findings from recent studies in humans indicating that children born from mothers that were overweight or obese before pregnancy have a higher risk of becoming overweight or obese during adolescence [25–27]. In contrast, non-overweight women losing weight before pregnancy have a higher risk of having small-for-gestational-age newborns [28], a feature that has been replicated to a certain extent in ruminant models of undernutrition. For instance, ewes subjected to undernutrition for 60 days before conception developed higher insulin sensitivity at 65 days of pregnancy [29], associated with lower growth rate of fetuses in late pregnancy compared with well-nourished control counterparts [29, 30]. Of clinical relevance is the fact that the impaired secretion pattern of blood analytes and the altered repertoire of cardiovascular and blood vessel function referred to in the aforementioned models of malnutrition have been associated with the metabolic syndrome and/or cardiovascular disease [11].

Maternal malnutrition before conception has been associated with impaired behavioral activity as well. In the above-mentioned murine low protein model of undernutrition it was also observed that offspring from underfed mice displayed abnormal anxiety-related behavior when subjected to open field tests [20]. Similarly, rats experiencing 50% calorie restriction, in relation to a control group fed *ad libitum*, for 3 days 1 week prior to conception produced offspring that exhibited greater anxiety-like behavior [31]. Unlike the low protein model [20], the calorie-restriction study found differences in postnatal growth, revealing that offspring from calorie-restricted dams were heavier than their control counterparts, with values showing statistical significance at 8 days after birth and persisting until 84 days post-partum [31]. In another model of undernutrition in which ewes were fed to achieve a 10–15% body weight reduction for 60 days before mating the resultant offspring showed fewer attempts to escape when subjected to an isolation stress test compared to lambs born from control dams [32]. The implications of these alterations in behavioral function for human well-being are unknown, but nevertheless they could be significant. For instance, compared to control individuals unexposed to the Holocaust, Holocaust survivors that experienced malnutrition and related stress showed alterations in cardiometabolic variables [33], and their offspring displayed higher levels of distress, including higher anxiety levels, lower self-esteem, and relational ambivalence than their comparison counterparts [34, 35], which were associated with a greater use of medication for psychotropic conditions and hypertension and lipid disorders [36].

The mechanisms behind the phenomenon of oocyte developmental programming via maternal challenge are complex and not fully understood. Substantial evidence generated in somatic cells of animal models indicates that such mechanisms share similarities with the human situation and include permanent structural changes, epigenetic modifications associated with permanent changes in gene expression, and mitochondrial dysfunction linked to cumulative oxidative damage [37]. Likewise, several endocrine, cellular, and molecular variables can be affected in the ovarian follicle and the enclosed oocyte during maternal challenges, but a cause–effect relationship has not been fully established [11].

Transgenerational oocyte developmental programming beyond the F1 generation

The above-discussed information indicates that environmental challenges taking place before conception, during the postnatal life of the mother (i.e., F0 generation), can affect the health of the resultant F1 offspring (Figure 30.1). However, growing evidence indicates that certain phenotypes induced by challenges imposed solely in the F0 generation can be transmitted beyond the F1 generation in animals and humans [12, 13, 38]. Indeed, it is known that female germ mutagens such as doxorubicin, a chemotherapeutic agent used for the treatment of human cancers, can cause physical and functional defects in mice offspring from F0 dams undergoing exposure prior to conception; with detrimental effects being observed up to the F6 generation [39]. Similarly, transgenerational non-genomic transmission of phenotypic changes to subsequent generations has been reported. For instance, in rodent models, several maternal challenges imposed during pregnancy in F0 dams can program the development of altered phenotypes that can persist to the F3 generation (Table 30.1). In this case the detrimental effect may be exerted via events occurring during the prenatal life, including primordial germ cell generation, oogonia differentiation, and oocyte formation (Figure 30.1). Interestingly, some of the adverse effects are not always transmitted to the F3 generation and it has been argued that transmission of induced phenotypes to the F2 generation may not be an epigenetic transgenerational phenotype [13, 40]. An F0 gestating female exposed to hazardous environments will expose her F1 embryo and the F2 germ line inside the developing F1 embryo. Hence any induced phenotype in the F1 and F2 generation will be the result of direct exposure to the environmental challenge in the F0 generation (Figure 30.2). The induced phenotype transmitted to the F2 generation could be due to an abnormality in the germ cell not caused by reprogramming of the germ line. The F3 offspring will be the first generation where progenitor cells are not exposed directly to hazardous environments. Any phenotypic change observed in the F3 generation will be the result of reprogramming of the germ line, and therefore, a truly epigenetic transgenerational phenotype [40].

Growing evidence suggests that adverse phenotypes may be induced through epigenetic transgenerational mechanisms via the maternal and/or paternal line [13, 38]. Indeed, environmental constraints in F0 females during pregnancy caused by toxicants [41] or malnutrition [42] can induce changes in the expression of the transcriptome for at least three generations. These studies suggest that maternal challenges occurring in the F0 mother capable of modifying the normal development and differentiation of germ cells in the growing F1 embryo can impact epigenetic programming and lead to transgenerational inheritance [41, 43]. The transmission of epigenetic changes

Table 30.1. Non-genomic transmission beyond the F1 generation of phenotypes induced during F0 pregnancy in rodents

Species	F0 generation challenge	Period of challenge	Phenotypic variables induced in subsequent generations	Generations affected beyond F1	Reference
Rat	Protein-restricted diet	Whole pregnancy	• Raised blood pressure • Impaired blood vessel function	F2	[60]
Mouse	Protein-restricted diet	Whole pregnancy	• Insulin resistance • Adipocyte hypertrophy	F2	[61]
Mouse	Protein-restricted diet	Whole pregnancy	• Reduced pancreatic volume • Altered pancreatic islet morphology	F2, F3	[55]
Rat	Fungicide[a]	E8–E14[b]	• Anemia • Kidney abnormalities	F2, F3	[56]
Rat	Environmental toxicants[c]	E8–E14[b]	• Early onset of puberty • Reduced primordial follicle pool size[d]	F2, F3	[41]
Rat	Environmental toxicants[e]	E8–E14[b]	• Increased number of ovarian cysts[f] • Reduced primordial follicle pool size[f]	F3	[57]
Rat	Feeding restriction[g]	Whole pregnancy	• Raised blood pressure • Impaired blood vessel function	F2, F3	[58]

[a] Intraperitoneal injections of vinclozolin.
[b] Embryonic day 8–14.
[c] Intraperitoneal injections of bisphenol A; bis(2-ethylhexyl) phthalate; dibutyl phthalate; *N,N*-diethylmeta-toluamide; 2,3,7,8-tetrachlorodibenzo-*p*-dioxin; jet propellant 8.
[d] Primordial follicle pool size was reported only in the F3 generation.
[e] Intraperitoneal injections of bisphenol A; vinclozolin; permethrin; bis(2-ethylhexyl) phthalate; dibutyl phthalate; *N,N*-diethylmeta-toluamide; 2,3,7,8-tetrachlorodibenzo-*p*-dioxin; jet propellant 8.
[f] Data from the F2 generation were not reported.
[g] 50% of the *ad libitum* intake of control counterparts.

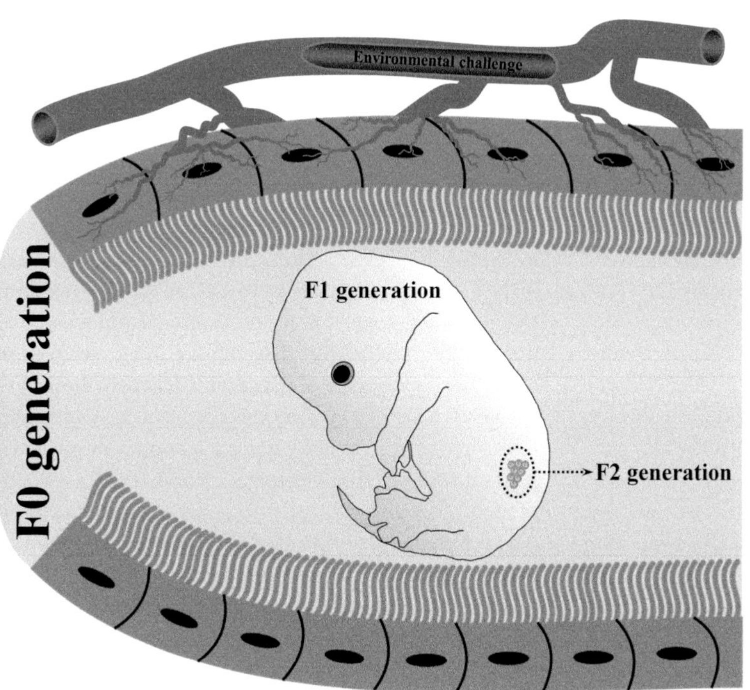

Figure 30.2 An F0 gestating female subjected to an environmental challenge will expose her F1 embryo and the F2 germ line inside the developing F1 embryo. Any induced phenotype in the F1 and F2 generation will be the result of direct exposure to the environmental challenge in the F0 generation, but may not constitute an epigenetic transgenerational phenotype (see text for details).

between generations in the absence of any direct environmental insult is known as epigenetic transgenerational inheritance, and as implied above, this term is applicable from the F3 generation onwards [41]. Importantly, epigenetic changes in comparison with genetic ones are potentially reversible. For instance, obesity in an animal model attributed to epigenetic modifications was reversed with a hypermethylating dietary supplement [44]. However, the study of epigenetic transgenerational inheritance is very much in its infancy and the underlying epigenetic mechanisms involved in developmental programming of NCDs in childhood and adulthood across generations remain to be fully determined.

Assisted reproductive technology (ART) and oocyte developmental competence

The maternal challenges discussed above usually take place during natural conception cycles where the offspring is conceived after spontaneous ovulation. However, worldwide availability of ART is rising and its application is in constant demand [45]. Increasing evidence supports the notion that ART may affect offspring health [46–49], most probably via epigenetic abnormalities induced in gametes and embryos [50, 51]. It has been suggested that the vascular dysfunction of the systemic and pulmonary circulation observed in children conceived by in vitro fertilization (IVF) procedures is not due to the ovarian stimulation per se, but to the in vitro microenvironment during fertilization and preimplantation embryo development used in ART [49]. Nevertheless, in the latter study only 16 children were included to investigate the effect of ovulation induction (OI) and the ovarian stimulation protocols used for oocyte retrieval by ovum-pick in ART cycles were not analyzed. Interestingly, with a sample of 4467 children born after OI, Klemetti *et al.* [52] reported that children born to women subjected to OI with or without intrauterine insemination had an increased risk for cerebral palsy, allergy, and asthma, along with long-term medication use, and long episodes of hospitalization compared to naturally conceived counterparts. Besides ovarian stimulation protocols for OI and oocyte retrieval in IVF cycles, other emerging ART-associated techniques with putative effects on oocyte developmental competence such as in vitro oocyte maturation, and ovarian tissue and oocyte cryopreservation should be addressed in future research investigating the health of offspring derived from ART. Given that human oocyte developmental competence can be potentially affected by lifestyle factors [53, 54] and the transgenerational oocyte developmental programming of NCDs found in animal models [55–58], the impact of past lifestyle of human donors in oocyte donation models should also be investigated. However, this is a challenging task due to difficulties in collecting accurate long-term preconception information on lifestyle habits and health status in human populations. Furthermore, the study of epigenetic transgenerational inheritance should not only take into account maternal challenges but also paternal influences. Indeed, a recent study reported that in vitro culture conditions during murine preimplantation development affected fertility and glucose metabolism exclusively in the male offspring for three generations (F0–F2) [59].

Conclusions

Evidence has indicated that environmental constraints taking place solely during folliculogenesis in the F0 generation can result in F1 offspring with compromised health status in the postnatal life. Several studies have also shown that the adverse phenotype in the F1 offspring induced in the intrauterine environment of the F0 generation can be transmitted to the F2 generation in the absence of subsequent environmental challenges. This adverse phenotype is probably programmed in events taking place during primordial germ cell generation, oogonia differentiation, and oocyte formation. However, the transmission of induced phenotypes up to the F2 generation may not be an epigenetic transgenerational phenotype as the adverse phenotype may be due to an abnormality in the germ cell not caused by reprogramming of the germ line, but by direct exposure to environmental insults in the F0 pregnancy. Examination of the F3 generation (e.g., first generation not directly exposed) is required to identify a truly epigenetic transgenerational phenotype associated to intrauterine exposure of F1 offspring to environmental insults. Although substantial evidence is now available demonstrating the effects of in vitro microenvironments during fertilization and preimplantation embryo development on offspring health, less effort has been put into analyzing the effects of assisted reproduction on oocyte developmental competence. The underlying mechanisms involved in developmental programming of NCDs in childhood and adulthood across generations are complex and far from being properly understood. Research is necessary to develop strategies for therapeutic intervention. The above-discussed information suggests that such strategies should be implemented before conception.

Acknowledgments

The authors are grateful for research funding and support from BBSRC, MRC, NICHD, EU (FP7 and COST Gemini) to T. P. F. in recent years.

References

1. Mathers CD, Loncar D. Projections of global mortality and burden of disease from 2002 to 2030. *PLoS Med* 2006; **3**: e442.
2. Gluckman PD, Hanson MA, Cooper C, Thornburg KL. Effect of in utero and early-life conditions on adult health and disease. *N Engl J Med* 2008; **359**: 61–73.
3. McMillen IC, MacLaughlin SM, Muhlhausler BS, *et al.* Developmental origins of adult health and disease: the role of periconceptional and foetal nutrition. *Basic Clin Pharmacol Toxicol* 2008; **102**: 82–9.
4. Watkins AJ, Fleming TP. Blastocyst environment and its influence on offspring cardiovascular health: the heart of the matter. *J Anat* 2009; **215**: 52–9.
5. Langley-Evans SC, McMullen S. Developmental origins of health and disease. *Med Princ Pract* 2010; **19**: 87–98.
6. Zhang S, Rattanatray L, McMillen IC, Suter CM, Morrison JL. Periconceptional nutrition and the early programming of a life of obesity or adversity. *Prog Biophys Mol Biol* 2011; **106**: 307–14.
7. Fleming TP, Lucas ES, Watkins AJ, Eckert JJ. Adaptive responses of the embryo to maternal diet and consequences for post-implantation development. *Reprod Fertil Dev* 2012; **24**: 35–44.
8. Lewis RM, Cleal JK, Hanson MA. Review: Placenta, evolution and lifelong health. *Placenta* 2012; **33**: S28–32.
9. Fleming TP, Velazquez MA, Eckert JJ, Lucas ES, Watkins AJ. Nutrition of females during the peri-conceptional period and effects on foetal programming and health of offspring. *Anim Reprod Sci* 2012; **130**: 193–7.
10. Eichenlaub-Ritter U, Peschke M. Expression in in-vivo and in-vitro growing and maturing oocytes: focus on regulation of expression at the translational level. *Hum Reprod* 2002; **8**: 21–41.
11. Velazquez MA, Fleming TP. Maternal diet, oocyte nutrition and metabolism, and offspring health. In: Coticchio G, Albertini DF, De Santis L, eds. *Oogenesis.* London: Springer. 2013; 329–51. SBN 978-0-85729-825-6.
12. Lucas ES, Fleming TP. Developmental programming and epigenetics: DNA methylation makes its mark. *Cell Tissue Biol Res* 2009; **1**: 15–23.
13. Hanson M, Godfrey KM, Lillycrop KA, Burdge GC, Gluckman PD. Developmental plasticity and developmental origins of non-communicable disease: theoretical considerations and epigenetic mechanisms. *Prog Biophys Mol Biol* 2011; **106**: 272–80.
14. Stanhope R, Adams J, Jacobs HS, Brook CGD. Ovarian ultrasound assessment in normal children, idiopathic precocious puberty, and during low dose pulsatile gonadotrophin releasing hormone treatment of hypogonadotrophic hypogonadism. *Arch Dis Child* 1985; **60**: 116–19.
15. Terasawa E, Fernandez DL. Neurobiological mechanisms of the onset of puberty in primates. *Endocr Rev* 2001; **22**: 111–51.
16. Baerwald AR, Adams GP, Pierson RA. Ovarian antral folliculogenesis during the human menstrual cycle: a review. *Hum Reprod Update* 2012; **18**: 73–91.
17. Zuccotti M, Merico V, Cecconi S, Redi CA, Garagna S. What does it take to make a developmentally competent mammalian egg? *Hum Reprod Update* 2011; **17**: 525–40.
18. Mermillod P, Dalbiès-Tran R, Uzbekova S, *et al.* Factors affecting oocyte quality: who is driving the follicle? *Reprod Domest Anim* 2008; **43**(Suppl 2): 393–400.
19. Velazquez MA. The role of nutritional supplementation on the outcome of superovulation in cattle. *Anim Reprod Sci* 2011; **126**: 1–10.
20. Watkins AJ, Wilkins A, Cunningham C, *et al.* Low protein diet fed exclusively during mouse oocyte maturation leads to behavioural and cardiovascular abnormalities in offspring. *J Physiol* 2008; **586**: 2231–44.
21. Watkins AJ, Lucas ES, Wilkins A, Cagampang FRA, Fleming TP. Maternal periconceptional and gestational low protein diet affects mouse offspring growth, cardiovascular and adipose phenotype at 1 year of age. *PLoS One* 2011; **6**: e28745.
22. Torrens C, Snelling TH, Chau R, *et al.* Effects of pre- and periconceptional undernutrition on arterial function in adult female sheep are vascular bed dependent. *Exp Physiol* 2009; **94**: 1024–33.

23. Bytautiene E, Tamayo E, Kechichian T, *et al.* Prepregnancy obesity and sFlt1-induced preeclampsia in mice: developmental programming model of metabolic syndrome. *Am J Obstet Gynecol* 2011; **204**: 398.e1–8.

24. Rattanatray L, Maclaughlin SM, Kleemann DO, *et al.* Impact of maternal periconceptional overnutrition on fat mass and expression of adipogenic and lipogenic genes in visceral and subcutaneous fat depots in the postnatal lamb. *Endocrinology* 2010; **151**: 5195–205.

25. Kitsantas P, Pawloski LR, Gaffney KF. Maternal prepregnancy body mass index in relation to Hispanic preschooler overweight/obesity. *Eur J Pediatr* 2010; **169**: 1361–8.

26. Pirkola J, Pouta A, Bloigu A, *et al.* Risks of overweight and abdominal obesity at age 16 years associated with prenatal exposures to maternal prepregnancy overweight and gestational diabetes mellitus. *Diabetes Care* 2010; **33**: 1115–21.

27. Jääskeläinen A, Pussinen J, Nuutinen O, *et al.* Intergenerational transmission of overweight among Finnish adolescents and their parents: a 16-year follow-up study. *Int J Obes (Lond)* 2011; **35**:1289–94.

28. Diouf I, Charles MA, Thiebaugeorges O, *et al.* The EDEN Mother–Child Cohort Study Group. Maternal weight change before pregnancy in relation to birth weight and risks of adverse pregnancy outcomes. *Eur J Epidemiol* 2011; **26**: 789–96.

29. Jaquiery AL, Oliver MH, Rumball CWH, Bloomfield FH, Harding JE. Undernutrition before mating in ewes impairs the development of insulin resistance during pregnancy. *Obstet Gynecol* 2009; **114**: 869–76.

30. Rumball CWH, Bloomfield FH, Oliver MH, Harding JE. Different periods of periconceptional undernutrition have different effects on growth, metabolic and endocrine status in fetal sheep. *Pediatr Res* 2009; **66**: 605–13.

31. Levay EA, Paolini AG, Govic A, *et al.* Anxiety-like behaviour in adult rats perinatally exposed to maternal calorie restriction. *Behav Brain Res* 2008; **191**: 164–72.

32. Hernandez CE, Matthews LR, Oliver MH, Bloomfield FH, Harding JE. Effects of sex, litter size and periconceptional ewe nutrition on offspring behavioural and physiological response to isolation. *Physiol Behav* 2010; **101**: 588–94.

33. Yehuda R, Bierer LM, Andrew R, Schmeidler J, Seckl JR. Enduring effects of severe developmental adversity, including nutritional deprivation, on cortisol metabolism in aging Holocaust survivors. *J Psychiatr Res* 2009; **43**: 877–83.

34. Scharf M. Long-term effects of trauma: psychosocial functioning of the second and third generation of Holocaust survivors. *Dev Psychopathol* 2007; **19**: 603–22.

35. Gangi S, Talamo A, Ferracuti S. The long-term effects of extreme war-related trauma on the second generation of Holocaust survivors. *Violence Vict* 2009; **24**: 687–700.

36. Flory JD, Bierer LM, Yehuda R. Maternal exposure to the holocaust and health complaints in offspring. *Dis Markers* 2011; **30**: 133–9.

37. Warner MJ, Ozanne SE. Mechanisms involved in the developmental programming of adulthood disease. *Biochem J* 2010; **427**: 333–47.

38. Gluckman PD, Hanson MA, Beedle AS. Non-genomic transgenerational inheritance of disease risk. *Bioessays* 2007; **29**: 145–54.

39. Kujjo LL, Chang EA, Pereira RJG, *et al.* Chemotherapy-induced late transgenerational effects in mice. *PLoS One* 2011; **6**: e17877.

40. Skinner MK. What is an epigenetic transgenerational phenotype? F3 or F2. *Reprod Toxicol* 2008; **25**: 2–6.

41. Manikkam M, Guerrero-Bosagna C, Tracey R, Haque MM, Skinner MK. Transgenerational actions of environmental compounds on reproductive disease and identification of epigenetic biomarkers of ancestral exposures. *PLoS One* 2012; **7**: e31901.

42. Hoile SP, Lillycrop KA, Thomas NA, Hanson MA, Burdge GC. Dietary protein restriction during F0 pregnancy in rats induces transgenerational changes in the hepatic transcriptome in female offspring. *PLoS ONE* 2011; **6**: e21668.

43. Daxinger L, Whitelaw E. Understanding transgenerational epigenetic inheritance via the gametes in mammals. *Nat Rev Genet* 2012; **13**: 153–62.

44. Waterland RA, Travisano M, Tahiliani KG, Rached MT, Mirza S. Methyl donor supplementation prevents transgenerational amplification of obesity. *Int J Obes (Lond)* 2008; **32**: 1373–9.

45. International Committee for Monitoring Assisted Reproductive Technology (ICMART): de Mouzon J, Lancaster P, Nygren KG, *et al.* World collaborative report on Assisted Reproductive Technology, 2002. *Hum Reprod* 2009; **24**: 2310–20.

46. Ceelen M, van Weissenbruch MM, Vermeiden JPW, van Leeuwen FE, Delemarre-van de Waal HA. Cardiometabolic differences in children born after in vitro fertilization: follow-up study. *J Clin Endocrinol Metab* 2008; **93**: 1682–8.

47. Sakka SD, Malamitsi-Puchner A, Loutradis D, Chrousos GP, Kanaka-Gantenbein C. Euthyroid

hyperthyrotropinemia in children born after in vitro fertilization. *J Clin Endocrinol Metab* 2009; **94**: 1338–41.

48. Davies MJ, Moore VM, Willson KJ, *et al.* Reproductive technologies and the risk of birth defects. *N Engl J Med* 2012; **366**: 1803–13.

49. Scherrer U, Rimoldi SF, Rexhaj E, *et al.* Systemic and pulmonary vascular dysfunction in children conceived by assisted reproductive technologies. *Circulation* 2012; **125**: 1890–6.

50. Huntriss J, Picton HM. Epigenetic consequences of assisted reproduction and infertility on the human preimplantation embryo. *Hum Fertil (Camb)* 2008; **11**: 85–94.

51. van Montfoort APA, Hanssen LLP, de Sutter P, *et al.* Assisted reproduction treatment and epigenetic inheritance. *Hum Reprod Update* 2012; **18**: 171–97.

52. Klemetti R, Sevón T, Gissler M, Hemminki E. Health of children born after ovulation induction. *Fertil Steril* 2010; **93**: 1157–68.

53. Anderson K, Nisenblat V, Norman R. Lifestyle factors in people seeking infertility treatment – A review. *Aust N Z J Obstet Gynaecol* 2010; **50**: 8–20.

54. Toledo E, Lopez-del Burgo C, Ruiz-Zambrana A, *et al.* Dietary patterns and difficulty conceiving: a nested case-control study. *Fertil Steril* 2011; **96**: 1149–53.

55. Frantz EDC, Aguila MB, Pinheiro-Mulder Ada R, Mandarim-de-Lacerda CA. Transgenerational endocrine pancreatic adaptation in mice from maternal protein restriction in utero. *Mech Ageing Dev* 2011; **132**: 110–16.

56. Nilsson EE, Anway MD, Stanfield J, Skinner MK. Transgenerational epigenetic effects of the endocrine disruptor vinclozolin on pregnancies and female adult onset disease. *Reproduction* 2008; **135**: 713–21.

57. Nilsson E, Larsen G, Manikkham M, *et al.* Environmentally induced epigenetic transgenerational inheritance of ovarian disease. *PLoS ONE* 2012; **7**: e36129.

58. Ponzio BF, Carvalho MHC, Fortes ZB, do Carmo Franco M. Implications of maternal nutrient restriction in transgenerational programming of hypertension and endothelial dysfunction across F1-F3 offspring. *Life Sci* 2012; **90**: 571–7.

59. Calle A, Miranda A, Fernandez-Gonzalez R, *et al.* Male mice produced by in vitro culture have reduced fertility and transmit organomegaly and glucose intolerance to their male offspring. *Biol Reprod* 2012; **87**: 34.

60. Torrens C, Poston L, Hanson MA. Transmission of raised blood pressure and endothelial dysfunction to the F2 generation induced by maternal protein restriction in the F0, in the absence of dietary challenge in the F1 generation. *Br J Nutr* 2008; **100**: 760–6.

61. Peixoto-Silva N, Frantz EDC, Mandarim-de-Lacerda CA, Pinheiro-Mulder A. Maternal protein restriction in mice causes adverse metabolic and hypothalamic effects in the F1 and F2 generations. *Br J Nutr* 2011; **106**: 1364–73.

Section 5 Pathology

Chapter 31

Obesity and oocyte quality

Rebecca L. Robker and Robert J. Norman

Introduction

Obesity has become one of the most urgent nutritional and health issues of our time. Globally, the number of obese people is at a historical high with the incidence continuing to rise. Obesity is prevalent in young women [1] and latest predictions indicate that in the USA and UK 40–50% of women will be obese by 2030 [2]. A neglected complication of obesity is female infertility as well as increased risk of polycystic ovary syndrome (or PCOS), a prevalent endocrine disorder which manifests with both metabolic symptoms including insulin resistance and dyslipidemia, as well as reproductive complications such as anovulation. Entering pregnancy in an obese condition predisposes both mother and fetus to significant health problems that can complicate an already risky pregnancy.

It is increasingly evident that obesity is a self-perpetuating transgenerational disease that is transmitted from mothers to the next generation. While obesity alters body metabolism and leads to consequences in multiple aspects of the reproductive system, this chapter will summarize the available data from experimental animal models and clinical studies showing an impact on oocyte developmental potential. This rapidly accumulating evidence, particularly from animal models, demonstrates that obesity affects oocyte maturation and the earliest stages of embryo development; alterations that have lasting consequences on the metabolism and developmental programming of the progeny.

Effects of obesity on oocytes in animal models

In experimental animal models obesity is not strictly defined but typically refers to animals with increased body fat compared to controls; for instance those with increased fatness due to high fat diet or genetic mutations leading to appetite dysregulation. Considerable research, in such animal models, has begun to investigate how obesity impacts the oocyte and shows considerable effects on blastocyst and subsequent fetal development.

Impaired oocyte developmental competence in rodent models of obesity

A number of laboratories have independently reported that obesity causes distinct defects in oocytes that manifest as alterations in subsequent embryo development. In one of the earliest studies, female mice fed a high fat diet for 16 weeks were "obese," hyperinsulinemic, and dyslipidemic; and exhibited altered oocyte developmental competence [3]. Specifically, zygotes isolated following mating and monitored in vitro exhibited slower development to the 4- to 8-cell stage that was maintained to the blastocyst stage [3]; demonstrating that oocytes from an obese animal, even when removed from the systemic environment and cultured in vitro, possess intrinsic differences that influence subsequent embryo development. The cell type distribution of the resultant embryos was also disrupted, with blastocysts from oocytes of obese females having a lower inner cell mass to trophectoderm ratio, a phenotype that is predictive of smaller size at birth and altered postnatal health [4–6]. In other studies preovulatory follicles of female mice fed a high fat diet for 16 weeks had smaller oocytes that were delayed in undergoing germinal vesicle breakdown (GVBD) [7]. Female mice fed a high fat diet for 4 weeks and mated following gonadotropin stimulation exhibited reduced fertilization rates [8]. Female mice fed an obesogenic

Biology and Pathology of the Oocyte, 2nd edn., ed. Alan Trounson, Roger Gosden, and Ursula Eichenlaub-Ritter. Published by Cambridge University Press.

diet for 6 weeks and mated following gonadotropin stimulation exhibited reduced zygote progression to the blastocyst stage in vivo [9]. Rats obese from overfeeding for 4 weeks produced blastocysts with dramatically different gene expression profiles, particularly for inflammatory and mitochondrial genes, compared to non-obese rats [10]. Thus, in a number of experimental dietary paradigms obesity is associated with poor oocyte developmental competence.

As cumulus cells are integral to oocyte health, are coupled to the ooycte, and are key regulators of oocyte metabolism and maturation, investigators have also examined the function of these cells in response to obesity. Cumulus cells directly control the amount of glucose in oocytes [11] and cumulus cells from mice fed a high fat diet for 4 weeks exhibited impaired insulin-stimulated glucose uptake [12]. To investigate the role of insulin resistance in mediating the effects of obesity on oocyte developmental competence, obese female mice were treated with an insulin sensitizer for just 4 days prior to mating and embryo development from the zygote stage was monitored in vitro [3]. Treatment with rosiglitazone, a PPARγ transcription factor agonist, corrected hyperinsulinemia and glucose metabolism and reduced circulating triglycerides; but also normalized the delayed blastocyst development and altered embryo cell allocation, effectively rendering embryos from oocytes of obese females identical to those from oocytes of females on the control diet [3]. Thus, acute treatment with a specific insulin sensitizer prior to conception can reverse defects in oocyte developmental competence caused by obesity, confirming that oocyte developmental competence is responsive to systemic metabolic cues prior to ovulation, while still contained in the preovulatory ovarian follicle. However, it is not known whether the beneficial effects of insulin sensitizers on oocyte developmental competence in obese mice are mediated through direct actions on the oocyte or via alterations in insulin sensitivity in cumulus cells or even systemically. Thus, functional changes in cumulus cells, such as metabolism, must also be considered in order to understand more completely how female oocyte quality is dysregulated during the obese metabolic condition.

Oocytes and ovarian cells exhibit lipotoxicity in response to obesity

Lipotoxicity is a cellular response to lipid overload which has been well characterized in a number of cell types, particularly myocytes, pancreatic β-cells, and hepatocytes; and is likely involved in the pathogenesis of obesity (reviewed in [13]). Lipotoxicity is characterized by intracellular lipid accumulation which damages organelle membranes, inducing endoplasmic reticulum stress (ER stress), mitochondrial dysfunction, and reactive oxygen species (ROS) production; cellular stresses which, if not resolved, culminate in apoptosis [14].

Increasing evidence indicates that oocytes as well as their surrounding cumulus and granulosa cells initiate lipotoxic mechanisms in response to obesity. Oocytes (and cumulus cells) of female mice fed a high fat diet for 4 weeks contain markedly more neutral lipid than oocytes from non-obese mice fed a control diet [8]. Similarly, oocytes from ob/ob mice, which are obese due to lack of the satiety-regulating hormone leptin, show lipid droplet accumulation as well as the absence of microvilli through the zona pellucida [15].

Cellular stress and dysfunction is evidenced by increased levels of ER stress marker genes *Atf4* and *Hspa5* in cumulus–oocyte complexes of obese mice [8]. Mitochondrial abnormalities have also been observed in oocytes from obese mice; namely altered mitochondrial membrane potential [8, 9], and increased generation of ROS [9], indicative of mitochondrial stress. Mitochondrial DNA copy number, as well as expression of nuclear genes encoding mitochondrial DNA transcription factors, was also increased in oocytes from preovulatory follicles of obese mice but these differences were not maintained in zygotes following fertilization [9]. Oocytes from obese ob/ob mice show mitochondrial structural abnormalities by electron microscopy [15]. Mitochondrial alterations, such as those in oocytes from obese mice, are likely to lead to functional changes in metabolic activity, although to date this has not been directly demonstrated.

Increased lipid content and mitochondrial alterations in oocytes and ovarian cells of obese mice are consistently associated with increased rates of apoptosis in the follicular somatic cells. This includes observations of high rates of apoptosis in ovarian cells of the severely obese db/db mutant mouse model which lacks functional leptin receptor [16] as well as increased granulosa and cumulus cell apoptosis in ovaries of female mice with diet-induced obesity [7, 8]. This increased incidence of cell death is indicative of poor follicular health which would be detrimental to the

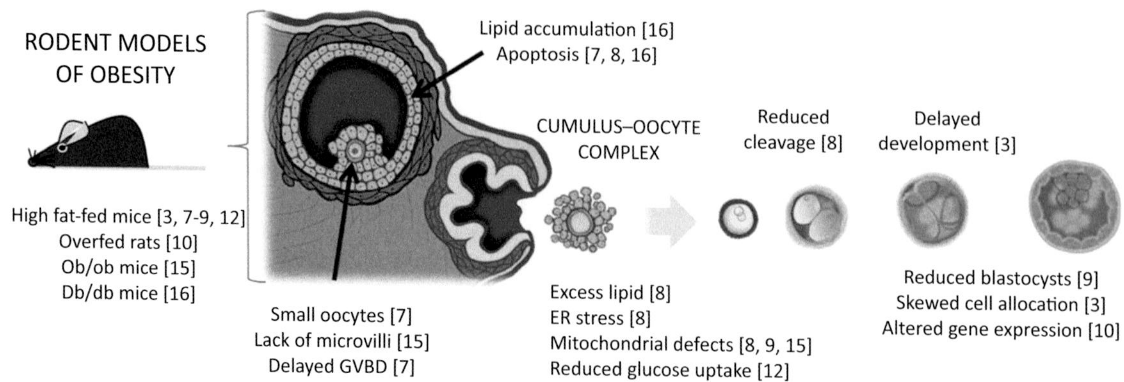

Figure 31.1 Alterations in ovarian cells, oocytes, and embryo, of rodent models of obesity. Experimental models include high fat diet-fed mice and overfed rats as well as mutant mice lacking genes for the satiety hormone leptin (ob/ob) or its receptor (db/db). Defects have been observed within the ovaries, cumulus–oocyte complexes (COC), and resultant embryos of obese rodents by the indicated citations. GVBD, germinal vesicle breakdown; ER, endoplasmic reticulum.

oocyte; however the casual basis for the association of lipid accumulation and apoptosis has not been resolved.

In summary, a number of studies using genetic and diet-induced obesity rodent models (see Figure 31.1) demonstrate that obesity and its associated metabolic perturbations change oocyte structure, lipid content, and mitochondrial activity. These alterations in oocytes are associated with the induction of lipotoxicity – namely ER stress, oxidative stress, and apoptosis in follicular cells. Ultimately these cellular defects contribute to reduced oocyte developmental competence – namely reduced fertilization rates and poor blastocyst development, but the exact mechanisms mediating these negative outcomes are only just emerging.

Lipotoxicity mechanisms in oocytes

In vitro oocyte maturation systems are beginning to shed light on the mechanisms by which lipotoxicity causes poor oocyte quality. Several studies have used the saturated fatty acid palmitic acid, which at high doses is considered a classic stimulator of lipotoxicity. In vitro studies using bovine cumulus–oocyte complexes have demonstrated that palmitic acid is detrimental to oocytes, causing impaired cumulus expansion; increased cumulus cell apoptosis; and impaired oocyte nuclear maturation, fertilization, and blastocyst development rates [17, 18]. Mouse cumulus–oocyte complexes treated with palmitic acid exhibited a dose-dependent increase in ER stress marker gene expression (*Atf4*, *Atf6*, *Xbp1s*, and *Hspa5*) and decreased protein secretion by cumulus cells [19], consistent with impaired ER function. Oocytes matured in high dose palmitic acid also had significantly altered mitochondrial membrane potential and dramatically impaired developmental competence that were specifically due to ER stress since inclusion of an ER stress inhibitor in the oocyte maturation medium completely reversed each of the defects [19]. Thus palmitic acid-induced lipotoxicity in the maturing cumulus–oocyte complex impairs the subsequent earliest stages of embryo development via induction of ER stress; but these effects are reversible.

Palmitic acid is one of the most prevalent fatty acids in human follicle fluid [20] but it is currently unclear how its levels are regulated and whether any physiological conditions lead to elevated concentrations. Serum fatty acids increase with obesity, yet follicular fluid fatty acid and palmitic acid levels are not strictly related to body mass index (BMI) ([20]; R. Robker and R. Norman unpublished data, 2012). In contrast, in cows it is clear that palmitic acid levels are altered under different physiological contexts; for instance palmitic acid is elevated in follicular fluid of dairy cows which are known to have very poor conception rates during lactation [21].

There is therefore abundant evidence from animal models, particularly mice, that obesity alters oocyte developmental potential to form embryos; with defects occurring in the context of altered follicular development, including increased granulosa/cumulus cell stress and apoptosis in preovulatory follicles. There is intense interest in determining whether similar obesity-induced defects occur in human ovaries and oocytes as this would have profound implications for the future health of embryos of obese women.

Effects of obesity on oocyte quality in humans

Obesity is clinically defined by the World Health Organization (WHO) standards of body mass index (or BMI), calculated from an individual's weight and height and measured in the units kg/m^2. A BMI of 18.5–24.9 is classified as normal, 25–29.9 as overweight, and ≥30 as obese. Less commonly, waist circumference and waist:hip ratio (WHR) are used as indicators for the assessment of obesity and its co-morbidities such as metabolic syndrome and cardiovascular disease.

Obesity reduces pregnancy rates

In normally cycling healthy women, increased BMI is associated with reduced conception rates [22, 23]; suggesting that, as in animal models, obesity affects critical periconception events, such as oocyte and/or embryo quality. The effects of obesity on the fertility of women undergoing assisted reproduction mirror those of women conceiving naturally in that obesity significantly reduces pregnancy rates, increases miscarriage rates, and decreases live birth rates (see [24, 25] for systematic reviews). Thus it is clear that obesity is associated with poorer pregnancy and neonatal outcomes in women undergoing assisted reproduction and in women conceiving naturally; however, whether defects in the oocyte are responsible is an issue of great debate.

Effects of obesity on human oocyte quality and developmental potential

To investigate more directly the effects of obesity on oocyte quality a number of studies have examined oocytes and embryos of women undergoing in vitro fertilization (IVF), which requires close inspection of oocytes and their fertilization and subsequent embryonic development. Overweight women and obese women often have significantly fewer oocytes retrieved (Table 31.1), likely due to decreased gonadotropin responsiveness, which leads to the requirement for higher gonadotropin doses, yet increased cycle cancellation rates (reviewed in [26, 27]). Inconsistent observations regarding BMI effects on oocyte number likely relate to differences in gonadotropin stimulation regimen. This is illustrated when two protocols are directly compared – obese women undergoing a "long stimulation protocol" had fewer oocytes than normal while obese women undergoing a "short protocol" did not [28]. Additional studies which report reductions in oocyte number are reviewed elsewhere [26, 27].

Oocyte maturity has been directly assessed using graded scoring systems in only a few studies (Table 31.1). Wittemer *et al.* determined whether each of the oocytes was "good quality" (at metaphase I or metaphase II [MII]) or "bad quality" (at germinal stage, post-mature, or with fractured zona) and found that the ratio of good quality to bad quality oocytes was significantly reduced in women with BMI ≥25 compared to those with BMI 20–25 [28]. Subsequent studies also found that fewer mature MII oocytes were retrieved from obese women (BMI >30) [29] and morbidly obese women (BMI ≥40) [30] compared to women with lower BMIs. More recent studies, however, have reported no differences in oocyte maturity with BMI (Table 31.1). When oocytes of women with PCOS were assessed (n = 116 cycles), there was no effect of BMI (n = 25 cycles in women with BMI [30] on the ability of oocytes to undergo maturation in vitro (IVM) [31]. Interestingly, oocytes from obese women were reported to be significantly smaller than oocytes from non-obese women [32]; and another report suggests that oocytes of overweight and obese women are more likely to have a "granular cytoplasm" [33].

Fertilization rates are more commonly reported and several have documented reduced fertilization rates in obese women (Table 31.1). One study reports a 45% reduction in fertilization rates of oocytes from obese women compared to those of moderate weight [34]. However, just as many clinics report seeing no differences in fertilization rates in oocytes of obese women compared to non-obese (Table 31.1).

Increasingly, clinics are assessing the effects of obesity on oocyte developmental potential since early studies that investigated mean embryo grade found that it was decreased in women with a BMI of >30 (Table 31.1). Carrell *et al.* found that embryo quality based on blastomere morphology was significantly reduced on the day of transfer (72 hours after oocyte retrieval) in obese women compared to women with a BMI of 20–30 [29]. Another study assessed embryos on shape of blastomeres, texture

Table 31.1. Studies analyzing oocytes and embryos in obese women. "Obesity" was not always defined as body mass index (BMI) ≥30, and thus often included overweight women

Reference	"Obese"/Total patients or *cycles*	"Obese" BMI	Oocyte no.	Oocyte maturity	Fertilization rate	Embryo quality	Pregnancy rate
Lewis, 1990 [47]	36/368	27.6	↓		↔		
Lashen, 1999 [48]	76/333	27.9	↔		↔		↔
Fedorcsak, 2000 [49]	79/383	25	↓		↔		↓
Wittemer, 2000 [28]	48/398	28	↓[a]	↓			↔
Carrell, 2001 [29]	34/247	30	↔	↓[b]		↓	↓
Salha, 2001 [50]	50/100	26	↓		↓		↓
Fedorcsak, 2004 [51]	241/2660	30	↓		↔		↓
Van Swieten, 2005 [34]	29/162	30	↔		↓		↔
Dechaud, 2006 [52]	36/573	30	↔		↔		↔
Dokras, 2006 [30]	315/1293	30	↔	↓[c]	↔		↔
Metwally, 2007 [35]	72/426	≥30	↔		↔	↓[d]	↔
Esinler, 2008 [53]	102/775 *147/1113*	≥30	↓	↔	↔		↔
Martinuzzi, 2008 [54]	52/417	≥30	↔		↔		↔
Matalliotakis, 2008 [39]	138/278 *291/582*	24	↓		↓[e]		↔
Orvieto, 2009 [55]	397 *78/516*	30	↓[b]		↓		↓
Robker, 2009 [41]	32/96	≥30	↓		↔	↔	↔
Bellver, 2010 [36]	*419/6500*	≥30	↔	↔	↔	↔	↓
Li, 2010 [56]	153/1107	≥24	↔		↔		↔
Zhang, 2010 [57]	27/2628	30	↓[b]		↓	↓[b]	↔
Depalo, 2011 [33]	108/268	25	↔	↔	↔	↔	↓[g]
Hill, 2011 [58]	21/117	≥30	↔	↔	↔		↔
Shah, 2011 [59]	310/1721	≥30	↔	↔	↓[f]	↔	↓[c]
Vilarino, 2011 [60]	191 *71/208*	25	↔		↔	↔	↔

[a] Long stimulation protocol only.
[b] Trend, not statistically significant.
[c] > BMI 40 only.
[d] <35 years old only.
[e] No difference in cleavage rate.
[f] > BMI 35 only.
[g] Implantation rate.
↓, decreased; ↔, not different, in overweight/obese compared to normal weight patients.

of cytoplasm, and degree of fragmentation on day 2 following oocyte retrieval and found that mean embryo grade was significantly poorer in obese women [35]. Conversely, a large retrospective study of 6500 IVF/ICSI (intracytoplasmic sperm injection) cycles, of which 419 [6.4%) were in obese women, found pregnancy and live birth rates were reduced with increasing BMI, but no indication of reduced oocyte maturity or altered embryo quality, in terms of blastomere number or fragmentation on day 2 or day 3 [36]. A retrospective study of >45000 embryo transfers, however, in which 16.5% were transfers to obese women, found that pregnancy and live birth rates were reduced with increasing BMI, but that the use of donor oocytes normalized pregnancy rates in obese women [37], suggesting that aspects of oocyte quality are impaired by obesity. Age, however, is another important cofactor for oocyte quality and at least three studies [35, 37, 38] have reported that BMI dramatically impairs IVF outcomes in women less than

35 years old, but has a minimal impact on IVF outcomes in women over 36 years old.

These studies are complicated by continuously evolving laboratory techniques, the diversity of patient factors, and retrospective analysis of poor quality data. Thus additional and larger studies are very much needed to clarify the conflicting observations of reduced oocyte maturity and poor embryo growth in obese women. Cumulative observations to date, however, suggest that alterations in oocytes and embryos in response to obesity may contribute to the decreased pregnancy rates and higher early miscarriage rates observed in obese women.

Alterations in ovarian cells and oocytes of obese women

A number of laboratories have begun to investigate how obesity impacts critical functions of the ovary in order to better understand the mechanisms by which obesity impacts oocyte developmental competence and early embryo growth. Obesity is associated with reduced numbers of large follicles even in women treated clinically with gonadotropins [39, 40]. Other studies have analyzed cellular functions and biomarkers known to be dysregulated by obesity in other tissues, for instance inflammatory markers, oxidative stress, and lipotoxicity. C-reactive protein (CRP), a classic marker of inflammation, is dramatically increased in follicular fluid of obese women [41]. Levels of the adipokine leptin also increase in follicular fluid with increasing BMI and adiposity [42, 43], similar to changes in blood.

A marker of oxidative stress, oxidized low-density lipoprotein (oxLDL), is elevated in follicular fluid of obese women [44]. Expression of LOX-1, an oxLDL scavenger receptor which activates NFkB signaling and inflammatory cytokine production, is increased in granulosa cells of obese women compared to non-obese women, but this difference is seen only in women treated with relatively low doses of follicle-stimulating hormone (FSH) [45]. Another scavenger receptor, SRBI, was also observed to be modestly increased in granulosa cells of obese women [41]. Antioxidant detoxification systems appear to be amplified in the ovarian follicles of obese women as well since both catalase and glutathione peroxidase enzyme activity were significantly higher in follicular fluids from obese women than non-obese women [44].

Obesity is associated with a dramatic increase in follicular fluid triglyceride levels [41] that are correlated with increased levels of free fatty acids [46]. Free fatty acid levels have in turn been shown to be associated with poor cumulus morphology [20]. ER stress is emerging as a key response to lipotoxicity and inflammatory reactions that occur in response to obesity. ATF4 mRNA, a marker of ER stress, was increased in granulosa cells of obese women compared to granulosa cells of non-obese women [8]. Both oxidative stress and ER stress culminate in cellular apoptosis if not resolved [14] and increased numbers of dead cells were observed in follicular fluid of obese women compared to non-obese women [45].

How these obesity-induced increases in lipotoxicity, inflammation, and oxidative stress within the ovarian follicular environment impact subsequent oocyte developmental potential is not yet clear but is an important area of investigation.

Conclusions

Obesity is prevalent in young women and rates are increasing dramatically in all countries. There is clear evidence from animal models that obesity is harmful to oocytes and has subsequent long-term effects and transgenerational consequences for offspring. Thus there is intense interest in delineating the effects of obesity on human oocytes and embryos in order to better understand how obesity leads to poorer pregnancy outcomes both in natural conceptions as well as following IVF, so that effective intervention strategies can be developed. In light of increasing rates of obesity in young women this information has great implications for subsequent generations.

References

1. Vahratian A. Prevalence of overweight and obesity among women of childbearing age: results from the 2002 National Survey of Family Growth. *Matern Child Health J* 2009; **13**(2): 268–73.
2. Wang YC, McPherson K, Marsh T, *et al.* Health and economic burden of the projected obesity trends in the USA and the UK. *Lancet* 2011; **378**(9793): 815–25.
3. Minge CE, Bennett BD, Norman RJ, *et al.* Peroxisome proliferator-activated receptor-gamma agonist rosiglitazone reverses the adverse effects of diet-induced obesity on oocyte quality. *Endocrinology* 2008; **149**(5): 2646–56.

4. Kwong WY, Wild AE, Roberts P, *et al.* Maternal undernutrition during the preimplantation period of rat development causes blastocyst abnormalities and programming of postnatal hypertension. *Development* 2000; **127**(19): 4195–202.
5. Lane M, Gardner DK. Differential regulation of mouse embryo development and viability by amino acids. *J Reprod Fertil* 1997; **109**(1): 153–64.
6. Williams CL, Teeling JL, Perry VH, *et al.* Mouse maternal systemic inflammation at the zygote stage causes blunted cytokine responsiveness in lipopolysaccharide-challenged adult offspring. *BMC Biol* 2011; **9**: 49.
7. Jungheim ES, Schoeller EL, Marquard KL, *et al.* Diet-induced obesity model: abnormal oocytes and persistent growth abnormalities in the offspring. *Endocrinology* 2010; **151**(8): 4039–46.
8. Wu LL, Dunning KR, Yang X, *et al.* High-fat diet causes lipotoxicity responses in cumulus-oocyte complexes and decreased fertilization rates. *Endocrinology* 2010; **151**(11): 5438–45.
9. Igosheva N, Abramov AY, Poston L, *et al.* Maternal diet-induced obesity alters mitochondrial activity and redox status in mouse oocytes and zygotes. *PLoS One* 2010; **5**(4): e10074.
10. Shankar K, Zhong Y, Kang P, *et al.* Maternal obesity promotes a proinflammatory signature in rat uterus and blastocyst. *Endocrinology* 2011; **152**(11): 4158–70.
11. Wang Q, Chi MM, Schedl T, *et al.* An intercellular pathway for glucose transport into mouse oocytes. *Am J Physiol Endocrinol Metab* 2012; **302**(12): E1511–18.
12. Purcell SH, Chi MM, Moley KH. Insulin-stimulated glucose uptake occurs in specialized cells within the cumulus oocyte complex. *Endocrinology* 2012; **153**(5): 2444–54.
13. Malhotra JD, Kaufman RJ. Endoplasmic reticulum stress and oxidative stress: a vicious cycle or a double-edged sword? *Antioxid Redox Signal* 2007; **9**(12): 2277–93.
14. Breckenridge DG, Germain M, Mathai JP, *et al.* Regulation of apoptosis by endoplasmic reticulum pathways. *Oncogene* 2003; **22**(53): 8608–18.
15. Serke H, Nowicki M, Kosacka J, *et al.* Leptin-deficient (ob/ob) mouse ovaries show fatty degeneration, enhanced apoptosis and decreased expression of steroidogenic acute regulatory enzyme. *Int J Obes (Lond)* 2012; **36**(8): 1047–53.
16. Garris DR. Ovarian follicular lipoapoptosis: structural, cytochemical and metabolic basis of reproductive tract atrophy following expression of the hypogonadal diabetes (db/db) syndrome. *Reprod Toxicol* 2005; **20**(1): 31–8.
17. Aardema H, Vos PL, Lolicato F, *et al.* Oleic acid prevents detrimental effects of saturated fatty acids on bovine oocyte developmental competence. *Biol Reprod* 2011; **85**(1): 62–9.
18. Leroy JL, Vanholder T, Mateusen B, *et al.* Non-esterified fatty acids in follicular fluid of dairy cows and their effect on developmental capacity of bovine oocytes in vitro. *Reproduction* 2005; **130**(4): 485–95.
19. Wu LL, Russell DL, Norman RJ, *et al.* Endoplasmic reticulum (ER) stress in cumulus-oocyte complexes impairs pentraxin-3 secretion, mitochondrial membrane potential (DeltaPsi m), and embryo development. *Mol Endocrinol* 2012; **26**(4): 562–73.
20. Jungheim ES, Macones GA, Odem RR, *et al.* Associations between free fatty acids, cumulus oocyte complex morphology and ovarian function during in vitro fertilization. *Fertil Steril* 2011; **95**(6): 1970–4.
21. Bender K, Walsh S, Evans AC, *et al.* Metabolite concentrations in follicular fluid may explain differences in fertility between heifers and lactating cows. *Reproduction* 2010; **139**(6): 1047–55.
22. van der Steeg JW, Steures P, Eijkemans MJ, *et al.* Obesity affects spontaneous pregnancy chances in subfertile, ovulatory women. *Hum Reprod* 2008; **23**(2): 324–8.
23. Gesink Law DC, Maclehose RF, Longnecker MP. Obesity and time to pregnancy. *Hum Reprod* 2007; **22**(2): 414–20.
24. Maheshwari A, Stofberg L, Bhattacharya S. Effect of overweight and obesity on assisted reproductive technology – a systematic review. *Hum Reprod Update* 2007; **13**(5): 433–44.
25. Rittenberg V, Seshadri S, Sunkara SK, *et al.* Effect of body mass index on IVF treatment outcome: an updated systematic review and meta-analysis. *Reprod Biomed Online* 2011; **23**(4): 421–39.
26. Robker RL. Evidence that obesity alters the quality of oocytes and embryos. *Pathophysiology* 2008; **15**(2): 115–21.
27. Wu LL, Norman RJ, Robker RL. The impact of obesity on oocytes: evidence for lipotoxicity mechanisms. *Reprod Fertil Dev* 2011; **24**(1): 29–34.
28. Wittemer C, Ohl J, Bailly M, *et al.* Does body mass index of infertile women have an impact on IVF procedure and outcome? *J Assist Reprod Genet* 2000; **17**(10): 547–52.
29. Carrell DT, Jones KP, Peterson CM, *et al.* Body mass index is inversely related to intrafollicular HCG concentrations, embryo quality and IVF outcome. *Reprod Biomed Online* 2001; **3**(2): 109–11.

30. Dokras A, Baredziak L, Blaine J, *et al.* Obstetric outcomes after in vitro fertilization in obese and morbidly obese women. *Obstet Gynecol* 2006; **108**(1): 61–9.

31. Shalom-Paz E, Marzal A, Wiser A, *et al.* Effects of different body mass indices on in vitro maturation in women with polycystic ovaries. *Fertil Steril* 2011; **96**(2): 336–9.

32. Marquard KL, Stephens SM, Jungheim ES, *et al.* Polycystic ovary syndrome and maternal obesity affect oocyte size in vitro fertilization/intracytoplasmic sperm injection cycles. *Fertil Steril* 2011; **95**(6): 2146–9, 2149.e1.

33. Depalo R, Garruti G, Totaro I, *et al.* Oocyte morphological abnormalities in overweight women undergoing in vitro fertilization cycles. *Gynecol Endocrinol* 2011; **27**(11): 880–4.

34. van Swieten EC, van der Leeuw-Harmsen L, Badings EA, *et al.* Obesity and clomiphene challenge test as predictors of outcome of in vitro fertilization and intracytoplasmic sperm injection. *Gynecol Obstet Invest* 2005; **59**(4): 220–4.

35. Metwally M, Cutting R, Tipton A, *et al.* Effect of increased body mass index on oocyte and embryo quality in IVF patients. *Reprod Biomed Online* 2007; **15**(5): 532–8.

36. Bellver J, Ayllon Y, Ferrando M, *et al.* Female obesity impairs in vitro fertilization outcome without affecting embryo quality. *Fertil Steril* 2010; **93**(2): 447–54.

37. Luke B, Brown MB, Stern JE, *et al.* Female obesity adversely affects assisted reproductive technology (ART) pregnancy and live birth rates. *Hum Reprod* 2011; **26**(1): 245–52.

38. Sneed ML, Uhler ML, Grotjan HE, *et al.* Body mass index: impact on IVF success appears age-related. *Hum Reprod* 2008; **23**(8): 1835–9.

39. Matalliotakis I, Cakmak H, Sakkas D, *et al.* Impact of body mass index on IVF and ICSI outcome: a retrospective study. *Reprod Biomed Online* 2008; **16**(6): 778–83.

40. Awartani KA, Nahas S, Al Hassan SH, *et al.* Infertility treatment outcome in sub groups of obese population. *Reprod Biol Endocrinol* 2009; **7**: 52.

41. Robker RL, Akison LK, Bennett BD, *et al.* Obese women exhibit differences in ovarian metabolites, hormones, and gene expression compared with moderate-weight women. *J Clin Endocrinol Metabol* 2009; **94**(5): 1533–40.

42. Hill MJ, Uyehara CF, Hashiro GM, *et al.* The utility of serum leptin and follicular fluid leptin, estradiol, and progesterone levels during an in vitro fertilization cycle. *J Assist Reprod Genet* 2007; **24**(5): 183–8.

43. Mantzoros CS, Cramer DW, Liberman RF, *et al.* Predictive value of serum and follicular fluid leptin concentrations during assisted reproductive cycles in normal women and in women with the polycystic ovarian syndrome. *Hum Reprod* 2000; **15**(3): 539–44.

44. Bausenwein J, Serke H, Eberle K, *et al.* Elevated levels of oxidized low-density lipoprotein and of catalase activity in follicular fluid of obese women. *Mol Hum Reprod* 2010; **16**(2): 117–24.

45. Vilser C, Hueller H, Nowicki M, *et al.* The variable expression of lectin-like oxidized low-density lipoprotein receptor (LOX-1) and signs of autophagy and apoptosis in freshly harvested human granulosa cells depend on gonadotropin dose, age, and body weight. *Fertil Steril* 2010; **93**(8): 2706–15.

46. Yang X, Wu LL, Chura LR, *et al.* Exposure to lipid-rich follicular fluid is associated with endoplasmic reticulum stress and impaired oocyte maturation in cumulus-oocyte complexes. *Fertil Steril* 2012; **97**(6): 1438–43.

47. Lewis CG, Warnes GM, Wang XJ, *et al.* Failure of body mass index or body weight to influence markedly the response to ovarian hyperstimulation in normal cycling women. *Fertil Steril* 1990; **53**(6): 1097–9.

48. Lashen H, Ledger W, Bernal AL, *et al.* Extremes of body mass do not adversely affect the outcome of superovulation and in vitro fertilization. *Hum Reprod* 1999; **14**(3): 712–15.

49. Fedorcsak P, Storeng R, Dale PO, *et al.* Obesity is a risk factor for early pregnancy loss after IVF or ICSI. *Acta Obstet Gynecol Scand* 2000; **79**(1): 43–8.

50. Salha O, Dada T, Sharma V. Influence of body mass index and self-administration of hCG on the outcome of IVF cycles: a prospective cohort study. *Hum Fertil (Camb)* 2001; **4**(1): 37–42.

51. Fedorcsak P, Dale PO, Storeng R, *et al.* Impact of overweight and underweight on assisted reproduction treatment. *Hum Reprod* 2004; **19**(11): 2523–8.

52. Dechaud H, Anahory T, Reyftmann L, *et al.* Obesity does not adversely affect results in patients who are undergoing in vitro fertilization and embryo transfer. *Eur J Obstet Gynecol Reprod Biol* 2006; **127**(1): 88–93.

53. Esinler I, Bozdag G, Yarali H. Impact of isolated obesity on ICSI outcome. *Reprod Biomed Online* 2008; **17**(4): 583–7.

54. Martinuzzi K, Ryan S, Luna M, *et al.* Elevated body mass index (BMI) does not adversely affect in vitro fertilization outcome in young women. *J Assist Reprod Genet* 2008; **25**(5): 169–75.

55. Orvieto R, Meltcer S, Nahum R, *et al.* The influence of body mass index on in vitro fertilization outcome. *Int J Gynaecol Obstet* 2009; **104**(1): 53–5.

56. Li Y, Yang D, Zhang Q. Impact of overweight and underweight on IVF treatment in Chinese women. *Gynecol Endocrinol* 2010; **26**(6): 416–22.

57. Zhang D, Zhu Y, Gao H, *et al.* Overweight and obesity negatively affect the outcomes of ovarian stimulation and in vitro fertilisation: a cohort study of 2628 Chinese women. *Gynecol Endocrinol* 2010; **26**(5): 325–32.

58. Hill MJ, Hong S, Frattarelli JL. Body mass index impacts in vitro fertilization stimulation. *ISRN Obstet Gynecol* 2011; **2011**: 929251.

59. Shah DK, Missmer SA, Berry KF, *et al.* Effect of obesity on oocyte and embryo quality in women undergoing in vitro fertilization. *Obstet Gynecol* 2011; **118**(1): 63–70.

60. Vilarino FL, Christofolini DM, Rodrigues D, *et al.* Body mass index and fertility: is there a correlation with human reproduction outcomes? *Gynecol Endocrinol* 2011; **27**(4): 232–6.

Section 5 Pathology

Chapter 32

Safety of ovarian stimulation

Dominic Stoop, Ellen Anckaert, and Johan Smitz

Introduction

Ovarian stimulation exposes the body to supraphysiological levels of steroid hormones. The most serious complication related to that stimulation is the ovarian hyperstimulation syndrome (OHSS) characterized by the shift of protein-rich fluid from the intravascular space to the third space, mainly the abdominal cavity. Two main clinical forms of OHSS, the early and the late, are distinguished by their time of onset and by the origin of the human chorionic gonadotropin (hCG) triggering that induces this complication. Early OHSS usually occurs within 9 days of oocyte retrieval in response to exogenous hCG, while endogenous hCG of early pregnancy or exogenous hCG for luteal phase support mainly causes the late OHSS.

According to the literature, the incidence of moderate cases of OHSS is about 5%, whereas in 2% (on average) of cycles hospitalization is required [1, 2]. Apart from the physical discomfort, the disorder constitutes a serious health risk and may even be fatal. Reports on maternal mortality rates from the Netherlands and the UK indicate an incidence of about 3 deaths per 100 000 cycles performed [3, 4]. In view of the rapid expansion of assisted reproductive treatments, the total number of maternal deaths related to OHSS may be far greater than initially expected [5]. In this chapter, we give an overview of the approaches available to limit or even completely prevent the occurrence of this complication.

This chapter further discusses long-term risks that might be associated with ovarian stimulation, such as the effect on ovarian functioning and potential oncological risks.

Table 32.1. Risk factors/predictive factors for OHSS

Risk factor	Threshold of risk
Primary risk factors (patient-related)	
High basal AMH	Cut-off level of 3.36 ng/ml has a sensitivity of 90.5% and specificity of 80% in predicting OHSS
High AFC	AFC >14 may predict hyper-response
Age	<33 years
Previous OHSS	Moderate or severe cases especially when hospitalization is required
PCOS characteristics	≥12 antral follicles 2–8 mm in diameter is predictive
Secondary risk factors (ovarian response-related)	
No. follicles on day of hCG	≥14 follicles diameter of 11 mm or >11 follicles with diameter of 10 mm
Absolute level or rate of increase of serum E_2	Poorly predictive for OHSS
VEGF levels	Not applicable
Elevated inhibin β levels	Elevated levels on day 5 of gonadotropin stimulation, at OPU and 3 days before OPU appear to correlate with development of OHSS

AFC, antral follicle count; AMH, anti-Müllerian hormone; E2, estradiol; OPU, oocyte pickup; PCOS, polycystic ovary syndrome; VEGF, vascular endothelial growth factor.
Adapted from Humaidan *et al.* [6].

Identification of risk factors

Risk factors for OHSS are either related to the patient characteristics (primary) or related to ovarian response (secondary) [6]. The latter type of risk factor becomes apparent during ovarian stimulation in patients with no known predisposing factors. Although these risk factors have a variable sensitivity and specificity, they may guide the clinician in the tailoring of the ovarian stimulation (Table 32.1).

Biology and Pathology of the Oocyte, 2nd edn., ed. Alan Trounson, Roger Gosden, and Ursula Eichenlaub-Ritter.
Published by Cambridge University Press.

1. Patient-related risk factors
   Careful ovarian stimulation is mandatory in women of young age, previous OHSS, and in the presence of polycystic ovary syndrome (PCOS). Ovarian reserve tests such as anti-Müllerian hormone (AMH) and the antral follicle count (AFC) are reported to be predictors of ovarian hyper-response and OHSS.
2. Ovarian response-related risk factors
   Papanikolaou *et al.* found that the number of follicles can discriminate the patients who are at risk for developing OHSS, whereas estradiol (E_2) concentrations are less reliable for the purpose of prediction [7]. According to this study, a threshold of $\geq$18 follicles and/or E_2 of $\geq$5000 ng/l yields a 83% sensitivity rate with a specificity as high as 84% for the severe OHSS cases. Other factors have been suggested to better identify women at risk, such as vascular endothelial growth factor (VEGF), inhibin β, or interleukins; their predictive value, however, remains to be determined.

Which types of ovarian stimulation are safer?

Use of gonadotropins

The role of FSH and LH in determining follicle number

In the natural cycle follicle-stimulating hormone (FSH) and luteinizing hormone (LH) complement each other and this cooperation leads to the process of follicle selection [8, 9]. As FSH concentrations decrease, by the feedback of estrogens to the hypothalamo-pituitary axis, the smaller follicles, which are not yet expressing an LH receptor on the granulosa, experience a shortage of cAMP. Those follicles which express an LH receptor survive as the concentrations of LH will increase and provide cAMP to the granulosa via LH receptor activation. It is this subtle balance between FSH and LH and the expression dynamics of the LH receptor on the granulosa of the growing follicle (larger than 10 mm in human) which plays a role in the survival of the group of early antral follicles recruited by the inter-cycle FSH rise.

The stimulated ovulatory cycle

In the early follicular phase the action of FSH induces LH receptor on granulosa cells. LH receptor is continuously present on theca cells of the small antral follicle and drives the androgen production in the follicle. When LH is present at high concentrations from the early follicular phase it will increase the thecal androgen production. In the presence of an increased androgen/estrogen ratio the follicle could become atretic [8, 10–12].

In the late follicular phase the FSH drive progressively suppresses the androgen receptor, hence providing an "escape" mechanism for the potential increase of androgen levels. FSH concentrations also decrease (by estrogen feedback), but nevertheless continue to stimulate estrogen production and the growth of the follicles. As soon as LH receptors are expressed on the granulosa cells (on follicles of >10 mm) the presence of LH will potentiate FSH's induction of aromatase induction, but as long as LH concentration remains low, the cAMP generation also remains low. It has been demonstrated by Yong *et al.* [10, 11] that the single second messenger cAMP can mediate different actions in granulosa cells, depending on its concentration. Low cAMP favors cell growth, while high levels of cAMP lead to inhibition of cell growth by arresting the proliferation of the granulosa cells. When LH concentrations become increased, these will lead to a high cAMP tonus.

LH is more efficient (than FSH) in increasing cAMP by binding to its receptor on the granulosa cells. When LH is present in high amounts: the increased cAMP levels will trigger the "high cAMP sensitive" genes. The mechanisms of LH being a possible disruptor of ongoing follicular growth during superovulation treatments were suggested from experiments in animal models: sheep and rat. Baird and Campbell suggested that the underlying mechanism for this effect was induced by androgen action in the follicle that ultimately causes growth arrest of the follicle [13]. The largest follicle(s), still lacking full aromatase activity, can cope with an increased androgen production, because their increased capacity is converted into estrogen. However, secondary follicles (i.e., the cohort following the "leading" follicles) have lower levels of aromatase activity, so that the androgens are instead reduced to dihydrotestosterone by 5α-reductase and this might hasten follicular atresia [10, 11].

Treatment of the World Health Organization (WHO) anovulation type I and II requires the use of exogenous gonadotropins, and such patients are prone to developing similar side-effects and complications with gonadotropin treatment. Depending on the chosen strategy to treat the anovulatory patient two practices are considered; in anovulatory patients the therapy aims to drive the growth of ovarian follicles and to obtain one or two large follicles, which are triggered to ovulate by a large hCG dose. However, in ovarian stimulation for in vitro fertilization (IVF) the aim is to recruit a larger group of follicles, so that many oocytes can be retrieved under ultrasound-guided control without the danger of multiple pregnancy, as supernumerary embryos can be cryopreserved.

The unwanted side-effect for ovulation induction is multiple pregnancy by multiple hCG-induced ovulations and clinical hyperstimulation syndrome (OHSS). The feared complication during ovarian stimulation in assisted reproduction is mainly hyperstimulation syndrome (OHSS), as the danger for multiple pregnancy is very much reduced, because of single embryo transfer.

Although Hillier, Lunenfeld, and Baird and Campbell pointed out in the early 1990s the potential use of LH for its tempering effect on progression of follicle growth, there was no way at that time to actually test the "ideal" experiments in the human to prove their concept, because recombinant LH (rLH) was not available [9, 13, 14]. Only purified urinary menotrophin preparations (hMGs) were on the market. Hence induction of ovulation at that time had LH (or hCG) molecules in combination with FSH present from the beginning of the stimulation protocols [15]. Nevertheless, Hillier, Baird and Campbell, and Lunenfeld had expressly stated that "once the pure FSH and LH would be available," the use of LH in high doses might bring a solution for the problem of multiple folliculogenesis in ovulation induction [9, 13, 14]. This concept was further explored clinically by Filicori, who emphasized the role of LH (via hCG administration) in ovarian stimulation [16].

Subsequent large prospective studies also found that stimulation for IVF had uniformly one or two oocytes less with highly purified hMG (HP-hMG), which besides highly purified urinary FSH also contains hCG and a small amount of LH, in comparison to recombinant FSH (rFSH) [17–21]. However, despite a decrease in the number of retrieved oocytes in IVF, the embryo quality as well as the endocrine parameters were improved, leading to an increase in live birth rates [22, 23]. The marginal (4– 5%) but significant superiority in those large clinical studies was also accompanied by a significantly lower number of clinical corrective actions for OHSS (i.e., use of albumin IV to avoid overt development of OHSS, reduction of FSH dosage, hospitalization for intravascular fluid control) when HP-hMG was used instead of rFSH [21]. Hence HP-hMG may be considered a safer alternative to pure FSH protocols for superovulation treatment for IVF [18, 19, 21] and in ovulation induction for PCOS [24]. Meta-analyses and Cochrane database results have also reported the superiority of hMG or HP-hMG protocols in IVF [25, 26].

The higher ongoing pregnancy rate and live birth rates suggest that increasing circulating LH/hCG levels during the stimulation phase are associated with improved pregnancy outcomes [19, 27]. However, determining the optimal dosage of hCG for controlled ovarian stimulation (COS) is a complex issue which may be influenced by inter-patient variations in liver and kidney metabolism.

The concept of LH ceiling

Hillier's experiments in animal models suggested that developing follicles have an upper limit regarding their requirement for LH [9]. Exceeding this "LH ceiling" might interfere with normal follicular maturation. The concept of an LH ceiling has been studied clinically in WHO II anovulatory women with doses of 225 or 450 IU rLH [28]. However, as only a few patients were included in the pilot trial, the results cannot be considered robust.

In a later study, the question of LH ceiling dose was re-addressed by Hugues *et al.* on a larger group of patients. Hugues assessed the minimal effective dose required to induce atresia of secondary follicles in WHO II anovulatory patients being stimulated for artificial insemination, while supporting the growth of a dominant follicle to a preovulatory stage [29]. These data suggested that 30 μg rLH was the most appropriate dose for follicle reduction, without inducing a premature luteinization. A dose of 60 μg rLH consistently increased progesterone and decreased pregnancy outcomes. Calculating that 30 μg rLH is equivalent to 660 IU of LH bioactivity, such a high dose can only be reached theoretically by administration of more than eight ampoules of hMG (containing 75 IU of FSH/amp). Administration of more than eight ampoules (75 IU of FSH/amp) is an unrealistically high dose to be used in IVF protocols [30]. Alternatively, combinations of rFSH and rLH or rhCG could be prepared for clinical use.

A pilot study in IVF patients addressing the question of the ceiling effect by hCG was first published by Thuesen *et al.* [31]. Daily doses of 100 IU and 150 IU of hCG had a trend to reduce the number of small and medium follicles, while sustaining the growth of the large follicles, without any obvious negative effect on ongoing pregnancy rates. With a dose of 150 IU of hCG, a slight but significant increase in the plasma progesterone concentration was observed in association with a leveling off of E_2 concentrations. However, even with the high dose of 150 IU/day of hCG, the progesterone value remained lower than the currently accepted alarm value (1.3 ng/ml or 4 nmol/l) [31].

In conclusion, endogenous serum LH concentrations during ovarian stimulation treatment were not predictive of live birth in anovulatory WHO group II patients undergoing ovulation induction with rFSH or HP-hMG. On the other hand, the exogenous hCG activity in HP-hMG stimulation was positively associated with treatment outcome. The ceiling level, defined as a level of LH bioactivity causing detrimental effects on stimulation, could only be eventually reached when extremely high doses of gonadotropins are injected (more than eight ampoules of 75 IU/day). The consistent presence of LH bioactivity in highly purified hMG (mainly under the bioactive form of hCG) reduced the explosive responses in patients with a normal follicular reserve.

The most recent clinical recommendations are that in patients with a high serum AMH concentration the use of either HP-hMG preparations or combined rLH/rhCG-rFSH protocols from day 1 of stimulation is a safer option than using an FSH-alone regimen. The preliminary value of basal serum AMH or the basal follicle count is important to decide the starting dose of FSH or hMG therapy [32, 33].

Long-acting corifollitropin alfa

This is a recombinant fusion protein that is able to initiate and sustain follicular growth for 1 week so that a single injection can replace the first seven daily injections of FSH/hMG. It has been demonstrated that repeated ovarian stimulation with this fusion protein does not raise concerns about immunogenicity [34]. In view of its equivalence and safety profile, corifollitropin alfa in combination with daily gonadotropin-releasing hormone (GnRH) antagonist seems to be an alternative to daily rFSH injections in normal responding patients [35]. The incidence of OHSS in corifollitropin alfa-stimulated cycles appears to be comparable to that in rFSH-stimulated cycles. However, a meta-analysis by Mahmoud Youssef *et al.* found that a significantly higher number of cycles were cancelled due to overstimulation in corifollitropin alfa cycles as compared to controls, with all studies only including expected normally responding patients [35].

GnRH analogs

Two meta-analyses have demonstrated that GnRH antagonist protocols are associated with a lower incidence of OHSS [36, 37]. A Cochrane review not only found a significant reduction in OHSS (relative risk [RR], 0.61; 95% confidence interval [CI] 0.42–0.89; P = 0.01) but also found a higher incidence of coasting and cycle cancellations in GnRH agonist cycles [36]. The second meta-analysis noted a significant reduction of OHSS-related hospital admissions in GnRH antagonist protocols (odds ratio [OR], 0.46; 95% CI 0.26–0.93; P = 0.01) [37].

Modification of final triggering of oocyte maturation

Although a GnRH antagonist can reduce the risk of OHSS, early OHSS cannot be excluded as long as hCG is being used for the final oocyte maturation. A randomized study comparing triggering with either 5000 IU or 10 000 IU of hCG demonstrated that both appear effective as far as the oocyte recovery is concerned, but both doses can result in severe OHSS [38].

A GnRH agonist can effectively induce final oocyte maturation in GnRH antagonist protocols, replacing the need for hCG. The elimination of hCG appears to prevent entirely the occurrence of OHSS [39]. The short half-life of LH compared to hCG in combination with pituitary desensitization results in rapid, complete, and irreversible luteolysis [40]. This approach can completely prevent OHSS after an ovarian stimulation in GnRH antagonist protocols [5].

However, several randomized trials found disappointing clinical outcomes in GnRH agonist-triggered cycles [41, 42]. Humaidan *et al.* described a reduction in clinical pregnancy rate from 36% to 6% in a group of 122 normogonadotropic patients [41]. Another randomized trial by Kolibianakis *et al.* had to be discontinued because of the dramatic difference in ongoing pregnancy rate in the GnRH agonist arm [42]. Both authors hypothesized that this poor outcome was caused by a luteal phase insufficiency induced by GnRH agonist trigger, which cannot be overcome with conventional luteal support regimens. The GnRH agonist trigger significantly reduces the circulating LH levels owing to a difference in profile and duration of the surge elicited by the GnRH agonist. As the idea of an "OHSS-free" ovarian stimulation remains appealing, several approaches have been suggested to overcome the limitation of reduced implantation.

Agonist triggering and enhanced luteal support (ELS)

An intensive luteal phase supplementation strategy has been suggested because the use of a standard luteal phase support after a GnRH agonist trigger is inadequate. Engmann *et al.* studied a modified luteal support using a combination of 50 mg intramuscular (IM) progesterone (P_4) daily and 0.3 mg transdermal E_2 patches on alternate days, starting the day after oocyte retrieval and continued until 10 weeks of gestation [43]. Serum E_2 and P_4 levels were monitored on days 3 and 7 after oocyte retrieval and then weekly, until 10 weeks of gestation. The IM P_4 dose was increased to 75 mg daily, if required, to maintain serum P_4 >20 pg/ml, and the dose of transdermal E_2 patches was increased to a maximum of 0.4 mg with oral micronized E_2 added, if necessary, to maintain serum E_2 >200 pg/ml. This randomized controlled trial, performed in high-risk patients, found no difference in ongoing pregnancy rates compared to conventional hCG triggering (16/30 [53.3%] vs. 14/29 [48.3%]). Although the ELS approach appears to result in excellent clinical results, a more recent study suggests that these clinical outcomes are related to cycle characteristics [39]. Kummer *et al.* found that the implantation rate (34.4 vs. 25.3; P = 0.02) and clinical pregnancy rate (53.6 vs. 38.1%; P = 0.02) were significantly higher in patients with peak E_2 levels ≥ 4000 pg/ml.

Agonist triggering and low dose hCG (dual trigger)

A pilot study performed by Humaidan *et al.* found that the administration of a single bolus of low dose hCG (1500 IU) immediately after oocyte retrieval could normalize the pregnancy rates after GnRH agonist triggering in normal-responding women [44]. These excellent implantation rates were later confirmed in high-risk patients; however, one patient developed a moderate late-onset OHSS [45]. A large randomized controlled trial comparing hCG trigger with a GnRH agonist + 1500 IU hCG trigger did not find a significant difference in live birth rates (31% and 24% respectively) [46]. No OHSS case was observed in the GnRH agonist group as compared to 2% in the hCG-triggered group.

The combination of GnRH agonist trigger with a low dose hCG injection can also be performed on the same day, as a "dual trigger," as opposed to administering the hCG on the day of oocyte retrieval [47]. A retrospective comparison of three GnRH antagonist protocols, with either an agonist trigger alone, a dual trigger, or the previously described enhanced luteal support, found that both latter approaches resulted in a better clinical outcome [47]. In this study, the dual trigger approach, however, did not entirely prevent OHSS. Based on the available literature, we can conclude that the GnRH agonist trigger with low dose hCG approach eliminates the severe early-onset OHSS and reduces the risk of a late-onset OHSS [48].

Agonist triggering and freeze-all approach (segmentation)

The introduction of the oocyte and embryo vitrification technique (see Chapter 36) has produced a revolution in artificial reproductive technologies (ARTs) because of the excellent survival and implantation rates after oocyte and embryo cryopreservation. Cryopreservation gained importance with the evolution of single embryo transfer (SET) to prevent multiple gestation. A "freeze-all" approach (all embryos developing from an ovarian stimulation cycle) may now become the next obvious step to minimize the complications of OHSS. This complete separation of the timing of ovarian stimulation and embryo transfer, the so-called segmentation model, is the only approach that completely eliminates the risks of early-onset and late-onset OHSS [5, 49].

Freeze all embryos (embryo segmentation)

The vitrification technique enables the efficient cryopreservation of all stages of embryos [50]. Several embryo segmentation studies have been performed at different stages of embryo development. Shapiro *et al.* performed randomized trials evaluating a freeze-all approach at the blastocyst stage and in normal and in high responders [51, 52]. The authors demonstrate that the freeze-all approach can effectively increase the treatment outcome by circumventing the possible impaired endometrial receptivity after ovarian stimulation.

Freeze all oocytes (oocyte segmentation)

Recent studies have demonstrated a retention of viability of vitrified oocytes compared to controls in terms of their rates of fertilization, embryo development, and ongoing pregnancy rate [53, 54].

Alternatively, ovulation triggering could also be performed by the administration of rLH that would mimic the natural LH surge. However, reduced pregnancy rates and a poor cost/benefit ratio make this option less applicable in daily practice.

Case reports by Martinez *et al.* indicate that in patients undergoing IVF with a long protocol at high risk for severe OHSS the cycle can still be rescued by withdrawing the agonist and replacing it with an antagonist. This conversion allows the triggering by a GnRH agonist, leading to a reduction of the risk for OHSS [55].

Specific treatment modalities

Oocyte donation

Oocyte donation has become an increasingly used fertility treatment. The safety of ovarian stimulation is of paramount importance as the treatment relies on treating young healthy women with superovulatory doses of gonadotropins. The use of GnRH agonist triggering in a GnRH-antagonist protocol in combination with the absence of a possible pregnancy eliminates the risk of OHSS [5].

Caution to prevent excessive ovarian response is still mandatory as ovarian torsion may still complicate ovarian stimulation. Although the AMH level is associated with the number of oocytes retrieved, it appears to have a modest ability in discriminating women with low or excessive ovarian response [56].

In contrast to the well-known medical risks and burdens related to donation, data on the effect of ovarian stimulation on the future reproductive health of oocyte donors are scarce. A study by Stoop *et al.* found a low incidence of need for fertility treatment in past donors (5.0%). The cross-sectional survey concluded that the short-term reproductive health of donors does not seem to be affected by previous ovarian stimulations and oocyte retrievals [57].

In vitro maturation (IVM)

IVM is an artificial reproductive technology where oocytes are collected from antral follicles, typically from unstimulated or minimally stimulated ovaries, and collected, matured, and fertilized in vitro (see Chapter 18). Apart from the patient friendliness, this approach eliminates all the complications related to ovarian stimulation.

Low estrogen stimulation

In the last decade, an increasing focus in the field of reproductive medicine has been the preservation of fertility for patients facing potential sterility as a consequence of cancer treatment. In women with an estrogen-sensitive tumor, the elevation of circulating E_2 levels during conventional ovulation stimulation with gonadotropins may be undesirable. Alternative protocols have been suggested such as natural cycle IVF, aromatase inhibitors, or selective estrogen receptor modulators (SERMs) [58].

Prepubertal stimulation

Pediatric female patients with cancer typically undergo ovarian tissue cryopreservation, while adults preferentially undergo ovarian stimulation with oocyte or embryo cryopreservation. Reichman *et al.* did, however, perform a successful ovarian stimulation allowing the cryopreservation of 18 mature oocytes in a 13-year-old premenarcheal girl [59]. Because the efficiency of GnRH agonist triggering has not been assessed in premenarcheal girls who have an immature hypothalamic–pituitary–gonadal axis, reduced-dose hCG triggering could be considered as a safe alternative.

Long-term risks

Ovarian reserve

It is believed that repeated ovarian stimulation is unlikely to reduce significantly the ovarian pool of primordial follicles given that these follicles do not express FSH receptors. The short-term effects of repetitive oocyte donation were assessed in 284 oocyte donors who had at least two repetitive cycles of donation [60]. No significant difference was observed in the numbers of retrieved oocytes up to nine consecutive cycles of superovulation in the same donor. The study also found that the pregnancy rate in the oocyte recipients was maintained throughout the consecutive cycles. A retrospective cohort analysis by Bukulmez *et al.*, did not find a decrease in serum AMH levels over repetitive oocyte donation cycles, which may imply that accelerated ovarian aging may not occur after ovarian stimulation [61].

Oncological risks

The risk of cancer among infertile women has been repeatedly studied for many cancer types, with inconsistent and sometimes contradictory results. Most of these studies focused on hormonal-related gynecological and breast cancers. A large Dutch cohort study by van Leeuwen *et al.* concluded that ovarian stimulation for IVF may increase the risk of ovarian malignancies, especially borderline ovarian tumors [62]. In line with some small case reports, the authors noted a particularly strong elevation in the first year after IVF. Since the induction period of ovarian cancer with respect to established risk factors amounts to 25 years or more, much longer follow-up is needed to fully evaluate the effects of gonadotropins [62]. A second large study was performed by linking the Finnish Cancer Registry to a cohort of women who purchased drugs for IVF and their age- and residence-matched controls [63]. The authors did not find a general cancer risk increase or an increase of hormonal-related cancers by IVF (Table 32.2). A significantly lower incidence of cervical cancer (OR: 0.51, 95% CI: 0.30–0.85) was found in IVF women, but women that have undergone IVF had more skin cancers other than melanoma (OR: 3.11, 95% CI: 1.02–9.6).

The authors of both studies conclude that future studies need to include treatment characteristics such as the different medications used and their dosage [62, 63]. Studies that analyze infertile women as one group cannot reliably determine risk as conditions causing impaired fertility have different risk potential for a given cancer.

Table 32.2. Cancer cases among IVF women and controls (matched for age and residence)

	IVF women (n = 9175)	Control women (n = 9175)	OR (CI)
Any cancer	178	193	1.01 (0.80–1.27)
Breast cancer	55	60	0.93 (0.62–1.40)
Invasive ovarian cancer	9	3	2.57 (0.69–9.63)
Borderline tumors of the ovary	4	4	1.68 (0.31–9.27)
Cervical cancer	34	67	0.51 (0.30–0.85)
Uterine cancer	4	2	2.0 (0.37–10.9)[a]
Pulmonary cancer	0	5	NC[b]
Thyroid cancer	10	8	1.27 (0.31–5.2)
Melanoma	12	9	1.27 (0.34–4.8)
Other skin cancer	24	10	3.11 (1.02–9.6)[c]
Tumors in central nervous system	9	7	9.4 (0.56–159.5)
Gastrointestinal tract tumors	12	10	1.88 (0.52–6.8)
Leukemia or lymphoma	4	5	0.34 (0.04–3.06)

[a] Crude OR due to small case number
[b] Non-calculable
[c] Statistically significant ($P < 0.05$)
Adapted from Yil-Kuha *et al.* [63].

Epigenetic safety

There is concern that ovarian stimulation might interfere at the epigenetic level and, in particular, with genomic imprinting. Imprinted genes are differently marked by epigenetic modifications such as DNA methylation in the parental alleles so that only one of the alleles is expressed [64, 65]. A balanced uniparental expression of imprinted genes is important for development, growth, and neurobehavior and these genes are involved in human syndromes such as Beckwith–Wiedemann syndrome (BWS) and in cancer [66].

Erasure of previous somatic imprints occurs in primordial germ cells when the bulk of DNA is demethylated [67], allowing imprints to be reset during gametogenesis in a sex-specific manner. For most of the imprinted genes, DNA methylation at imprinting control centers (ICRs) is acquired at the maternal allele during oocyte growth after the transition from primordial to antral follicle stages [68–70].

To allow full-term development, imprints should not only be accurately established during gametogenesis, but also correctly maintained in the presence of genome-wide DNA de- and remethylation waves after fertilization. Several oocyte-expressed genes, such as *Dnmt1o*, *Zfp57*, *Stella*, and *Mbd3* are known to be required for this imprinting maintenance [71–74]. Consequently, it might be anticipated that ovarian stimulation could interfere with the establishment and/or maintenance of imprinting.

ART-related studies on imprinting in the human

Several studies have suggested a possible link between ART and rare imprinting syndromes such as BWS [75], although other studies did not find any association [76, 77]. Nearly all of the BWS cases were associated with a loss of DNA methylation at the maternally methylated *KvDMR1*, while this epigenetic abnormality is found in only half of sporadic BWS patients [78, 79], suggesting that epigenetic mechanisms might be affected in ART.

Moreover, an array-based study in 10 ART children suggested more widespread epigenetic alterations involving also non-imprinted genes implicated in chronic metabolic disorders such as type II diabetes and obesity [80]. As an array of techniques are used, such as IVF and embryo culture (which have been associated with aberrant imprinting in animal models) [81], and there are other confounding factors such as infertility (also associated with aberrant imprinting [77, 81]), no really useful conclusions can be drawn on the effect of ovarian stimulation from the studies in ART children cited above.

Only a few studies are available on the establishment of imprinting in human oocytes obtained from ART cycles. Sato *et al.* found abnormal DNA methylation at the maternally methylated *MEST* and the paternally methylated *H19* genes in immature oocytes retrieved after ovarian stimulation [82]. However, the underlying infertility or advanced maternal age might have contributed to the abnormal findings. Another confounding factor is that (low quality) oocytes that failed to mature after ovarian stimulation were used in the studies [82]. In contrast, Borghol *et al.* described normal DNA methylation at *H19* differentially methylated regions (DMR) in five immature human oocytes retrieved after ovarian stimulation [83]. A third study found that in vitro matured oocytes from natural cycle PCOS patients displayed a slightly (6%) higher methylation at *KvDMR1* compared to in vitro matured oocytes from stimulated cycles, suggesting that ovarian stimulation might interfere with imprinting establishment at *KvDMR1*, at least for oocytes that failed to mature after ovarian stimulation and were subsequently in vitro matured [84].

Ovarian stimulation for related studies in the mouse model

Global DNA methylation patterns of 2-cell mouse embryos differed between stimulated and non-stimulated females and were associated with reduced preimplantation development in vitro [85]. However, studies on the effect of ovarian stimulation on establishment of imprinting in mouse oocytes have shown conflicting results. Sato *et al.* described aberrant hypermethylation at *H19* in equine (e)CG/hCG stimulated BDF and ICR mouse metaphase II (MII) oocytes, while *Mest*, *Lit1*, and *Zac* were unaffected [82]. But a recent study found normal imprinting for *H19* and maternally imprinted genes (*Snrpn*, *Peg3*) in MII oocytes from stimulated B6(CAST7p6)x B6 mice (6.5 or 10 IU of eCG/hCG [86]). Likewise, unaltered DNA methylation was described at *H19*, *Snprn*, and *Igf2r* in 2-cell embryos derived from stimulated mice [87].

The contrasting findings between these studies might be due to the fact that sequential doses were used in Sato's study, or to the fact that different mouse strains were used [82]. Alternatively, a bias due to cumulus cell contamination in the oocyte samples from Sato's study should be considered as only the latter two studies applied elegant measures to exclude this bias. Finally, an in vitro follicle culture system in the mouse showed that supraphysiological doses of rFSH had no effects on DNA methylation at *Snrpn*, *Igf2r*, and *H19* in MII oocytes [88], confirming two of the in vivo studies cited above [86, 87].

Although the majority of mouse studies found no effects on imprinting establishment, more concern has been raised about the possible effects of ovarian stimulation on imprinting maintenance during preimplantation development.

It has been shown that ovarian stimulation leads to a higher proportion of mouse blastocysts without detectable *H19* expression compared to controls [89] and to aberrant biallelic expression of *Snrpn* and *H19* in placentas [90]. In a recent study, ovarian stimulation resulted in a dose-dependent loss of methylation at the maternally methylated *Snrpn*, *Peg3*, and *Kcnq1ot1* loci; and a dose-dependent gain at the paternally methylated *H19* in mouse blastocysts [91]. For *Snrpn*, abnormalities in blastocysts were occurring at a rate as high as 4 in 10 blastocysts for the low dose (6.25 IU) and 9/10 for the high (10 IU) eCG/hCG dose. Finally, abnormal methylation was reported for

H19 or *Peg3* (but not for *Snrpn*) in liver and brain tissue in three out of eight mice derived from stimulated oocytes [92].

Collectively, studies in the mouse suggest that ovarian stimulation might interfere with the capacity of oocytes to maintain imprinting during preimplantation development. Although future studies are necessary to unravel the exact mechanisms, it might be that ovarian stimulation interferes with oocyte-expressed genes, such as *Dnmt1o*, that are required for imprinting maintenance after fertilization.

Of further concern are possible transgenerational epigenetic effects because it has been suggested that ovarian stimulation in mice results in altered methylation levels at *H19*, *Mest*, and *Snrpn* in sperm of first and second generation male offspring [93].

Conclusion on effects of stimulation on imprinting

The studies in the human do not allow the drawing of conclusions on the epigenetic safety of ovarian stimulation due to a number of confounding factors described. However, studies in mice suggest that ovarian stimulation might interfere with the maintenance of imprinting after fertilization. Clearly, more studies in animal models and well-designed studies in humans will be needed to assess the epigenetic safety of ovarian stimulation and to select those stimulation protocols with minimal epigenetic risk.

General conclusion

OHSS is a severe iatrogenic complication related to an excessive ovarian response to hormonal stimulation. Although the condition is often difficult to predict, early OHSS and even late OHSS are entirely preventable. GnRH agonist triggering in a GnRH antagonist protocol removes the exogenous hCG necessary to induce early OHSS. A "freeze-all" protocol allows the introduction of the segmentation of ART, which can rule out the risk of a late OHSS. Alternatively, implantation chances appear to be successfully safeguarded by modifying the luteal support or by the addition of low dose hCG at the time of GnRH agonist trigger (dual trigger) or at the time of oocyte retrieval.

In patients with PCO and PCOS the risk for OHSS can be predicted by hormonal measurements and ovarian ultrasound. A new promising technique avoiding ovarian stimulation is IVM of oocytes (see Chapter 18), which totally avoids OHSS. Further studies on follow-up of patients after ovarian stimulation are needed to exclude with high confidence the potential for cancer and rare imprinting syndromes.

References

1. Papanikolaou EG, Tournaye H, Verpoest W, *et al.* Early and late ovarian hyperstimulation syndrome: early pregnancy outcome and profile. *Hum Reprod* 2005; **20**: 636–41.
2. Delvigne A. Symposium: Update on prediction and management of OHSS. Epidemiology of OHSS. *Reprod Biomed Online* 2009; **19**: 8–13.
3. Lyons G. Saving mothers' lives: confidential enquiry into maternal and child health 2003–5. *Int J Obstet Anesth* 2008; **17**: 103–5.
4. Braat DDM, Schutte JM, Bernardus RE, *et al.* Maternal death related to IVF in the Netherlands 1984–2008. *Hum Reprod* 2010; **25**: 1782–6.
5. Devroey P, Polyzos NP, Blockeel C. An OHSS-free clinic by segmentation of IVF treatment. *Hum Reprod* 2011; **26**: 2593–7.
6. Humaidan P, Quartarolo J, Papanikolaou EG. Preventing ovarian hyperstimulation syndrome: guidance for the clinician. *Fertil Steril* 2010; **94**: 389–400.
7. Papanikolaou EG, Pozzobon C, Kolibianakis EM, *et al.* Incidence and prediction of ovarian hyperstimulation syndrome in women undergoing gonadotropin-releasing hormone antagonist in vitro fertilization cycles. *Fertil Steril* 2006; **85**: 112–20.
8. Hillier SG. Ovarian manipulation with pure gonadotrophins. *J Clin Endocrinol* 1990; **127**: 1–4.
9. Hillier SG. Ovarian stimulation with recombinant gonadotrophins: LH as an adjunct to FSH. In: Jacobs HS, ed. *The New Frontier in Ovulation Induction* Carnforth, UK: Parthenon. 1993; 39–47.
10. Yong EL, Baird DT, Yates R, *et al.* Hormonal regulation of the growth and steroidogenic function of human granulosa cells. *J Clin Endocrinol Metab* 1992; **74**: 842–9.
11. Yong ET, Baird DT, Hillier SG. Mediation of gonadotrophin-stimulated growth and differentiation of human granulosa cells by adenosine-3′,5′-monophosphate: one molecule, two messages. *Clin Endocrinol* 1992; **37**: 51–8.
12. Andersen CY, Ziebe S. Serum levels of free androstenedione, testosterone and oestradiol are lower in the follicular phase of conceptional than of non-conceptional cycles after ovarian stimulation with a gonadotrophin-releasing hormone agonist protocol. *Hum Reprod* 1992; **7**: 1365–70.
13. Baird DT, Campbell BK. Supplementation with recombinant LH to reduce multiple folliculogenesis

and ovarian hyperstimulation. In: Filicori M, Flamigni C, eds. *Ovulation Induction Update 1998,* The Proceedings of the 2nd World Conference on Ovulation Induction, Bologna, Italy, 12–13 September 1997. Canforth, Lancs, UK: The Parthenon Publishing Group. 1998; 159–64.

14. Lunenfeld B. Stimulations de l'ovulation: une nouvelle approche basée sur desdonnées physiologiques et cliniques récentes. Perspectives d'avenir.*Contraception, Fertilité, Sexualité* 1993; **2** (Suppl. 4): 1–7.
15. Stokman PG, de Leeuw R, van den Wijngaard HA, *et al.* Human chorionic gonadotropin in commercial human menopausal gonadotropin preparations. *Fertil Steril* 1993; **60**: 175–8.
16. Filicori M, Cognigni GE, Tabarelli C, *et al.* Stimulation and growth of antral ovarian follicles by selective LH activity administration in women. *J Clin Endocrinol Metab* 2002; **87**: 1156–61.
17. Wolfenson C, Groisman J, Couto AS, *et al.* Batch-to-batch consistency of human-derived gonadotrophin preparations compared with recombinant preparations. *Reprod Biomed Online* 2005; **10**: 442–54.
18. Andersen AN, Devroey P, Arce JC. Clinical outcome following stimulation with highly purified hMG or recombinant FSH in patients undergoing IVF: arandomized assessor-blind controlled trial. *Hum Reprod* 2006; **21**: 3217–27.
19. Smitz J, Andersen AN, Devroey P, *et al.* Endocrine profile in serum and follicular fluid differs after ovarian stimulation with HP-hMG or recombinant FSH in IVF patients. *Hum Reprod* 2007; **22**: 676–87.
20. Platteau P, Nyboe Andersen A, Loft A, *et al.* Highly purified HMG versus recombinant FSH for ovarian stimulation in IVF cycles. *Reprod Biomed Online* 2008; **17**: 190–8.
21. Devroey P, Pellicer A, Nyboe AA, *et al.* A randomized assessor-blind trial comparing highly purified hMG and recombinant FSH in a GnRH antagonist cycle with compulsory single-blastocyst transfer. *Fertil Steril* 2012; **97**: 561–71.
22. Platteau P, Smitz J, Albano C, *et al.* Exogenous luteinizing hormone activity may influence the treatment outcome in in vitro fertilization but not in intracytoplasmic sperm injection cycles. *Fertil Steril* 2004; **81**: 1401–4.
23. Ziebe S, Lundin K, Janssens R, *et al.* Influence of ovarian stimulation with HP-hMG or recombinant FSH on embryo quality parameters in patients undergoing IVF. *Hum Reprod* 2007; **22**: 2404–13.
24. Platteau P, Nyboe Andersen A, Balen A, *et al.* Similar ovulation rates, but different follicular development with highly purified menotrophin compared with recombinant FSH in WHO Group II anovulatory infertility: a randomized controlled study. *Hum Reprod* 2006; **21**: 1798–804.
25. van Wely M, Kwan I, van der Veen F, *et al.* Recombinant FSH versus urinary gonadotrophins for ovarian hyperstimulation in IVF or ICSI cycles. A systematic review and meta-analysis. *Hum Reprod* 2009; Suppl 1: i134.
26. van Wely M, Kwan I, Burt AL, *et al.* Recombinant versus urinary gonadotrophin for ovarian stimulation in assisted reproductive technology cycles. *Cochrane Database Syst Rev* 2011; **2**: CD005354.
27. Arce JC, Smitz J. Exogenous hCG activity, but not endogenous LH activity, is positively associated with live birth rates in anovulatory infertility. *Hum Fertil (Camb)* 2011; **14**: 192–9.
28. Loumaye E, Engrand P, Shoham Z, *et al.* Clinical evidence for an LH 'ceiling' effect induced by administration of recombinant human LH during the late follicular phase of stimulated cycles in World Health Organization type I and type II anovulation. *Hum Reprod* 2003; **18**: 314–22.
29. Hugues JN, Soussis J, Calderon I, *et al.* Does the addition of recombinant LH inWHO group II anovulatory women over-responding to FSH treatment reduce the number of developing follicles? A dose-finding study. *Hum Reprod* 2005; **20**: 629–35.
30. Land JA, Yarmolinskaya MI, Dumoulin JC, *et al.* High-dose human menopausal gonadotropin stimulation in poor responders does not improve in vitro fertilization outcome. *Fertil Steril* 1996; **65**: 961–5.
31. Thuesen LL, Loft A, Egeberg AN, *et al.* A randomized controlled dose-response pilot study of addition of hCG to recombinant FSH during controlled ovarian stimulation for in vitro fertilization. *Hum Reprod* 2012 **27**: 3074–84.
32. Nelson SM, Yates RW, Lyall H, *et al.* Anti-Müllerian hormone-based approach to controlled ovarian stimulation for assisted conception. *Hum Reprod* 2009 **24**: 867–75.
33. Anckaert E, Smitz J, Schiettecatte J, *et al.* The value of anti-Mullerian hormone measurement in the long GnRH agonist protocol: association with ovarian response and gonadotrophin-dose adjustments. *Hum Reprod* 2012; **27**: 1829–39.
34. Norman RJ, Zegers-Hochschild F, Salle BS, *et al.* Repeated ovarian stimulation with corifollitropin alfa in patients in a GnRH antagonist protocol: no concern for immunogenicity. *Hum Reprod* 2011; **26**: 2200–8.
35. Mahmoud Youssef MA, van Wely M, Aboulfoutouh I, *et al.* Is there a place for corifollitropin alfa in IVF/ICSI

cycles? A systematic review and meta-analysis. *Fertil Steril* 2012; **97**: 876–85.

36. Al-Inany HG, Abou-Setta AM, Aboulghar M. Gonadotrophin-releasing hormone antagonists for assisted conception. *Cochrane Database Syst Rev* 2006; **3**: CD001750.

37. Kolibianakis EM, Collins J, Tarlatzis BC, *et al.* Among patients treated for IVF with gonadotrophins and GnRH analogues, is the probability of live birth dependent on the type of analogue used? A systematic review and meta-analysis. *Hum Reprod Update* 2006; **12**: 651–71.

38. Kolibianakis EM, Papanikolaou EG, Tournaye H, *et al.* Triggering final oocyte maturation using different doses of human chorionic gonadotropin: a randomized pilot study in patients with polycystic ovary syndrome treated with gonadotropin-releasing hormone antagonists and recombinant follicle-stimulating hormone. *Fertil Steril* 2007; **88**: 1382–8.

39. Kummer N, Benadiva C, Feinn R, *et al.* Factors that predict the probability of a successful clinical outcome after induction of oocyte maturation with a gonadotropin-releasing hormone agonist. *Fertil Steril* 2011; **96**: 63–8.

40. Kol S. Luteolysis induced by a gonadotropin-releasing hormone agonist is the key to prevention of ovarian hyperstimulation syndrome. *Fertil Steril* 2004; **81**: 1–5.

41. Humaidan P, Bredkjaer HE, Bungum L, *et al.* GnRH agonist (buserelin) or hCG for ovulation induction in GnRH antagonist IVF/ICSI cycles: a prospective randomized study. *Hum Reprod* 2005; **20**: 1213–20.

42. Kolibianakis EM, Schultze-Mosgau A, Schroer A, *et al.* A lower ongoing pregnancy rate can be expected when GnRH agonist is used for triggering final oocyte maturation instead of HCG in patients undergoing IVF with GnRH antagonists. *Hum Reprod* 2005; **20**: 2887–92.

43. Engmann L, DiLuigi A, Schmidt D, *et al.* The use of gonadotropin-releasing hormone (GnRH) agonist to induce oocyte maturation after cotreatment with GnRH antagonist in high-risk patients undergoing in vitro fertilization prevents the risk of ovarian hyperstimulation syndrome: a prospective randomized controlled study. *Fertil Steril* 2008; **89**: 84–91.

44. Humaidan P, Bungum L, Bungum M, *et al.* Rescue of corpus luteum function with peri-ovulatory HCG supplementation in IVF/ICSI GnRH antagonist cycles in which ovulation was triggered with a GnRH agonist: a pilot study. *Reprod Biomed Online* 2006; **13**: 173–8.

45. Humaidan P. Luteal phase rescue in high-risk OHSS patients by GnRHa triggering in combination with low-dose HCG: a pilot study. *Reprod Biomed Online* 2009; **18**: 630–4.

46. Humaidan P, Ejdrup Bredkjaer H, Westergaard LG, *et al.* 1,500 IU human chorionic gonadotropin administered at oocyte retrieval rescues the luteal phase when gonadotropin-releasing hormone agonist is used for ovulation induction: a prospective, randomized, controlled study. *Fertil Steril* 2010; **93**: 847–54.

47. Shapiro BS, Daneshmand ST, Garner FC, *et al.* Comparison of "triggers" using leuprolide acetate alone or in combination with low-dose human chorionic gonadotropin. *Fertil Steril* 2011; **95**: 2715–7.

48. Humaidan P. Agonist trigger: what is the best approach? Agonist trigger and low dose hCG0. *Fertil Steril* 2012; **97**: 529–30.

49. Garcia-Velasco JA. Agonist trigger: what is the best approach? Agonist trigger with vitrification of oocytes or embryos. *Fertil Steril* 2012; **97**: 527–8.

50. Cobo A, de Los Santos MJ, Castellò D, *et al.* Outcomes of vitrified early cleavage-stage and blastocyst-stage embryos in a cryopreservation program: evaluation of 3,150 warming cycles. *Fertil Steril* 2012; **98**: 1138–46.

51. Shapiro BS, Daneshmand ST, Garner FC, *et al.* Evidence of impaired endometrial receptivity after ovarian stimulation for in vitro fertilization: a prospective randomized trial comparing fresh and frozen-thawed embryo transfer in normal responders. *Fertil Steril* 2011; **96**: 344–8.

52. Shapiro BS, Daneshmand ST, Garner FC, *et al.* Evidence of impaired endometrial receptivity after ovarian stimulation for in vitro fertilization: a prospective randomized trial comparing fresh and frozen-thawed embryo transfers in high responders. *Fertil Steril* 2011; **96**: 516–18.

53. Rienzi L, Romano S, Albricci L, *et al.* Embryo development of fresh "versus" vitrified metaphase II oocytes after ICSI: a prospective randomized sibling-oocyte study. *Hum Reprod* 2010; **25**: 66–73.

54. Cobo A, Meseguer M, Remohí J, *et al.* Use of cryo-banked oocytes in an ovum donation programme: a prospective, randomized, controlled, clinical trial. *Hum Reprod* 2010; **25**: 2239–46.

55. Martínez F, Rodríguez DB, Buxaderas R, *et al.* GnRH antagonist rescue of a long-protocol IVF cycle and GnRH agonist trigger to avoid ovarian hyperstimulation syndrome: three case reports. *Fertil Steril* 2011; **95**: 2432.e17–9.

56. Polyzos NP, Stoop D, Blockeel C, *et al.* Anti-Müllerian hormone for the assessment of ovarian response in GnRH-antagonist-treated oocyte donors. *Reprod Biomed Online* 2012; **24**: 532–9.

57. Stoop D, Vercammen L, Polyzos NP, *et al.* Effect of ovarian stimulation and oocyte retrieval on

reproductive outcome in oocyte donors. *Fertil Steril* 2012; **97**: 1328–30.

58. Reddy J, Oktay K. Ovarian stimulation and fertility preservation with the use of aromatase inhibitors in women with breast cancer. *Fertil Steril* 2012; **98**: 1363–9.

59. Reichman DE, Davis OK, Zaninovic N, *et al.* Fertility preservation using controlled ovarian hyperstimulation and oocyte cryopreservation in a premenarcheal female with myelodysplastic syndrome. *Fertil Steril* 2012; **98**: 1225–8.

60. Caligara C, Navarro J, Vargas G, *et al.* The effect of repeated controlled ovarian stimulation in donors. *Hum Reprod* 2001; **16**: 2320–3.

61. Bukulmez O, Li Q, Carr BR, *et al.* Repetitive oocyte donation does not decrease serum anti-Müllerian hormone levels. *Fertil Steril* 2010; **94**: 905–12.

62. van Leeuwen FE, Klip H, Mooij TM, *et al.* Risk of borderline and invasive ovarian tumours after ovarian stimulation for in vitro fertilization in a large Dutch cohort. *Hum Reprod* 2011; **26**: 3456–65.

63. Yil-Kuha A-N, Gissler M, Klemetti R, *et al.* Cancer morbidity in a cohort of 9175 Finnish women treated for infertility. *Hum Reprod* 2012; **27**: 1149–55.

64. Li E. Chromatin modification and epigenetic reprogramming in mammalian development. *Nat Rev Genet* 2002; **3**: 662–73.

65. Reik W, Walter J. Genomic imprinting: parental influence on the genome. *Nat Rev Genet* 2001; **2**: 21–32.

66. Hirasawa R, Feil R. Genomic imprinting and human disease. *Essays Biochem* 2010; **48**: 187–200.

67. Feng S, Jacobsen SE, Reik W. Epigenetic reprogramming in plant and animal development. *Science* 2010; **330**: 622–7.

68. Obata Y, Kono T. Maternal primary imprinting is established at a specific time for each gene throughout oocyte growth. *J Biol Chem* 2002; **277**: 5285–9.

69. Lucifero D, Mann MR, Bartolomei MS, *et al.* Gene-specific timing and epigenetic memory in oocyte imprinting. *Hum Mol Genet* 2004; **13**: 839–49.

70. Hiura H, Obata Y, Komiyama J, *et al.* Oocyte growth-dependent progression of maternal imprinting in mice. *Genes Cells* 2006; **11**: 353–61.

71. Howell CY, Bestor TH, Ding F, *et al.* Genomic imprinting disrupted by a maternal effect mutation in the DnmtI gene. *Cell* 2001; **104**: 829–38.

72. Li X, Ito M, Zhou F, *et al.* A maternal-zygotic effect gene, Zfp57, maintains both maternal and paternal imprints. *Dev Cell* 2008; **15**: 547–57.

73. Nakamura T, Arai Y, Umehara H, *et al.* PGC7/Stella protects against DNA demethylation in early embryogenesis. *Nat Cell Biol* 2007; **9**: 64–71.

74. Reese KJ, Lin S, Verona RI, *et al.* Maintenance of paternal methylation and repression of the imprinted H19 gene requires MBD3. *PLoS Genet* 2007; **3**: e137.

75. van Montfoort APA, Hanssen LLP, de Sutter P, *et al.* Assisted reproduction treatment and epigenetic inheritance. *Hum Reprod Update* 2012; **18**: 171–97.

76. Lidegaard O, Pinborg A, Andersen AN. Imprinting diseases and IVF: Danish National IVF cohort study. *Hum Reprod* 2005; **20**: 950–4.

77. Doornbos ME, Maas SM, McDonnell J, *et al.* Infertility, assisted reproduction technologies and imprinting disturbances: a Dutch study. *Hum Reprod* 2007; **22**: 2476–80.

78. Lee MP, DeBaun MR, Mitsuya K, *et al.* Loss of imprinting of a paternally expressed transcript, with antisense orientation to KVLQTI, occurs frequently in Beckwith-Wiedemann syndrome and is independent of insulin-like growth factor II imprinting. *Proc Natl Acad Sci USA* 1999; **96**: 5203–8.

79. Engel JR, Smallwood A, Harper A, *et al.* Epigenotype-phenotype correlations in Beckwith-Wiedemann syndrome. *J Med Genet* 2000; **37**: 921–6.

80. Katari S, Turan N, Bibikova M, *et al.* DNA methylation and gene expression differences in children conceived in vitro or in vivo. *Hum Mol Genet* 2009; **18**: 3769–78.

81. Denomme MM, Mann MRW. Genomic imprints as a model for the analysis of epigenetic stability during assisted reproductive technologies. *Reproduction* 2012; **144**: 393–409.

82. Sato A, Otsu E, Negishi H, *et al.* DNA methylation of imprinted loci in superovulated oocytes. *Hum Reprod* 2007; **22**: 26–35.

83. Borghol N, Lornage J, Blachere T, *et al.* Epigenetic status of the H19 locus in human oocytes following in vitro maturation. *Genomics* 2006; **87**: 417–26.

84. Khoueiry R, Ibala-Rhomdane S, Méry L, *et al.* Dynamic CpG methylation of the KCNQIOTI gene during maturation of human oocytes. *J Med Genet* 2008; **45**: 583–8.

85. Shi W, Haaf T. Aberrant methylation patterns at the two-cell stage as an indicator of early developmental failure. *Mol Reprod Dev* 2002; **63**: 329–34.

86. Denomme MM, Zhang L, Mann MR. Embryonic imprinting perturbations do not originate from superovulation-induced defects in DNA methylation acquisition. *Fertil Steril* 2011; **96**: 734–8.e2.

87. El Hajj N, Trapphoff T, Linke M, *et al.* Limiting dilution bisulfite (pyro)sequencing reveals parent-specific methylation patterns in single early mouse embryos and bovine oocytes. *Epigenetics* 2011; **6**: 1176–88.

88. Anckaert E, Adriaenssens T, Romero S, *et al.* Unaltered imprinting establisment of key imprinted genes in mouse oocytes after follicle culture under variable follicle-stimulating hormone exposure. *Int J Dev Biol* 2009; **53**: 541–8.

89. Fauque P, Jouannet P, Lesaffre C, *et al.* Assisted reproductive technology affects developmental kinetics, H19 imprinting control region methylation and H19 gene expression in individual mouse embryos. *BMC Dev Biol* 2007; **7**: 116.

90. Fortier AL, Lopes FL, Darricarrère N, *et al.* Superovulation alters the expression of imprinted genes in the midgestation mouse placenta. *Hum Mol Genet* 2008; **17**: 1653–65.

91. Market-Velker BA, Zhang L, Magri LS, *et al.* Dual effects of superovulation: loss of maternal and paternal imprinted methylation in a dose-dependent manner. *Hum Mol Genet* 2010; **19**: 36–51.

92. de Waal E, Yamazaki Y, Ingale P, *et al.* Gonadotropin stimulation contributes to an increased incidence of epimutations in ICSI-derived mice. *Hum Mol Genet* 2012; **21**: 4460–72.

93. Stouder C, Deutsch S, Paoloni-Giacobino A. Superovulation in mice alters the methylation pattern of imprinted genes in the sperm of the offspring. *Reprod Toxicol* 2009; **28**: 536–41.

Section 5 Pathology

Chapter 33

Oocyte epigenetics and the risks for imprinting disorders associated with assisted reproduction

Serge McGraw and Jacquetta M. Trasler

Introduction

As a treatment for female infertility, assisted reproductive technology (ART) commonly uses a number of treatments and manipulations, including hormonal stimulation of follicular development and ovulation, cryopreservation, in vitro maturation (IVM), in vitro fertilization (IVF)/intracytoplasmic sperm injection (ICSI) and embryo culture, all of which could adversely affect oocyte development or function during early embryogenesis. Over the last decade, concern has been raised about possible increases in the occurrence of rare genomic imprinting disorders, in particular Beckwith–Wiedemann syndrome (BWS) and Angelman syndrome (AS), in ART-conceived children. The genomic imprinting disorders seen in children conceived using ART were accompanied in many cases by a loss of maternal DNA methylation at imprinted loci. Genomic imprinting refers to the acquisition of a unique epigenetic profile in a small subset of genes during gametogenesis. This differential epigenetic mark in the gametes results in a parent-of-origin-specific expression of these imprinted genes in the offspring. Most imprinted genes exist in clusters in the genome and their allele-specific expression is regulated by sequence elements called imprinting control regions (ICRs). Genomic imprinting is under the control of epigenetic mechanisms including DNA methylation at ICRs, also known as differentially methylated domains or regions (DMDs, DMRs). One of the best studied epigenetic mechanisms, DNA methylation, is heritable and reversible and susceptible to being perturbed during development. At most ICRs, DNA methylation occurs in the female germ line and is inherited from the mother. Following fertilization, male and female gametic imprints must be maintained through preimplantation development and into adulthood. Thus any factor that affects the ability of oocytes to acquire imprints or normal epigenetic patterns during oogenesis or maintain these patterns after fertilization could potentially predispose to imprinting disorders in the offspring. This chapter reviews current data on the effects of ART on genomic imprinting in humans, along with the human and animal research that is beginning to help explain how perturbations in oocyte biology may be linked to the etiology of ART-associated epigenetic dysregulation and abnormalities in genomic imprinting.

Genomic imprinting disorders and assisted reproduction

In the initial reports, the two imprinting disorders linked to ARTs were BWS and AS. BWS patients show variable phenotypes that can include overgrowth, exomphalos, macroglossia, fetal hypoglycemia, umbilical and abdominal wall defects, and increased susceptibility to the development of childhood tumors. In the imprinted region on chromosome 11p15 five genes have been implicated in the pathogenesis of BWS including, in the distal ICR1 cluster, insulin-like growth factor 2 (*IGF2*) and in the proximal ICR2 cluster, cyclin-dependent kinase inhibitor 1c (*CDKN1C*), potassium voltage-gated channel KQT-like subfamily member 1 (*KCNQ1*) and *KCNQ1* overlapping transcript 1 (*KCNQ1OT1*, previously called *LIT1*) [1]. *IGF2* and *KCNQ1OT1* are both paternally expressed while *H19*, *CDKN1C*, and *KCNQ1* are maternally expressed. About 50% of sporadic BWS cases result from promoter hypomethylation at ICR2 or *KvDMR1*, within

Biology and Pathology of the Oocyte, 2nd edn., ed. Alan Trounson, Roger Gosden, and Ursula Eichenlaub-Ritter.
Published by Cambridge University Press.

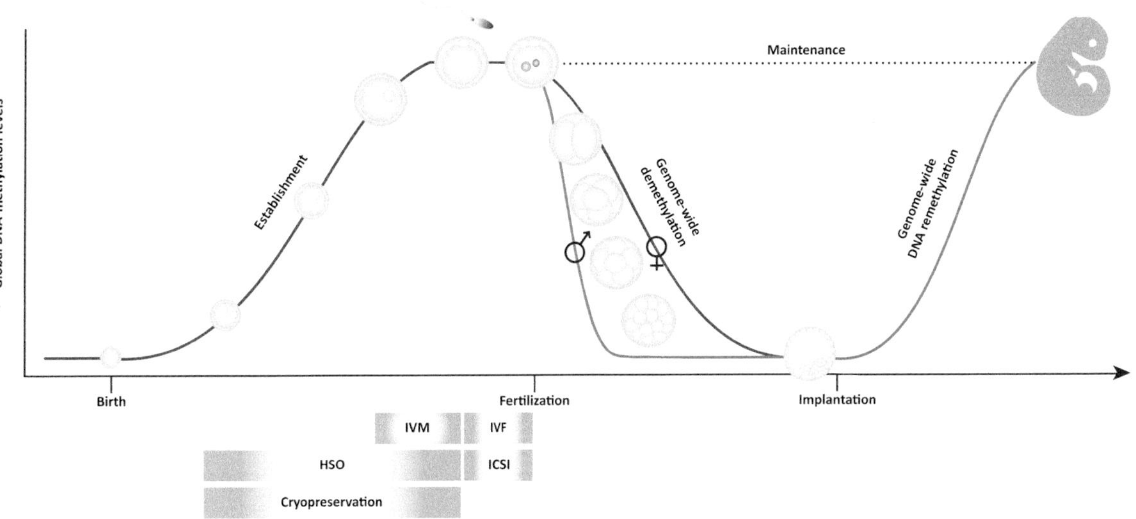

Figure 33.1 Assisted reproductive technologies and female germ cell susceptibility to imprinting errors. In female germ cells, the establishment of new DNA methylation marks, including those on maternally methylated imprinted genes, takes place during the oocyte growth phase. Following fertilization, while much of the genome is globally demethylated, and then remethylated after implantation, DNA methylation patterns on imprinted genes must be maintained during preimplantation development (dotted line). During oocyte growth, and the time leading up to sperm–egg fusion, various treatments associated with assisted reproduction expose the oocyte to environments not normally encountered in vivo. These treatments include hormonal stimulation of ovulation (HSO), cryopreservation, in vitro maturation (IVM), in vitro fertilization (IVF), and intracytoplasmic sperm injection (ICSI). Exposure of growing oocytes to ARTs could either interfere with the normal acquisition of DNA methylation patterns or affect the quality of the oocyte such that methylation on imprinted genes is not properly maintained in the preimplantation embryo. (Adapted from [66, 67]).

KCNQ1OT1. Loss of maternal methylation at *KvDMR1* leads to biallelic expression of *KCNQ1OT1* and silencing of *KCNQ1* and *CDKN1C*. Another epigenetic defect, the hypermethylation of the *H19* promoter and/or ICR1 region resulting in silencing of *H19* and biallelic expression of *IGF2*, is found in about 2–7% of BWS patients. AS involves an imprinted region on chromosome 15q11–q13 and results in loss of maternal expression of the *UBE3A* gene. Patients with AS have mental retardation, microcephaly, movement disorders including ataxia, seizure disorders, abnormal behavior, and limited development of speech and language. In contrast to BWS, only a small proportion, about 3–5%, of AS cases are the result of methylation defects in the 15q11–q13 region [2].

The initial studies linking ARTs and genomic imprinting disorders suggested an increased risk of developing BWS amongst ART-conceived as compared to naturally conceived children, from three countries [3–5] (reviewed in [6]). Following these reports, a number of further studies have linked ARTs and BWS [7–9] (reviewed in [10]). The mechanisms suggested to underlie the ART-associated BWS were either related to the techniques used or the underlying infertility of the parents. Some reports postulated that BWS is linked to more specific procedures such as IVF/ICSI [11] or ovarian stimulation [12]. In many cases the BWS was associated with maternal hypomethylation of *KvDMR1*, the imprinting center on chromosome 11p15 that is normally hypomethylated in about 50–60% of cases of BWS [13]. Lim and colleagues [14] reported that for 24 out of 25 cases of BWS following ARTs, the molecular basis of the disease was maternal hypomethylation. The higher proportion of BWS cases associated with maternal *KvDMR1* hypomethylation following ARTs suggests that maternal imprints were either not acquired normally during oogenesis or were not maintained post-fertilization (Figure 33.1). Interestingly, in BWS patients with *KvDMR1* hypomethylation, two groups reported additional imprinted gene epigenetic defects [14, 15]. One of the studies found higher frequencies of loss of methylation at DMRs outside the BWS chromosome 11p15 region in ART cases than in non-ART cases [14]. The results suggest the presence of more extensive, potentially multi-locus, epigenetic defects following ARTs.

Thus, a number of studies among children identified as having BWS have consistently reported a higher prevalence of those conceived with ARTs [3–5, 9, 11, 12]. Larger follow-up studies of children conceived using ARTs have assessed the numbers of children with BWS in their cohorts. Two cohort studies, one from Sweden [16] and another from Denmark [17], did not find an increased risk of BWS among ART-conceived children. However, a French IVF follow-up cohort study reported 6 BWS cases amongst 15 162 IVF children; considering the rarity of BWS of about 1 in 13 000 births, these results provided further support for an increased risk of BWS associated with ART [18]. With the rarity of the syndrome, it is likely a large international study comparing the prevalence of BWS among naturally conceived and ART-conceived children would be required to accurately assess the potential connection between ARTs and BWS. Nonetheless, considering an approximate threefold risk, an estimate of the overall prevalence of BWS is about 1 in 4000 ART births, a low risk, but one that should be mentioned in preconception counseling.

There is less compelling evidence that AS is also associated with ARTs. As for BWS, the underlying molecular mechanism appears to be demethylation; in the case of AS, within the DMR of the imprinted gene *SNRPN* [10, 11, 19, 20]. Furthermore, an increased prevalence of imprinting defects was reported in AS patients born to subfertile couples, suggesting that underlying infertility and techniques might interact [21]. Another study found a higher risk of AS children amongst parents with fertility problems where ovulation induction was used, providing further support for an interaction between infertility and a specific technique used in ART [8]. Negative reports have also appeared in the literature. For example, a study in 92 children born after ICSI found no evidence of methylation defects at *SNRPN* [22]. However, it should be noted that much larger samples would likely be needed to detect an increased prevalence of imprinting defects. To date, there have been reports of four cases of AS with an epigenetic basis associated with ARTs. Given the rarity of AS (1/10 000–1/20 000 births) and the fact that hypomethylation is the molecular cause in only a small proportion (~6%) of cases [23], further studies are warranted.

More recently, another imprinting disorder, Silver–Russell syndrome (SRS), has been linked to ARTs. SRS patients show heterogeneous clinical features but generally include severe intrauterine growth restriction, poor postnatal growth, characteristic craniofacial features, and body asymmetry. The clinical heterogeneity of SRS may be due to the fact that several different chromosomes have been linked to the disease, suggesting that there are multiple different disorders that have been grouped into this single category. Two imprinted genes have been implicated in SRS: growth receptor bound protein 10 (*GRB10*) at chromosome 7p11.2–p13 and *IGF2* on chromosome 11p15. *H19–IGF2* epimutations have been linked to SRS, following the identification of patients carrying maternal uniparental disomy for chromosome 11p15 showing characteristics of SRS. When further examination of the methylation at the *H19* ICR was undertaken, hypomethylation was observed in 38–63% of cases (reviewed in [24]). Since *H19* and *IGF2* are tightly linked, when the *H19* ICR is hypomethylated, reduced expression of *IGF2* occurs, leading to growth defects. SRS is extremely rare, with an incidence of 1 in 100 000 live births [25]. While the link between SRS and ARTs is tenuous, four cases of SRS have been described following ARTs, two in which the molecular etiology was unknown [17, 26, 27] and two cases with DNA methylation defects, one of which was the hypomethylation of *H19* [28, 29]. Given the rarity of SRS, and the evidence of hypomethylation at *H19*, the association of SRS with ARTs is currently only suggestive.

Epigenetic abnormalities in children conceived using ARTs

Although fewer than 100 have been identified to date, estimates suggest there may be about 200 imprinted genes in the human genome [30]. Imprinted genes play critical roles in growth and development and when abnormally expressed can contribute to carcinogenesis. In particular, many imprinted genes are expressed in the placenta and play a role in its normal function, in turn contributing to fetal development and size [31]. Although ART has been associated with abnormalities at only a few imprinted regions to date, there is concern that other regions important for postnatal development or capable of contributing to cancer only later in life might be affected [32]. Thus, investigators are beginning to search for imprinting defects at multiple loci in cohorts of children conceived using ART.

One study examined whether abnormalities in genomic imprinting might underlie the increased proportion of small-for-gestational-age (SGA) babies following ART [33]. Methylation patterns were assessed at six imprinted loci in DNA from buccal cells of 19 SGA babies conceived with ICSI as compared to 29 naturally conceived children of normal birth weight. No major difference in imprints was found between the two groups. One ICSI-conceived SGA child showed hypermethylation of the paternal copy of the *KCNQ1OT1* DMR but the significance of this finding was unclear; such a defect would be predicted to be due to a lack of erasure of the maternal methylation mark in the paternal germ line, something that has been noted in male infertility [34], but could also be due to an abnormal gain in methylation during early embryo development as has been seen in some animal studies. In a study of 18 ART-conceived and 30 spontaneously conceived clinically normal children, Gomes *et al.* found a higher frequency of *KvDMR1* hypomethylation in children conceived by ART as compared to spontaneously conceived children [35]. A larger study examined DNA methylation at 10 DMRs in 185 phenotypically normal children, 77 conceived by ICSI, 35 by IVF, and 73 conceived spontaneously; except for a slightly more variable *MEST* DMR methylation in the IVF group, methylation was similar across all groups [36]. The number of ART-conceived children examined to date for imprinting abnormalities is still small. In addition, the studies have been limited to a small number of genes and regions. The recent advent of sensitive whole genome epigenomic profiling techniques will allow more comprehensive studies to be done. More attention should also be paid to epigenetic studies in those ART-conceived fetuses lost early in gestation that might have more epigenetic abnormalities. However, the presence of both positive and negative findings to date suggest that larger numbers of ART-conceived children need to be studied with more imprinted genes targeted for analysis as well as additional tissues examined.

A more comprehensive study [37] used an array-based approach to examine methylation over about 1500 CpG sites in the promoters of 700 genes including sites in all known imprinted genes. DNA methylation was compared in placenta and cord blood samples between 10 children conceived using IVF without ICSI and 13 children conceived naturally (in vivo). The results were used to examine gene expression profiles in a larger group of children. Overall, lower levels of methylation in the placenta and higher levels in cord blood were found in the IVF group. The methylation differences correlated with altered expression of a small number of adjacent genes. Together the results provided evidence that methylation abnormalities associated with ARTs can extend beyond imprinted genes, although the significance of such changes for the offspring is unknown. The finding of altered methylation and expression in the placenta is notable as placental function might be affected and contribute to decreased birth weight in ART-conceived children.

Potential mechanisms underlying imprinting defects in ARTs

The genomic imprinting disorders seen in children conceived using ART were accompanied in many cases by a loss of maternal DNA methylation at imprinted loci. The fact that genomic DNA methylation patterns are acquired and dynamic during germ cell development and the preimplantation period [38], times that could be affected by techniques used in assisted reproduction, provided biological plausibility for the potential for ARTs to perturb genomic imprinting (Figure 33.1). However, infertility of the parents was proposed as an alternate explanation for the genomic imprinting disorders amongst ART-conceived children, and received support from a number of studies reporting DNA methylation defects in imprinted genes in the sperm of infertile men (reviewed in [34]). It was also suggested that subfertility and ARTs might interact to predispose children to genomic imprinting disorders [21, 39]. Thus perturbation of several male and female factors, separately or in combination, could potentially contribute to imprinting or other epigenetic defects in the offspring following ART. Here, evidence that ARTs can either alter the acquisition of DNA methylation imprints in oocytes or result in the production of oocytes with altered ability to maintain imprints in the early embryo will be reviewed. As the availability of human samples is limited, examples of results from animal models that may help inform follow-up human studies will be included. The use of animal models is beginning to define which gamete and embryo developmental stages may be most susceptible to perturbation by ARTs in the absence of the complicating factor of subfertility or infertility.

Perturbations to normal oocyte physiology and the etiology of imprinting disorders in ARTs

Perturbing imprints during oogenesis

Studies in mouse models have defined the normal timing of DNA methylation in female germ cells. Following erasure of DNA methylation in primordial germ cells, in the female germ line, gametic methylation is only acquired postnatally, after pachytene and during the oocyte growth phase [40, 41]. Bisulfite sequencing studies, in particular, have been useful in characterizing the acquisition of DNA methylation on the DMRs of imprinted genes in oocytes. DNA methylation is acquired progressively during oocyte growth with some imprinted genes becoming methylated early (e.g., *Snrpn*) and others later (e.g., *Peg1/Mest*) in the oocyte growth phase [40, 42]. Imprinted genes with paternally methylated DMRs such as *H19* are unmethylated in fully grown oocytes. Most studies of human oocytes have reported that imprinted genes such as *SNRPN* and the chromosome 11p15 *KvDMR* are methylated in fully grown oocytes, emphasizing evolutionary conservation with the mouse [43–45].

A few human studies with small numbers of oocytes have examined whether ARTs affect methylation imprints in oocytes. To assess the normality of methylation of imprinted genes in oocytes, investigators have examined the DMRs of maternally methylated imprinted genes (normally 100% methylated) and paternally methylated imprinted genes (normally 0% methylated). Techniques that could potentially interfere with imprint acquisition include ovulation induction with hormones, IVM of oocytes, and cryopreservation or vitrification. An important caveat of these studies is that oocyte abnormalities associated with age or underlying female subfertility or infertility may contribute to the findings.

Considering maternally methylated DMRs first, in one study ovarian stimulation was associated with low levels of methylation of the *PEG1/MEST* DMR in a subset of human oocytes [45]. A further study found that the *KCNQ1OT1 KvDMR1* in DNA from germinal vesicle (GV) and metaphase I (MI) oocytes was more methylated when obtained from natural cycles than from patients receiving gonadotropin stimulation; the authors suggested that ovarian stimulation recruits immature follicles in which the methylation of imprinted genes is not yet completed [46]. In contrast, other reports suggested that the DMRs of *SNRPN* [43] and *KCNQ1OT1* [44] were unaffected by ovulation induction in the majority of oocytes.

There are only a few paternally methylated imprinted genes, and the *H19* and *DLK1/MEG3* DMRs have been the subject of most DNA methylation studies. One study found evidence of abnormal methylation of *H19* in two of six human oocytes after ovarian stimulation [45]. In contrast, the *H19* DMR was appropriately unmethylated in all five superovulated oocytes examined in another study [47]. Similarly, the *DLK1/MEG3* DMR was for the most part unmethylated in GV and MI stage oocytes obtained following ovarian stimulation [48].

In mouse studies, Sato and colleagues [45] examined the methylation of three maternally methylated genes (*Peg1*, *Zac*, *Kcnq1ot1*) and one paternally methylated gene (*H19*) in oocytes following superovulation. All of the maternally methylated genes had normal methylation after superovulation; however, interestingly, *H19* gained methylation. The results suggested that the acquisition of maternal methylation imprints was unaffected but that the oocyte quality was affected such that abnormal methylation was acquired on *H19* during oogenesis. A recent careful study involving a large number of mouse oocytes examined the effects of low and high dose ovarian hormone stimulation on the methylation patterns of the DMRs of *Snrpn*, *Kcnq1ot1*, *Peg3*, and *H19* and detected no evidence of alterations [49]. The latter study provided evidence that superovulation did not affect the acquisition of DNA methylation patterns at imprinted loci nor perturb *H19* in oocytes.

IVM of human oocytes is used clinically to avoid exposure to ovarian stimulation. There is the possibility that not all methylation of imprinted genes is completely acquired in the immature oocytes subjected to IVM. Both positive and negative findings have been reported in human studies. While the methylation of the DMRs of *SNRPN* and *KCNQ1OT1* was unaffected following IVM of GV and MI oocytes in one study [43, 44], a second reported that the methylation of the *KCNQ1OT1* DMR was lower in IVM-derived versus in vivo-derived oocytes [46]. For paternal methylation imprints following IVM, while methylation was appropriately absent on the *DLK1/MEG3* DMR [48], abnormally high levels of methylation were found for *H19* in about 25% of oocytes examined [47]. Mouse studies allow the effects of gamete manipulations on oocyte imprints to be examined in the absence of female infertility, a potential confounder. In one study loss of *Peg1* DMR methylation was observed in mouse oocytes after IVM [50]. However, several other mouse studies have shown that maternal and paternal methylation imprints are normal in GV and MII oocytes following a combination of in vitro manipulations including in vitro growth, IVM, and vitrification [51–53].

For ovarian stimulation and other oocyte manipulations, in both the human and mouse studies, the methylation of a limited number of imprinted genes has been examined and the functional consequences for the offspring have not been evaluated in detail. Growth, development, and health of the offspring and the potential for transgenerational passage of epimutations can be best studied in animal models. Examining the offspring in animal and human studies using genome-wide epigenomic profiling will allow more comprehensive epigenetic studies, extending to all imprinted genes as well as other sequences in the genome; inter-species comparisons will help separate out effects of infertility from those of the techniques used in assisted reproduction.

Altering oocyte quality and the maintenance of imprints in early embryos

In the mouse and human, a second phase of epigenetic reprogramming takes place during preimplantation development. The precise biochemical events and epigenetic mechanisms, including DNA methylation, chromatin modifications, and small RNAs, a number of which could potentially be affected by ART, are still being defined [54]. Preimplantation DNA methylation events have been the best characterized to date. In the zygote, following fertilization, 5-methylcytosine residues within the paternal genome are rapidly converted to 5-hydroxymethylcytosine [55]; the maternal genome is more gradually demethylated over the course of preimplantation development [38, 56, 57]. Unlike many of the sequences in the genome, imprinted sequences retain their gamete-derived methylation throughout the preimplantation stages and into adulthood. Several factors contributed by the oocyte are important for the maintenance of DNA methylation imprints during preimplantation development; these include the DNA methyltransferase enzymes DNMT1s and DNMT1o as well as proteins involved in chromatin, such as ZFP57, PGC7, and ELP3 (reviewed in [54]). As a potential mechanism to explain imprinting defects associated with ART, a number of mouse studies have indicated that ART may disrupt maternal-effect gene products required for imprint maintenance during preimplantation development. A few examples involving superovulation are reviewed here.

Fauque *et al.* observed decreased levels of expression of *H19* in blastocysts after superovulation [58]; the results could be explained by an alteration in oocyte quality affecting *H19* epigenetic marking or a delay in embryo development since *H19* is usually first expressed at the blastocyst stage. A detailed examination of the DNA methylation status of four imprinted genes in individual blastocysts following low and high dose superovulation regimens was reported recently. In this study a dose-dependent loss of DNA methylation at the DMRs of the maternally methylated imprinted genes *Snrpn*, *Peg3*, and *Kcnq1ot1* and a gain of methylation of *H19* were found [59]. Following publication of their study [49] indicating that the same regimens of superovulation do not disrupt acquisition of methylation imprints during oocyte growth, the authors concluded that the superovulation was instead altering the oocyte's ability to maintain imprints during preimplantation development. Effects of superovulation have also been examined at later times in development. A low dose superovulation protocol was shown to alter the expression of maternally and paternally methylated imprinted genes in the midgestation mouse placenta, suggesting that trophectoderm-derived tissues may be more susceptible to disruption of imprinted genes than the embryo proper [60]. Studies of live offspring from superovulated females showed evidence of altered expression and/or methylation of imprinted genes in somatic tissues in a subset of the pups [61]. Further mouse studies are necessary to understand what aspects of oocyte biology or maternal gene products are affected by gonadotropin treatments. Together, the mouse studies support the use of ovulation protocols that preserve the function of oocyte factors needed for normal epigenetic reprogramming during preimplantation development.

Assisted reproduction and other potential epigenetic effects

ARTs have been linked to other phenomena that may be related to the underlying epigenetic etiology of the reported ART-associated imprinting disorders. A higher rate of monozygotic twinning, about 2–12 times that for spontaneous births, has been reported in association with ARTs [62]. In a recent meta-analysis, blastocyst transfer was associated with a higher male:female sex ratio and an increased risk of monozygotic twins amongst the offspring [63]. While it has been suggested that the increased risk of twins following ART is likely due to embryo manipulation or effects of culture, it may also be due to perturbation of epigenetic events during preimplantation development. BWS has been reported in naturally conceived monozygotic twins in which the twins were discordant for BWS. The BWS in the affected twin was associated with hypomethylation of *KvDMR1* and, in most such cases, the twins were female [64]. The authors proposed that a failure to appropriately maintain DNA methylation, through the DNMT1o DNA methyltransferase, at the "susceptible" BWS locus on chromosome 11p15, at a key time in preimplantation development, could explain the epigenetic asymmetry between the twins as well as the predominance of females [64, 65]. To explain the association between ART and imprinting syndromes, it is plausible that ART, through ovulation of poor quality or immature oocytes or embryo culture, could prevent the maintenance of key DNA methylation patterns during preimplantation development, resulting in imprinting defects and altered sex ratio. Such a possibility could best be tested in animal models.

Table 33.1. Summary of methylation defects associated with ART procedures (as reviewed in this chapter)

Gene/locus Human	Methylation defect	ART treatment(s)	Reference
KCNQ1OT1	Hyper	ICSI	[34]
(*LIT1*,	Hypo	IVF	[4, 8, 9, 14, 35]
KvDMR1)		ICSI	[4, 5, 8, 14, 35]
		ART*	[3, 9, 11]
		HSO	[8, 46]
		AI	[8]
H19	Hyper	ART*	[3, 9]
		HSO	[45]
		HSO + IVM	[47]
	Hypo	ICSI	[28]
PEG1 (*MEST*)	Hyper	IVF	[29]
	Hypo	IVF	[14]
		ICSI	[14]
		HSO	[45]
SNRPN	Hypo	ICSI	[14, 19–21]
		HSO	[21]
		AID	[11]
ZAC	Hypo	ICSI	[14]
Mouse			
Kcnq1ot1 (*Lit1*, *Kvdmr1*)	Hypo	HSO	[59]
H19	Hyper	HSO	[45, 59]
		HSO + IVF	[58]
		IV-FG	[50]
	Hypo	ICSI	[61]
		HSO + IVF	[58]
		HSO	[59, 61]
Peg1 (*Mest*)	Hypo	IV-FG	[50]
Snrpn	Hypo	HSO	[59]
Igf2r	Hypo	IV-FG	[50]
Peg3	Hypo	ICSI	[61]
		HSO	[59, 61]

Hyper, DNA hypermethylation; Hypo, DNA hypomethylation; ICSI, intracytoplasmic sperm injection; IVF, in vitro fertilization; ART, assisted reproductive technology; HSO, hormonal stimulation of ovulation; AI, artificial insemination; IVM, in vitro maturation; AID, artificial insemination by donor; IV-FG, in vitro follicular growth.
*ART, various combinations of ART used or insufficient details on specific techniques.

Conclusions

Data from animal models indicate that the developmental DNA methylation events occurring during oogenesis and early embryogenesis can be perturbed by ARTs, while the human studies suggest a link between ART and imprinting errors (Table 33.1). Thus, further studies in the human as well as other species are warranted. There is a need for well-designed prospective long-term follow-up studies to monitor health outcomes in ART-conceived children. Such studies will need to be continued into adulthood to determine if there is an increased risk of cancer or other adult-onset diseases. Outcomes should be linked to clinical records with precise details of the type(s) of infertility treatment used. To begin to tease out the effects of ART versus subfertility or infertility, consideration of appropriate comparison groups will be important, including the children of infertile/subfertile couples who conceived naturally as well as those of couples who used ART in the absence of infertility. Collecting biological samples including the placenta and DNA from the mother, father, and child will allow high-resolution genomic and epigenomic studies to be performed using next generation sequencing techniques and genome-wide profiling. Additional research is also required to better understand the genetic and epigenetic causes of female and male infertility.

Acknowledgments

Research in the Trasler laboratory is supported by a grant from the Canadian Institutes of Health Research (CIHR). J. M. T. is a James McGill Professor of McGill University. J. M. T is a member of the Research Institute of the McGill University Health Centre, which is supported in part by the Fonds de la recherché en Santé du Québec (FRSQ).

References

1. Enklaar T, Zabel BU, Prawitt D. Beckwith-Wiedemann syndrome: multiple molecular mechanisms. *Expert Rev Mol Med* 2006; **8**: 1–19.
2. Horsthemke B, Wagstaff J. Mechanisms of imprinting of the Prader-Willi/Angelman region. *Am J Med Genet A* 2008; **146A**: 2041–52.
3. DeBaun MR, Niemitz EL, Feinberg AP. Association of in vitro fertilization with Beckwith-Wiedemann syndrome and epigenetic alterations of LIT1 and H19. *Am J Hum Genet* 2003; **72**: 156–60.
4. Gicquel C, Gaston V, Mandelbaum J, *et al.* In vitro fertilization may increase the risk of Beckwith-Wiedemann syndrome related to the abnormal imprinting of the KCN1OT1 gene. *Am J Hum Genet* 2003; **72**: 1338–41.
5. Maher ER, Brueton LA, Bowdin SC, *et al.* Beckwith-Wiedemann syndrome and assisted reproduction technology (ART). *J Med Genet* 2003; **40**: 62–4.
6. Gosden R, Trasler J, Lucifero D, *et al.* Rare congenital disorders, imprinted genes, and assisted reproductive technology. *Lancet* 2003; **361**: 1975–7.
7. Bowdin S, Allen C, Kirby G, *et al.* A survey of assisted reproductive technology births and imprinting disorders. *Hum Reprod* 2007; **22**: 3237–40.
8. Doornbos ME, Maas SM, McDonnell J, *et al.* Infertility, assisted reproduction technologies and imprinting disturbances: a Dutch study. *Hum Reprod* 2007; **22**: 2476–80.
9. Halliday J, Oke K, Breheny S, Algar E, Amor DJ. Beckwith-Wiedemann syndrome and IVF: a case-control study. *Am J Hum Genet* 2004; **75**: 526–8.
10. Owen CM, Segars JH, Jr. Imprinting disorders and assisted reproductive technology. *Semin Reprod Med* 2009; **27**: 417–28.
11. Sutcliffe AG, Peters CJ, Bowdin S, *et al.* Assisted reproductive therapies and imprinting disorders – a preliminary British survey. *Hum Reprod* 2006; **21**: 1009–11.
12. Chang AS, Moley KH, Wangler M, *et al.* Association between Beckwith-Wiedemann syndrome and assisted reproductive technology: a case series of 19 patients. *Fertil Steril* 2005; **83**: 349–54.
13. Weksberg R, Shuman C, Smith AC. Beckwith-Wiedemann syndrome. *Am J Med Genet C Semin Med Genet* 2005; **137C**: 12–23.
14. Lim D, Browdin SC, Tee L, *et al.* Clinical and molecular genetic features of Beckwith-Wiedemann Syndrome associated with assisted reproductive technologies. *Hum Reprod* 2009; **24**: 741–7.
15. Rossignol S, Steunou V, Chalas C. The epigenetic imprinting defect of patients with Beckwith-Wiedemann syndrome born after assisted reproductive technology is not restricted to the 11p15 region. *J Med Genet* 2006; **43**: 902–7.
16. Lidegaard O, Pinborg A, Andersen AN. Imprinting diseases and IVF: Danish National IVF cohort study. *Hum Reprod* 2005; **20**: 950–4.
17. Kallen B, Finnstrom O, Nygren KG, *et al.* In vitro fertilization (IVF) in Sweden: infant outcome after different IVF fertilization methods. *Fertil Steril* 2005; **84**: 611–17.
18. Viot G, Epelboin S, Olivennes F. Is there an increased risk of congenital malformations after ART: results from a prospective French long-term survey of a cohort of 15,162 children. *Hum Reprod* 2010; **25** Suppl 1: 154–5.
19. Cox GF, J Burger, Lip V, *et al.* Intracytoplasmic sperm injection may increase the risk of imprinting defects. *Am J Hum Genet* 2002; **71**: 162–4.
20. Orstavik KH, Eiklid K, van der Hagen CB, *et al.* Another case of imprinting defect in a girl with Angelman syndrome who was conceived by intracytoplasmic semen injection. *Am J Hum Genet* 2003; **72**: 218–19.
21. Ludwig M, Katalinic A, Gross S, *et al.* Increased prevalence of imprinting defects in patients with Angelman syndrome born to subfertile couples. *J Med Genet* 2005; **42**: 289–91.
22. Manning M, Lissens W, Bonduelle M, *et al.* Study of DNA methylation patterns at chromosome

15q11-q13 in children born after ICSI reveals no imprinting defects. *Mol Hum Reprod* 2000; **6**: 1049–53.

23. Williams CA. Neurological aspects of the Angelman syndrome. *Brain Dev* 2005; **27**: 88–94.
24. Eggermann T. Silver-Russell and Beckwith-Wiedemann syndromes: opposite (epi)mutations in 11p15 result in opposite clinical pictures. *Horm Res* 2009; **71** Suppl 2: 30–5.
25. Perkins RM, Hoang-Xuan MT. The Russell-Silver syndrome: a case report and brief review of the literature. *Pediatr Dermatol* 2002; **19**: 546–9.
26. Svensson J, Björnstahl A, Ivarsson SA. Increased risk of Silver-Russell syndrome after in vitro fertilization? *Acta Paediatr* 2005; **94**: 1163–5.
27. Kallen B, Finnstrom O, Lindam A, *et al.* Congenital malformations in infants born after in vitro fertilization in Sweden. *Birth Defects Res A Clin Mol Teratol* 2010; **88**: 137–43.
28. Bliek J, Terhal P, van den Bogaard MJ, *et al.* Hypomethylation of the H19 gene causes not only Silver-Russell syndrome (SRS) but also isolated asymmetry or an SRS-like phenotype. *Am J Hum Genet* 2006; **78**: 604–14.
29. Kagami M, Nagai T, Fukami M, *et al.* Silver-Russell syndrome in a girl born after in vitro fertilization: partial hypermethylation at the differentially methylated region of PEG1/MEST. *J Assist Reprod Genet* 2007; **24**: 131–6.
30. Luedi PP, Dietrich FS, Weidman JR, *et al.* Computational and experimental identification of novel imprinted genes. *Genome Res* 2007; **17**: 1723–30.
31. Coan PM, Burton GJ, Ferguson-Smith AC. Imprinted genes in the placenta – a review. *Placenta* 2005; **26** (Suppl A) S10–20.
32. Wilkins-Haug L. Epigenetics and assisted reproduction. *Curr Opin Obstet Gynecol* 2009; **21**: 201–6.
33. Kanber D, Buiting K, Zeschnigk M, *et al.* Low frequency of imprinting defects in ICSI children born small for gestational age. *Eur J Hum Genet* 2009; **17**: 22–9.
34. Filipponi D, Feil R. Perturbation of genomic imprinting in oligospermia. *Epigenetics* 2009; **4**(1): 27–30.
35. Gomes MV, Huber J, Ferriani RA, *et al.* Abnormal methylation at the KvDMR1 imprinting control region in clinically normal children conceived by assisted reproductive technologies. *Mol Hum Reprod* 2009; **15**: 471–7.
36. Tierling S, Souren NY, Gries J, *et al.* Assisted reproductive technologies do not enhance the variability of DNA methylation imprints in human. *J Med Genet* 2010; **47**: 371–6.
37. Katari S, Turan N, Bibikova M, *et al.* DNA methylation and gene expression differences in children conceived *in vitro* or *in vivo*. *Hum Mol Genet* 2009; **18**: 3769–78.
38. Reik W, Dean W, Walter J. Epigenetic reprogramming in mammalian development. *Science* 2001; **293**: 1089–93.
39. Horsthemke B, Ludwig M. Assisted reproduction: the epigenetic perspective. *Hum Reprod Update* 2005; **11**: 473–82.
40. Lucifero D, Mann MRW, Bartolomei M, *et al.* Gene-specific timing and epigenetic memory in oocyte imprinting. *Hum Mol Genet* 2004; **3**: 839–49.
41. Obata Y, Kono T. Maternal primary imprinting is established at a specific time for each gene throughout oocyte growth. *J Biol Chem* 2002; **277**: 5285–9.
42. Hiura H, Obata Y, Komiyama J, *et al.* Oocyte growth-dependent progression of maternal imprinting in mice. *Genes Cells* 2006; **11**: 353–61.
43. Geuns E, De Rycke M, Van Steirteghem A, *et al.* Methylation imprints of the imprint control region of the SNRPN-gene in human gametes and preimplantation embryos. *Hum Mol Genet* 2003; **12**: 2873–9.
44. Geuns E, Hilver P, Van Steirteghem A, *et al.* Methylation analysis of KVDMR1 in human oocytes. *J Med Genet* 2007; **44**: 144–7.
45. Sato A, Otsu E, Negishi H, *et al.* Aberrant DNA methylation of imprinted loci in superovulated oocytes. *Hum Reprod* 2007; **22**: 26–35.
46. Khoueiry R, Ibala-Rhomdane S, Méry L, *et al.* Dynamic CpG methylation of the KCNQ1OT1 gene during maturation of human oocytes. *J Med Genet* 2008; **45**(9): 583–8.
47. Bourghol N, Lornage J, Blachère T, Garret AS, Lefèvre A. Epigenetic status of the H19 locus in human oocytes following in vitro maturation. *Genomics* 2006; **87**: 417–6.
48. Geuns E, De Temmerman N, Hilven P, *et al.* Methylation analysis of the intergenic differentially methylated region of DLK1-GTL2 in human. *Eur J Hum Genet* 2007; **15**: 352–61.
49. Denomme MM, Zhang L, Mann MR. Embryonic imprinting perturbations do not originate from superovulation-induced defects in DNA methylation acquisition. *Fertil Steril* 2011; **96**: 734–8.
50. Kerjean A, Couvert P, Hearns T, *et al.* In vitro follicular growth affects oocyte imprinting establishment in mice. *Eur J Hum Genet* 2003; **11**: 493–6.

51. Anckaert E, Adriaenssens T, Romero S, *et al.* Unaltered imprinting establishment of key imprinted genes in mouse oocytes after in vitro follicle under variable follicle stimulating hormone exposure. *Int J Dev Biol* 2009; **53**: 541–8.

52. Anckaert E, Adriaenssens T, Romero S, *et al.* Ammonium accumulation and use of mineral oil overlay do not alter imprinting establishment at three key imprinted genes in mouse oocytes grown and matured in a long-term follicle culture. *Biol Reprod* 2009; **81**: 666–73.

53. Trapphoff T, El Hajj N, Zechner U, *et al.* DNA integrity, growth pattern, spindle formation, chromosomal constitution and imprinting patterns of mouse oocytes from vitrified pre-antral follicles. *Hum Reprod* 2010; **25**: 3025–42.

54. van Montfoort AP, Hanssen LL, de Sutter P, *et al.* Assisted reproduction treatment and epigenetic inheritance. *Hum Reprod Update* 2012; **18**: 171–9.

55. Wossidlo M, Nakamura T, Lepikhov K, *et al.* 5-Hydroxymethylcytosine in the mammalian zygote is linked with epigenetic reprogramming. *Nat Commun* 2011; **2**:241.

56. Smith ZD, Chan MM, Mikkelsen TS, *et al.* A unique regulatory phase of DNA methylation in the early mammalian embryo. *Nature* 2012; **484**: 339–44.

57. Santos F, Hyslop L, Stojkovic P, *et al.* Evaluation of epigenetic marks in human embryos derived from IVF and ICSI. *Hum Reprod* 2010; **25**: 2387–95.

58. Fauque P, Jouannet P, Lesaffre C, *et al.* Assisted reproductive technology affects developmental kinetics, H19 imprinting control region methylation and H19 gene expression in individual mouse embryos. *BMC Dev Biol* 2007; **7**: 116

59. Market-Velker BA, Zhang L, Magri LS, *et al.* Dual effects of superovulation: loss of maternal and paternal imprinted methylation in a dose-dependent manner. *J Hum Mol Genet* 2010; **19**: 36–51.

60. Fortier AL, Lopes FL, Darricarrere N, *et al.* Superovulation alters the expression of imprinted genes in the midgestation mouse placenta. *Hum Mol Genet* 2008; **17**: 1653–65.

61. De Waal E, Yamazaki Y, Ingale P, *et al.* Gonadotropin stimulation contributes to an increased incidence of epimutations in ICSI-derived mice. *Hum Mol Genet* 2012; **21**: 4460–72.

62. Aston KI, Peterson CM, Carrell DT. Monozygotic twinning associated with assisted reproductive technologies: a review. *Reproduction* 2008; **136**: 377–86.

63. Chang HJ, Lee JRL, Jee BC, *et al.* Impact of blastocyst transfer on offspring sex ratio and monozygotic twinning rate: a systematic review and meta-analysis. *Fertil Steril* 2009; **91**: 2381–90.

64. Weksberg R, Shuman C, Caluseriu O, *et al.* Discordant KCNQ1OT1 imprinting in sets of monozygotic twins discordant for Beckwith-Wiedemann syndrome. *Hum Mol Genet* 2002; **11**: 1317–25.

65. Bestor TH. Imprinting errors and developmental asymmetry. *Phil Trans Royal Soc Lond B Biol Sci* 2003; **358**: 1411–15.

66. Reik W, Walter J. Genomic imprinting: parental influence on the genome. *Nat Rev Genet* 2001; **2**(1): 21–32.

67. Smallwood SA, Kelsey G. De novo DNA methylation: a germ cell perspective. *Trends Genet* 2012; **28**(1): 33–42.

Chapter 34

Genetic basis for primary ovarian insufficiency

Luca Persani, Stephanie Sherman, and Lawrence Nelson

Introduction

Approximately 1% of women under the age of 40 years and 0.1% under the age of 30 years experience "premature menopause" [1]. "Premature menopause" or "premature ovarian failure" (POF) has generally been defined as 4–6 months of amenorrhea in women under the age of 40 years associated with serum gonadotropin concentrations in the postmenopausal range and hypoestrogenism (hypergonadotropic hypogonadism). Depending on the age of onset, the disorder can manifest as failure to enter pubertal development and the associated primary amenorrhea (PA), or secondary amenorrhea (SA) after the onset of menarche and the associated pubertal development [2, 3]. Substantial published evidence has demonstrated that POF may have a long and variable clinical course with the possibility of spontaneous remission and even pregnancy many years after the diagnosis. Therefore, the term primary ovarian insufficiency (POI) is now generally accepted as a less stigmatizing term to young women. It is, as well, a more scientifically accurate definition, to describe more clearly a continuum of intermittent and unpredictable ovarian function [4, 5]. The continuum is divided into two categories of clinical states: (1) POI that is overt, meaning that menstrual cycles have become irregular, and (2) POI that is occult (oPOI), meaning that the menstrual cycles are still regular but other evidence supports a conclusion that ovarian function is impaired [5].

POI generates two orders of consequences, hypoestrogenism and infertility at an early age. Hypoestrogenism can nowadays be acceptably treated by hormone replacement therapy, generally given until the age of physiological menopause. In contrast, fertility cannot be recovered when follicle-stimulating hormone (FSH) is in the menopausal range and the diagnosis of overt POI is made. Also, fertility may well be compromised in the phase of the disease when the clinical manifestations are absent (oPOI). The relevance of this disorder is growing dramatically in recent years because women tend to postpone their conception due to economic reasons or working opportunities.

Pathogenetic mechanisms and genetic origin of POI

The possible mechanisms at the origin of POI can be (a) an initial deficient primordial follicle pool; (b) an accelerated follicular atresia; or (c) an altered maturation/recruitment of primordial follicles. However, in most of the cases in which a pathogenesis has been defined, ovarian insufficiency occurs because of a dramatic reduction in the size of the primordial follicular pool. The etiological causes that may activate such mechanisms are highly heterogeneous and include chromosomal, genetic, autoimmune, metabolic, infectious, and iatrogenic factors [6–8]. At present, about 25% of all forms of POI can be classified as iatrogenic and related to cancer treatment, but more than 50% of the cases remain idiopathic, so that the origins of POI are still largely unknown.

Several observations support a prevalent role of genetic mechanisms in the pathogenesis of idiopathic POI [9]. One important clue is the role of familial trends in the determination of menopausal age. Epidemiological evidence supports the inheritance of menopausal age between mothers and daughters [9–11] and recent genome-wide studies found loci that were significantly associated with age at natural menopause [12]. In a large series of women with POI, the incidence of familial forms ranges from 4% to 31%, depending on the population studied but this percentage can increase further if a familia

Biology and Pathology of the Oocyte, 2nd edn., ed. Alan Trounson, Roger Gosden, and Ursula Eichenlaub-Ritter.
Published by Cambridge University Press.

Table 34.1. List of genetic defects associated with POI and their estimated frequencies

X chromosome defects	**Estimated frequency in POI**	**References**
Turner syndrome and related defects	4–5%	[7, 14, 22]
Fragile X syndrome (*FMR1* premutation)	3–15%	[63]
DIAPH2 disruption (translocation)	Unknown	[7, 14]
BMP15 variants	1.5–12%	[8, 62]
PGRMC1 variants	1.5%	[81]
Autosomal defects Complex diseases		
Galactosemia (*GALT*), BPES (*FOXL2*), APECED (*AIRE*), mitochondrial (*POLG*), Demirhan syndrome (*BMPR1B*), PHP1a (*GNAS*), ovarioleukodystrophy (*EIF2B*), ataxia telangiectasia (*ATM*)	Rare	[7, 8]
Isolated disease		
FSH/LH resistance (*FSHR and LHR*)	0–1%	[72]
INHA variants	0–11%	[79, 80]
GDF9 variants	1.4%	[8, 62]
FOXO3 variants	2.2%	[87]
NOBOX variants	0–6%	[89, 90]
NR5A1 variants	8% in 25 Europeans	[84]
Meiotic gene variants	Rare	[82]
FIGLA variants	2% (in 100 Chinese)	[91]

history of early menopause (EM) between 40 and 45 years of age is considered [13]. Pedigree analysis demonstrates different modes of inheritance, but the more frequent maternal transmission would be consistent with an X-linked inheritance with incomplete penetrance [6, 14, 15]. However, the presence of women with PA, POI, or EM in the same pedigree indicates that POI may be a genetic disease with a highly variable expressivity [16], thus supporting the view of POI as a complex multifactorial disease probably involving the contribution of stochastic events, several alleles, and/or epigenetics. In the next section, we illustrate the main genes involved in the pathogenesis of POI (Table 34.1), either when ovarian insufficiency arises apparently isolated (nonsyndromic forms) or when this defect is part of a complex phenotype involving other organs and tissues (syndromic forms).

Syndromic POI

Turner syndrome

Turner syndrome (TS) is the consequence of complete or partial absence of one X chromosome in a phenotypic female, usually associated with short stature and infertility. In about 50% of the cases there is complete loss of one X chromosome, whereas the remaining patients with TS harbor mosaicism or structural abnormalities of the X chromosome, resulting in a milder phenotype. The prevalence of the disorder is about 1:2500 live female births [17]. In women with 45,X karyotype, oocyte loss occurs in the early stages of meiotic prophase, resulting in gonadal dysgenesis and primary amenorrhea with elevated FSH levels even in early childhood [18]. However, spontaneous menarche and pregnancy have been reported not only in patients with mosaic karyotype, but also in a few women with nonmosaic 45,X [19, 20]. The TS phenotype may be explained by several mechanisms, including the defective pairing of X chromosomes at meiosis [21], but the most substantiated one is the haploinsufficiency of X-linked genes (such as *SHOX*) that physiologically escape X chromosome inactivation and are needed in two copies for ovarian function [22]. The requirement for a double dosage of certain X-linked genes is supported by the observation that complete spontaneous puberty can be reached in 30–40% of patients with 45,X/46,XX mosaics [19]. Consistently, subjects with 45,X have FSH levels already in the postmenopausal range during infancy, whereas FSH levels are frequently normal in patients with mosaic Turner of the same age [18].

Many forms of familial as well as sporadic POI implicate X chromosome aberrations that range from numerical defects, such as the X monosomy and trisomy X, to structural defects, such as deletions, isochromosomes, and balanced X to autosome translocations [14]. Cytogenetic and molecular analysis of women with POI carrying a balanced X to autosome translocation allowed the identification of a "critical region" for ovarian development and function on the long arm of the X chromosome from Xq13.3 to q27. This region could be split into two functionally different portions: Xq13–21 and Xq23–27 [14]. In balanced tranlocations, most breakpoints involve the region Xq13–21, while only interstitial deletions in Xq23–27 were found associated with POI. Alternative mechanisms proposed for the explanation of the ovarian defect account for the size of the critical Xq region [14]. They include the direct disruption of relevant loci or a "position effect" caused by the rearrangements on contiguous genes, which might cause changes in gene transcription. Transcriptional characterization of breakpoint regions led to the identification of five genes interrupted by translocations: the *XPNPEP2* (MIM *300145) gene in Xq25, the *POF1B* (MIM *300603) gene in Xq21.2, the *DACH2* (MIM *300608) gene in Xq21.3, the *CHM* (MIM *300390) gene in Xq21.2, and the *DIAPH2* (MIM *300108) gene in Xq22 [14, 15]. However, breakpoints described in women with POI were frequently mapped in Xq21, outside of genic regions, consistent with models for POI associated with X to autosome translocations that involve extra-X-chromosome effects. Recently, heterochromatin rearrangements of the Xq13–21 region were reported to down-regulate oocyte-expressed genes during oocyte and follicle maturation, indicating that X-linked POI may be an epigenetic disorder [23]. Another model suggests that some translocations adversely affect X chromosome structure leading to defective meiotic pairing that might increase apoptosis of germ cells at meiotic checkpoints [24], thereby leading to POI.

Autoimmune polyendocrinopathy syndrome type I (APS1)

APS1 (Phenotype MIM #240300) is caused by mutation in the autoimmune regulator gene (*AIRE* MIM #607358). The syndrome is characterized by having two of three major clinical findings: Addison disease, and/or hypoparathyroidism, and/or chronic mucocutaneous candidiasis. Generally in this syndrome, the Addison disease has its onset in childhood or early adulthood. APS1 is frequently associated with chronic active hepatitis, malabsorption, juvenile-onset pernicious anemia, alopecia, and primary hypogonadism. Insulin-dependent diabetes mellitus and autoimmune thyroid disease are infrequent in APS1. In 1980 Neufeld *et al.* suggested the presence of three types of autoimmune polyendocrinopathy syndromes [25]. APS2 (MIM #269200) is also known as Schmidt syndrome, the genetics of which has yet to be well defined. APS2 includes patients who have Addison disease in association with autoimmune thyroid disease and/or insulin-dependent diabetes mellitus. APS3 includes patients with autoimmune thyroid disease and another autoimmune disorder other than Addison disease.

In 1990 Ahonen *et al.* reported on 68 patients from 54 families with APS1 [26]. Candidiasis was the presenting symptom in 60% of the patients. POI was present in 60% of the girls and women over the age of 13 years. Hypoparathyroidism was present in 79% and adrenocortical insufficiency in 72%.

Two independent laboratories isolated the gene responsible for APS1 in 1997 and designated it *AIRE* (autoimmune regulator) [27, 28]. The gene is located at 21q22.3. The AIRE protein contains motifs suggestive of a transcription factor, including two zinc finger motifs. AIRE is involved in the induction of tolerance to self-antigens by inducing the expression of numerous peripheral tissue self-antigens in thymic stromal cells. Normally, this promotes the clonal deletion of differentiating T cells that recognize these self-antigens. In the absence of AIRE protein, many tissue-specific self-antigens fail to be expressed in the thymus. This leads to multi-organ autoimmunity because of the faulty negative selection of auto-reactive T cells [29]. Negative selection normally causes death of T cells which have receptors that are highly specific for self-peptides. If these auto-reactive T cells are left unchecked autoimmunity may result. More than 45 mutations in *AIRE* have been identified. Most are inherited in an autosomal recessive manner.

Soderbergh *et al.* in their study of a cohort of 90 patients with APS1 found that the presence of antibodies to 21-hydroxylase (P450 c21) and side chain cleavage enzyme (P450scc) were associated with Addison disease, with odds ratios of 7.8 and 6.8, respectively [30]. In the same report hypogonadism was exclusively associated with antibodies against P450 scc, with an odds ratio of 12.5. Recent evidence has clearly associated antibodies to MATER [31] (also known as NALP5) with the presence of autoimmune POI in women with APS1 [32]. This is intriguing because MATER was first discovered by screening an ovarian cDNA library with immune sera from mice with autoimmune oophoritis generated in the neonatally thymectomized mouse model [33, 34]. MATER protein expression in the ovary is specific to the oocyte [35]. The specific function of MATER has yet to be clearly defined but it appears to play a role in oocyte cytoplasmic lattice formation [36]. Evidence suggests that the autoimmunity to MATER plays a role in the pathogenesis of the disorder rather than as a mere epiphenomenon. Transgenic expression of MATER in antigen-presenting cells induces antigen-specific tolerance with a significant reduction in ovarian autoimmunity in the animal model [37]. Lack of complete disease protection by induction of tolerance to MATER suggests that other oocyte antigens also play a pathogenetic role in the ovarian autoimmunity. Jasti *et al.* examined the fertility and ovarian function of *Aire*-deficient mice and found that only 16% were able to produce two litters [38]. By 20 weeks of age approximately half of these mice exhibited ovarian follicle depletion. This was associated with ovarian infiltration of proliferating CD3+ T lymphocytes and the presence of serum antibodies against oocytes as well as stromal and luteal cells. Taken together the findings are consistent with the hypothesis that ovarian follicular dysfunction and eventual follicular depletion are mechanisms of infertility in *Aire*-deficient mice. The findings have important implications for the pathogenesis of ovarian autoimmunity in women. Interestingly, MATER (NALP5) is also expressed in the human parathyroid and is significantly associated with hypoparathyroidism in APS1 as well as with POI [32].

Women with POI related to steroidogenic cell autoimmunity have lymphocytic autoimmune oophoritis as the mechanism of their POI (Figures 34.1 and 34.2) [39]. Reato *et al.* investigated the prevalence of POI in women with autoimmune Addison disease [40]. In this specific clinical setting they found POI in 41% of women with APS1 and 16% of women with APS2. Overall, 20% of women with Addison disease in this series also had POI. Falorni *et al.* examined the prevalence of steroidogenic cell autoantibodies in women with POI who also had adrenal autoimmunity [41]. They found that women with Addison disease-related POI were in most cases positive for 17-hydroxylase and/or P450scc autoantibodies. Bakalov *et al.* assessed the association between serum adrenal cortex autoantibodies and histologically confirmed autoimmune lymphocytic oophoritis in women who had POI as the presenting complaint and with no history of Addison disease [39]. They assessed serum adrenal cortex antibodies by indirect immunofluorescence and found a statistically significant association between adrenal cortex autoantibodies and histologically confirmed autoimmune lymphocytic oophoritis. Overall, they found that only 4% of women with POI as a presenting complaint tested positive for adrenal cortex antibodies. All four women with histologically confirmed autoimmune lymphocytic oophoritis had serum antibodies against the 21-hydroxylase and P450scc enzymes.

Ovarian antibodies detected by indirect immunofluoresence lack specificity and testing for them is not warranted [42]. Pelvic ultrasound in some cases will identify enlarged multifollicular ovaries which may undergo torsion. Ovarian biopsy does not provide information that helps management and therefore is not indicated outside of an investigational protocol. There is a 50% risk of developing adrenal insufficiency in women who have evidence of adrenal autoimmunity in association with their POI [43]. Patients with POI and evidence for adrenal autoimmunity should be evaluated annually with an adrenocorticotrophic hormone (ACTH) stimulation test. Theoretically, one would expect adrenal-cell antibodies to be present when the ovarian insufficiency develops if the mechanism is steroidogenic cell autoimmunity. However, all patients with POI should be educated regarding the symptoms of adrenal insufficiency and should undergo assessment of adrenal function if symptoms develop.

Blepharophimosis, ptosis, and epicanthus inversus syndrome (BPES)

BPES (MIM #110100) is an autosomal dominant eyelid malformation characterized by BPES and telecanthus. When the condition is associated with POI it is considered type I BPES. When not associated with POI it is considered type II BPES. *FOXL2* (forkhead transcription factor L2) (MIM *605597) is the only gene currently known to be associated with BPES [44]. Animal models of human BPES, including the goat with polled/intersex syndrome (PIS) and the *Foxl2* knockout mice, were shown to replicate the findings in humans [45, 46]. Extensive histological studies showed that FOXL2 can be implicated in the squamous-to-cuboidal transformation of granulosa cells and also in the oocyte activation process. The *FOXL2* gene encodes a nuclear protein, the role of which has not been elucidated yet. More than 125 *FOXL2* variants have been described in individuals with BPES types I and II, demonstrating that phenotypic features

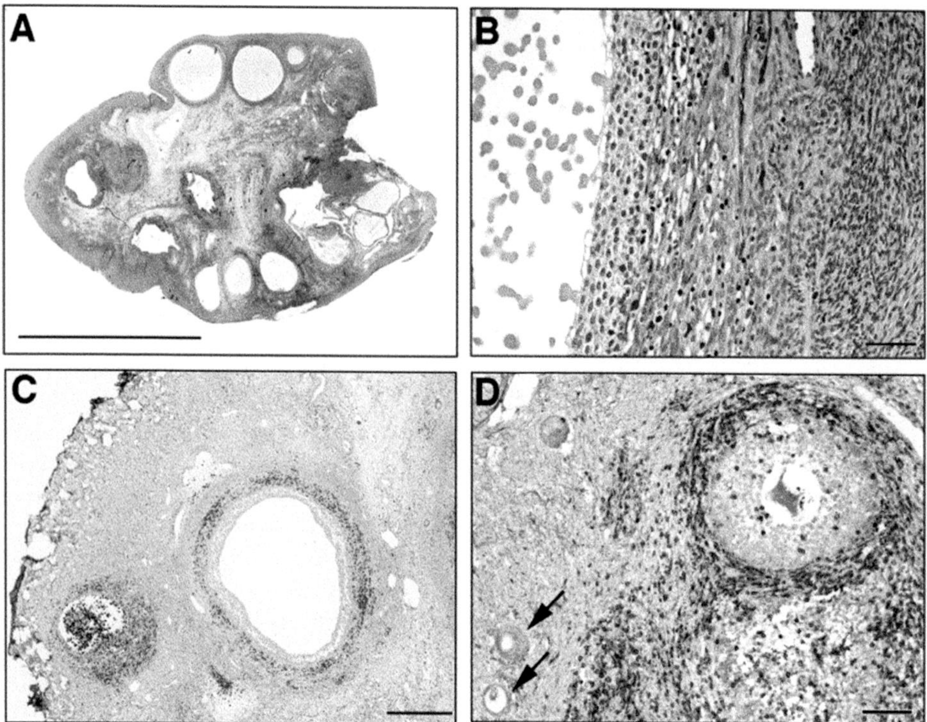

Figure 34.1 Autoimmune lymphocytic oophoritis. Hematoxylin and eosin staining shows multiple antral follicles are present (A), bar = 1 cm. Higher magnification shows lymphocytic infiltration of the theca of an antral follicle and luteinized granulosa cells (B), bar = 50 μm. Immunoperoxidase staining for CD3 highlights infiltration of lymphocytes into the theca in this patient (C), bar = 500 μm. Immunoperoxidase staining for CD3 demonstrates infiltration of lymphocytes into the theca of a preantral follicle and presence of earlier stage follicles free of lymphocytic infiltration (arrows) (D), bar = 100 μm.

are caused by the pleiotropic effect of a single gene (FOXL2 mutation database at http://medgen.ugent.be/foxl2) [47]. Intragenic mutations of all types represent about 80% of the genetic defects found in BPES cohorts. Genomic rearrangements comprising deletions encompassing *FOXL2* entire gene or located outside its transcription unit represent 12% and 5% of all genetic defects, respectively [47].

A genotype–phenotype correlation for intragenic mutations was proposed: mutations predicted to result in proteins with truncation before the poly-Ala tract might be associated with BPES type I, whereas poly-Ala expansions might rather lead to BPES type II. These correlations were based on the classification of intragenic mutations into seven groups according to their effect on the predicted protein that is likely to be produced [47]. A recent model of FOXL2 protein proposed that mutants can be sorted into two classes: those that potentially alter protein–protein interactions and those that might disrupt the interactions with DNA [48]. However, recently reported cases emphasize the importance of long-term clinical follow-up of ovarian function also in patients with a poly-Ala expansion [8].

Recently, the first functional study supporting a role of FOXL2 mutations in non-syndromic POI was reported [49]. Nevertheless, FOXL2 sequence variants in POI cases without BPES appear to be a rare event.

Galactosemia and carbohydrate-deficient glycoprotein syndromes (CDGs)

Galactosemia (MIM #230400) is a hereditary disorder of galactose metabolism caused by deficiency of GALT (MIM *606999) enzyme (galactose-1-phosphatase uridyltransferase). The incidence of disease in Europe and North America is about 1:30 000–1:50 000 [50]). Galactosemia presents with the worst complications in organs with high GALT expression, such as liver, kidney, ovary and heart. More than 220 mutations have been described in *GALT* gene [51]; however, two

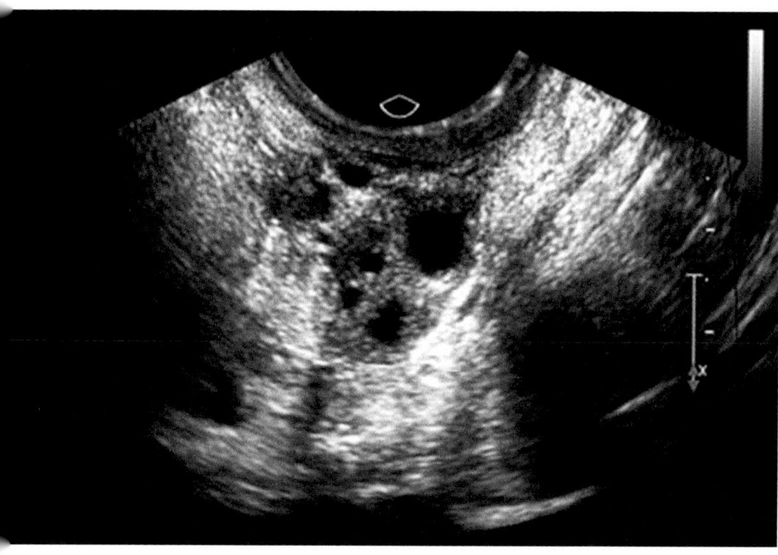

Figure 34.2 Transvaginal ultrasound scan from a patient with spontaneous 46,XX primary ovarian insufficiency who had follicle dysfunction due to autoimmune oophoritis. The ovary appears normal, with the presence of multiple follicles, despite amenorrhea, estrogen deficiency, and menopausal-level gonadotropins. Autoimmune oophoritis with thecal infiltration by lymphocytes was confirmed histologically by means of an ovarian biopsy performed when the patient was 26 years of age.

ommon mutations (Q188R and K285N) account or more than 70% of cases associated with impaired ALT function [52]. POI occurs in almost all women omozygous for mutations in the *GALT* gene that artially or completely abolish GALT activity and are ssociated with a severe phenotype [53]. FSH levels an be increased from birth to puberty and the timing f the damage to the ovary can vary, but is frequently ssociated with primary amenorrhea [50]. Pathoenetic mechanisms at the origin of galactosemia are ot well understood. Spontaneous pregnancies have een reported in a few women with galactosemia, ven when biochemical markers (undetectable anti-Müllerian hormone [AMH] and estradiol, and high onadotropins) were indicative of ovarian failure [54].

Genetic defects of enzymes providing glycosylaion of proteins (CDG syndromes) are rare an complex iseases generally characterized by severe systemic isorders, and ovarian defects may be seen indicating hat glycosylation of ovarian glycoproteins is critical or ovarian function.

seudo-hypoparathyroidism ype 1a (PHP1A)

he first intracellular element downstream of onadotropin receptors is Gsα, the G protein whose ctivation couples the stimulation of FSH and uteinizing hormone (LH) receptors (FSHR and LHR) o their enzymatic effector, adenylate cyclase. This rotein is encoded by a gene locus (*GNAS1*) (MIM +139320) on chromosome 20q13 that is subject to parental imprinting. *GNAS1* loss-of-function variants inherited from the mother are known to cause a generalized form of hormone resistance named pseudo-hypoparathyroidism type 1a (PHP1a). The presence of gonadotropin resistance and POI in these patients is justified by the preferential expression of a mutant maternal allele in gonads as in other target tissues of peptide hormones acting through the same G protein-coupled receptor (GPCR)–Gsα–cAMP pathway [55].

Progressive external ophthalmoplegia (PEO)

The *POLG* gene (MIM *174763) encodes for DNA polymerase gamma, the enzyme which replicates the human mitochondrial DNA. Mutations in this gene are causative of the autosomal dominant (MIM #157640) or recessive (MIM #258450) progressive external ophthalmoplegia (PEO), a disease characterized by weakness of the ocular muscles and fatigue secondary to the depletion of mitochondria in specific tissues. It is a genetically heterogeneous disease: dominant POLG mutations cluster in the polymerase (*pol*) domain while the recessive ones affect the proofreading (exonuclease, *exo*) domain. Luoma *et al.* described co-segregation of POI and parkinsonism with POLG *pol*-domain mutations in three families with PEO [56]. The POI manifestations were variable from PA to SA at 44 years of age, frequently anticipating the other manifestations. Pagnamenta *et al.* described dominantly maternally inherited POI in a three-generation pedigree in association with PEO and parkinsonism [57].

Ovarioleukodystrophy

Ovarian leukodystrophy is the name used by Schiffmann *et al.* to describe an unusual association of POI with vanishing white matter (VWM) disease observed in four patients on MRI [58]. VWM disease (MIM #603896) is characterized by slowly progressive neurological deterioration, but the onset is extremely variable, including prenatal period until adult age. Also the ovarian insufficiency onset is different among affected females and it could result in PA or SA. Moreover, the age at onset of neurological degeneration correlated positively with the severity of ovarian dysfunction [59]. The basic defect of VWM disease is associated with variations in any of the five subunits of eukaryotic translation initiation factor EIF2B. This factor has an important role in preventing accumulation of denatured proteins during cellular stress.

Ataxia telangiectasia

The *ATM* (ataxia telangiectasia mutated) gene (MIM *607585) encodes a protein kinase that is involved in cell-cycle regulation [60] and is also required for processing the DNA strand breaks that occur during meiosis, immune system maturation, and for telomere maintenance. Mutations in the *ATM* gene generally result in the total loss of the protein and are the underlying causes of ataxiatelangiectasia (AT; MIM #208900), an autosomal recessive neurodegenerative disorder characterized by uncoordinated movements and ocular telangiectases, chromosome instability, radiosensitivity, immunodeficiency, and a predisposition to cancer. Some patients with AT present ovarian insufficiency due to gonadal hypoplasia with a complete absence of mature gametes. The mouse phenotype closely resembles the human phenotype. *Atm*-deficient mutant female mice lack primordial and mature follicles, and oocytes, resulting in extremely small ovaries [8].

Demirhan syndrome

Demirhan *et al.* reported the case of a 16-year-old girl with acromesomelic chondrodysplasia, genital anomalies, amenorrhea, and hypergonadotropic hypogonadism due to a homozygous deletion in *BMPR1B*, the gene coding for bone morphogenetic protein receptor 1B (MIM *603248) [61]. Acromesomelic chondrodysplasias are hereditary skeletal disorders characterized by short stature, very short limbs, and hand/foot malformations. *BMPR1B* variants can occur naturally also in animals and are associated with the hyperprolific Booroola phenotype in sheep, while the female knockout mice present with brachydactyly and infertility [62].

Non-syndromic POI

Fragile X mental retardation 1 (*FMR1*)

The *FMR1* gene is located on the X chromosome and includes a trinucleotide repeat sequence, (CGG)n, in its 5′ untranslated region. Common alleles include 6–44 CGG repeats, typically with AGG interspersions every 9 or 10 repeats. When expanded to 55–200 repeats, this "premutation" is unstable when transmitted and has the potential to expand to over 200 repeats in one generation. This resulting "full" mutation leads to the silencing of the *FMR1* gene due to hypermethylation of the repeat and regulatory regions and causes fragile X syndrome, the most common inherited form of intellectual and developmental disabilities. The premutation is carried by about 1/250 women. Among women who carry the premutation, approximately 15–24% have POI [63], the disorder referred to as fragile X-associated primary ovarian insufficiency (FXPOI). About 11.5% (95% CI: 5.4–20.8%) of women with familial POI and 3.2% (95% CI: 1.4–6.2%) of those with sporadic POI carry the premutation [63]. Thus, the *FMR1* premutation has emerged as the leading known heritable cause of both sporadic and familial POI.

Studies of the hormonal profile of women with the premutation who are still cycling are consistent with the normal hypothalamic–pituitary–gonadal axis of an aging ovary: increased FSH and decreased inhibin β in the follicular phase and decreased inhibin α and progesterone in the luteal phase [64]. Recent studies have shown reduced levels of AMH among premutation carriers compared with non-carriers, again consistent with an aging ovary (e.g., [65]).

Two factors have surfaced as potential predictors of risk and severity of FXPOI, namely repeat size (e.g., [66]) and mean age at menopause of first-degree relatives (e.g., [67]). With respect to repeat size, a non-linear relationship with severity of FXPOI has been established: premutation carriers with the highest risk for FXPOI turn out to be those with about 80–100 repeats, not those with >100 repeats. Consistently, among those with 80–100 repeats, the onset of FXPOI was earliest, sometimes as early as the adolescent years. More work is needed to better define which repeat size alleles impose the highest risk and why. The second established risk factor is mean age at menopause of first-degree relatives (e.g., [67]). Thus, modifying genes play a substantial role in the variability of age at menopause among premutation carriers.

The mechanism leading to FXPOI is understudied. It is known that as the premutation repeat size increases, the level of *FMR1* transcripts containing a large repeat tract increases and the level of FMRP, the resulting protein, decreases (e.g., [68]). The toxic effect of the premutation could have its influence at several levels. FMR1 mRNA studies in the mouse (e.g., [69]) and FMRP expression studies in fetal ovaries [70] indicate that FMRP is highly expressed in the germ cells of the fetal ovary. Thus, FMRP may play a role in oogonia proliferation and the development of a woman's initial ovarian reserve. Interestingly, several studies have indicated that FMRP is expressed in granulosa cells in maturing follicles only, not those in the early stage (e.g., [69, 71]). Schuettler *et al.* suggested that this cellular shift of FMRP expression to granulosa cells during follicle maturation after birth indicates a role for FMRP in the maturation of an oocyte [71].

Based on the knowledge that FMRP regulates mRNA translation through a suppression mechanism, perhaps increased levels of FMRP at specific times during development could lead to haploinsufficiency of proteins needed in oocyte development or for follicle development and survival. Alternatively, the large CGG repeat track in the mRNA produced by the premutation allele may cause a cumulative toxic effect in granulosa cells, leading to an increased rate of follicular atresia later in a woman's reproductive life.

Gonadotropin receptors

FSH and LH receptors are glycoprotein hormone receptors belonging to the GPCR family [72]. Together with their binding hormones, LH and FSH, these receptors are essential for the normal reproductive function in both sexes. Loss-of-function mutations affecting these receptors cause gonadotropin resistance with hypergonadotropic hypogonadism. However, such mutations are rare. A linkage analysis in the Finnish population revealed a significant association between a locus on 2p21, which contains both of the genes encoding FSHR and LHR, and ovarian dysgenesis (MIM #233300). The analysis of the *FSHR* gene (MIM *136435) revealed a homozygous missense mutation that determines the p.A189V substitution in the extracellular domain of the receptor. This type of POI follows a classical recessive transmission with homozygous female carriers affected by PA and ovarian failure. From in vitro studies, this mutant receptor is retained inside the cells thus causing a complete FSH resistance. The p.A189V mutation appears to be particularly frequent only in the Finnish population and it was not found in most other populations [72]. Other mutations in different regions of the *FSHR* gene have nowadays been reported in women with the classical biochemical phenotype of POI (FSH higher than LH levels). Complete FSH resistance is associated with absent pubertal development and PA and partial forms are characterized by post-pubertal POI and SA. However, both the complete and partial forms undergo a typical recessive inheritance [72].

Biallelic inactivating variants of the *LHR* gene (MIM +152790) are a rare cause of POI in women who have a 46,XX karyotype. They represent a particular form of the disease characterized by LH levels higher than those of FSH. Evidence for a particular phenotype of ovarian insufficiency in women with LH resistance was obtained by the pedigree studies of males affected with Leydig cell hypoplasia [73]. Differently from male patients, the degree of LH resistance must be severe to cause the POI phenotype which is in general characterized by oligoamenorrhea or SA with evidence of multiple antral follicles on ultrasound. Ovarian biopsies reveal all stages of follicular development until the pre-ovulatory stage, but typically ovulation fails to occur.

Ligands of transforming growth factor beta (TGFβ)

Several TGFβ-like factors are expressed in the ovarian follicle, either by the oocyte or by granulosa cells [74]. These factors are known to promote growth and differentiation (GDFs) in the tissues where they are expressed and include GDFs, bone morphogenetic proteins (BMPs), as well as inhibins, activins, or AMH.

TGFβs are commonly translated as pre-pro-proteins. The pro-region typically regulates post-translational processing and dimerization of mature peptide, forming either hetero- or homodimeric proteins which finally exert the biological activity at the target cell. The follicular paracrine action of several of these factors has been shown to be required for correct folliculogenesis and the encoding genes have been investigated in the case of POI [8, 62].

Bone morphogenetic protein 15 (BMP15)

The *BMP15* gene (MIM *300247) encodes an oocyte-derived growth and differentiation factor which is involved in follicular development as a critical regulator of many granulosa cell processes [62, 74]. The main roles of BMP15 include: (a) the promotion of follicle maturation from the primordial gonadotropin-independent phases of folliculogenesis; (b) regulation of follicular granulosa cell sensitivity to FSH action; (c) prevention of granulosa cell apoptosis; (d) promotion of oocyte developmental competence; and (e) regulation of ovulation quota [74, 75]. The relevance of BMP15 action in ovarian folliculogenesis was initially shown by experimental and natural models. All together, the data so far collected in different mammalian species indicate that the role of BMP15 may be more critical in mono-ovulating species (such as sheep and human) than in the poly-ovulating ones (mice). Natural missense mutations in several strains of ewes cause a hyperprolificacy phenotype in the heterozygous state and a female infertility with complete block of folliculogenesis in the homozygous state [62, 74, 75]. *BMP15* maps to a locus on the short arm of the X chromosome (Xp11.2) within a "POF critical region" where several of the Turner syndrome traits are located, including POI [15, 22]. In humans, mutations in the *BMP15* gene have been found in association with both PA and SA in several worldwide POI cohorts, with a variable prevalence between 1.5% and 12% [8]. The first heterozygous mutation of the *BMP15* gene (p.Y235C) was reported in two Italian sisters with hypergonadotropic ovarian insufficiency characterized by PA and ovarian dysgenesis, who inherited the genetic alteration from the unaffected father [76]. This mutation was located in a residue highly conserved among species and generated aberrant high-molecular-weight products in vitro. Since then, other variants have been identified with variable frequency in patients from Europe, USA, North Africa, India, China, and Asia [62]. Almost all of these are missense variations found in the heterozygous state. These variations are also located in the gene sequence encoding the pro-region of the protein and generate hampered processing and a significant reduction of their biological effects [77]. Importantly, some of the missense variations in the *BMP15* gene have also been found in a low percentage of the control populations, a finding that may question or diminish their pathogenetic role. In light of these findings, one could hypothesize that BMP15 variations might play a predisposing role in a context of POI considered as a complex multifactorial disorder, in contrast with the view of POI as a monogenic disorder.

Growth differentiation factor 9 (GDF9)

GDF9 (MIM *601918) is the homologous gene of *BMP15* (also named *GDF9b*). *GDF9* is also expressed in the oocyte and its products can form non-covalent heterodimers acting in a synergistic manner on ovarian function on surrounding follicular granulosa cells. From experimental animals, GDF9 function is more critical in poly-ovulating species such as mice where GDF9 is required for folliculogenesis [62, 74]. Natural *GDF9* gene mutations with ovarian effects similar to those seen in BMP15 mutants were also detected in Cambridge and Belclare sheep [75]. GDF9 human variations described so far in different ethnicities are all missense and heterozygous, affect exclusively the pro-region with a prevalence of 1.4%, and were not detected in the control samples [62]. Some rare insertion/deletion and missense variations in *GDF9* gene have also been associated with spontaneous dizygotic twinning; the reported frequency of these variants is around 4%, confirming a possible role of this factor in the determination of ovulation quota also in humans.

Inhibin α (INHA)

INHA is another candidate gene for mutational studies in humans, given its important role in regulating ovarian function either as a negative modulator of pituitary FSH synthesis or as a paracrine factor. *INHA* gene knockout mice lack the bioactive inhibin dimers thus resulting in raised FSH levels, infertility, and sex cord stromal tumors at an early age with nearly 100% penetrance, demonstrating that inhibin functions in vivo as a tumor suppressor in the gonads of mice [78]. The first evidence of a genetic association between inhibin and

POI came from a woman with POI with the translocation 46,XX,t(2;15)(q32.3;q13.3). The translocation breakpoint on chromosome 2 interrupted the inhibin α (*INHA*; MIM *147380) subunit locus (2q33–36); therefore, further investigations have been aimed at the mutational screening of this gene [79]. One missense variation of the *INHA* gene (p.A257T) has been associated with POI in several populations, with a prevalence of 0–11% depending on the ethnicity of the population studied. A more recent study in a large cohort of Italian and German subjects found no differences in variant frequency was detected between POI cases and controls [80]. However, a meta-analysis of the random effects on the risk of POI in carriers of the *INHA* variant from the most relevant studies revealed a combined risk difference of 0.04 with 95% confidence interval (−0.03 to 0.11) [79]. On these bases, it is plausible that the *INHA* variant allele might confer a susceptibility to develop POI.

Progesterone receptor membrane component 1 (PGRMC1)

The *PGRMC1* (MIM *300435) gene was recently described as a new candidate thanks to the finding of an X/autosome translocation in a mother and daughter both diagnosed with POI that maps within the X "critical region" for POI at Xq13–26. The subsequent screening of the entire gene has been performed on a cohort of 67 women with idiopathic POI and revealed one patient with sporadic POI that was heterozygous for a single missense substitution (p. H165R) located in the intracellular C-terminus, within a domain which is essential for the non-transcriptional regulation of cytochrome P450. The missense variation of PGRMC1 would impair the anti-apoptotic action of progesterone in the developing ovary, resulting in the premature loss of ovarian follicles and, ultimately, in ovarian insufficiency [81].

Meiotic genes

Since animal models affected by a disrupted expression of meiotic genes showed a rapid depletion of germ cells in the ovaries, a recent study investigated whether variations in such genes may be associated with POI [82]. The authors analyzed genes involved in meiosis, including *DMC1* or *LIM15* (MIM *602721), *MSH4* (MIM *602105), MSH5 (MIM *603382), and *SPO11* (MIM *605114). The sequencing of genomic DNA from 41 women with POI led to the identification of a single heterozygous missense substitution in *MSH5* (p. P29S) in two White women. This variant was not found in 36 controls. Another woman with POI, of African origin, showed a homozygous change in *DMC1* gene (p. M200V). This study needs further confirmation in larger cohorts of patients and controls and functional studies evaluating the consequence of the variants.

Transcription factors

Steroidogenic factor 1 (SF1) or NR5A1

The *NR5A1* (MIM +184757) gene encodes a nuclear receptor expressed in bipotential gonads from early human embryonic development. NR5A1 is a key transcriptional regulator of genes involved in the hypothalamic–pituitary–steroidogenic axis [83], including *STAR*, *CYP11A1*, *CYP17A1*, *CYP19A1*, *LH/CGR*, and *INHA*. Mutations of *NR5A1* were described in cases of 46,XY disorders of sex development (DSD), with or without adrenal failure. Recently, NR5A1 mutations were also detected in members of four families with histories of both 46,XY DSD and 46,XX POI and also in 2/25 women with isolated ovarian insufficiency but in none of 700 control alleles [84]. Mutations were associated with a range of ovarian anomalies, including gonadal dysgenesis with PA or SA. Functional analysis revealed that each mutant protein had altered transactivational properties on gonadal promoters important for follicle growth and maturation.

Forkhead transcription factors

The family of forkhead transcription factors comprises over 100 members involved in several developmental processes, including the mediation of TGFβ superfamily signals by binding to members of the Smad family proteins. Similarly to FOXL2, a small subfamily of forkhead transcription factors consisting of *FOXO3a* (MIM *602681), *FOXO1a* (MIM *136533), and *FOXO4* (MIM *300033) also has a key role in ovarian function. Foxo3a knockout female mice exhibit a marked age-dependent decline in reproductive fitness due to a premature follicular development leading to oocyte death and early depletion of follicles, which results in infertility [85]. In contrast, the constitutive expression of Foxo3a in the oocytes of transgenic mice leads to a delayed follicular development and oocyte growth, causing infertility. Furthermore, constitutive expression of Foxo3a determines a significant reduction in BMP15 expression, suggesting a regulatory action of Foxo3a on this factor [86]. The ovarian phenotype of mouse models resembles the human POI phenotype, thus suggesting that *FOXO3a* could be a candidate gene for POI in women. The first mutation screening in POI patients revealed two potentially pathogenic variations that were absent in controls (p. S421L and p. R506H) in 2 out of 90 POI cases from New Zealand and Slovenia (2.2%) [87]. A subsequent analysis on 50 patients of a French cohort identified only one amino acid substitution (p. Y593S) probably with no deleterious impact on protein function [88].

Oocyte-specific transcription factors

NOBOX (Newborn ovary homeobox) (MIM *610934) and *FIGLA* (factor in germline alpha) (MIM *608697) encode two oocyte-specific transcription factors that regulate genes unique to oocytes. *NOBOX* is a homeobox gene that is critical for specifying an oocyte-restricted gene expression pattern. *Nobox* deletion in knockout mice accelerates postnatal oocyte loss, with follicles replaced by fibrous tissue, resulting in a phenotype similar to non-syndromic POI in women. Causative mutations in this gene have been investigated recently in several populations. A missense variant (p. R355H), which disrupts the binding of the NOBOX homeodomain to DNA, has been reported in 1 of 96 White women with POI from the United States [89]; though two studies failed to find causative mutations in Japanese and Chinese series [8], a French group identified a 6.2% prevalence of NOBOX mutations in a large series of women with POI suggesting one should consider *NOBOX* as the first autosomal candidate gene involved in this syndrome [90].

FIGLA is a basic helix-loop-helix transcription factor that regulates the expression of zona pellucida genes. Female *Figla*$^{-/-}$ mice show rapid oocyte loss after birth and no primordial follicle formation. The ovarian phenotype in knockout mice thus suggested that *FIGLA* variations might contribute to human POI. A mutational study identified two heterozygous deletions in 2 unrelated cases among 100 Chinese subjects with POI. These variants were not detected among 304 ethnically matched controls. Molecular analyses showed that these variants may indeed have a pathogenic role [91].

Conclusions

The prevalence of known genetic alterations in women with POI can nowadays be estimated as ranging from 20% to 25% of the cases originally classified as idiopathic. Therefore, the pathogenetic mechanism still remains unknown in most of the cases. However, when a genetic alteration is found in a woman it can be useful for family counseling by predicting the woman's relatives that are at higher risk for POI and fertility loss at young age. The women carriers will thus be able to program their conception before ovarian insufficiency occurs. This possibility is becoming more and more important as women throughout the world tend to conceive more frequently while in their thirties and forties, when the risk of POI in the general population is about 1–10%. At present, a facility involved in the counseling on female infertility should screen women with POI for the most prevalent genetic alterations, that is, X chromosome abnormalities and the *FMR1* premutation. The finding of these abnormalities has obvious implications for family counseling beyond fertility including the risk of X-linked male mental retardation associated with *FMR1* full mutation. More recent works may suggest the possibility of including the investigation of the *BMP15* gene and, if the initial studies are confirmed, *FIGLA, NOBOX,* and *NR5A1* genes should be added. The aim of several groups around the world is to increase in the near future the sensitivity of genetic screening and possibly develop a test for the prediction of menopausal age. This may indeed open the possibility of an efficient counseling service for infertility in women and establish "ad hoc" interventions for the prevention of the consequences of POI [8].

Acknowledgments

The authors are supported by the following grants Telethon Foundation Italy, grant: GGP09126A to L. P. NIH P30 HD24064 to S. S.; the Intramural Research Program, National Institute of Child Health and Human Development, National Institutes of Health to L. N.

References

1. Coulam CB, Adamson SC, Annegers JF. Incidence of premature ovarian failure. *Obstet Gynecol* 1986; **67**: 604–6.

2. Timmreck LS, Reindollar RH. Contemporary issues in primary amenorrhea. *Obstet Gynecol Clin North Am* 2003; **30**: 287–302.
3. Beck-Peccoz P, Persani L. Premature ovarian failure. *Orphanet J Rare Dis* 2006; **1**: 9.
4. Welt CK. Primary ovarian insufficiency: a more accurate term for premature ovarian failure. *Clin Endocrinol* 2008; **68**: 499–509.
5. Nelson LM. Clinical practice. Primary ovarian insufficiency. *N Engl J Med* 2009; **360**: 606–14.
6. Goswami D, Conway GS. Premature ovarian failure. *Hum Reprod Update* 2005; **11**: 391–410.
7. Simpson JL. Genetic and phenotypic heterogeneity in ovarian failure: overview of selected candidate genes. *Ann NY Acad Sci* **1135**: 146–54.
8. Persani L, Rossetti R, Cacciatore C. Genes involved in human ovarian failure. *J Mol Endocrinol* 2010; **45**: 257–79.
9. Cramer DW, Xu H, Harlow BL. Family history as a predictor of early menopause. *Fertil Steril* 1995; **64**: 740–5.
10. Torgerson DJ, Thomas RE, Reid DM. Mothers and daughters menopausal ages: is there a link? *Eur J Obstet Gynecol Reprod Biol* 1997; **74**: 63–6.
11. Murabito JM, Yang Q, Fox C, Wilson PW, Cupples LA. Heritability of age at natural menopause in the Framingham Heart Study. *J Clin Endocrinol Metab* 2005; **90:** 3427–30.
12. Stolk L, Perry JR, Chasman DI, *et al.* Meta-analyses identify 13 loci associated with age at menopause and highlight DNA repair and immune pathways. *Nat Genet* 2012; **44**: 260–8.
13. Vegetti W, Grazia Tibiletti M, Testa G, *et al.* Inheritance in idiopathic premature ovarian failure: analysis of 71 cases. *Hum Reprod* 1998; **13:** 1796–800.
14. Toniolo D. X-linked premature ovarian failure: a complex disease. *Curr Opin Genet Dev* 2006; **16**: 293–300.
15. Persani L, Rossetti R, Cacciatore C, Bonomi M. Primary ovarian insufficiency: X chromosome defects and autoimmunity. *J Autoimmun* 2009; **33**: 35–41.
16. Tibiletti MG, Testa G, Vegetti W, *et al.* The idiopathic forms of premature menopause and early menopause show the same genetic pattern. *Hum Reprod* 1999; **14**: 2731–4.
17. Sybert VP, McCauley E. Turner's syndrome. *N Engl J Med* 2004; **351**: 1227–38.
18. Fechner PY, Davenport ML, Qualy RL, *et al.* Toddler Turner Study Group. Differences in follicle-stimulating hormone secretion between 45,X monosomy Turner syndrome and 45,X/46,XX mosaicism are evident at an early age. *J Clin Endocrinol Metab* 2006; **91**: 4896–902.
19. Pasquino AM, Passeri F, Pucarelli I, Segni M, Municchi G. Spontaneous pubertal development in Turner's syndrome. Italian Study Group for Turner's Syndrome. *J Clin Endocrinol Metab* 1997; **82**: 1810–13.
20. Livadas S, Xekouki P, Kafiri G, *et al.* Spontaneous pregnancy and birth of a normal female from a woman with Turner syndrome and elevated gonadotropins. *Fertil Steril* 2005; **83**: 769–72.
21. Ogata T, Matsuo N. Turner syndrome and female sex chromosome aberrations: deduction of the principal factors involved in the development of clinical features. *Hum Genet* 1995; **95**: 607–29.
22. Zinn AR, Ross JL. Turner syndrome and haploinsufficiency. *Curr Opin GenetDev* 1998; **8**: 322–7.
23. Rizzolio F, Pramparo T, Sala C, *et al.* 2009 Epigenetic analysis of the critical region I for premature ovarian failure: demonstration of a highly heterochromatic domain on the long arm of the mammalian X chromosome. *J Med Genet* 1998; **46**: 585–92.
24. Schlessinger D, Herrera L, Crisponi L, *et al.* Genes and translocations involved in POF. *Am J Med Genet* 2002; **111**: 328–33.
25. Neufeld M, Maclaren N, Blizzard RM. Autoimmune polyglandular syndromes. *Pediatr Ann* 1980; **9**: 43–53.
26. Ahonen P, Myllarniemi S, Sipila I, Perheentupa J. Clinical variation of autoimmune polyendocrinopathy-candidiasis-ectodermal dystrophy (APECED) in a series of 68 patients. *N Engl J Med* 1990; **322**: 1829–36.
27. Nagamine K, Peterson P, Scott HS, *et al.* Positional cloning of the APECED gene. *Nat Genet* 1997; **17**(4): 393–8.
28. Finnish-German APECED Consortium. An autoimmune disease, APECED, caused by mutations in a novel gene featuring two PHD-type zinc-finger domains. *Nat Genet* 1997; **17**(4): 399–403.
29. Anderson MS, Venanzi ES, Klein L, *et al.* Projection of an immunological self shadow within the thymus by the aire protein. *Science* 2002; **298**(5597): 1395–401.
30. Soderbergh A, Myhre AG, Ekwall O, *et al.* Prevalence and clinical associations of 10 defined autoantibodies in autoimmune polyendocrine syndrome type I. *J Clin Endocrinol Metab* 2004; **89**(2): 557–62.
31. Tong ZB, Bondy CA, Zhou J, Nelson LM. A human homologue of mouse Mater, a maternal effect gene essential for early embryonic development. *Hum Reprod* 2002; **17**(4): 903–11.
32. Alimohammadi M, Bjorklund P, Hallgren A, *et al.* Autoimmune polyendocrine syndrome type 1 and

NALP5, a parathyroid autoantigen. *N Engl J Med* 2008; **358**(10): 1018–28.

33. Tong ZB, Nelson LM. A mouse gene encoding an oocyte antigen associated with autoimmune premature ovarian failure. *Endocrinology* 1999; **140**(8): 3720–6.
34. Tong ZB, Gold L, Pfeifer KE, *et al.* Mater, a maternal effect gene required for early embryonic development in mice. *Nat Genet* 2000; **26**(3): 267–8.
35. Tong ZB, Gold L, De Pol A *et al.* Developmental expression and subcellular localization of mouse MATER, an oocyte-specific protein essential for early development. *Endocrinology* 2004; **145**(3): 1427–34.
36. Kim B, Kan R, Anguish L, Nelson LM, Coonrod SA. Potential role for MATER in cytoplasmic lattice formation in murine oocytes. *PLoS One* 2010; **5**(9): e12587.
37. Otsuka N, Tong ZB, Vanevski K, *et al.* Autoimmune oophoritis with multiple molecular targets mitigated by transgenic expression of mater. *Endocrinology* 2011; **152**(6): 2465–73.
38. Jasti S, Warren BD, McGinnis LK, *et al.* The autoimmune regulator prevents premature reproductive senescence in female mice. *Biol Reprod* 2012; **86**(4): 110.
39. Bakalov VK, Anasti JN, Calis KA, *et al.* Autoimmune oophoritis as a mechanism of follicular dysfunction in women with 46,XX spontaneous premature ovarian failure. *Fertil Steril* 2005; **84**(4): 958–65.
40. Reato G, Morlin L, Chen S, *et al.* Premature ovarian failure in patients with autoimmune Addison's disease: clinical, genetic, and immunological evaluation. *J Clin Endocrinol Metab* 2011; **96**(8): E1255–61.
41. Falorni A, Laureti S, Candeloro P, *et al.* Steroid-cell autoantibodies are preferentially expressed in women with premature ovarian failure who have adrenal autoimmunity. *Fertil Steril* 2002; **78**(2): 270–9.
42. Novosad JA, Kalantaridou SN, Tong ZB, Nelson LM. Ovarian antibodies as detected by indirect immunofluorescence are unreliable in the diagnosis of autoimmune premature ovarian failure: a controlled evaluation. *BMC Womens Health* 2003; **3**(1): 2.
43. Betterle C, Volpato M, Rees SB, *et al.* I. Adrenal cortex and steroid 21-hydroxylase autoantibodies in adult patients with organ-specific autoimmune diseases: markers of low progression to clinical Addison's disease. *J Clin Endocrinol Metab* 1997; **82**(3): 932–8.
44. Crisponi L, Deiana M, Loi A, *et al.* The putative forkhead transcription factor FOXL2 is mutated in blepharophimosis/ptosis/epicanthus inversus syndrome. *Nat Genet* 2001; **27**: 159–66.
45. Schmidt D, Ovitt CE, Anlag K, *et al.* The murine winged-helix transcription factor Foxl2 is required for granulosa cell differentiation and ovary maintenance. *Development* 2004; **131**: 933–42.
46. Uda M, Ottolenghi C, Crisponi L, *et al.* Foxl2 disruption causes mouse ovarian failure by pervasive blockage of follicle development. *Hum Mol Genet* 2004; **13**: 1171–81.
47. Beysen D, De Paepe A, De Baere E. Mutation update: *FOXL2* mutations and genomic rearrangements in BPES. *Hum Mutat* 2009; **30**: 158–69.
48. Nallathambi J, Laissue P, Batista F, *et al.* Differential functional effects of novel mutations of the transcription factor FOXL2 in BPES patients. *Hum Mutat* 2008; **29**: E123–31.
49. Laissue P, Lakhal B, Benayoun BA, *et al.* Functional evidence implicating FOXL2 in non syndromic premature ovarian failure and in the regulation of the transcription factor OSR2. *J Med Genet* 2009; **46**: 455–7.
50. Rubio-Gozalbo ME, Gubbels CS, Bakker JA, *et al.* Gonadal function in male and female patients with classic galactosemia. *Hum Reprod Update* 2010; **16**: 177–88.
51. Calderon FRO, Phansalkar AR, Crockett DK, Miller M, Mao R. Mutation database for the galactose-1-phosphate uridyltransferase (GALT) gene. *Hum Mutat* 2007; **28**: 939–43.
52. Tyfield L, Reichardt J, Fridovich-Keil J, *et al.* Classical galactosemia and mutations at the galactose-1-phosphate uridyl transferase (GALT) gene. *Hum Mutat* 1999; **13:** 417–30.
53. Waggoner DD, Buist NR, Donnell GN. Long-term prognosis in galactosaemia: results of a survey of 350 cases. *J Inherit Metab Dis* 1990; **13**: 802–18.
54. Gubbels CS, Land JA, Rubio-Gozalbo ME. Fertility and impact of pregnancies on the mother and child in classic galactosemia. *Obstet Gynecol Surv* 2008; **63**: 334–43.
55. Mantovani G, Spada A. Mutations in the Gs alpha gene causing hormone resistance. *Best Pract Res Clin Endocrinol Metab* 2006; **20**: 501–13.
56. Luoma P, Melberg A, Rinne JO, *et al.* Parkinsonism, premature menopause, and mitochondrial DNA polymerase gamma mutations: clinical and molecular genetic study. *Lancet* 2004; **364**: 875–82.
57. Pagnamenta AT, Taanman JW, Wilson CJ, *et al.* Dominant inheritance of premature ovarian failure associated with mutant mitochondrial DNA polymerase gamma. *Hum Reprod* 2006; **21**: 2467–73.

58. Schiffmann R, Tedeschi G, Kinkel RP, *et al.* Leukodystrophy in patients with ovarian dysgenesis. *Ann Neurol* 1997; **41**: 654–61.

59. Boltshauser E, Barth PG, Troost D, Martin E, Stallmach T. "Vanishing white matter" and ovarian dysgenesis in an infant with cerebro-oculo-facio-skeletal phenotype. *Neuropediatrics* 2002; **33**: 57–62.

60. Kastan MB, Bartek J. Cell-cycle checkpoints and cancer. *Nature* 2004; **432**: 316–23.

61. Demirhan O, Türkmen S, Schwabe GC, *et al.* A homozygous BMPR1B mutation causes a new subtype of acromesomelic chondrodysplasia with genital anomalies. *J Med Genet* 2005; **42**: 314–17.

62. Persani L, Rossetti R, Cacciatore C, Fabre S. Genetic defects of ovarian TGF-β-like factors and premature ovarian failure. *J Endocrinol Invest* 2011; **34**: 244–51.

63. Sherman SL, Taylor K, Allen EG. FMR1 premutation: a leading cause of inherited ovarian dysfunction. In: Arrieta I, Penagarikano O, Telez M, eds. *Fragile Sites: New Discoveries and Changing Perspectives.* Hauppauge, NY: Nova Science Publishers, Inc. 2006; 290–320.

64. Welt CK, Smith PC, Taylor AE. Evidence of early ovarian aging in fragile X premutation carriers. *J Clin Endocrinol Metab* 2004; **89**(9): 4569–74.

65. Rohr J, Allen EG, Charen K, *et al.* Anti-Mullerian hormone indicates early ovarian decline in fragile X mental retardation (FMR1) premutation carriers: a preliminary study. *Hum Reprod* 2008; **23**(5): 1220–5.

66. Allen EG, Sullivan AK, Marcus M, *et al.* Examination of reproductive aging milestones among women who carry the FMR1 premutation. *Hum Reprod* 2007; **22**: 2142–52.

67. Hunter JE, Epstein MP, Tinker SW, Charen KH, Sherman SL. Fragile X-associated primary ovarian insufficiency: evidence for additional genetic contributions to severity. *Genet Epidemiol* 2008; **32**(6): 553–9.

68. Tassone F, Hagerman RJ, Taylor AK, *et al.* Elevated levels of FMR1 mRNA in carrier males: a new mechanism of involvement in the fragile-X syndrome. *Am J Hum Genet* 2000; **66**(1): 6–15.

69. Bachner D, Manca A, Steinbach P, *et al.* Enhanced expression of the murine FMR1 gene during germ cell proliferation suggests a special function in both the male and the female gonad. *Hum Mol Genet* 1993; **2**(12): 2043–50.

70. Rife M, Nadal A, Mila M, Willemsen R. Immunohistochemical FMRP studies in a full mutated female fetus. *Am J Med Genet A* 2004; **124**(2): 129–32.

71. Schuettler J, Peng Z, Zimmer J, *et al.* Variable expression of the Fragile X Mental Retardation 1 (FMR1) gene in patients with premature ovarian failure syndrome is not dependent on number of (CGG)n triplets in exon 1. *Hum Reprod* 2011; **26**(5): 1241–51.

72. Themmen APN, Huhtaniemi IT. Mutations of gonadotropins and gonadotropin receptors: elucidating the physiology and pathophysiology of pituitary-gonadal function. *Endocr Rev* 2000; **21**: 551–83.

73. Latronico AC, Anasti J, Arnhold IJ, *et al.* Brief report: testicular and ovarian resistance to luteinizing hormone caused by inactivating mutations of the luteinizing hormone-receptor gene. *N Engl J Med* 1996; **334**: 507–12.

74. Shimasaki S, Moore RK, Otsuka F, Erickson GF. The bone morphogenetic protein system in mammalian reproduction. *Endocr Rev* 2004; **25**: 72–101.

75. Fabre S, Pierre A, Mulsant P, *et al.* Regulation of ovulation rate in mammals: contribution of sheep genetic models. *Reprod Biol Endocrinol* 2006; **4**: 20.

76. Di Pasquale E, Beck-Peccoz P, Persani L. Hypergonadotropic ovarian failure associated with an inherited mutation of human bone morphogenetic protein-15 (BMP15) gene. *Am J Hum Genet* 2004; **75**: 106–11.

77. Rossetti R, Di Pasquale E, Marozzi A, *et al.* BMP15 mutations associated with primary ovarian insufficiency cause a defective production of bioactive protein. *Hum Mutat* 2009; **30**: 804–10.

78. Matzuk MM, Finegold MJ, Su JG, Hsueh AJ, Bradley A. Alpha-inhibin is a tumour-suppressor gene with gonadal specificity in mice. *Nature* 1992; **360**: 313–19.

79. Chand AL, Harrison CA, Shelling AN. Inhibin and premature ovarian failure. *Hum Reprod Update* 2010; **16**: 39–50.

80. Corre T, Schuettler J, Bione S, *et al.* Italian Network for the study of Ovarian Dysfunctions. A large-scale association study to assess the impact of known variants of the human INHA gene on premature ovarian failure. *Hum Reprod* 2009; **24**: 2023–8.

81. Mansouri MR, Schuster J, Badhai J, *et al.* Alterations in the expression, structure and function of progesterone receptor membrane component-1 (PGRMC1) in premature ovarian failure. *Hum Mol Genet* 2008; **17**: 3776–83.

82. Mandon-Pépin B, Touraine P, Kuttenn F, *et al.* Genetic investigation of four meiotic genes in women with

premature ovarian failure. *Eur J Endocrinol* 2008; **158**: 107–15.

83. Luo X, Ikeda Y, Parker KL. A cell-specific nuclear receptor is essential for adrenal and gonadal development and sexual differentiation. *Cell* 1994; **77**: 481–90.

84. Lourenço D, Brauner R, Lin L, *et al.* Mutations in NR5A1 associated with ovarian insufficiency. *N Engl J Med* 2009; **360**: 1200–10.

85. Castrillon DH, Miao L, Kollipara R, Horner JW, DePinho RA. Suppression of ovarian follicle activation in mice by the transcription factor Foxo3a. *Science* 2003; **301**: 215–18.

86. Liu L, Rajareddy S, Reddy P, *et al.* Infertility caused by retardation of follicular development in mice with oocyte-specific expression of Foxo3a. *Development* 2007; **134**: 199–209.

87. Watkins WJ, Umbers AJ, Woad KJ, *et al.* Mutational screening of FOXO3A and FOXO1A in women with premature ovarian failure. *Fertil Steril* 2006; **86**: 1518–21.

88. Vinci G, Christin-Maitre S, Pasquier M, *et al.* FOXO3a variants in patients with premature ovarian failure. *Clin Endocrinol* 2008; **68**: 495–7.

89. Qin Y, Choi Y, Zhao H, *et al.* NOBOX homeobox mutation causes premature ovarian failure. *Am J Hum Genet* 2007; **81**: 576–81.

90. Bouilly J, Bachelot A, Broutin I, Touraine P, Binart N. Novel NOBOX loss-of-function mutations account for 6.2% of cases in a large primary ovarian insufficiency cohort. *Hum Mutat* 2011; **32**: 1108–13.

91. Zhao H, Chen ZJ, Qin Y, *et al.* Transcription factor FIGLA is mutated in patients with premature ovarian failure. *Am J Hum Genet* 2008; **82**: 1342–8.

Chapter 35

Polar body screening for aneuploidy in human oocytes

Luca Gianaroli, M. Cristina Magli, and Anna P. Ferraretti

Introduction

Aneuploidy is the most common chromosome abnormality in humans, and is the main genetic cause of miscarriage and congenital birth defects following both natural conception and in vitro fertilization (IVF). It is now known that the majority of chromosome errors originate in maternal meiosis I (MI), maternal age is a risk factor for most human aneuploidies, and defects in recombination are strictly related to meiotic nondisjunction [1].

The possible reason for the increased predisposition to aneuploidy in oocytes when compared with sperm [2] resides in the profound dissimilarity between male and female gametogenesis. While male meiosis is a continuous process, females are born with a complete set of immature oocytes in a quiescent state, and terminate the maturation process in adulthood.

In both genders, the first step of meiosis is DNA replication followed by two rounds of cell division that lead to the formation of haploid gametes. In prophase I, homologous chromosomes align, form chiasmata, and recombination occurs. At the end of MI, homologs segregate, whereas sister chromatids separate in meiosis II (MII), the second meiotic division. In spermatogenesis, this process initiates after puberty and continues throughout male lifetime, whilst in the female, meiosis begins during fetal development, arrests at prophase I before birth, and resumes prior to ovulation at the luteinizing hormone (LH) surge. For some oocytes, this last phase may never happen, whereas for others it will only occur after several years, or even decades later. It is postulated that the long time interval of oocyte quiescence, elapsing between meiotic arrest in the fetus and each ovulation cycle, could be responsible for the increased incidence of aneuploidy.

The frequency of aneuploidy in human embryos

As already learned from natural pregnancy data, studies on human male and female gametes have confirmed that oogenesis is by far more error-prone than spermatogenesis [2]. The evaluation of aneuploidy in spermatozoa has shown that the incidence of aneuploidy for the 24 chromosomes is around 5%, although in severely pathological samples this proportion can be four- to fivefold higher [3]. As distinct from natural conceptions, the possibility exists that in cases of severe male factor infertility (including azoospermia with spermatozoa retrieved from the genital tract) intracytoplasmic sperm injection (ICSI)-derived embryos have a higher incidence of inherited paternal aneuploidy [4, 5].

For oocytes, there is a consensus average figure of approximately 20% aneuploidy that is supported by the analysis of oocytes derived from natural ovulatory cycles [6]. Similar findings derived from the study of oocytes, obtained after induction of multiple follicular growth in women attending infertility clinics, support data from PGS (preimplantation genetic screening) of polar bodies that can be used as a source of information regarding the meiotic process occurring during oogenesis. The data obtained in this way correlate well with the 20% aneuploidy rate, but with a wide range in a close correlation between advancing maternal age and increasing aneuploidy rates. Percentages of aneuploid oocytes exceeding 50% are commonly observed using fluorescence *in situ* hybridization (FISH), in women over the age of 40 years [7–9].

Biology and Pathology of the Oocyte, 2nd edn., ed. Alan Trounson, Roger Gosden, and Ursula Eichenlaub-Ritter.
Published by Cambridge University Press.

It has been estimated that about 30% of human zygotes are aneuploid, and this figure increases significantly in women aged 38 years or more [10]. The same age-related trend is observed when analyzing preimplantation embryos generated in vitro, with 50–70% incidence of chromosomal abnormalities, depending on maternal age [11]. The total frequency of aneuploidy in blastocysts appears to be lower than at the embryonic cleavage stages, but values of approximately 50% are still detected using FISH in patients of 37–38 years mean age [12]. This finding is in agreement with other reports demonstrating that chromosomal aneuploidy is still common even in morphologically normal blastocysts [13, 14].

This high proportion of aneuploid embryos gives rise to clinical consequences and approximately one-third of all miscarriages (fetal loss before the twentieth week of pregnancy) being chromosomally abnormal in origin [15]. Although the vast majority of aneuploid pregnancies culminate in early abortion and possibly failed implantation, some trisomies, namely 13, 18, 21, and those involving the sex chromosomes, are potentially compatible with viability. These concepti may result in the birth of babies with congenital defects and/or mental retardation, which in many cases are destined for early death.

Based on these considerations and especially on the preponderance of chromosomal errors in the oocyte that determine the condition of euploidy or aneuploidy in the resulting embryo, PGS on polar bodies was proposed in the 1990s as a tool to predict the oocyte chromosomal status [16, 17]. This was done with the aim of selecting against embryos for transfer those originating from aneuploid oocytes, in an effort to improve live birth rates of normal babies after assisted conception cycles.

The chromosomal status of the oocyte

Following resumption of meiosis at the time of the LH surge, bivalents separate and migrate to the opposite poles of the meiotic spindle. One set of chromosomes, each comprising two chromatids, enters the first polar body (PB1) while the other set remains in the ooplasm. If this process occurs correctly, each set contains 23 chromosomes and 46 chromatids, which are held together by specific cohesion proteins. This phase corresponds to the second meiotic arrest that terminates after the penetration of the sperm, induction of oocyte activation, and the extrusion of the second polar body (PB2). At this point, sister chromatids are separated and one of each chromatid migrates into the PB2, while the other remains in the oocyte (Figure 35.1A).

However, errors can occur during this process, resulting in an unbalanced distribution of chromosomes mainly due to (1) non-disjunction of the entire chromosome (Figure 35.1B) [18], or (2) the premature separation and random segregation of sister chromatids (Figure 35.1C) [19]. Recent studies suggest that different mechanisms can be responsible for erroneous segregation. Some could be associated with failure to crossover, others with the position of the chiasmata (too close to or too far away from the centromere), and others may be attributable to some abnormalities such as the loss of sister chromatid cohesion, or defects in spindle assembly/disassembly [1].

Two more mechanisms have been proposed as a possible cause of aneuploidy. The first one is anaphase lagging, which is due to chromosome lag and misalignment during MI [20]. In this case, the chromosome left behind and unattached to the meiotic plate would be degraded in the ooplasm, making the resulting oocyte euploid. The second mechanism is gonadal mosaicism, for which aneuploid oogonia originate during early mitoses [21]. Following the study of a group of oocytes and corresponding PB1s, the latter mechanism was recently proposed to be more frequent than originally expected. The presence of aneuploid oogonia could actually explain the occurrence of some non-complementary aneuploid results when comparing oocytes and the corresponding PB1s [22, 23].

Maternal age, which is the only factor indisputably associated with aneuploidy, probably affects differently each mechanism responsible for aneuploidy. In addition to female age, there is some evidence supporting an increased incidence of aneuploidy in embryos derived from women with a history of recurrent miscarriage [24, 25], or with repeated implantation failures [8, 26].

The study of aneuploidy in polar bodies

As a result of meiosis, the polar bodies contain the chromosomes and chromatids, which are discarded during both meiotic divisions to give a haploid status to the oocyte. Therefore, as depicted in Figure 35.1, normal polar bodies are the exact mirror image of the oocyte. Based on this observation, preimplantation genetic diagnosis for aneuploidy, now

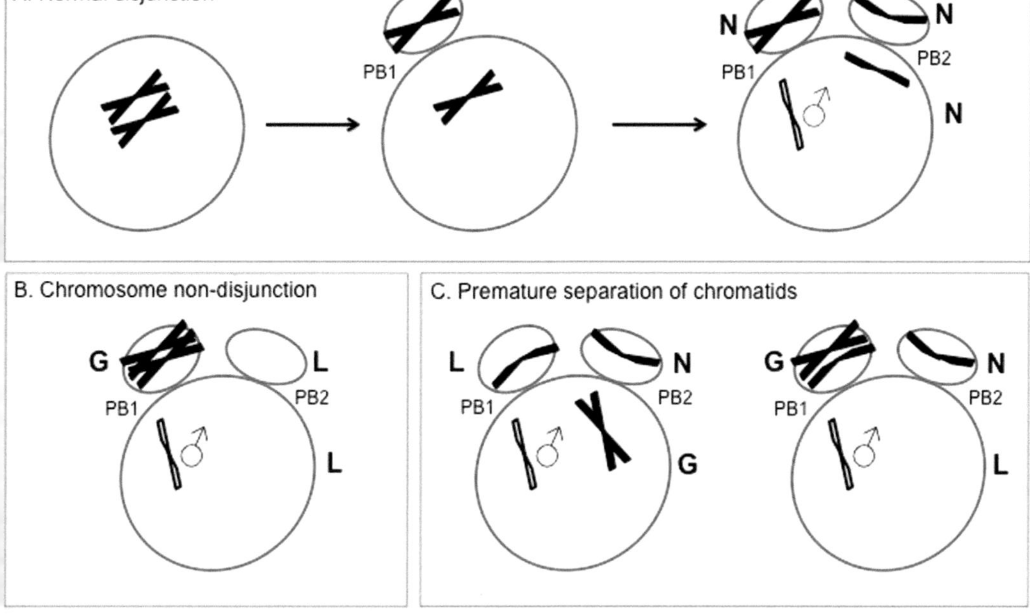

igure 35.1 Diagram representing copy number segregation patterns resulting from normal disjunction (A), whole chromosome on-disjunction (B), and premature separation of sister chromatids in a malsegregating chromosome (C). Only a few examples of the possible egregation patterns are represented. The segregation pattern is indicated as normal (N), gain (G), or loss (L), for the first polar body (PB1), the econd polar body (PB2), and the corresponding oocyte.

known as PGS, was proposed on polar bodies with the ntention of having the complete view of the chromo-omal meiotic process in the oocyte [16, 17]. Although PGS could only investigate the chromosomal status of he oocyte without including a contribution of aneu-ploidy of sperm and of embryonic mitotic origin, an advantage of this technique was that it left intact the embryonic cell mass, and used only polar bodies, the neiotic by-products.

FISH was the first technique to be used for PGS. By hybridizing probes specific for some chromosomes, and labeled with fluorescent dyes, FISH permitted the counting of the corresponding chromatids in each polar body. The analyses of these results were used to nfer the oocyte chromosomal status. As FISH only permits the analysis of a restricted number of chromo-omes, due to the limited availability of fluorochromes, priority was generally given to those chromosomes which are involved in aneuploid implantations, namely 13, 16, 18, 21, and 22, as indicated by data from clin-ical pregnancies. This imposed an evident limitation to the identification of the actual euploidy of oocytes, as no information was available for the remaining chromosomes. With the introduction of comparative genomic hybridization (CGH), the complete cytoge-netic analysis of PB1 and PB2 can be performed for the evaluation of the entire chromosome content of the oocyte [27]. The data obtained provide a unique insight into the process of meiosis, revealing different mechanisms responsible for aneuploidy during MI and MII, as well as the frequency for each chromosome variation.

Results from PGS on polar bodies

Most of the results published so far on the chromosomal status of the oocyte derive from the application of FISH for the chromosomes 13, 16, 18, 21, and 22. The application of this technique provided both clinical and biological data including the birth of several hundred babies [28]. Additional data are now coming from the more recently introduced techniques in the field of reproductive medicine, such as CGH, which has widened the spectrum of the studied chromosomes to the complete set typical of the human species.

Fluorescence *in situ* hybridization (FISH)

FISH studies on polar bodies from several thousands of human oocytes obtained in IVF clinics have indicated that approximately half of patients with 4
advanced reproductive age carry aneuploidies originating either from MI, MII, or from both MI and MII

[7]. It is recognized that some errors in estimation could be due to the limitations of the FISH technique, including the artifactual chromosome loss during cell fixation, and failure of hybridization. The data were, however, considered to be reasonably reliable when follow-up was performed in the resulting embryos [7]. In addition, the clear trend correlating maternal age and the incidence of chromosomal abnormalities was in total agreement with the clinical data derived from spontaneous pregnancies [7, 15].

There is no doubt that the accuracy of FISH in the PGS program should be kept under strict control and periodically monitored through the evaluation of the error rate, which represents the only measure of accuracy in PGS. Review of the literature demonstrates that each laboratory has different error rates, which may be caused by technical problems dependent on the level of skill and on the quality control system used [11]. The reliability of the FISH diagnosis on polar bodies was confirmed in a study where both polar bodies and the corresponding oocytes were tested for the same chromosomes [29]. In this study the prediction of euploidy or aneuploidy from polar bodies was confirmed in 98% of the 143 oocytes following their direct analysis. Therefore, the majority of the abnormalities detected in polar bodies were assumed to represent true errors reflected in the corresponding oocytes. The few cases of non-concordance could be explained by considering that aneuploidy can also derive, as mentioned earlier, from the sperm chromosomal contribution and by biological events such as anaphase lagging.

Clearly, the evaluation of the results regarding aneuploidy type and frequency must take into consideration that IVF patients may not necessarily represent the general female population, because the analyzed oocytes come from infertile women whose ovaries were treated by exogenous hormonal hyperstimulation for the retrieval of multiple oocytes. The largest experience on polar body chromosomal analysis comes from the group of Kuliev and Verlinsky [10], who pioneered this technique in the early 1980s. In 2004, they published the results from the FISH analysis for chromosomes 13, 16, 18, 21, and 22 on more than 8000 oocytes [7]. According to their report, similar error rates occurred in MI and MII oocytes (42% and 37%, respectively) with almost two-thirds of all oocytes with MII errors. The most frequent errors were complex chromosomal abnormalities.

The vast majority of MI abnormalities were due to chromatid errors, and while MI errors predominantly resulted in the presence of an extra chromatid or chromosome in oocytes, a random distribution of extra and missing chromatids was detected after MII. Reciprocal errors were found to be present in approximately one-third of all aneuploid oocytes. In these cases, the aneuploidy for one chromosome in MI was compensated by the opposite error for the same chromosome in the second meiotic division, resulting in zygotes with a euploid status for that chromosome. However, the follow-up of the corresponding embryos revealed that the great majority were chromosomally abnormal for the same or different chromosomes, or were mosaics suggesting a possible predisposition to mitotic errors [7]. It was postulated that mosaicism, which occurs at high frequency during embryonic cleavage, could originate in those oocytes with compensated errors occurring during meiosis. Should this be confirmed the testing of polar bodies could have an important clinical value for selecting euploid embryos for transfer.

The analysis of aneuploidy rates for individual chromosomes showed significant differences, with a higher incidence of errors for chromosome 21 and 22. In addition, errors for the chromosomes 18, 13, and 21 were shown to originate mostly at MI, while chromosome 16 and 22 errors derived more frequently from MII. This finding confirmed that the origin of aneuploidy for the individual chromosomes is not random although the data from trisomic pregnancies suggested that the majority of trisomies for chromosome 22 and all trisomies for chromosome 16 originate at MI [1]. It might be speculated that embryonic viability is associated with the origin of aneuploidy, for which trisomies 16 and 22 can implant only if they are generated at MI.

Complex aneuploidies involving two or more chromosomes, or the same chromosome in both meiotic divisions appear to occur in approximately 50% of aneuploidies [10]. The frequency of complex aneuploidies at MI was found to be particularly high in in vitro matured oocytes from superovulated cycles (62%); these oocytes had an incidence of total aneuploidy that was higher than that detected in in vivo matured oocytes (70% vs. 40%, respectively) [30]. This could explain, at least partially, the low viability of in vitro matured oocytes from stimulated cycles.

More information on the origin of aneuploidy could be drawn by a meticulous analysis of the chromosomal status of IVF-generated oocytes in relation to patients' characteristics, their reproductive history, the type of hormonal stimulation, and their response to induction of multiple follicular stimulation with exogenous gonadotropin. In a study evaluating more than 4000 oocytes involving the analysis of PB1s for chromosomes 13, 15, 16, 18, 21, and 22, it was reported that the proportion of normal oocytes was directly correlated with the number of mature oocytes recovered after superovulation and the establishment of a clinical pregnancy [8]. Conversely, an inverse correlation was found with the patients' age, the causes of female infertility (specifically endometriosis, repeated abortion, ovulatory disturbance), poor prognosis indications for IVF success (number of previous treatment cycles, or the presence of multiple poor prognosis indications, that is, the combination of one or more factors that negatively affect the chances of pregnancy, such as advanced age, repeated IVF failures, and repeated abortions), and number of follicle-stimulating hormone (FSH) units used for superovulation for each oocyte and for each mature oocyte recovered [8]. These findings suggested that the type of infertility is strictly associated with the onset of errors at the first meiotic division and the incidence was significantly higher in the presence of female pathological conditions (an ovulatory factor or endometriosis) or in women who experienced repeated abortions. It was also shown that aneuploidy events, namely the occurrence of a specific abnormality or a specific chromosome alteration, are related not to a specific variable, but to multiple variables, with the aneuploidy being of any type [8]. In other words, the mechanisms responsible for aneuploidy and the frequency of a single chromosome variation do not depend on a specific variable (age, for example), but on groups of variables, suggesting that no correlation exists between a specific type of aneuploidy and any of the female infertility indications [8]. Therefore, chromosomal errors seem to be correlated to generalized oocyte disorganization and not to a single, specific oocyte alteration.

One of the major limitations of the FISH analysis resides in the reduced number of chromosomes that can be tested. Intuitively, this was clear from the beginning of PGS and applied both on polar body and for blastomeric analyses. In some cases, especially for blastomeres, the addition of extra probes was adopted in successive rounds of hybridization, but this strategy was not common for polar bodies. With the aim of evaluating the possible contribution of other chromosomes to the clinical outcome, a study was performed on a group of pregnant and non-pregnant patients, who had completed an ICSI cycle in combination with PGS on PB1 for the chromosomes 13, 15, 16, 18, 21, and 22 [29]. These patients had been treated in the same period and their clinical outcome (either no pregnancy, term pregnancy, or abortion) was known. The corresponding PB1s, which had been stored after completion of the treatment cycle, were rehybridized with the probes for the chromosomes 1, 4, and 6, and the information derived from the testing of the nine chromosomes was related to the clinical outcome. The results demonstrated that the presence of aneuploidy for chromosomes 1, 4, and 6 was not compatible with implantation, while no effect was detected on the occurrence of early abortion [29]. In other words, an abnormal condition for such large chromosomes does not allow implantation to occur or, should it happen, embryonic absorption would follow so quickly that the pregnancy would be undetected. These results have been confirmed by other studies [9, 31].

At this point, the introduction of a technique permitting the testing of all chromosomes was desirable; although the frequent occurrence of complex abnormalities made it apparent that a linear increase of the aneuploidy rate was not the expected outcome [7]. The 24-color FISH painting technique using the combination of five fluorochromes was proposed as spectral karyotyping, known as SKY, for the cytogenetic analysis of oocytes and polar bodies [32, 33]. The reported results confirmed the previous findings in FISH studies on the incidence of aneuploidy and on the occurrence of chromatid predivision involving especially the smaller chromosomes [33]. Unfortunately, the difficulty of obtaining high quality chromosome spreading and the low limits of resolution made this technique of scarce applicability in clinical settings.

Impact of FISH on clinical success rates

The clinical impact of PGS FISH analyses demonstrates a low repeatability of the technique that is effective in some clinics and not in others. This could be due to systematic technical problems, for example low levels of accuracy, or to patient selection, as it is clear that the technique is not effective for all cases. Besides the adequate technical skill, an improved implantation is actually dependent on the availability of a minimum number of oocytes or embryos to be analyzed, as only in this case is selection possible [11]. Several randomized clinical trials (RCTs) performed on embryos biopsied at the cleavage stage and analyzed by FISH have documented no differences in comparison with a control group, or even a worse outcome [34]. Nevertheless, none of these RCTs has applied optimal methodology, the main shortcomings being a poor consideration of the critical relevance of cell biopsy, and low accuracy levels of FISH results [11]. In other words, there is still the need of methodologically correct studies to evaluate properly the clinical performance of PGS using FISH. Having these results would be very convenient in many situations, as the high cost of microarrays still makes FISH attractive, especially in those cases where an appropriate and tailored strategy seems to favor the clinical outcome [35].

Comparative genomic hybridization (CGH)

Since the introduction of CGH as a technique able to detect aneuploidy in single cells [36, 37], there has been considerable optimism that this technique will have important clinical applications in identifying the viable embryos for transfer and to markedly increase success rates of assisted reproduction that could not be achieved with FISH analysis. Besides covering the complete set of chromosomes, CGH avoids the need of spreading polar bodies on a microscope slide, removing a step that may cause errors due to artifactual loss of chromosomes that would overestimate chromosomal aneuploidy rates. The idea behind the testing of polar bodies for the whole chromosome set was that the transfer of the resulting euploid embryos could increase the chances of implantation, thus leading to an increased success rate for assisted conception, the replacement of fewer embryos in each ovulatory cycle, and a consequent reduction of the incidence of multiple gestations.

Given that a cell only contains approximately 6 pg of DNA, while CGH protocols necessitate approximately 1 μg, the method requires amplification of the cell DNA. The amplified product is then differentially labeled (the test sample is traditionally labeled with a green fluorochrome, the chromosomally normal reference with a red fluorochrome) and set to competitive hybridization to normal metaphase chromosomes fixed on a slide. The ratio of green to red fluorescence along the length of each chromosome is analyzed by specific software, and the given values indicate any possible gain or loss of DNA in the test sample.

This formulation, known as metaphase-CGH, is labor intensive and requires as many as 4 days to obtain the results. For this reason, performing CGH on the PB1 on the day of oocyte retrieval, and even on both polar bodies on the following day, was regarded as a promising approach that was compatible with fresh embryo transfer [27, 31].

Further development of the methodology was achieved by combining CGH with microarrays and this approach, known as array-CGH, made it possible to drastically reduce the experimental time to less than 24 hours. Obviously, the possibility of testing oocytes by array-CGH on polar bodies in a clinical setting was very appealing. The approach that was designed permitted the completeness of CGH covering the entire 23 chromosomes present in the polar body with the ability offered by FISH to provide a result within a time frame compatible with fresh embryo transfer.

As for metaphase-CGH, the first step consists of whole genomic amplification (WGA) of the test DNA (from the polar body in this case) and of the genomic DNA extracted from a normal control, followed by the labeling with different fluorochromes: red for the test DNA and green for the control DNA (Figure 35.2). The two labeled DNAs are mixed and allowed to compete for hybridization to thousands of specific DNA sequences attached to a microarray. If the test DNA is euploid for a given chromosome, it will equally compete with the control to bind the sequences on the array specific for that chromosome; therefore, the resulting color on the array will be yellow (combination of red and green). Conversely, hyperhaploidy of that chromosome will result in an excess of red, while hypohaploidy will result in an excess of green. Microarrays are scanned and the resulting images are evaluated by specific software where gains and losses are plotted in relation to the reference DNA (Figure 35.3). However, a screening method selected for clinical application must be highly efficient and accurate. The first data on oocytes and polar bodies reported variable diagnostic efficiency rates ranging from 64% to 78% that were unacceptably low and not reproducible enough to substantiate array-CGH for clinical use [31, 38]. The critical analysis of these results led to some relevant and practical conclusions that were helpful for further improvement. It became evident that there was a learning curve in the processing of polar bodies for CGH, that they are very fragile and susceptible to non-optimal storage conditions, such as long transport after biopsy and before WGA, and storage in freezers that do not reach temperatures of −80°C

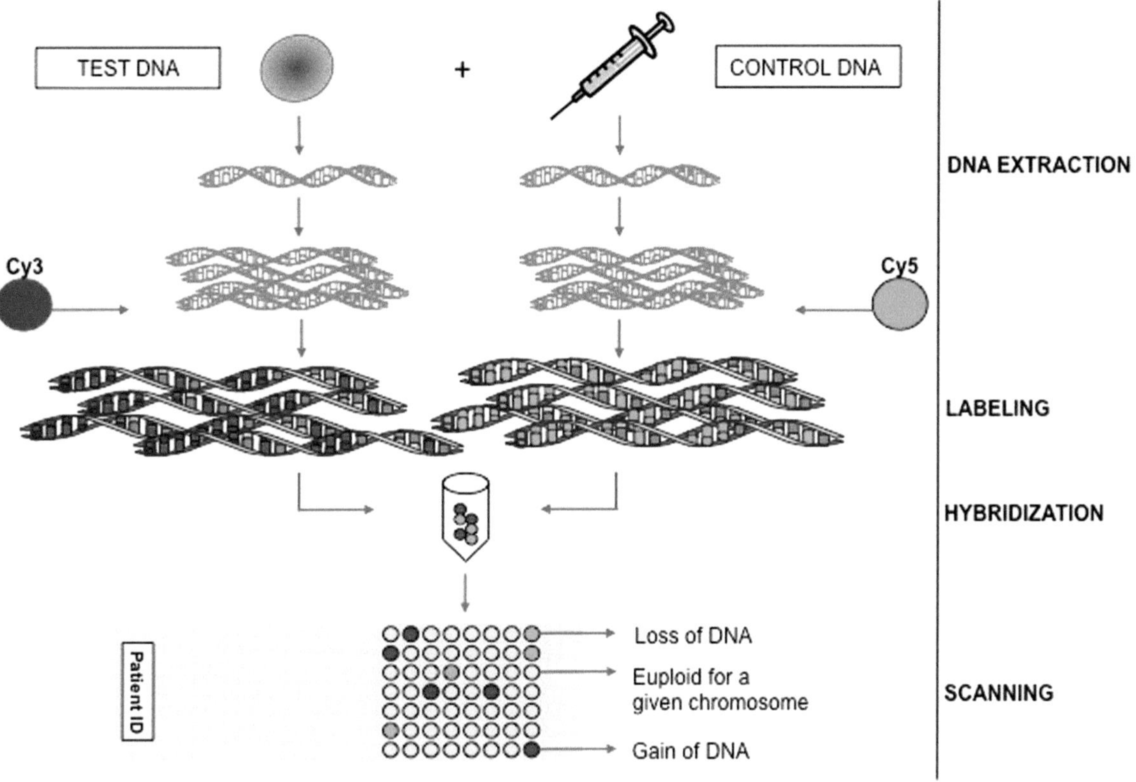

Figure 35.2 Diagram representing the workflow for array-CGH. See the text for details.

−20°C freezers are insufficient to maintain polar body DNA integrity) [38].

With the aim to standardize the array-CGH technique, the European Society of Human Reproduction and Embryology (ESHRE) undertook a proof-of-principle study to investigate the feasibility and reliability of the technique on both polar bodies from fertilized oocytes [39]. The aims of this study were: (1) to show that the analysis of polar bodies could be completed within 12 hours, and (2) to ensure the reliable identification of the chromosomal status in at least 90% of the biopsied oocytes. The rate of reliability was determined by comparing the results of the oocyte chromosomal complements that were not clinically used with those from their corresponding polar bodies. By using bacterial artificial chromosome (BAC) array technology, the workflow could actually take 12–13 hours provided that there were no more than six cells for analysis, corresponding to three zygotes. One extra hour should be considered for each six additional cells. The experimental protocol was flexible enough to extend some steps in a way of having an overnight procedure, so that the entire method can be accommodated during normal working hours. During the study, some technical details were found to be of special relevance for the success of the procedure, with significant reference to the time of polar body biopsy, which seemed to be directly correlated to the amplification efficiency of PB2 [40].

The ploidy status could be predicted in 195 of the 226 biopsied oocytes (86%), which originated from 42 cycles with a mean maternal age of 40 years [38]. In all, 72% of oocytes were found to be aneuploid based on polar body testing. The analysis of the results indicated that 76% of the detected aneuploidies would have been identified also by using the conventional FISH probe set for the chromosomes 13, 16, 18, 21, and 22. Assuming a 100% technical accuracy of FISH, array-CGH avoided the transfer of 38 chromosomally abnormal embryos whose aneuploidy events were due to chromosomes which are not tested by conventional FISH. The rate of concordance, evaluated on 138 trios (PB1, PB2, and corresponding oocyte), was 94%. Notably, in seven of the eight discordant cases, the

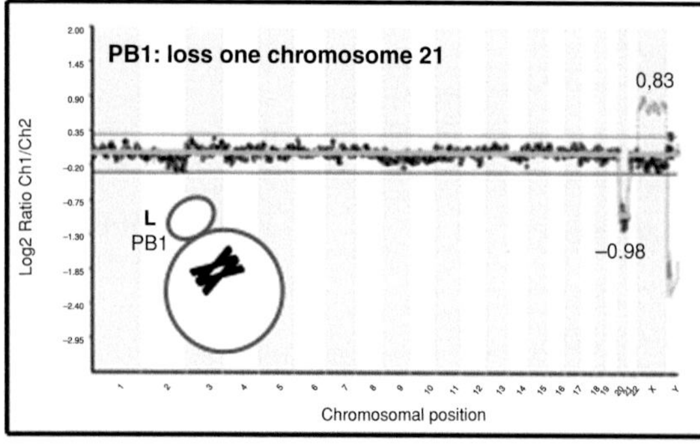

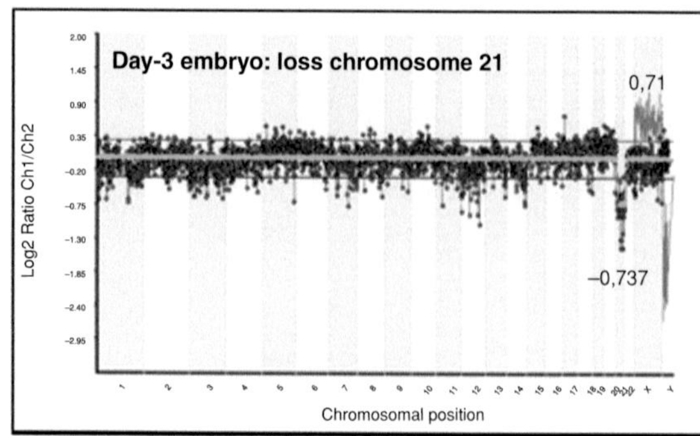

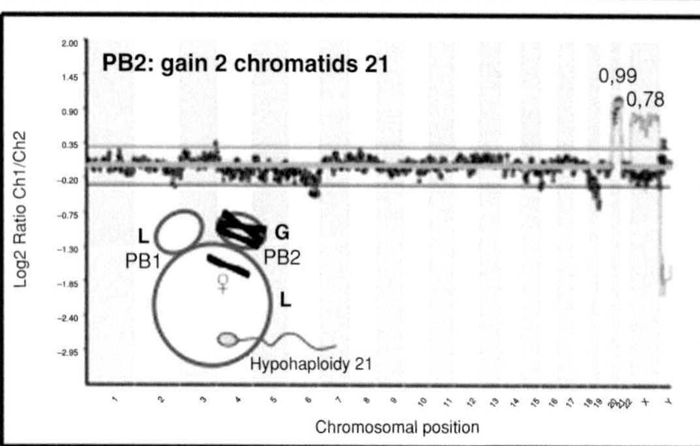

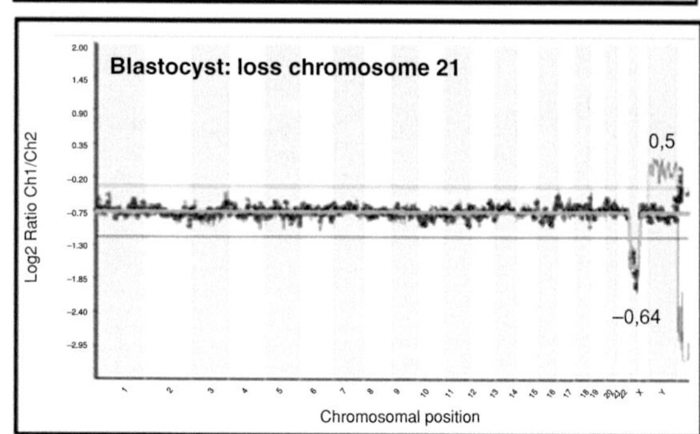

Figure 35.3 Array-CGH ratio plots for the first and second polar bodies (PB1 and PB2), corresponding day-3 embryo, and blastocyst. There is one error in meiosis I and one in meiosis II for chromosome 21. As represented in the diagram, the segregation patterns indicate meiosis I non-disjunction for chromosome 21, while the meiosis II errors resulted in loss in the zygote due to the extrusion of one chromosome and one chromatid in PB2. The fertilizing spermatozoon was possibly hypohaploid for chromosome 21; therefore, the resulting embryo and blastocyst are monosomic for chromosome 21. The two horizontal lines either side of log2 ratio 0.0 represent the 95% confidence interval for normal copy number.

oocyte was found to be euploid irrespective of anomalies detected in one or both polar bodies. It can be postulated that the detected discordances could be derived from the sperm (Figure 35.3) or from anaphase lagging. In the latter case, as already mentioned, the chromosomes left behind would be degraded, especially when occurring at MII, making the resulting oocyte euploid for that chromosome. The results obtained in the ESHRE proof-of-principle study opened up to a randomized control trial on PGS on polar bodies involving seven different centers. This study, which is currently ongoing, has two primary aims among women with advanced maternal age: (1) to assess the prediction value of having no euploid oocytes in future ART cycles, when no euploid oocytes are detected in the first attempt; and (2) to improve live birth rate following the transfer of embryos derived from euploid oocytes.

Several observations derived from the proof-of-principle study were in full agreement with FISH results: (1) premature separation of sister chromatids rather than non-disjunction of whole chromosomes caused the vast majority of errors (97%) in the first meiotic division; (2) more aneuploid events in the aneuploid oocytes were caused by errors in MII although the incidence of aneuploid PB1 was more frequent than aneuploid PB2; (3) there was a trend towards losses from the polar bodies in both divisions; (4) most abnormal oocytes had multiple aneuploidies (58%), with an incidence that was age dependent; (5) the most frequent aneuploid events involved small chromosomes, including 16 and 22, followed by 21, 19, and 15 [41]. Comparable results were reported by other studies [9, 26].

Another finding in agreement with different reports is the occurrence of reciprocal gains and losses [7, 9, 26, 42]. As already mentioned, the clinical use of these oocytes was not recommended even though they were euploid. It was reported that the compensation of the anomaly at MI with that occurring at MII predisposed the derived embryos to mitotic abnormalities [7]. However, there has been a recent case report that has documented the birth of a healthy baby from an oocyte whose PB1 was found to be missing a single chromatid of chromosome 21 and whose PB2 possessed an extra chromatid of the same chromosome [43]. Before transfer, a trophectoderm biopsy from the resulting blastocyst was analyzed by single nucleotide polymorphism (SNP) microarray-based comprehensive chromosome screening (CCS), and compensation of the meiotic error by deletion of the additional chromosome that existed was verified. These data demonstrate the developmental potential of an oocyte with reciprocal aneuploidies in polar bodies, questioning the previous reports. The same group is investigating the ploidy of other embryos derived from oocytes with reciprocal gains and losses in polar bodies, and the prevalence of euploidy in the corresponding embryos deserves further research [44].

As already suggested by PGS results on embryos, other groups of patients, beside those with a maternal age factor, are at higher risk of generating aneuploid oocytes or embryos. This seems to be the case especially for couples with recurrent pregnancy loss or repeated implantation failures, which together with advanced maternal age, are the factors predisposing women to reduced chances of achieving or maintaining a pregnancy to term. In a recent study, the highest aneuploidy rates were detected in women with advanced reproductive age (77.2%) and repeated implantation failures (72.8%), when compared with patients with recurrent miscarriages (54.8%) [9]. Unfortunately, the three studied categories had a similar maternal age, adding some confusion to the interpretation of results. However, the same group studied the chromosomal status in PB1 and corresponding oocytes from young, non-infertile donors (mean age 22 years) and in this case the rate of aneuploidy was only 3% [38]. Even when considering that PB2s were not analyzed, it is clear that maternal age is strongly linked to aneuploidy [8]. This is especially evident when results are stratified for maternal age, with total aneuploidies and complex abnormalities following the same trend [7, 9, 10, 26].

Some evidence suggests that there is a difference in the mechanisms leading to meiotic errors in the different categories of poor prognosis patients. FISH on PB1 has already shown this, where the advanced-age group had a stronger prevalence at MI of chromatid predivision in comparison with the recurrent implantation failure group [45], and this was confirmed by CGH [9].

Finally, array-CGH permits detection of partial rearrangement aneuploidies that arise because of *de novo* chromosome breakage taking place during either MI or MII. This phenomenon was seen in 4–10% of the investigated oocytes, and generally affected the larger chromosomes [9, 41]. In the ESHRE proof-of-principle study, for 17 of these cases, results were available for PB1, PB2, and the corresponding oocytes. This revealed that the structural abnormality detected in polar bodies was confirmed in nine oocytes; in three cases the abnormality in PB1 was compensated by the opposite abnormality in PB2, whereas in the remaining five cases there was no evidence in the oocytes of the structural abnormality found in the corresponding polar bodies (ESHRE proof-of-principle study, unpublished). The clinical significance of partial aneuploidies is unknown and certainly depends on the size of the involved chromosome region. More research is expected to elucidate this matter.

Conclusions

Given that data from clinical pregnancies have proven the preponderance of maternal aneuploidy at conception, it was logical to postulate that most chromosomal anomalies originate in the oocyte and that such abnormalities should be transmitted to every cell of the resulting embryos. For this reason, performing PGS on polar bodies seemed to be a useful approach, having the advantage of leaving the embryonic cell mass intact. The clinical relevance of this strategy is still not clear as not much is known about the mechanisms controlling cell division that lead to the formation of viable embryos. Much remains to be known about oocyte and embryo ploidy, and about the time and modality that regulate the cell commitment to the developing embryo. Quite obscure is also the process controlling aneuploidy rescue, as well as the onset of mosaicism at cleavage stages and in the blastocyst. In other words, a great deal of research is still needed, but the progress made in recent years should engender further research to determine the nature of aneuploidy in humans. The reality is that most of the current understanding on female meiosis has stemmed from the application of PGS on polar bodies, which provided unique information concerning the processes of chromosome duplication, pairing, recombination, and segregation during MI and MII, disclosing findings of critical clinical and biological significance.

References

1. Hassold T, Hall H, Hunt P. The origin of human aneuploidy: where we have been, where we are going. *Hum Mol Genet* 2007; **16**: R203–8.
2. Gianaroli L, Magli MC, Ferraretti AP. Sperm and blastomere aneuploidy detection in reproductive genetics and medicine. *J Histochem Cytochem* 2005; **53**: 261–8.
3. Gianaroli L, Magli MC, Cavallini G, *et al.* Frequency of aneuploidy in spermatozoa from patients with extremely severe male factor infertility. *Hum Reprod* 2005; **20**: 2140–52.
4. Bernardini L, Costa M, Bottazzi C, *et al.* Sperm aneuploidy and recurrent pregnancy loss. *Reprod Biomed Online* 2004; **9**: 312–20.
5. Magli MC, Gianaroli L, Ferraretti AP, *et al.* Paternal contribution to aneuploidy in preimplantation embryos. *Reprod Biomed Online* 2009; **18**: 536–42.
6. Volarcik, K. Sheean L, Goldfarb J, *et al.* The meiotic competence of in-vitro matured human oocytes is influenced by donor age: evidence that folliculogenesis is compromised in the reproductively aged ovary. *Hum Reprod* 1998; **13**: 154–60.
7. Kuliev A, Verlinsky Y. Meiotic and mitotic non-disjunction: lessons from preimplantation genetic diagnosis. *Hum Reprod Update* 2004; **10**: 401–7.
8. Gianaroli L, Magli MC, Cavallini G, *et al.* Predicting aneuploidy in human oocytes: key factors which affect the meiotic process. *Hum Reprod* 2010; **25**: 2374–86.
9. Fragouli E, Alfarawati S, Goodall N, *et al.* The cytogenetics of polar bodies: insights into female meiosis and the diagnosis of aneuploidy. *Mol Hum Reprod* 2011; **17**: 286–95.
10. Kuliev A, Cieslak J, Verlinsky Y. Frequency and distribution of chromosome abnormalities in human oocytes. *Cytogenet Genome Res* 2005; **111**: 193–8.
11. Munné S, Wells D, Cohen J. Technology requirements for preimplantation genetic diagnosis to improve assisted reproduction outcomes. *Fertil Steril* 2010; **94**: 408–30.
12. Schoolcraft WB, Treff NR, Stevens JM, *et al.* Live birth outcome with trophectoderm biopsy, blastocyst vitrification, and single-nucleotide polymorphism microarray-based comprehensive chromosome screening in infertile patients. *Fertil Steril* 2011; **96**: 638–40.
13. Magli MC, Jones GM, Gras L, *et al.* Chromosome mosaicism in day 3 aneuploid embryos that develop to morphologically normal blastocysts in vitro. *Hum Reprod* 2000; **15**: 1781–6.
14. Wells D, Fragouli E, Stevens J, *et al.* High pregnancy rate after comprehensive chromosomal screening of blastocysts. *Fertil Steril* 2008; **90**: S80.
15. Hassold T, Hunt P. To err (meiotically) is human: the genesis of human aneuploidy. *Nat Rev Genet* 2001; **2**: 280–91.
16. Verlinsky Y, Cieslak J, Freidine M, *et al.* Pregnancies following pre-conception diagnosis of common aneuploidies by fluorescent in-situ hybridization. *Hum Reprod* 1995; **10**: 1923–7.
17. Verlinsky Y, Cieslak J, Freidine M, *et al.* Polar body diagnosis of common aneuploidies by FISH. *J Assist Reprod Genet* 1996; **13**: 157–62.
18. Zenzes MT, Casper RF. Cytogenetics of human oocytes, zygotes and embryos after in vitro fertilisation. *Hum Genet* 1992; **88**: 367–75.
19. Angell RR. Predivision in human oocytes at meiosis I: a mechanism for trisomy formation in man. *Hum Genet* 1991; **86**: 383–7.
20. Jin F, Hamada M, Malureanu L, *et al.* Cdc20 is critical for meiosis I and fertility of female mice. *PLoS Genet* 2010; **30**(6): pii:e1001147.
21. Cozzi J, Conn CM, Harper JC, *et al.* A trisomic germ cell line and precocious chromatid separation causes repeated trisomic conceptions. *Hum Genet* 1999; **104**: 23–8.
22. Hultén MA, Jonasson J, Nordgren A, *et al.* Germinal and somatic trisomy 21 mosaicism: how common is it, what are the implications for individual carriers and how does it come about? *Curr Genomics* 2010; **11**: 409–19.
23. Obradors A, Rius M, Cuzzi J, *et al.* Errors at mitotic segregation early in oogenesis and at first meiotic division in oocytes from donor females: comparative genomic hybridization analyses in metaphase II oocytes and their first polar body. *Fertil Steril* 2010; **93** 675–9.
24. Rubio C, Simòn C, Vidal F, *et al.* Chromosomal abnormalities and embryo development in recurrent miscarriage couples. *Hum Reprod* 2003; **18**: 182–8.
25. Garrisi JG, Colls P, Ferry KM, *et al.* Effect of infertility maternal age, and number of previous miscarriages on the outcome of preimplantation genetic diagnosis for idiopathic recurrent pregnancy loss. *Fertil Steril* 2009; **92**: 288–95.
26. Fragouli E, Katz-Jaffe M, Alfarawati S, *et al.* Comprehensive chromosome screening of polar bodies and blastocysts from couples experiencing repeated implantation failure. *Fertil Steril* 2010; **94**: 875–87.
27. Wells D, Escudero T, Levy B, *et al.* First clinical application of comparative genomic hybridization and

polar body testing for preimplantation genetic diagnosis of aneuploidy. *Fertil Steril* 2002; **78**: 543–9.

28. Kuliev A, Zlatopolsky Z, Kirillova I, *et al.* Polar body based PGD for genetic and chromosomal disorders. *Reprod Biomed Online* 2012; Suppl 2: S31–8.
29. Magli MC, Gianaroli L, Crippa A, *et al.* Aneuploidies of chromosomes 1, 4 and 6 are not compatible with human embryos' implantation. *Fertil Steril* 2010; **94**: 2012–6.
30. Magli MC, Ferraretti AP, Crippa A, *et al.* First meiosis errors in immature oocytes generated by stimulated cycles. *Fertil Steril* 2006; **86**: 629–35.
31. Gutiérrez-Mateo C, Wells D, Benet J, *et al.* Reliability of comparative genomic hybridization to detect chromosome abnormalities in first polar bodies and metaphase II oocytes. *Hum Reprod* 2004; **19**: 2118–25.
32. Márquez C, Cohen J, Munné S. Chromosome identification in human oocytes and polar bodies by spectral karyotyping. *Cytogenet Cell Genet* 1998; **81**: 254–8.
33. Sandalinas M, Márquez C, Munné S. Spectral karyotyping of fresh, non-inseminated oocytes. *Mol Hum Reprod* 2002; **8**: 580–5.
34. Mastenbroek S, Twisk M, van der Veen F, *et al.* Preimplantation genetic screening: a systematic review and meta-analysis of RCTs. *Hum Reprod Update* 2011; **17**: 454–66.
35. Munné S, Fragouli E, Colls P, *et al.* Improved detection of aneuploid blastocysts using a new 12-chromosome FISH test. *Reprod Biomed Online* 2010; **20**: 92–7.
36. Voullaire L, Slater H, Williamson R, *et al.* Chromosome analysis of blastomeres from human embryos by using comparative genomic hybridization. *Hum Genet* 2000; **106**: 210–17.
37. Wells D, Delhanty JDA. Comprehensive chromosomal analysis of human preimplantation embryos using whole genome amplification and single cell comparative genomic hybridization. *Mol Hum Reprod* 2000; **6**: 1055–62.
38. Fragouli E, Escalona A, Gutiérrez-Mateo C, *et al.* Comparative genomic hybridization of oocytes and first polar bodies from young donors. *Reprod Biomed Online* 2009; **19**: 228–37.
39. Geraedts J, Montag M, Magli MC, *et al.* Polar body array CGH for prediction of the status of the corresponding oocyte. Part I: clinical results. *Hum Reprod* 2011; **26**: 3173–80.
40. Magli MC, Montag M, Köster M, *et al.* Polar body array CGH for prediction of the status of the corresponding oocyte. Part II: technical aspects. *Hum Reprod* 2011; **26**: 3181–5.
41. Handyside AH, Montag M, Magli MC, *et al.* Multiple meiotic errors caused by predivision of chromatids in women of advanced maternal age undergoing in vitro fertilisation. *Eur J Hum Genet* 2012; **20**: 742–7.
42. Magli MC, Grugnetti C, Castelletti E, *et al.* Five chromosome segregation in polar bodies and the corresponding oocyte. *Reprod Biomed Online* 2012; **24**: 331–8.
43. Scott RT, Jr., Treff NR, Stevens J, *et al.* Delivery of a chromosomally normal child from an oocyte with reciprocal aneuploid polar bodies. *J Assist Reprod Genet* 2012; **29**: 533–7.
44. Forman EJ, Treff NR, Stevens JM, *et al.* Embryos whose polar bodies contain isolated reciprocal chromosome aneuploidy are almost always euploid. *Hum Reprod* 2012; **28**: 502–8.
45. Vialard F, Lombroso R, Bergere M, *et al.* Oocyte aneuploidy mechanisms are different in two situations of increased chromosomal risk: older patients and patients with recurrent implantation failure after in vitro fertilization. *Fertil Steril* 2007; **87**: 1333–9.

Chapter 36 Cryopreservation of oocytes

Alan Trounson and Laura Rienzi

Introduction

Oocyte cryopreservation is a major issue in human reproductive medicine. The need to cryopreserve oocytes rather than embryos is not limited to countries with restrictive legislation. In fact, all the major clinical applications rely on fertility preservation for both medical and non-medical reasons [1–4] and for oocyte donation programs [5–7].

The first success in freezing human oocytes was reported by Chen [8] using a slow-cooling method in dimethyl sulfoxide (DMSO) as the cryoprotectant. The technique was essentially a modification of that used for cryopreservation of human embryos, which in turn had evolved from methods applied for freezing mouse and cattle embryos. Out of 40 thawed oocytes, the reported survival, fertilization, and cleavage rates were 80%, 83%, and 60%, respectively. Despite the technique resulting in a twin pregnancy, its adoption in human reproductive medicine was delayed, due to the failure to reproduce the results reported. Concerns were expressed about the difficulty in dehydrating and cooling human oocytes due to their large volume, the sensitive nature of the metaphase nucleus, premature cortical granule release, and interruption to intercellular ultrastructure [9, 10].

Interest in the cryopreservation of unfertilized oocytes began to increase in the 1990s with the observation that oocytes could be slow cooled in the cryoprotectant 1,2-propanediol (PROH) and by adding sucrose as an extracellular solute, with improved results if the thawed oocytes were subsequently inseminated using intracytoplasmic sperm injection (ICSI) [11]. In a study reported by Tucker *et al.* [12], in 22 cycles of oocyte thawing the cryosurvival rate was 24%, and 5 pregnancies were established. They also reported that 44% of germinal vesicle (GV) stage oocytes survived cryopreservation and a term pregnancy was obtained after thawing, in vitro maturation, and ICSI. This certainly set the stage for an increased interest in the cryopreservation of human oocytes.

Another milestone in the history of oocyte cryopreservation was the report of the birth of a healthy baby girl after oocyte vitrification [13]. Out of 17 oocytes rewarmed, 11 (64.7%) survived and were inseminated, 5 (45%) fertilized correctly, and 3 embryos were transferred to three patients. One term pregnancy was achieved. The result promoted new efforts in further research to explore the potential benefits of vitrification as a new and more effective method for human oocyte cryopreservation.

But the real impetus for clinical application of oocyte crypreservation occurred in Italy in 2004, when the Italian government forbad the production of more than three embryos per in vitro fetilization (IVF) treatment cycle (and thus the insemination of more than three oocytes) and outlawed embryo selection and freezing. As a consequence, Italian embryologists were forced to cryopreserve all supernumerary oocytes or to discard them. The data collected by the Italian National Register from 2005 to 2007 involving 193 IVF clinics were reported by Scaravelli *et al.* [14]. Out of 42 917 thawed oocytes, 22 005 (51.3%) survived and were suitable for ICSI, producing 14 966 (68%) transferable embryos. The reported pregnancy rate was 12.5% for cryopreserved oocytes and was lower than those arising from fresh and frozen embryo cycles (24.9% and 16.4%, respectively). Similarly, the implantation rate (only 6.9%) was lower when compared to those obtained with the transfer of freshly derived and frozen–thawed embryos – 13.5% and 8.8%, respectively. There were 582 babies born from 505 deliveries

Biology and Pathology of the Oocyte, 2nd edn., ed. Alan Trounson, Roger Gosden, and Ursula Eichenlaub-Ritter.

The overall take home baby rate per thawed oocyte was only 1.36% (582/42 917) [14]. The results were rather disappointing and the data collected clearly underlined the need to improve and optimize the existing cryopreservation protocols, positively stimulating further research in this area.

Cryopreservation methods

All the cryopreservation methods adopted so far include the use of cryoprotectant agents (CPAs) in order to protect the cells from damage caused by the formation and growth of intracellular ice crystals. CPAs are classified as "permeating" and "non-permeating." Permeating CPAs, such as PROH and DMSO, pass through the cell membrane and substitute for the exit of intracellular water. These compounds form hydrogen bonds with any intracellular water molecules and prevent intracellular ice crystallization. On the contrary, non-permeating CPAs, such as sucrose, are extracellular solutes which contribute to cell dehydration by providing an osmotic gradient for water removal, without entering the cell. However, it is important to note that, if not used correctly, CPAs themselves can be cytotoxic at increasing concentrations. It is therefore fundamental to balance the need for dehydration (in order to avoid the formation of intracellular ice crystals) and the necessity to prevent cytotoxic side-effects of CPAs. Freezing by slow-cooling methods and vitrification attempt to solve these problems in different ways.

Cryopreservation of oocytes by slow-cooling methods

Slow-cooling methods evolved from the studies on freezing mammalian embryos [15] based on the demonstration by Mazur and colleagues [16–19] that cleavage stage embryos could be slowly cooled to low subzero temperatures in a small number of appropriate intracellular cryoprotectants, which effectively dehydrated the cells. The principle underlying slow-cooling methods consists of gradual cell dehydration that is enabled by slow-cooling rates, typically less than 0.5 °C/min. Oocytes are first equilibrated in one or more solutions containing low CPA concentrations, typically 1.5 M of CPA in a pH buffered isotonic salt solution (such as phosphate buffered saline) with or without sucrose (0.1–0.3 M), and serum or protein to prevent cell adhesion to plastic or glass surfaces. The presence of solutes in the extracellular space determines an osmotic gradient for the extraction of intracellular water. Since the cell membrane is more permeable to water than CPAs, at first the water efflux is not balanced by permeating CPA influx, resulting in cell shrinkage and gradual cell re-expansion as the CPA enters the cell. A second step includes the exposure to both intracellular and extracellular CPAs that re-establish the osmotic gradient and induce additional dehydration. Finally, oocytes are loaded into plastic straws or glass vials and are slowly cooled to a temperature below the freezing point of the medium (typically between −6 °C and −8 °C). At this stage, ice nucleation is manually induced by touching the straw or vial near the solution interface with a pre-cooled object, such as pincers. The temperature is then reduced slowly (0.3 to 0.1 °C/min) using a programmable freezing machine to −30 °C or lower. This slow-cooling process prevents the formation of intracellular ice crystals which destroy the cells. During the slow-cooling period, the cells are further dehydrated by the increasing extracellular solute concentration that occurs during ice formation and the extracted water is added to large innocuous ice crystals that are formed in the extracellular space. The intracellular compartment is super-cooled, with very few, if any, small ice crystals present. Cooling below −30 °C to −150 °C can be done rapidly and finally the straw or vial is plunged in liquid nitrogen at a temperature of −196 °C. The cells will remain stably dehydrated between the innocuous extracellular ice formations at −196 °C until rewarmed. Warming rates need to be fast enough to prevent intracellular ice formation and crystal growth. This is typically done by direct transfer of the straw or vial into a waterbath at 30–37 °C. It is then required to enable rehydration of the cell and allow the CPA to escape during the more rapid process of water re-entry. This is better managed by passing the cells through a graded concentration of an intracellular and an extracellular solute (such as sucrose) to keep the cell from excessively expanding in volume during the water entry phase of rehydration.

Cryopreservation of oocytes using vitrification

It is possible to design aqueous solutions of cryoprotectants which do not freeze during cooling to low subzero temperatures and subsequent warming. The liquid solidifies at low temperatures far below the normal freezing point, forming glass rather than ice. The physical properties of glass formation and the chemical aspects of solutes required for the design of vitrification of biological specimens have been reviewed by others [20, 21]. The principle underlying vitrification consists in the exposure of cells to high permeating (40% or more w/w) and non-permeating CPA concentrations followed by a single-step ultra-rapid cooling to −196 °C. In these conditions, cell dehydration is completed before cooling. The probability of vitrification depends upon the cooling and rewarming rates, the viscosity of the solutions used, and the volume of the sample. Fast cooling rates were thought to be important to prevent ice nucleation. This is coupled to the use of highly viscous solutions obtained by increasing the concentrations of extracellular solutes. Glass formation occurs because the equilibrium freezing point of water is depressed so far that ice crystal growth is very slow and may be bypassed. Temperature diffusivity is an important factor in ensuring glass formation and it is governed by the geometry of the sample, thermal conductivity and heat capacity, and quench temperature at the surface of the sample. Reducing the volume of the solution contributes to complete glass formation and enables faster cooling and warming rates. These data led to the design of vitrification devices that had a minimal volume of medium and maximum surface area for rapid heat exchange.

In the design of vitrification solutions, the chemistry is critical. Methylation can increase glass formation, and additional methyl groups enhance glass-forming properties of amides (used to reduce cell toxicity) and polols (e.g., glycerol and propanediol). These effects are likely due to increased association of these solutes with water molecules. High concentrations needed for vitrification cause cell and tissue toxicity and the neutralization of these effects is needed for successful vitrification [22]. Shortening the exposure to toxic cryoprotectant permeation for both influx and efflux can abolish the toxicity problem. Hence a careful balance between the glass-forming property of the solution and toxicity is essential for successful vitrification and cell survival. Using parameters predictive of glass-forming ability and low toxicity, Fahy *et al.* designed new cryoprotective solutions for vitrification and showed that mouse oocytes could be efficiently vitrified with >80% development to blastocysts after vitrification [23]. There has been interest in developing methods for introducing sugars into the intracellular environment because this is a mechanism used for some organisms to avoid intracellular ice formation [24]. However, this approach has waned with further progress on vitrification methods.

The main side-effect of vitrification is the cytotoxicity of the high CPA concentrations. As a consequence the design of new safer strategies was considered a priority. First of all, ethylene glycol (EG) and sucrose became standard CPAs in vitrification because of their lower cell toxicity. Later, multiple CPAs have been used in combination in order to reduce the individual CPA toxicity but maintaining, at the same time, the appropriate viscosity of the solutions. In this regard, EG and DMSO together with sucrose have evolved as the first choice CPAs. Moreover, gradual CPA addition represented a significant improvement for the technique. This is accomplished by pre-equilibrating the cells slowly in a solution containing relatively low CPA concentration followed by a brief exposure to higher more toxic CPA concentrations in the final vitrification solution.

A major concern for applying vitrification methods consists of the choice of an appropriate support device During the years, different devices have been proposed and used, such as traditional plastic 0.25 ml insemination straws, glass vials, open-pulled straws, hemi-straws, Cryotops, Cryoloops, Cryoleafs, and Flexipets. As a general rule, vitrification methods are classified as "open" if the support device directly exposes the sample solution to liquid nitrogen when plunged into liquid nitrogen, or "closed" if the device is sealed prior to plunging into liquid nitrogen. Open systems allow extremely high cooling and warming rates but have the hypothetical risk of pathogen contamination due to direct contact with non-sterile liquid nitrogen. While closed systems are safer for ensuring sterility than open system methods, thermal isolation of the samples in closed systems may influence negatively the cooling and, importantly, warming rates, potentially interfering with the stability of vitrification.

To date, the most popular method for vitrification appears to be that initially proposed by Kuwayama [25, 26]. The procedure is performed at room temperature. The equilibration solution is composed of 7.5% EG and 7.5% DMSO, whereas the vitrification solution contains 15% EG, 15% DMSO, and 0.5 M sucrose. Oocytes are gradually equilibrated through the exposure to slightly increasing CPA concentrations for 10–12 minutes. They are then transferred to the vitrification solution and incubated for 1 minute. They are

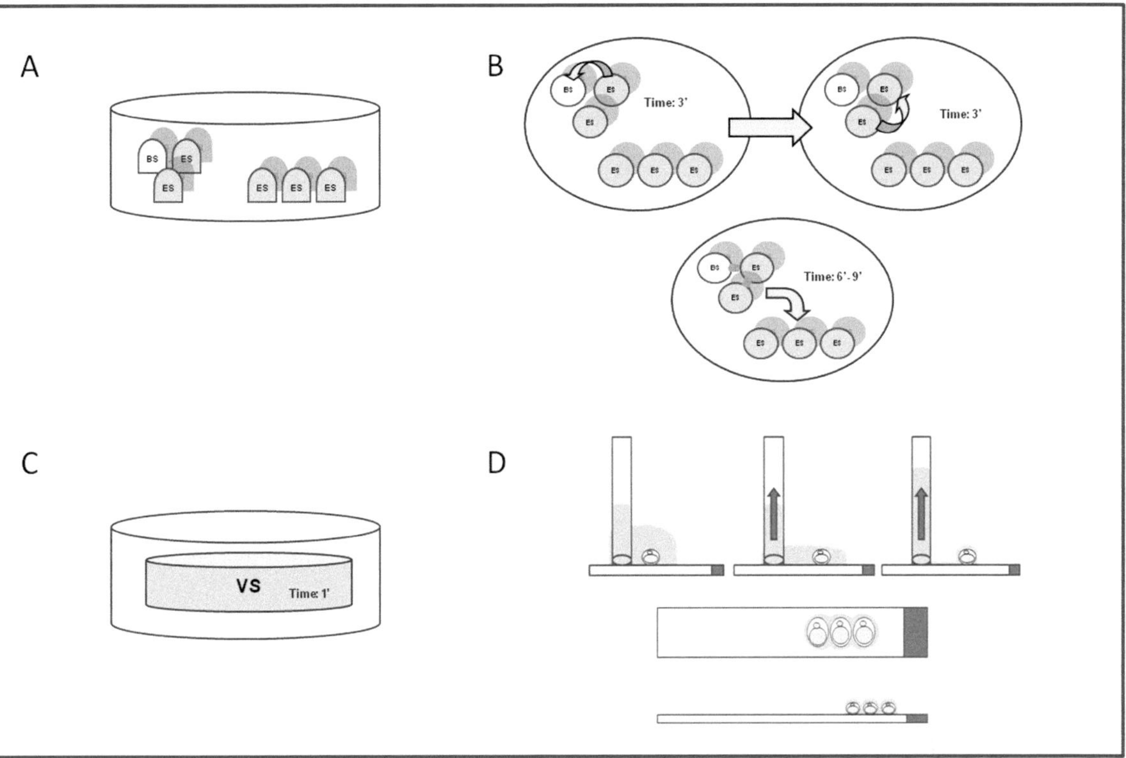

Figure 36.1 Vitrification protocol according to Kuwayama *et al.* [26] and adapted by Rienzi *et al.* [47]. The vitrification procedure is performed at room temperature. (A) Disposition of the vitrification drops (20 μl each) containing basic solution (BS) (HEPES buffered basic culture medium M199 with 20% synthetic serum substitute [SSS]) and equilibration solution (ES) (7.5% EG and 7.5% DMSO). (B) Oocytes are equilibrated in ES; to perform the equilibration gradually, the oocytes are first placed in BS and, immediately after, mixed with a second drop of ES. After 3 minutes' incubation, a third drop of ES solution is mixed. Finally, the oocytes are moved in a pure drop of ES and incubated for additional 6–9 minutes. (C) The oocytes (1 to 3, contemporaneously) are then transferred to 1 ml of vitrification solution (VS) containing 15% EG, 15% DMSO, and 0.5 M sucrose in M199 + 20% SSS for 1 minute. (D) The oocytes are then placed on the Cryotop strip in a single small drop of VS. Much care is taken to re-aspirate, as much as possible, the excess of VS in such a way as to leave just a thin layer around each oocyte.

then loaded on the support (Cryotop) paying attention to minimizing the volume of the solution, and finally they are plunged in liquid nitrogen (Figure 36.1).

A critical aspect for successful vitrification is the rewarming rate used. During this phase it is essential to prevent devitrification and the growth of small intracellular or extracellular ice crystals. When cooling to −196 °C, warming must be very rapid (>2200 °C/min). Seki and Mazur [27] showed convincingly that the successful vitrification of mouse oocytes in a solution containing 20% EG, 10% acetamide, 0.4 M sucrose, and 24% Ficoll, to −70 °C or to −196 °C, was dependent on rewarming rates. Later the same authors [28, 29] showed that the highest mouse oocyte survival (>80%) occurred at the highest rewarming rates (2950 °C/min), irrespective of the cooling rate. This indicates that the warming rate, rather that the cooling rate, is the primary determining factor in oocyte survival in vitrification cycles (Figure 36.2).

Reported outcomes of cryopreservating of oocytes

As a general rule, the critical evaluation of any cryopreservation outcomes should not be limited to the report of the survival rate of oocytes. It is very certain that cryopreservation will have some impact on oocyte physiology and predictably impair their subsequent development. The test of the method is to minimize these effects. Ultimately, the efficiency of the technique should be defined by the clinical results, namely pregnancy and implantation rates. Moreover, the reliability of the analysis should be assured by a direct comparison with fresh controls.

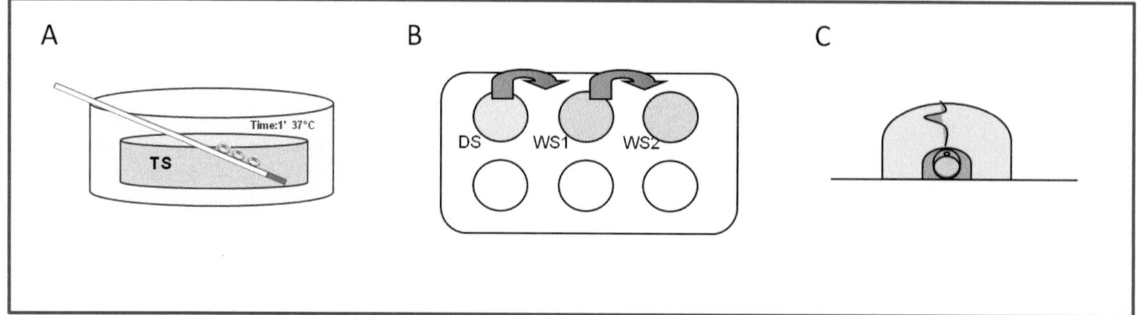

Figure 36.2 Warming procedure according to Kuwayama *et al.* [26] and adapted by Rienzi *et al.* [47]. (A) The first step of the warming procedure is performed at 37 °C. The cap is removed in liquid nitrogen and the Cryotop is immediately submerged in 1 ml of thawing solution (TS) containing 1.0 M sucrose in M199 + 20% SSS for 1 minute incubation. (B) After 1 minute, oocytes are placed in 1 ml of dilution solution (DS) containing 0.5 M sucrose, and incubated at room temperature (RT) for 3 minutes. Finally, the oocytes are washed at RT for 6 minutes in two different dishes containing 1 ml of washing solution (WS: basic medium M199 + 20% SSS) each, and transferred into 1 ml of culture medium. A gradient should be created in the passage between different solutions. Degenerated oocytes are removed from the cohort. (C) Schematic representation of the gradient to be created in the passage of the oocytes between different solutions. The previous solution is represented in dark pink, the new solution in light pink.

Outcome of freezing by slow cooling

During the years slow-cooling methods have been progressively modified in order to achieve better biological and clinical results. In particular, the original protocol with DMSO [8] was improved in the 1990s by substituting the cryoprotectant DMSO with PROH and adding sucrose at a concentration of 0.1 M, as mentioned previously. A number of studies have been performed applying this protocol [30–35] but unfortunately most of them did not compare the results with fresh oocyte controls, with the exception of a study conducted by Borini *et al.* [34]. They reported a 43.4% oocyte survival rate, and fertilization and embryo cleavage rates were 51.6% and 86%, respectively. The clinical pregnancy and implantation rates were 19.2% and 12.3%, much lower if compared to those obtained with fresh controls (30% and 22.6%, respectively). However, even if this study confirmed the inadequacy of the slow-cooling protocols, it nevertheless underlined the potential benefits offered in terms of the addition to overall cumulative pregnancy rate.

The disappointing results obtained with this method stimulated new suggestions, such as increasing sucrose concentration to 0.2 M or 0.3 M. Fabbri *et al.* [36] showed an enhancement of the oocyte survival rate in the presence of a higher sucrose concentration. The survival rate of oocytes was 34% in 0.1 M sucrose, increased to 60% in 0.2 M sucrose and to 82% in 0.3 M sucrose. Moreover, the survival rate could be improved by increasing the time of exposure to the equilibration solution from 5 minutes to >10 minutes. Similarly, Chen *et al.* [37] reported significantly higher survival, cleavage, and high quality embryo rates using 0.2 M sucrose (78.3%, 55.6%, 40.7%, respectively) when compared with 0.1 M sucrose (48.9%, 22.7%, 13.6%, respectively). These results suggest that 0.1 M sucrose did not allow sufficient cell dehydration. Unfortunately, neither study reported clinical results. Later some authors demonstrated that even if the survival and fertilization rates were higher in the case of 0.23 M and 0.3 M sucrose, the surviving oocytes may progress to embryos but with reduced developmental potential, since the reported pregnancy and implantation rates were lower when compared to those with 0.1 M sucrose [38, 39].

An alternative approach aimed at the improvement of the technique involved the use of choline as a substitute for sodium in the freezing solutions. It has been shown using mouse oocytes that extracellular choline may prevent the "solution effects" of high ionic concentrations during the freezing process [40]. However, despite encouraging results, the small sample sizes did not allow any categorical conclusions to be drawn [41, 42]. Moreover, it was not possible to demonstrate the superiority of the technique when compared to the conventional slow-cooling methods with standard freezing solutions even when using higher sucrose concentrations [43].

Vitrification outcomes

Comparisons were made between insemination straws, open-pulled straws and Cryotops for

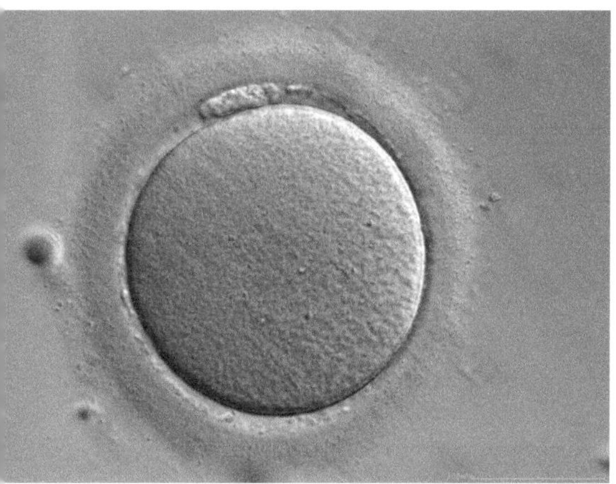

Figure 36.3 Human metaphase II oocyte after vitrification procedure (400 × magnification).

vitrification of bovine oocytes in EG (6.83 M) and sucrose (13 M) by Kuwayama *et al.* [25]. Oocytes were pre-equilibrated in 1.6 M EG for 5–15 minutes before they were transferred to the vitrification solution and loaded into each device (30 seconds), then plunged into liquid nitrogen. The best results were obtained with the Cryotop, despite the similarities seen for vitrification of mouse oocyte survival in straws and Cryotops [44]. The Cryotop is a specially constructed fine polythene strip attached to a plastic handle. Oocytes are vitrified in 1 μl of medium on this polythene strip. Twenty-three percent of blastocysts developed from Cryotop vitrification, compared with 5–7% in the other methods and 45% for fresh non-vitrified control oocytes. Reducing the concentration of EG to 5 M for human oocytes vitrified using the Cryotop was significantly better than 6.8 M and resulted in 50% blastocysts of 64 oocytes vitrified. Ten pregnancies (seven babies and three ongoing pregnancies) were obtained. This is a remarkable increase in the baby rate for cryopreserved oocytes (15.6%) (Figure 36.3). This method has now been reported to have resulted in more than 2000 babies from vitrified human oocytes [26, 45].

The adoption of this vitrification protocol designed by Kuwayama has enabled optimum biological and clinical outcomes to be achieved. Antinori *et al.* [46] demonstrated extremely high oocyte survival rate (99.4%) and these data were later confirmed by other authors; Cobo *et al.* [5] reported an oocyte survival rate of 96.9% and Rienzi *et al.* [47] a survival rate of 96.7%. Furthermore, the technique does not appear to impact significantly on the developmental competence of the oocytes, since fertilization rate, cleavage rate, and clinical outcomes in terms of clinical pregnancy and implantation rates were similar to those obtained with fresh oocyte controls [5, 46]. These results were confirmed recently in a prospective randomized controlled clinical trial for an oocyte donation program [7] and in a prospective randomized sibling–oocyte study in a standard infertility program [47, 48]. These latter reports clearly demonstrated the similarity of vitrified oocytes to fresh oocytes, with comparable outcomes for fertilization rate (79.2% vs. 83.3), cleavage rate of embryos (97.9 vs. 100%), and excellent quality embryo rate at day 2 (51.6% vs. 52%) [47]. In a subsequent study, the reported clinical results for vitrified oocytes were lower than those of fresh oocyte transfer cycles. However the "fresh" and "vitrified" oocyte groups may not be directly comparable because the former included all patients while the latter included only patients that did not became pregnant at the first embryo transfer attempt. Furthermore, fresh oocytes were transferred in superovulation cycles and the vitrified cycles were performed in normal hormonal cycles. As a consequence, the results may need to be considered in the larger context of cumulative ongoing pregnancy rate, which was high and comparable for transfer of fresh and cryopreserved embryos [48].

Recently an observational longitudinal cohort multicenter study was conducted in three European clinics (G.EN.E.R.A, Rome, Italy; Ca' Granda Ospedale Maggiore Policlinico, Milano, Italy; IVI, Valencia, Spain) in order to investigate the overall efficiency and consistency of oocyte cryopreservation by vitrification. A total of 486 warming cycles have been performed and the reported survival and fertilization were 84.7% and 75.2%, respectively. A total of 929 embryos have been transfered in 436 menstrual cycles, either at cleavage or blastocyst stage (83.2% and 16.7% respectively). A total of 166 clinical pregnancies were obtained (38.1% per transfer) and the delivery rate per transfer was 29.4%. These results further confirm that vitrification is a safe and efficient method for oocyte cryopreservation. Moreover, the same study investigated the predictive value of different infertility factors; delivery rate was not influenced by the stimulation protocol but the number of oocytes retrieved, the incubation period between retrieval and cryopreservation, maternal age, and the number of oocytes vitrified – all correlated to vitrification outcome. In particular, each year of maternal age

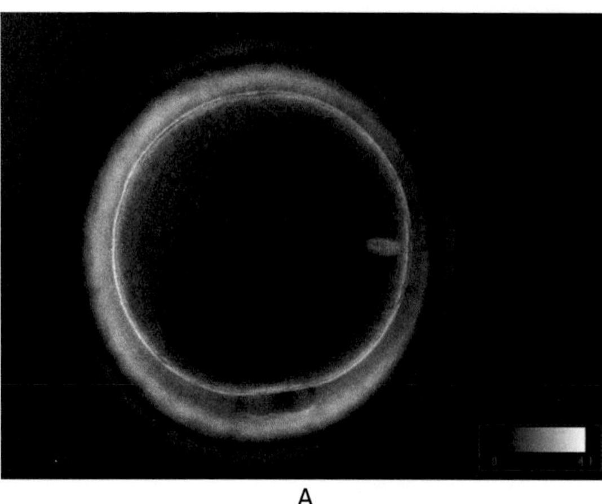

A

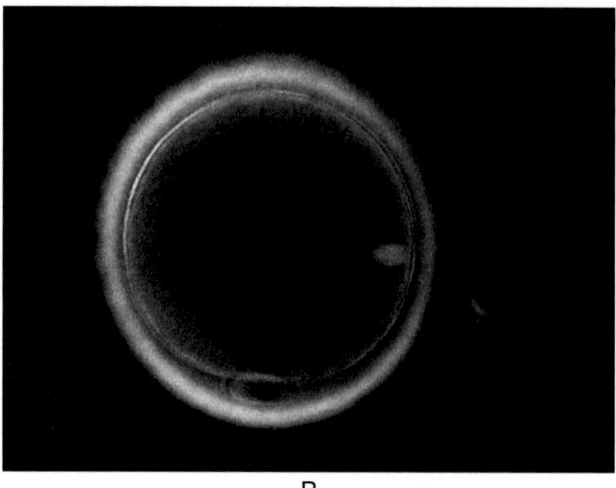

B

Figure 36.4 Human metaphase II oocyte prior (A) and after (B) vitrification procedure observed by polarized light microscopy (400× magnification). The meiotic spindle is clearly visible at 3 o'clock position.

decreased the delivery rate by 7%. Delivery rate doubled when more than eight oocytes were vitrified [49].

Vitrification versus slow cooling

The comparison of slow cooling with vitrification is difficult due to the existence of different protocols for both the methods. In particular, for slow cooling the sucrose concentration in the freezing and thawing solutions seems to be important for the success of the procedure. Similarly, the use of closed rather than open systems in vitrification, even if considered safer in terms of risk of pathogen cross-contamination, could impair the outcomes, reducing cooling and, particularly, rewarming rates.

Grifo and Noyes achieved better biological results with slow-cooled oocytes than with vitrified oocytes, but they did not draw any conclusion regarding the clinical outcomes [50, 51]. On the contrary, other authors reported better results from vitrification than from slow-cooling oocytes [52–54]. Moreover, it has been found that vitrified oocytes may have better ultrastructure and calcium function than the slow-cooled counterparts [55].

A recent meta-analysis on clinical application of oocyte vitrification [56] showed no difference between vitrified and fresh oocytes in terms of fertilization, embryo cleavage, top quality embryos, and ongoing pregnancy rates and it also suggests a superiority of vitrification over slow cooling. However, a retrospective cohort study by Bianchi and colleagues [57] reported satisfactory results using a 0.2–0.3 M sucrose concentration and slow-cooling protocol, concluding that slow cooling can still be a valid tool in IVF if a proper protocol is adopted.

Conclusions

Oocyte cryopreservation has represented a great challenge for assisted reproductive technologies and until recently it has been regarded as inconsistent and inefficient. A few years ago oocyte cryopreservation was still considered an experimental procedure [58]. However, the recent success reported with vitrified and frozen-oocyte cycles has changed this opinion such that oocyte vitrification is no longer considered an experimental procedure [59]. Conventional slow-cooling methods have been modified through the years, resulting in improved results, but the turning point is the introduction and development of vitrification protocols that allowed a significant enhancement of oocyte cryopreservation in terms of better laboratory and clinical outcomes. Survival rate is now >80% and fertilization, cleavage, pregnancy, and implantation rates are comparable to those obtained with fresh counterparts. However, it is important to note that, even if the cryopreservation protocol per se is fundamental for the success of the procedure, close attention must be paid in all quality control systems so that oocytes are not exposed to suboptimal culture conditions. For example, they should be frozen/vitrified immediately after denuding and inseminated not more than 2 hours after rewarming. Recently it has been postulated that this timing should be revised, since it has been demonstrated that the meiotic spindle repolymerizes (Figure 36.4) as soon as 1 hour after rewarming [60]. Moreover, denuding and oocyte selection for freezing should be performed in a controlled environment of gas composition (5–6% CO_2 and low O_2 tension) and humidification.

Finally, the debate about the safety of the cryopreservation procedures still remains. Despite reassuring preliminary data [61] we still need extensive obstetric data on babies born following oocyte cryopreservation. On the other hand, it is appropriate to formulate some considerations about the biosafety of the direct contact of the biological samples with non-sterile liquid nitrogen, in particular in the case of vitrification with open device systems. To date, there are no documented cases of cross-contamination in liquid nitrogen in the history of human reproductive medicine. However, research is needed to develop new devices that will allow the protection of cells while maintaining consistent and reproducible results. In this regard, the use of vapor storage tanks and the adoption of UV-sterilized liquid nitrogen may be valid approaches but more studies are needed to assure their reliability.

References

1. Cobo A, Domingo J, Perez S, *et al.* Vitrification: an effective new approach to oocyte banking and preserving fertility in cancer patients. *Clin Transl Oncol* 2008; **10**: 268–73.
2. Noyes N, Labella PA, Grifo J, Knopman JM. Oocyte cryopreservation: a feasible fertility preservation option for reproductive age cancer survivors. *J Assist Reprod Genet* 2010; **27**: 495–9.
3. Noyes N, Knopman JM, Melzer K, *et al.* Oocyte cryopreservation as a fertility preservation measure for cancer patients. *Reprod Biomed Online* 2011; **23**: 323–33.
4. Stoop D, Nekkebroeck J, Devroey P. A survey on the intentions and attitudes towards oocyte cryopreservation for non-medical reasons among women of reproductive age. *Hum Reprod* 2011; **26**: 655–61.
5. Cobo A, Kuwayama M, Perez S, *et al.* Comparison of concomitant outcome achieved with fresh and cryopreserved donor oocytes vitrified by the Cryotop method. *Fertil Steril* 2008; **89**:1657–64.
6. Nagy ZP, Chang CC, Shapiro DB, *et al.* Clinical evaluation of the efficiency on an oocyte donation program using egg cryo-banking. *Fertil Steril* 2009; **92**: 520–26.
7. Cobo A, Meseguer M, Remohi J, Pellicer A. Use of cyo-banked oocytes in an ovum donation programme: a prospective, randomized, controlled, clinical trial. *Hum Reprod* 2010; **25**: 2239–46.
8. Chen C. Pregnancy after human oocyte cryopreservation. *Lancet* 1986; **1**: 884–6.
9. Sathananthan AH, Trounson A, Freeman L. Morphology and fertilizability of frozen human oocytes. *Gamete Res* 1987; **16**: 343–54.
10. Sathananthan AH, Trounson A, Freeman L, Brady T. The effects of cooling human oocytes. *Hum Reprod* 1988; **3**: 968–77.
11. Mandelbaum J, Belaisch-Allart J, Junca AM, *et al.* Cryopreservation in human assisted reproduction is now routine for embryos but remains a research procedure for oocytes. *Hum Reprod* 1998; 13 Suppl **3**: 161–74.
12. Tucker MJ, Morton PC, Wright G, Sweitzer CL, Massey JB. Clinical application of human egg cryopreservation. *Hum Reprod* 1998; **13**: 3156–59.
13. Kuleshova L, Gianaroli L, Magli MC, Ferraretti A, Trounson A. Birth following vitrification of a small number of human oocytes: a case report. *Hum Reprod* 1999; **14**: 3077–9.
14. Scaravelli G, Vigiliano V, Mayorga JM, *et al.* Analysis of oocyte crypreservation in assisted reproduction: the Italian National Register data from 2005 to 2007. *Reprod Biomed Online* 2010; **21**: 496–500.
15. Saragusty J, Arav A. Current progress in oocyte and embryo cryopreservation by slow freezing and vitrification. *Reproduction* 2011; **141**: 1–19.
16. Leibo SP, Mazur P. The role of cooling rates in low-temperature preservation. *Cryobiology* 1971; **8**: 8447–52.
17. Whittingham DG, Leibo SP, Mazur P. Survival of mouse embryos frozen to −196 degrees and −269 degrees C. *Science* 1972; **178**: 411–14.
18. Leibo SP, Mazur P, Jackowski SC. Factors affecting survival of mouse embryos during freezing and thawing. *Exp Cell Res* 1974; **89**: 79–88.
19. Mazur P, Rall WF, Leibo SP. Kinetics of water loss and the likelihood of intracellular freezing in mouse ova. Influence of the method of calculating the temperature dependence of water permeability. *Cell Biophys* 1984; **6**: 197–213.
20. MacFarlane DR. Physical aspects of vitrification in aqueous solutions. *Cryobiology* 1987; **24**: 181–95.
21. Fahy GM, Levy DI, Ali SE. Some emerging principles underlying the physical properties, biological actions, and utility of vitrification solutions. *Cryobiology* 1987; **24**: 196–213.

22. Fahy GM. Cryoprotectant toxicity neutralization. *Cryobiology* 2010; **60**(3 Suppl): S45–53.

23. Fahy GM, Wowk B, Wu J, Paynter S. Improved vitrification solutions based on the predictability of vitrification toxicity. *Cryobiology* 2004; **48**: 22–35.

24. Wright DL, Eroglu A, Toner M, Toth TL. Use of sugars in cryopreserving human oocytes. *Reprod Biomed Online* 2004; **9**: 179–86.

25. Kuwayama M, Vajta G, Kato O, Leibo SP. Highly efficient vitrification method for the cryopreservation of human oocytes. *Reprod Biomed Online* 2005; **11**: 300–8.

26. Kuwayama M. Highly efficient vitrification for cryopreservation of human oocytes and embryos: the Cryotop method. *Theriogenology* 2007; **67**: 73–80.

27. Seki S, Mazur P. Effect of warming rate on the survival of vitrified mouse oocytes and on the recrystallization of intracellular ice. *Biol Reprod* 2008; **79**: 727–37.

28. Seki S, Mazur P .The dominance of warming rate over cooling rate in the survival of mouse oocytes subject to a vitrification procedure. *Cryobiology* 2009; **59**: 75–82.

29. Seki S, Mazur P. Stability of mouse oocytes at −80 °C: the role of recrystallization of intracellular ice. *Reproduction* 2011; **141**: 407–15.

30. Tucker M, Wright G, Morton P, *et al.* Preliminary experience with human oocyte cryopreservation using 1,2-propanediol and sucrose. *Hum Reprod* 1996; **11**: 1513–15.

31. Porcu E, Fabbri R, Seracchioli R, *et al.* Birth of a healthy female after intracytoplasmic sperm injection of cryopreserved human oocytes. *Fertil Steril* 1997; **68**(4): 724–6.

32. Chia CM, Chan WB, Quah E, Cheng LC. Triploid pregnancy after ICSI of frozen testicular spermatozoa into cryopreserved human oocytes: case report. *Hum Reprod* 2000; **15**: 1962–4.

33. Allan J. Case report: pregnancy from intracytoplasmic injection of a frozen-thawed oocyte. *Aust N Z J Obstet Gynaecol* 2004; **44**: 588.

34. Borini A, Lagalla C, Bonu MA, *et al.* Cumulative pregnancy rates resulting from the use of fresh and frozen oocytes: 7 years' experience. *Reprod Biomed Online* 2006; **12**: 481–6.

35. Magli C, Lappi M, Farretti AP, *et al.* Impact of cryopreservation on embryo development. *Fertil Steril* 2010; **93**: 510–16.

36. Fabbri R, Porcu E, Marsella T, *et al.* Human oocyte cryopreservation: new perspectives regarding oocyte survival. *Hum Reprod* 2001; **16**: 411–16.

37. Chen ZJ, Li M, Zhao LX, *et al.* Effects of sucrose concentration on the developmental potential of human frozen-thawed oocytes at different stages of maturity. *Hum Reprod* 2004; **19**: 2345–9.

38. Levi Setti PE, Albani E, Novara PV, Cesana A, Morreale G. Cryopreservation of supernumerary oocytes in IVF/ICSI cycles. *Hum Reprod* 2006; **21**: 370–5.

39. De Santis L, Cino I, Rabellotti E, *et al.* Oocyte cryopreservation: clinical outcome of slow-cooling protocols differing in sucrose concentration. *Reprod Biomed Online* 2007; **14**: 57–63.

40. Stackechi JJ, Cohen J, Willadsen GM. Detrimental effects of sodium during mouse oocyte cryopreservation. *Biol Reprod* 1998; **59**: 395–400.

41. Quintans CJ, Donaldson MJ, Bertolino MV, Pasqualini RS. Birth of two babies using oocytes that were cryopreserved in a choline-based freezing medium. *Hum Reprod* 2002; **17**: 3149–52.

42. Boldt J, Tidswell N, Sayers A, Kilani R, Cline D. Human oocyte cryopreservation: 5-year experience with a sodium-depleted slow freezing method. *Reprod Biomed Online* 2006; **13**: 96–100.

43. Gook DA, Edgar DH. Human oocyte cryopreservation *Hum Reprod Update* 2007; **13**: 591–605.

44. Mazur P, Seki S. Survival of mouse oocytes after being cooled in a vitrification solution to −196 °C at 95° to 70,000°C/min and warmed at 610° to 118,000 °C/min: a new paradigm for cryopreservation by vitrification. *Cryobiology* 2011; **62**(1): 1–7.

45. Kuwayama M. Vitrification of human oocytes. *Reprod Biomed Online* 2010; **20**(Suppl 3): S3 (Abstr.).

46. Antinori M, Licata E, Dani G, *et al.* Cryotop vitrification of human oocytes results in high survival rate and healthy deliveries. *Reprod Biomed Online* 2007; **14**: 72–9.

47. Rienzi L, Romano S, Albricci L, *et al.* Embryo development of fresh"versus" vitrified metaphase II oocytes after ICSI: a prospective randomized sibling-oocyte study. *Human Reprod* 2010; **25**: 66–73.

48. Ubaldi F, Anniballo R, Romano S, *et al.* Cumulative ongoing pregnancy rate achieved with oocyte vitrification and cleavage stage transfer without embryo selection in a standard infertility program. *Hum Reprod* 2010; **25**: 1199–205.

49. Rienzi L, Cobo A, Paffoni A, *et al.* Consistent and predictable delivery rates after oocytes vitrification: an observational longitudinal cohort multicentric study. *Hum Reprod* 2012; **27**(6): 1606–12.

50. Grifo JA, Noyes N. Delivery rate using cryopreserved oocytes is comparable to conventional in vitro fertilization using fresh oocytes: potential fertility preservation for female cancer patients. *Fertil Steril* 2010; **93**: 391–6.

51. Noyes N, Knopman J, Labella P, *et al.* Oocyte cryopreservation outcomes including pre-cryopreservation and post-thaw meiotic splindle evaluation following slow cooling and vitrification of human oocytes. *Fertil Steril* 2010; **94**: 2078–82.

52. Fadini R, Brambillasca R, Renzini MM, *et al.* Human oocyte cryopreservation: comparison between slow and ultrarapid methods. *Reprod Biomed Online* 2009; **19**: 171–80.

53. Cao YX, Xing Q, Li L, *et al.* Comparison of survival and embryonic development in human oocytes cryopreserved by slow-freezing and vitrification. *Fertil Steril* 2009; **92**: 1306–11.

54. Smith GD, Serafini PC, Fioravanti J, *et al.* Prospective randomized comparison of human oocyte cryopreservation with slow-rate freezing or vitrification. *Fertil Steril* 2010; **94**: 2088–95.

55. Gualtieri R, Mollo V, Barbato V, Fiorentino I, Iaccarino M. Ultrastructure and intracellular calcium response during activation in vitrified and slow-frozen oocytes. *Hum Reprod* 2011; **26**: 2452–60.

56. Cobo A, Diaz C. Clinical application of oocyte vitrification: a systematic review and meta-analysis of randomized controlled trials. *Fertil Steril* 2011; **96**: 277–85.

57. Bianchi V, Lappi M, Bonu MA, Borini A. Oocyte slow freezing using a 0.2–0.3 M sucrose concentration protocol: is it really the time to trash the cryopreservation machine? *Fertil Steril* 2012; **97**(5): 1101–7.

58. Practice Committees of American Society for Reproductive Medicine; Society for Assisted Reproductive Technology. Ovarian tissue and oocyte cryopreservation. *Fertil Steril* 2008 **90**(5 Suppl): S241–6.

59. Practice Committee of American Society for Reproductive Medicine; Practice Committee of Society for Assisted Reproductive Technology. Mature oocyte cryopreservation: a guideline. *Fertil Steril* 2013; **99**(1): 37–43.

60. Bromfield JJ, Coticchio G, Hutt K, *et al.* Meiotic spindle dynamics in human oocytes following slow-cooling cryopreservation. *Hum Reprod* 2009; **24**: 2114–23.

61. Noyes N, Porcu E, Borini A. Over 900 oocyte cryopreservation babies born with no apparent increase in congenital anomalies. *Reprod Biomed Online* 2009;**18**(6): 769–76.

Chapter 37

Transplantation of ovarian tissue or immature oocytes to preserve and restore fertility in humans

Sherman Silber, Natalie Barbey, and David Silber

Introduction

It is now possible to preserve and restore fertility, using ovary and egg freezing and ovary transplantation, in young women with cancer who are undergoing otherwise sterilizing chemotherapy and radiation. This approach can also be used for any woman who wishes to prolong her reproductive lifespan. This chapter is limited to the clinically proven therapeutic applications of this technology. Our clinical results with these new therapeutic approaches are adding to our understanding of the basic science of reproduction, and may eventually obviate the growing worldwide epidemic of female age-related decline in fertility.

The developed world is in the midst of a widespread infertility epidemic. Economies in Japan, the United States, southern Europe, and even China are threatened by a decreasing population of young people having to support an increasing population of elderly and retirees [1]. The most common reason to see a doctor in countries such as India and China, seemingly plagued with overpopulation, is for infertility. Infertility clinics are popping up throughout the world in huge numbers [2].

It is clear to all that the major reason for the world's growing infertility epidemic is that as women put off childbearing, their oocytes die off and those that survive are of poor quality [3–6]. In her teen years a woman has a 0.2% chance of being infertile, and by her early twenties it is up to 2%. By her early thirties, it is up to 20% [2, 7]. Many modern women today do not think of having a baby until their mid thirties, and by then over 25% are infertile, simply because of the aging and the decline in number of their oocytes. This is clearly demonstrated by the high pregnancy rate using donor oocytes from young women placed into the uterus of older women [2, 3, 7]. Yet fertility physicians struggle to make a pathological entity diagnosis to explain the infertility, which in truth in most cases is just a normal physiological response to oocyte aging [2, 3, 7].

Preserving fertility for women who wish to put off childbearing or who are about to undergo treatment with gonadotoxic drugs: using ovarian freezing and transplantation

Until recently oocyte freezing had very poor to no success, and so ovary tissue slow freezing was the only method we could rely upon for preservation. Of course, now we also have a favorable option of preserving oocytes after ovarian stimulation and egg retrieval using vitrification instead of slow freezing for cryopreservation [4, 8, 9] (see Chapter 36). Nonetheless ovarian tissue freezing and transplantation still has great advantages over oocyte freezing. There does not need to be a prior delaying stimulation cycle so ovarian tissue freezing will delay the cancer treatment by only a few days. Furthermore, one cycle of ovarian stimulation and egg freezing does not assure successful pregnancy as much as an entire ovary would, and finally, transplanting ovarian tissue back not only restores fertility but also restores endocrine function.

Biology and Pathology of the Oocyte, 2nd edn., ed. Alan Trounson, Roger Gosden, and Ursula Eichenlaub-Ritter. Published by Cambridge University Press.

Fresh series of identical twins with premature ovarian failure

Let us take the clinical evolution of this technology in logical order. The first successful fresh human ovary transplantation was reported between a pair of remarkable monozygotic twins discordant for premature ovarian failure (POF), using a cortical grafting technique [10]. This key event allowed us to assess the results of fresh transplantation unclouded by confusion that might have been caused by freezing. The first successful human frozen ovary auto-grafts were reported around the same time with tissue cryopreserved for cancer patients prior to their sterilizing bone marrow transplants [11, 12]. These followed similar results described in the sheep over a decade earlier [8]. The transplantation technique has subsequently been refined over a larger series of nine consecutive successful fresh ovary transplants in identical twins (plus two fresh allotransplants to be treated separately), with resumption of normal hormonal cycling and menstruation in all cases, eventually leading to 14 pregnancies and 11 healthy babies born from the nine fresh identical twin recipients [5, 13–15]. This unusual consecutive series of fresh ovary cortical transplants helped us also refine the techniques necessary for successful preservation of fertility for cancer patients using ovarian tissue freezing, with three additional successful pregnancies from three frozen transplants. This unusual series also helped to establish a method for distinguishing between the oocyte loss from transplant ischemia and the oocyte loss from cryopreservation. We now can report long-term follow-up (up to 8 years) of this original series of fresh transplants, and add to it our more recent experience with cryopreserved ovarian tissue. The results appear to be remarkably more robust than had originally been contemplated [6, 16].

The first such twin case inquired about the possibility of fresh ovary transplantation originally from researching an earlier testis transplant we had reported for anorchia [10, 17, 18]. From that point forward, patients in similar situations sought this treatment. All of them found the possibility of natural conception more attractive than in vitro fertilization (IVF) or oocyte donation. In most cases, the twins lived far apart (even in different countries) and the donors preferred to make a single visit for a one-time ovary donation, rather than go through multiple cycles of ovarian hyperstimulation. We knew when we began this series that there would be few clinical cases in the world like these that would warrant fresh ovarian transplantation. However, this series would allow us to learn how to more effectively freeze and transplant human ovarian tissue, which would have far reaching consequences and widespread application for preservation of fertility in cancer patients and for women who just need to delay childbearing for social reasons.

Despite risks, the evidence does not support a deleterious effect of unilateral oophorectomy either on fertility or on age at menopause [19, 20].

One entire ovary of the donor was therefore removed and the cortex dissected away from the medulla. The cortex of the non-functioning recipient ovary was removed in entirety, and the donor cortex slices were transplanted onto the exposed recipient medulla using 9-0 nylon interrupted sutures. A tiny piece of spare tissue of the donor, as well as the entire resected atrophied ovarian cortex of the recipient were examined histologically in all cases (Figures 37.1A and 37.1B).

Micro-hematoma formation under the graft was avoided by micro-bipolar cautery and micropressure stitches of 9-0 nylon. Constant pulsatile irrigation with heparinized saline prevented adhesions (Figure 37.2A–D).

Only one-third of the ovarian cortex was grafted fresh and two-thirds were frozen.

Ovarian cryopreservation

All of our fresh clinical transplant studies involved cryopreservation of spare tissue for future thawed transplants. We also have frozen the ovarian tissue of 68 cancer patients and 7 patients who simply wanted to delay childbearing, all with Institutional Review Board (IRB) approval. All of the frozen cases thus far transplanted back to the patient have utilized the slow freeze approach [8, 21, 22]. However, we now use vitrification exclusively for cryopreservation in humans because of the results of in vitro viability analysis in humans as well as in vivo transplant studies in the bovine [5, 23].

The goal of the in vitro study was to determine which method produced a higher cell survival rate: slow freezing, or vitrification. The high viability (92%) of oocytes in control (fresh) specimens indicated that disaggregation per se had caused only minimal damage to the oocytes [5]. Overall 2301 oocytes were examined from 16 specimens. Results within each of the three groups revealed no significant difference

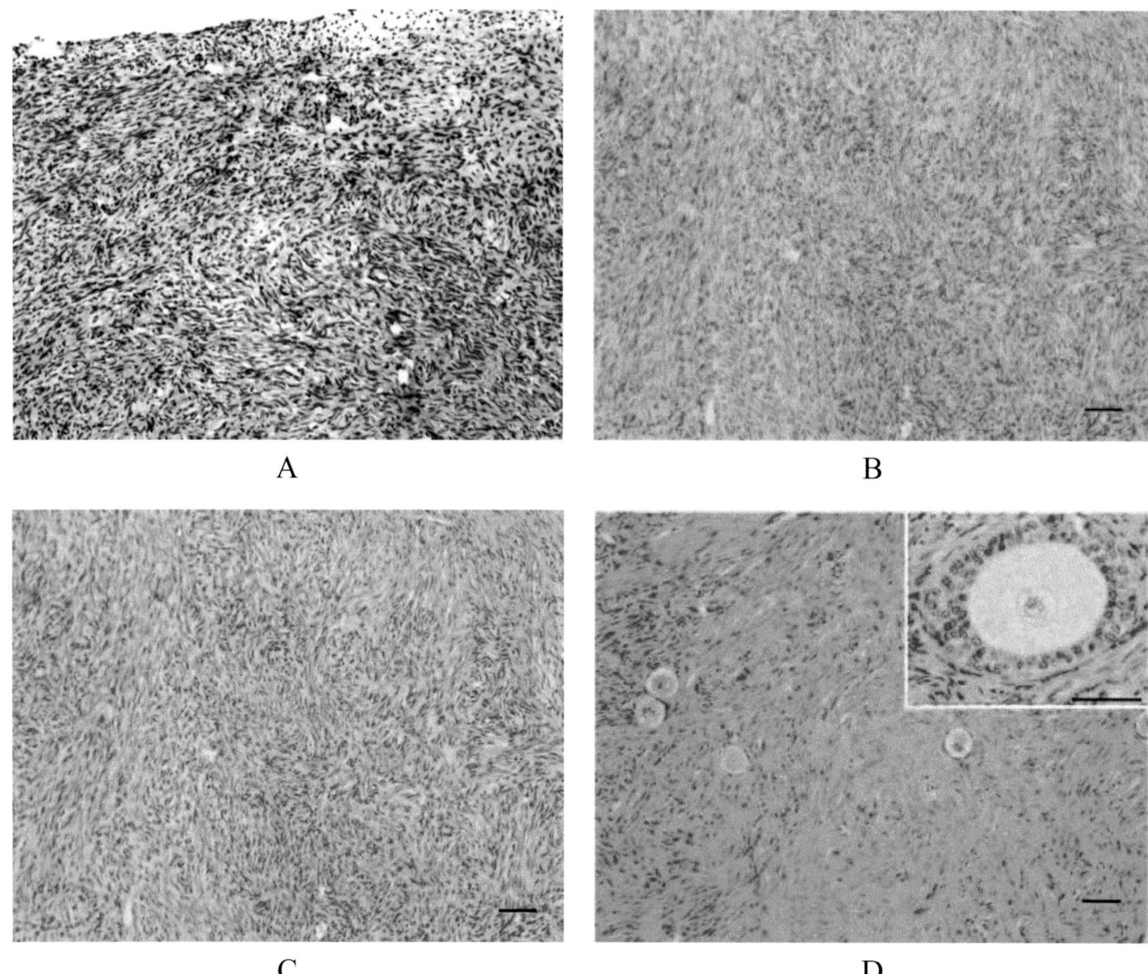

Figure 37.1 (A, B) Showing the absence of primordial or preantral follicles in ovarian biopsies of this candidate for ovarian transplantation compared with (C, D) that in her fertile sister.

between fresh and vitrified tissue, but the viability of slow freeze-cryopreserved tissue was less than one-half that of vitrified tissue or controls (42%) ($P < 0.01$). Transmission electron microscopy also has been used to analyze ovarian tissue that had been either cryopreserved by slow freezing or vitrified by ultra-rapid freezing, showing vitrification to be superior [24].

Standard hematoxylin and eosin (H&E) histology showed no difference between pre-freeze ovarian tissue and post-vitrification ovarian tissue (Figure 37.3A and 37.3B).

Finally, quantitative histological study of primordial follicles in the bovine after vitrification and transplantation back to the cow 2 months later remarkably showed no follicle loss.

The basic science concept of vitrification, whether for eggs, embryos, or tissue, is to avoid completely any ice crystal formation by using a very high concentration of cryoprotectant and a very rapid rate (virtually "instant") of cooling. This is quite different from classic slow-freeze cooling, which relies on a partial and very gradual removal of water from the cell by encouraging ice crystal formation preferentially on the outside of the cell, drawing water out.

Using the vitrification technique, cortex tissue of each ovary is cut into slices $1 \times 10 \times 10$ mm. The ultra-thinness of the tissue is crucial, not only for the cryopreservation, but also for rapid revascularization after grafting. Ovarian tissues are initially equilibrated in 7.5% ethylene glycol (EG) and 7.5% dimethyl

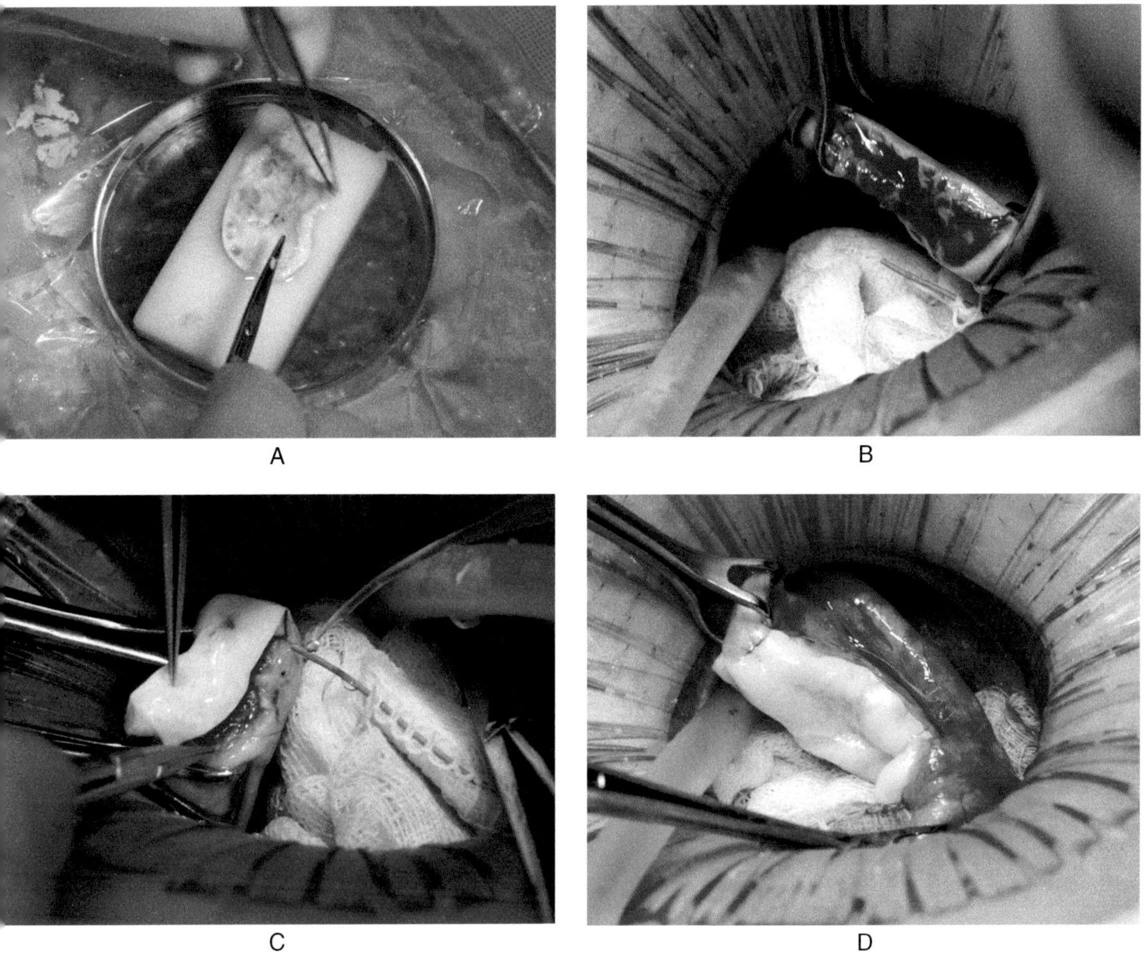

A B

C D

Figure 37.2 (A–D) Steps in the procedure of ovarian transplantation between monozygotic twin sisters: (A) preparation of donor ovarian cortex by dissection in a Petri dish on ice; (B) preparation of recipient ovarian medulla; (C) attaching donor cortical tissue to recipient ovarian medulla; (D) attaching thawed donor cortical tissue for re-transplant to the recipient medulla.

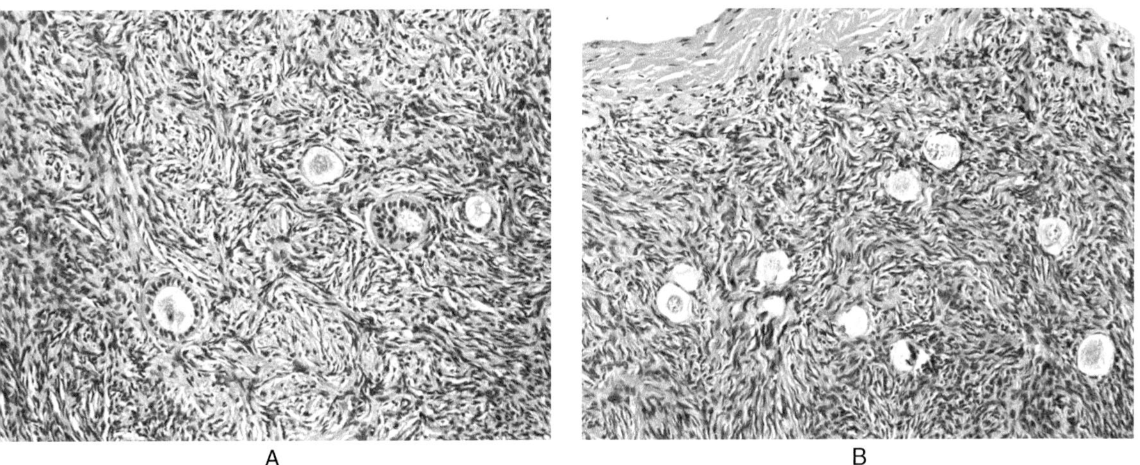

Figure 37.3 Histology pre (A) and post (B) vitrification of ovarian tissue.

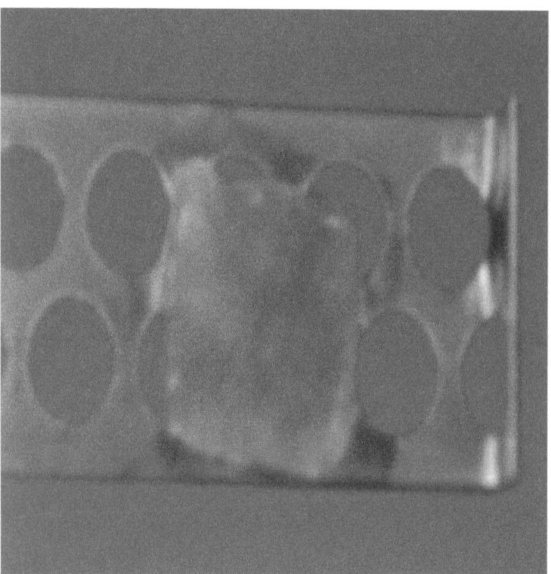

Figure 37.4 Ovarian tissue slice.

sulfoxide (DMSO) in handling medium (HM: HEPES-buffered TCM-199 solution supplemented with 20% [v/v] synthetic serum substitute [SSS; Irvine Scientific, Santa Ana, CA, USA]) for 25 minutes followed by a second equilibration in 20% EG and 20% DMSO with 0.5 M sucrose for 15 minutes. Ovarian tissues are then placed in a minimum volume of solution (virtually "dry") onto a thin metal strip (Cryotissue: Kitazato BioPharma, Fujinomiya, Japan), and submerged directly in sterile liquid nitrogen [25], following which the strip is inserted into a protective container and placed into a liquid nitrogen storage tank (Figure 37.4).

For thawing, the protective cover is removed and the Cryotissue metal strip is immersed directly in 40 ml of 37 °C HM solution supplemented with 1.0 M sucrose for 1 minute. Then, ovary tissues are transferred into 15 ml of 0.5 M sucrose HM solution for 5 minutes at room temperature, and washed twice in HM solution for 10 minutes before viability analysis, or transplantation. No ice crystal formation occurs during any of these vitrification procedures [23].

Intact whole ovary transplantation

Before we had long-term follow-up of the cortical tissue grafts, we had postulated, incorrectly we now believe, that we could lengthen graft survival and avoid ischemic loss of follicles by instead doing a whole intact ovary microvascular transplantation.

To transplant an intact whole ovary, the donor ovary is removed by clamping the infundibular pelvic ligament at its base in order to obtain maximum length. The veins (3–5 mm) are easily identified, but the ovarian artery (0.3 mm) is often not grossly visible. The entire specimen is placed in Leibovitz medium at 4 °C and two veins and one artery are dissected and isolated under the operating microscope. The recipient's infundibular pelvic ligament is clamped at the base and transected close to her non-functioning ovary. The donor's ovarian veins are then anastomosed to the recipient's with 9-0 nylon interrupted sutures and the ovarian arteries are anastomosed with 10-0 nylon interrupted sutures (Figure 37.5A–C).

When the microvascular clamps are removed, blood flow is confirmed by fresh bleeding from the surface of the ovary where a cortical slice had been taken for cryopreservation as a backup.

This patient is recipient number 8 in Table 37.1 and Figure 37.6. Her recovery of ovulatory menstrual cycling was similar to all of the cortical tissue slice transplants. She conceived spontaneously a healthy baby girl, delivered at term, and her graft functioned for greater than 4 years. However, we found that this intact whole ovary approach did not produce results superior to cortical tissue grafts, which were equally robust. The original concept behind whole intact ovary microvascular transplantation was to avoid the supposed ischemic damage that was incorrectly attributed to cortical grafting [26]. Current results seem to eliminate the need for whole ovary transplantation, as these fresh cortical ovarian tissue grafts have now also been shown to have a very long duration of function.

Results of fresh and frozen ovarian transplantation

Results are summarized in Table 37.1 and in Figures 37.6 and 37.7.

All nine identical twin pairs underwent their orthotopic ovarian isotransplantation between April 2004 and April 2008.

The recipients, for the most part, continued to cycle, from 2 years in two patients whose donor had low ovarian reserve to over 7 years in most cases. The two whose donors had low antral follicle counts (AFC) of fewer than ten, only functioned for 2 years. However, even these two cases had spare frozen cortical tissue that remains available for future transplants. Menstrual cycles began within 3 months in all patients,

Table 37.1. Ovarian transplant results for 14 babies (11 from 9 fresh; 3 from 3 frozen)

Patient no.	Age	Pre-op FSH	Post-op FSH	Initial post-op menses intervals	Preg	Babies delivered	Years of graft function
1	24	75	7.1	2nd baby: FROZEN	3	2	4
2	38	96	5.2	93, 42, 24, 27, 25 …	3	3	>7
3	25	112	6.8	76, 23, 30, 26, 25, 26, 21, 24, 27, 34, 25, 27, 51, 30, 27, 26, 28, 19 …	1	2	>6
4	34	58	9.4	81, 22, 47, 26, 21, 20, 27, 26 …	2	1	4
5	40	60	6.8	86, 29, 38, 34, 28, 28, 31, 35, 34, 28, 33, 35, 30 …	0	0	4
6	26	101	7.5	64, 20, 39, 40, 32, 26, 29, 26, 26, 41 …	1	1	2
7	34	86	4.4	83, 22, 29, 29 …	3	2	>6
8	37	86	7.4	100, 17, 39, 29, 27, 22, 23, 20, 34, 25, 26, 29 …	1	1	>4
9	35	54	4.2	128, 42, 18, 25 …	1	0	2
10	31	78	3.4	FROZEN	1	1	2
11	33	85	8.6	FROZEN	1	1	>1

Note: each graft represents only one-third of one ovary or one-sixth of the entire ovarian reserve.

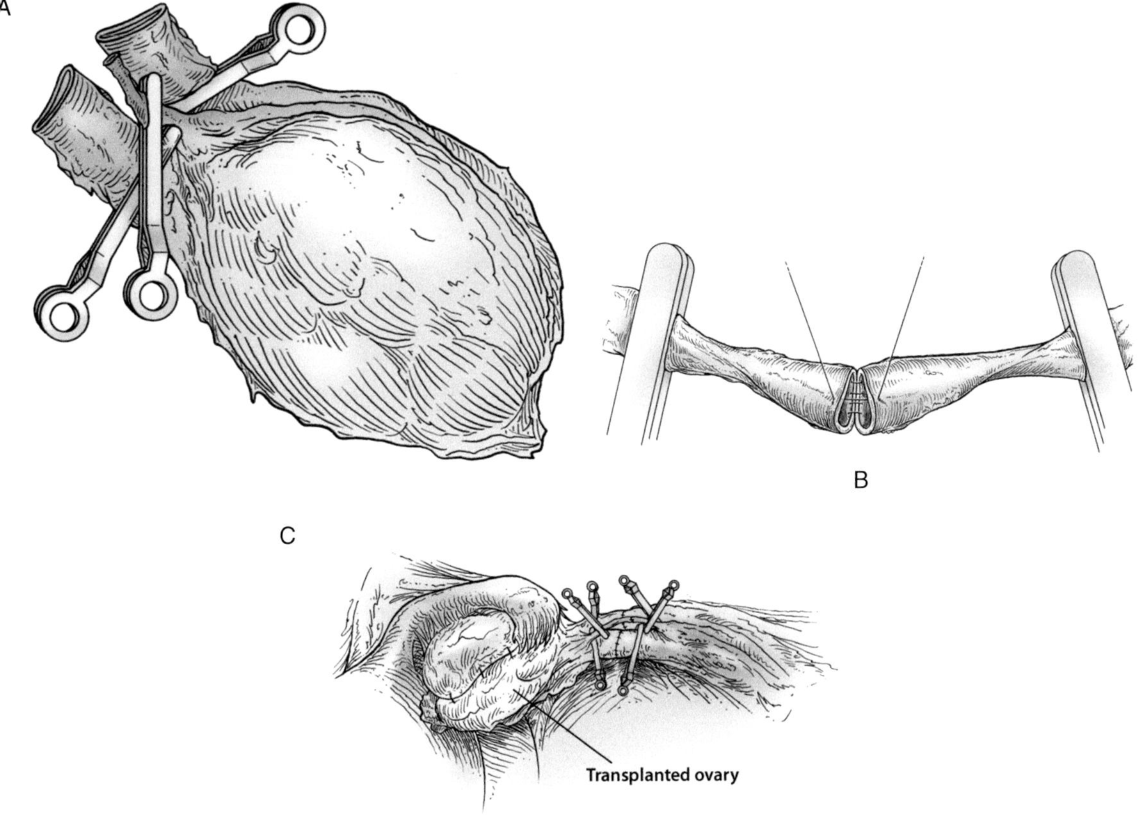

Figure 37.5 (A–C) Steps in the procedure of intact ovary microvascular transplantation: (A) microsurgical isolation of donor ovary blood supply; (B) end-to-end anastomosis of ovarian blood vessel; (C) completed anastomosis of ovarian artery and veins.

and day 3 follicle-stimulating hormone (FSH) levels returned to normal by 4.5 months and ovulation then resumed in all cases (Figure 37.6).

A total of 14 healthy babies resulted from the 12 ovary transplants, 11 from the 9 fresh transplants, and 3 from the 3 frozen transplants (Table 37.1).

One of our twin recipients became pregnant at 39 years of age without medical assistance after her fifth menses, 8 months after transplantation. She delivered a healthy baby girl at full-term and then conceived again at age 42, and delivered a healthy baby boy, again at full-term, 4 years after her transplant. Her ovary is still functioning to date after 7 years, and she conceived again at age 45 with another healthy boy, more than 7 years after her transplant.

One case of ovary transplant was an identical twin whose POF was caused by a bone marrow transplant with pelvic irradiation for leukemia, with her identical twin sister being the donor. She became spontaneously pregnant 5 months after her fresh ovary transplant from her sister, but miscarried. Then at 1.5 years she became pregnant again and had a healthy baby, and at 5 years after the transplant, she became pregnant again, and had a second healthy baby. Over 6 years later, her original transplant is still functioning, and she still has two-thirds of an ovary that remains frozen. It does not appear from this or from the frozen cases that pelvic radiation is incompatible with a healthy pregnancy, and in fact, it appears (contrary to expectations) that transplantation of ovarian cortical tissue using this technique is a very robust procedure.

This newly favorable experience with ovarian cortex grafting is not limited just to our center [27]. Equally robust results are being experienced in Belgium, France, Spain, Denmark, and Israel. Frozen ovarian grafts (even with the slow-freeze technique) in Denmark are lasting over 5 years and many spontaneous pregnancies have been reported, with no need for IVF or other ancillary treatment. At the time of this writing, 28 healthy babies have been born from ovarian tissue grafting, fresh and frozen, and most involved no IVF, and resulted from just regular intercourse with no special treatment (Table 37.2).

Frozen cortical ovarian transplantation

The most common benefit of ovarian transplant is not the unusual cases of fresh grafting in identical twins but rather to protect the fertility and future endocrine function of young women undergoing cancer

Table 37.2. Worldwide frozen ovarian cortex tissue transplant pregnancies

Case no.	Diagnosis	Babies	Where
1	Hodgkin's	1	Donnez
2	Neuro tumor	1	Donnez
3	Non-Hodgkin's	1	Meirow
4	Hodgkins	1	Demeestere
5	Ewings	1	Andersen
6	Hodgkin's	1	Andersen
7	POF	1	Silber
8	Hodgkin's	2	Silber
9	Polyangiitis	1	Piver
10	Breast cancer	2	Pellicer
11	Sickle cell	1	Piver
12	Hodgkin's	2	Revel
Totals: 12 patients		17 Babies	8 Centers
Fresh + Frozen		28 Babies	Silber – 14 Babies

treatment [5, 23, 28–34]. Since 1996, we have frozen ovary tissue for 68 young women with cancer or at risk for POF, of whom 16 had spare frozen tissue subjected to detailed viability testing before cryopreservation and after thawing. All 68 had histological review by a variety of pathologists. Only one had ovarian metastasis (and then only in the medulla), a young woman with widespread breast cancer metastasis throughout her entire body. Otherwise, none of our other 61 cancer cases had any tumor cells in their ovary. Andersen has also noted a complete lack of ovarian metastasis, even in the majority of leukemia cases. The reason for the remarkable absence of ovarian metastasis might possibly be due to the fibrous avascular nature of the ovarian cortex (C. Andersen, personal communication, 2007). In fact, the reason why fetal ovarian cords (which in the fetal male become seminiferous tubules) invade the fibrous cortex and become follicles is that the dense fibrous tissue of the cortex (which in the fetal and adult testis is just tunica albuginea) is needed to suppress the resting follicles from developing all at once prematurely. By analogy, in the male, leukemic cells do indeed routinely lodge in the testis proper, but not ever in the tunica albuginea of the testis. That same phenomenon protects these ovarian slices as well. In addition to these 61 pathological cases, 7 women have had ovarian tissue frozen simply to allow them the possibility of having children at an older age because they had to delay childbearing for strong personal or economic reasons.

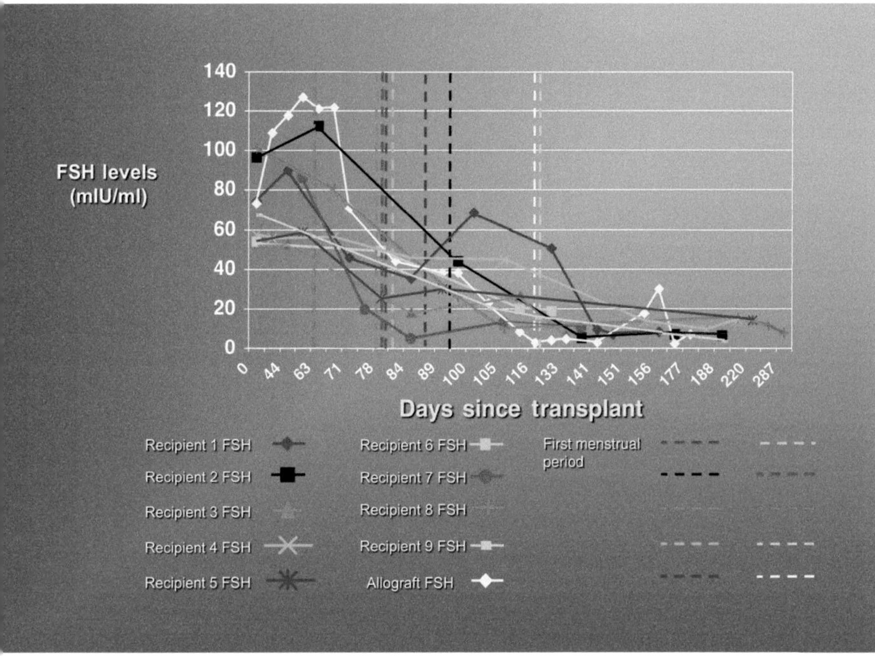

Figure 37.6 Recovery of ovarian function. The eight fresh transplant cases showed a dramatic decline in day 3 serum follicle-stimulating hormone (FSH) by 80–140 days post-operatively corresponding approximately to the resumption of menses. The results of the microvascular whole ovary transplant and the cortical tissue allotransplant are not significantly different from cortical isografts.

Thus far, only three of our frozen cases have had their frozen tissue transplanted back. In all three cases, the tissue was cryopreserved with slow freezing because this was before we adopted vitrification as our standard method in 2009. Of our three cases of frozen transplanted tissue thus far, even with slow freeze, all have had a robust return of ovulatory menstrual cycles within 4 months with spontaneous pregnancy eventually; although with slow-freezing cases this return of function was somewhat slower and the transplant duration was briefer (Figure 37.7).

The duration of function for these slow freeze grafts was about one-third or less than that of our fresh grafts. This could be an intrinsic problem with our slow-freezing technique. We hope that with vitrification, because we found no loss of oocyte viability, that the frozen grafts, once transplanted, will last as long as the fresh ones. It is clear from our fresh grafts that with proper microsurgical technique, ischemia time is not a serious problem for cortical grafting.

Genetics of non-cancer premature ovarian failure, and low ovarian reserve

Identical twins discordant for ovarian function present a true genetic puzzle [20]. The great majority of women enter menopause in their fifth or sixth decade of life, at an average of 51 years, but 1% undergo menopause quite prematurely, that is, before 40 years of age [35–37]. POF is assumed to have a genetic etiology (see Chapter 34) and menopausal age normally is strongly heritable judging by the greater concordance between monozygotic than dizygotic twins [38–41]. It was remarkable, therefore, to identify monozygotic twin pairs in which one sister had undergone menopause for unexplained reasons at a very early age, from 14 to 22 years, whereas the other was still fertile, with naturally conceived children as well as normal ovulatory cycles and ovarian reserve [10, 13–15].

We have not yet taken advantage of the unique opportunity these twins offered for studying the possible genetic or epigenetic origin of ovarian reserve, but genomic DNA and lymphoblastoid cell lines were prepared and carefully stored for future genetic and epigenetic studies. Details of the obstetric records on the original chorionicity at birth of these identical twin sisters revealed 50% were monochorionic–monoamniotic, which was surprisingly high since the incidence of mono/mono is normally only $\approx$2% ($P < 0.0005$). It is clear that late splitting, for whatever reason, predisposes otherwise identical twins to discordant germ cell deficiency [14, 42, 43].

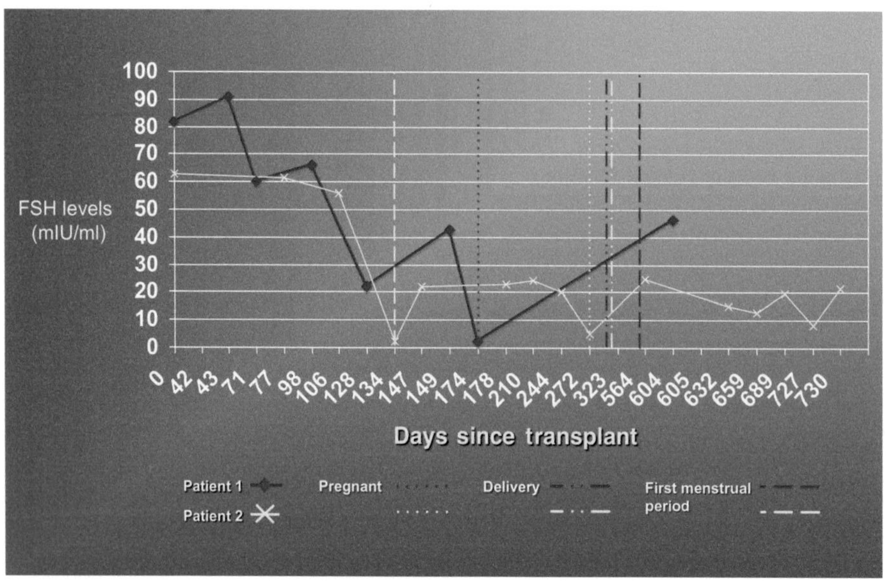

Figure 37.7 Transplant of thawed ovarian tissue. After a frozen cortical re-transplant, serum FSH declined again to normal levels, similar to those of fresh transplants.

Thus far the search for genes controlling ovarian reserve in the human has yielded meager results, the only modestly common candidate being the pre-mutation carrier status for fragile X (*FMR1*). The answer oddly enough may be found in the structural peculiarity of the Y chromosome actually, with its huge concentration of amplicons and palindromes, which are very difficult to sequence [44]. These regions of long sequence identity with many multicopy genes would not have been sequenced with routine methods and most would have been missed in the sequencing without special methodology. Similar regions on the X chromosome that did not undergo the very specialized type of sequencing used for the Y would therefore not have been elicited in the genome sequence yet. We now estimate that 12% of the X chromosome remains unsequenced, and in fact is ampliconic, making the X chromosome a very attractive place to find genes which control ovarian reserve (as well as spermatogenesis). But to sequence these ampliconic regions is a very slow and laborious task compared to sequencing the more conventional regions of the genome.

Future prospects for ovarian tissue transplantation

After ovarian transplantation, all patients were able to attempt natural conception every month without medical assistance, and heterotopic sites have produced no successful pregnancies to date. Our patients preferred the chance of natural conception anyway [45–48]. In fact, the commonly held view that egg freezing is a proven technique and ovary tissue transplantation is "experimental," is belied by the fact that all of the successful pregnancies resulting from fertility preservation in cancer patients thus far have been from frozen ovary tissue, and none at the date of this writing have come from frozen oocytes [27].

It is generally assumed that premature ovarian failure or low ovarian reserve is related to the number of primordial follicles the woman has at birth and this number is certainly heritable and is most likely genetically determined [43]. Many modern women are concerned about what is commonly referred to as their "biological clock" as they worry about the chances of conceiving by the time they have established their career and/or their marriage and their financial stability. Most of our cured cancer patients, who have "young" ovarian tissue frozen, feel almost grateful they had cancer, because otherwise they would share this same fear many modern, liberated women have about their "biological clock." But it is not only having a child that worries them.

The major application of ovarian tissue cryopreservation and transplantation is obviously for fertility preservation in cancer patients and possibly for women who need to delay childbearing. However, for patients who have already lost ovarian function

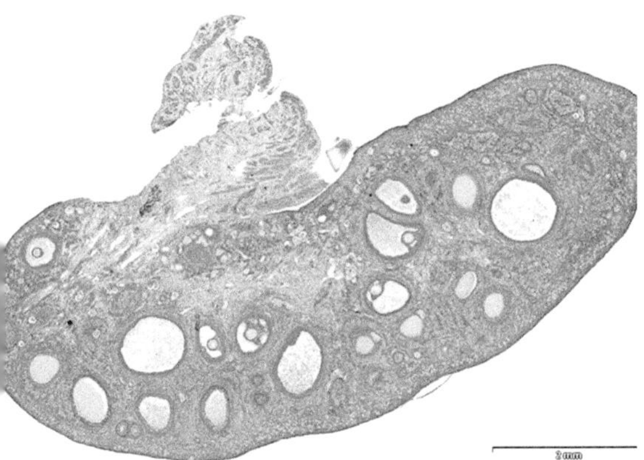

Figure 37.8 All the primordial follicles of the ovary are located in the outer 0.75 mm of the cortex. Therefore, very thin slices of cortex will contain all these follicles and allow rapid revascularization.

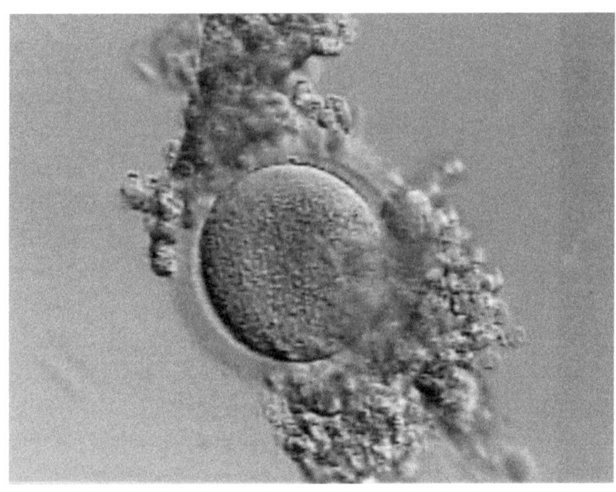

Figure 37.9 Partial cumulus denudation prior to vitrification of GV oocytes.

from bone marrow transplant, allografts may be an option. Allografts might be considered if ovarian tissue is available from a young woman who previously donated bone marrow to the same patient. However, it is very important not to attempt this without immune suppression if the graft recipient has any sign of graft-versus-host disease. Reassuringly, well-matched (HLA) kidney transplant recipients on immunosuppression have favorable obstetric outcomes [49].

At the time of this writing, we are aware of numerous other births after implanting ovarian tissue, for a total of 30 live births thus far [11, 12, 27, 50–53]. Thus, despite initial skepticism, this technique is now gaining worldwide acceptance, and is being enthusiastically received by young women of reproductive age with cancer. For pediatric cases, certainly, the only option is ovarian tissue freezing, because ovarian hyperstimulation is contraindicated. Although we are certain that one day in vitro maturation of primordial follicles for 3 months will be possible in human work, at the present time, in vivo maturation via transplantation is all we can hope for.

For leukemia patients, or any patients in whom transplantation of prior frozen ovarian tissue might create a risk of re-introducing cancer cells, we recommend that before the cortical tissue is dissected and frozen, all the antral follicles of the removed ovary be aspirated for germinal vesicle (GV) oocyte retrieval. Of course, as referred to earlier, even most leukemia patients do not have tumor cells in their dense fibrous ovarian cortex, but nonetheless this is still a concern for this particular cancer, which is why we suggest freezing GV oocytes as well. These GVs can then be partially denuded of cumulus cells, and vitrified just as for oocyte freezing (with one minor modification) (see Figures 37.8 and 37.9).

The vitrification media for partially denuded GV oocytes should contain 20% DMSO and 20% EG with 0.5% sucrose, instead of 15% DMSO and 15% EG, similar to the vitrification medium for ovarian tissue. This is because our studies showed poorer results with only partially demanded oocytes if the concentration of vitrification solution was not increased, similar to our results with ovarian tissue vitrification.

Egg and embryo vitrification

Vitrification for freezing eggs or embryos was first suggested in the mid 1980s [54, 55]. However, it was not until 2005 that a highly efficient method was published, which stimulated a huge wave of justified enthusiasm for this approach to egg and embryo freezing [4, 9, 56, 57]. The concept behind vitrification is not just its potential simplicity (e.g., no freezing machine is required) but that it could eliminate ice crystal formation completely. Instead of clinical IVF programs having to weigh carefully the risks to pregnancy rate posed by embryo freezing, embryos could now be frozen without concern in virtually any case in which there would be a clinical advantage. With the new vitrification methodology, there is no difference between fresh and frozen embryos. Furthermore vitrification of eggs and embryos offers an alternative to ovarian tissue freezing for preservation of fertility, giving the patient another option.

For vitrification the cryoprotectant solution is a combination of EG and DMSO (cat. no. 90133; Irvine Scientific, Santa Ana, CA, USA). The embryo is transferred initially into increasing concentrations of equilibration solution (7.5 M EG and 7.5% DMSO in 20% synthetic serum substitute [SSS]) for 10–15 minutes, followed by placement for 1 minute or longer in vitrification solution (15 M EG and 15 M DMSO in 20% SSS and 0.5 M sucrose). The embryo is not left in a droplet, as that would slow the cooling rate. All excess fluid is removed by pipette from the Cryotop platform so that there is only a thin film of fluid surrounding it, in order to allow for the most rapid temperature drop. The embryo is then directly immersed in liquid nitrogen. The Cryotop containing the embryo is then placed in a canister in the liquid nitrogen tank for storage.

In the warming step, embryos are placed in decreasing concentrations of sucrose solutions to remove the cryoprotectants. The Cryotops are first rapidly plunged into a 37 °C dish containing warming solution (1.0 M sucrose) for 1 minute. The embryos are then slowly introduced in a stepwise fashion to dilution solutions (0.5 M sucrose). A wash solution (without sucrose) is slowly added to embryos in the dilution solution and the final rinse for the embryos is in 100% wash solution [9]. This protocol was designed to avoid too rapid osmotic shifts that could be caused by such high concentrations of cryoprotectant. The high concentration of cryoprotectant is actually not toxic in itself to eggs, embryos or tissue, in the protocols described. The appearance of toxicity comes only from too rapid an osmotic shift. The ultra-rapid rate of cooling (−23 000 °C per minute) and the high end concentration of cryoprotectant lowers the freezing point dramatically and thus allows the ice crystallization phase to be completely avoided.

With vitrification, mature retrieved oocytes can be successfully frozen with 95% success. For embryos, there really is no difference at all between those fresh or frozen [4].

Conclusion

New technology in cryopreservation via vitrification allows us to remove ovary tissue and freeze it to protect it from sterilizing cancer treatment in young women, as well as to freeze individual mature (as well as immature) eggs. It also allows us to stop the aging of the ovary and eggs, which is the major cause of the current worldwide infertility epidemic. It will protect the future fertility potential of young women with cancer, and will also allow an expansion of the reproductive lifespan in any young woman who wishes to delay childbearing or delay her age of menopause.

References

1. Connolly MP, Pollard MS, Hoorens S, *et al.* Long-term economic benefits attributed to IVF-conceived children: a lifetime tax calculation. *Am J Manag Care* 2008; **14**(9): 598–604.
2. Silber SJ. *How to Get Pregnant: The Classic Guide to Overcoming Infertility, Completely Revised and Updated*, 2nd edn. Boston, MA: Little, Brown, 2007.
3. Baerwald AR, Adams GP, Pierson RA. Ovarian antral folliculogenesis during the human menstrual cycle: a review. *Hum Reprod Update* 2012; **18**(1): 73–91.
4. Homburg R, van der Veen F, Silber SJ. Oocyte vitrification – women's emancipation set in stone. *Fertil Steril* 2009; **91**: 1319–20.
5. Silber SJ, Kagawa N, Kuwayama M, Gosden R. Duration of fertility after fresh and frozen ovary transplantation. *Fertil Steril* 2010; **94**(6): 2191–6.
6. Silber SJ. Ovary cryopreservation and transplantation for fertility preservation. *Mol Hum Reprod* 2012; **18**(2): 59–67.
7. Mosher WD. Fecundity and infertility in the United States 1965–1982. *Adv Data* 1985; **1**: 1.
8. Gosden RG, Baird DT, Wade JC, Webb R. Restoration of fertility to oophorectomized sheep by ovarian autografts stored at −196 degrees C. *Hum Reprod* 1994; **9**(4): 597–603.
9. Kuwayama M, Vajta G, Kato O, Leibo SP. Highly efficient vitrification method for cryopreservation of human oocytes. *Reprod Biomed Online* 2005; **11**(3): 300–8.
10. Silber SJ, Lenahan KM, Levine DJ, *et al.* Ovarian transplantation between monozygotic twins discordant for premature ovarian failure. *N Eng J Med* 2005; **353**(1): 58–63.
11. Donnez J, Dolmans MM, Demylle D, *et al.* Livebirth after orthotopic transplantation of cryopreserved ovarian tissue. *Lancet* 2004; **364**(9443): 1405–10.
12. Meirow D, Levron J, Eldar-Geva T, *et al.* Pregnancy after transplantation of cryopreserved ovarian tissue in a patient with ovarian failure after chemotherapy. *N Engl J Med* 2005; **353**(3): 318–21.
13. Silber SJ, Gosden RG. Ovarian transplantation in a series of monozygotic twins discordant for ovarian failure. *N Eng J Med* 2007; **356**: 1382–4.

14. Silber SJ, DeRosa M, Pineda J, *et al.* A series of monozygotic twins discordant for ovarian failure: ovary transplantation (cortical versus microvascular) and cryopreservation. *Hum Reprod* 2008; **23**(7): 1531–7.

15. Silber SJ, Grudzinskas G, Gosden RG. Successful pregnancy after microsurgical transplantation of an intact ovary. *N Eng J Med* 2008; **359**(24): 2617–18.

16. Wallace WH, Critchley HO, Anderson RA. Optimizing reproductive outcome in children and young people with cancer. *J Clin Oncol* 2012; **30**(1): 3–5.

17. Bedaiwy MA, Falcone T. Harvesting and autotransplantation of vascularized ovarian grafts: approaches and techniques. *Reprod Biomed Online* 2007; **14**(3): 360–71.

18. Silber SJ. Transplantation of a human testis for anorchia. *Fertil Steril* 1978; **30**(2): 181–7.

19. Gosden RG, Telfer E, Faddy MJ, Brook DJ. Ovarian cyclicity and follicular recruitment in unilaterally ovariectomized mice. *J Reprod Fertil* 1989; **87**(1): 257–64.

20. Faddy MJ, Gosden RG, Gougeon A, Richardson SJ, Nelson JF. Accelerated disappearance of ovarian follicles in mid-life: implications for forecasting menopause. *Hum Reprod* 1992; **7**(10): 1342–6.

21. Gook DA, Edgar DH, Stern C. Effect of cooling rate and dehydration regimen on the histological appearance of human ovarian cortex following cryopreservation in 1,2-propanediol. *Hum Reprod* 1999; **14**(8): 2061–8.

22. Newton H, Aubard Y, Rutherford A, Sharma V, Gosden R. Low temperature storage and grafting of human ovarian tissue. *Hum Reprod* 1996; **11**(7): 1487–91.

23. Kagawa N, Silber S, Kuwayama M. Successful vitrification of bovine and human ovarian tissue. *Reprod Biomed Online* 2009; **18**(4): 568–77.

24. Keros V, Xella S, Hultenby K, *et al.* Vitrification versus controlled-rate freezing in cryopreservation of human ovarian tissue. *Hum Reprod* 2009; **24**(7): 1670–83.

25. Fuentes F, Dubettier R. *Air Separation Method and Plant*, United States Patent. 2004; Patent No. US 6,776,005 B2.

26. Baird DT, Webb R, Campbell BK, Harkness LM, Gosden RG. Long-term ovarian function in sheep after ovariectomy and transplantation of autografts stored at −196 °C. *Endocrinology* 1999; **140**(1): 462–71.

27. Donnez J, Silber S, Andersen CY, *et al.* Children born after autotransplantation of cryopreserved ovarian tissue. A review of 13 live births. *Ann Med* 2011; **43**(6): 437–50.

28. Bleyer WA. The impact of childhood cancer on the United States and the world. *CA Cancer J Clin* 1990; **40**(6): 355–67.

29. Ries LAG, Smith MA, Gurney JG, *et al.* (eds.) *Cancer Incidence and Survival Among Children and Adolescents: United States SEER Program, 1976–1995.* Bethesda: National Cancer Institute, 1999.

30. Jeruss JS, Woodruff TK. Preservation of fertility in patients with cancer. *N Engl J Med* 2009; **360**(9): 902–11.

31. Anderson RA, Themmen AP, Al-Qahtani A, Groome NP, Cameron DA. The effects of chemotherapy and long-term gonadotrophin suppression on the ovarian reserve in premenopausal women with breast cancer. *Hum Reprod* 2006; **21**(10): 2583–92.

32. Anderson RA, Cameron DA. Assessment of the effect of chemotherapy on ovarian function in women with breast cancer. *J Clin Oncol* 2007; **25**(12): 1630–1. Author reply 1632.

33. Larsen EC, Muller J, Schmiegelow K, Rechnitzer C, Andersen AN. Reduced ovarian function in long-term survivors of radiation- and chemotherapy-treated childhood cancer. *J Clin Endocrinol Metab* 2003; **88**(11): 5307–14.

34. Lee SJ, Schover LR, Partridge AH, *et al.* American Society of Clinical Oncology. American Society of Clinical Oncology recommendations on fertility preservation in cancer patients. *J Clin Oncol* 2006; **24**(18) 2917–31.

35. Coulam CB, Adamson SC, Annegers JF. Incidence of premature ovarian failure. *Obstet Gynecol* 1986; **67**(4): 604–6.

36. Riboli E, Hunt KJ, Slimani N, *et al.* European Prospective Investigation into Cancer and Nutrition (EPIC): study of populations and data collection. *Public Health Nutr* 2002; **5**(6B): 1113–24.

37. Luborsky JL, Meyer P, Sowers MF, Gold EB, Santoro N. Premature menopause in a multi-ethnic population study of the menopause transition. *Hum Reprod* 2003; **18**(1): 199–206.

38. Goswami D, Conway GS. Premature ovarian failure. *Hum Reprod Update* 2005; **11**(4): 391–410.

39. Snieder H, MacGregor AJ, Spector TD. Genes control the cessation of a woman's reproductive life: a twin study of hysterectomy and age at menopause. *J Clin Endocrinol Metab* 1998; **83**(6): 1875–80.

40. de Bruin JP, Bovenhuis H, van Noord PA, *et al.* The role of genetic factors in age at natural menopause. *Hum Reprod* 2001; **16**(9): 2014–18.

41. van Asselt KM, Kok HS, Pearson PL, *et al.* Heritability of menopausal age in mothers and daughters. *Fertil Steril* 2004; **82**(5): 1348–51.

42. Su LL. Monoamniotic twins: diagnosis and management. *Acta Obstet Gynecol Scand* 2002; **81**(11): 995–1000.

43. Gosden RG, Treloar SA, Martin NG, *et al.* Prevalence of premature ovarian failure in monozygotic and dizygotic twins. *Hum Reprod* 2007; **22**(2): 610–15.

44. Silber SJ. The Y chromosome in the era of intracytoplasmic sperm injection: a personal review. *Fertil Steril* 2011; **95**(8): 2439–48.

45. Oktay K, Buyuk E, Veeck L, *et al.* Embryo development after heterotopic transplantation of cryopreserved ovarian tissue. *Lancet* 2004; **363**(9412): 837–40.

46. Rosendahl M, Loft A, Byskov AG, *et al.* Biochemical pregnancy after fertilization of an oocyte aspirated from a heterotopic autotransplant of cryopreserved ovarian tissue: case report. *Hum Reprod* 2006; **21**(8): 2006–9.

47. Hilders CG, Baranski AG, Peters L, Ramkhelawan A, Trimbos JB. Successful human ovarian autotransplantation to the upper arm. *Cancer* 2004; **101**(12): 2771–8.

48. Kim SS, Hwang IT, Lee HC. Heterotopic autotransplantation of cryobanked human ovarian tissue as a strategy to restore ovarian function. *Fertil Steril* 2004; **82**(4): 930–2.

49. Armenti VT, Radomski JS, Moritz MJ, *et al.* Report from the National Transplantation Pregnancy Registry (NTPR): outcomes of pregnancy after transplantation. *Clin Transpl* 2000: 123–34.

50. Andersen CY, Rosendahl M, Byskov AG, *et al.* Two successful pregnancies following autotransplantation of frozen/thawed ovarian tissue. *Hum Reprod* 2008; **23**(10): 2266–72.

51. Demeestere I, Simon P, Emiliani S, Delbaere A, Englert Y. Fertility preservation: successful transplantation of cryopreserved ovarian tissue in a young patient previously treated for Hodgkin's disease. *Oncologist* 2007; **12**(12): 1437–42.

52. Sanchez-Serrano M, Crespo J, Mirabet V, *et al.* Twins born after transplantation of ovarian cortical tissue and oocyte vitrification. *Fertil Steril* 2010; **93**(1): 268.e11–13.

53. Piver P, Amiot C, Agnani G, *et al.* Two pregnancies obtained after a new technique of autotransplantation of cryopreserved ovarian tissue. *Hum Reprod* 2009; **24**(15): 10–35.

54. Rall WF. Factors affecting the survival of mouse embryos cryopreserved by vitrification. *Cryobiology* 1987; **24**(5): 387–402.

55. Fahy GM, MacFarlane DR, Angell CA, Meryman HT. Vitrification as an approach to cryopreservation. *Cryobiology* 1984; **21**(4): 407–26.

56. Kuwayama M. Highly efficient vitrification for cryopreservation of human oocytes and embryos: the Cryotop method. *Theriogenology* 2007; **67**(1): 73–80.

57. Katayama KP, Stehlik J, Kuwayama M, Kato O, Stehlik E. High survival rate of vitrified human oocytes results in clinical pregnancy. *Fertil Steril* 2003; **80**(1): 223–4.

Index

Printed in the United States
By Bookmasters